The Complete Vegetarian

The Food Series

*A list of books in the series appears
at the back of this book.*

The Complete Vegetarian

The Essential Guide to Good Health

Edited by
Peggy Carlson, MD

University of Illinois Press
Urbana and Chicago

Library of Congress Cataloging-in-Publication Data

The complete vegetarian : the essential guide to
good health / edited by Peggy Carlson.
    p.   cm. — (The food series)
Includes index.
ISBN-13 978-0-252-03251-6 (cloth : alk. paper)
ISBN-10
ISBN-13 978-0-252-07506-3 (pbk. : alk. paper)
ISBN-10
1. Vegetarianism—Popular works.   2. Nutrition—Popular works.
I. Carlson, Peggy.
TX392.C69   2007
641.5'636—dc22   2007030754

This book is dedicated to my mother,
who taught me to love animals,

and to Callie, Charcoal, Ginger, and Grizzie
who taught me that they love back.

—Peggy Carlson, MD

Contents

References   274

19. **Pregnancy and Lactation**   **277**
     Reed Mangels, PhD, RD, FADA

     Introduction   277
     Summary of the Scientific Literature   277
     Practical Aspects   282
     Conclusion   284
     References   284

20. **Optimal Nutrition for Active Vegetarians and
     Vegetarian Athletes**   **288**
     D. Enette Larson-Meyer, PhD, RD, FACSM
     Mary Helen Niemeyer, MD, MPH, FAAFP

     Introduction   288
     Summary of the Scientific Literature   289
     Practical Aspects   309
     Conclusion   310
     References   310

21. **Environmental and Food Safety Aspects of
     Vegetarian Diets**   **317**
     Carl V. Phillips, MPP, PhD
     Simon K. Emms, PhD
     Erin L. Kraker, MS, REHS

     Introduction   317
     Types of Animal Food Production   318
     A Variety of Environmental Impacts   318
     Summary of the Scientific Literature   319
     Practical Aspects   333
     Conclusion   334
     Acknowledgment   335
     References   335

22. **Planning Nutritious Vegetarian Diets**   **338**
     Cheryl Sullivan, MA, RD

     Introduction   338
     Summary of the Scientific Literature   338
     Practical Aspects   342
     Conclusion   343
     References   344

1

Introduction

Peggy Carlson, MD

There is a vast amount of research on the nutritional and health aspects of a vegetarian diet. Most of this literature has been published in the past 25 to 35 years, during which time the research has become progressively more sophisticated and rigorous. The scientific community is increasingly taking note. So, too, is much of the general public, which is beginning to realize the important effects that diet has on health.

The research being done on vegetarian diets is relevant to everyone. It is important not only to those who are now vegetarian, but also to those who are considering becoming vegetarian. Currently, a major reason that people give for adopting a vegetarian diet is the positive health effects it affords.

In addition to current and potential vegetarians, the research regarding vegetarian diets is important to nutritionists and other health professionals. The research shows that vegetarian diets can both help prevent and treat many diseases. Diet may very well be one of the most underutilized tools in the health practitioner's armamentarium.

The relevance of this research also spans a much broader context. The information learned

from research on vegetarian diets sheds light on many individual dietary factors and the roles they play in all diets, even nonvegetarian, for it is not just the absence of meat that characterizes a vegetarian diet. In general, vegetarian diets, when compared with nonvegetarian diets, have less total fat, less saturated fat, less cholesterol, less protein, more fiber, more unsaturated fats, more phytochemicals, more antioxidants, different sources of protein, and differences in amounts of some vitamins and minerals. Research that helps to elucidate the role of each of these factors in diet, as well as in health, broadens our knowledge about these factors in everyone's diet.

This book examines the current status of what we know about vegetarian diets. It starts with a look at the nutritional aspects of these diets, with special attention to protein, fats, fiber, iron, calcium, vitamin D, vitamin B12, zinc, and other vitamins and minerals. The second part of the book examines diseases that research shows may be affected by vegetarian diets. These include heart disease, cancer, high blood pressure, stroke, obesity, diabetes, osteoporosis, kidney disease, and many gastrointestinal disorders, among others. The last part discusses meal planning for vegetarians in general and then specifically for children, pregnant women, and athletes. A chapter on the important topic of the environmental impact of diets summarizes how our food choices affect the earth.

This book has information for everyone. Be smart, eat well, and be healthy!

Vegetarians

A *vegetarian diet*, by definition, is a diet without meat. This means no red meat, as well as no fish and no chicken or other poultry.

There are several different types of vegetarian diets. *Ovo-lacto vegetarians* do eat eggs (*ovo*) and dairy (*lacto*) products. *Lacto vegetarians* eat dairy products, but not eggs. The less common *ovo vegetarians* eat eggs, but not dairy products. *Vegans* are vegetarians who consume no animal products whatsoever. A vegan diet contains no meat, no dairy, and no eggs.

In a 2003 U.S. poll, 2.8% of those surveyed said they never eat meat, poultry, or fish/seafood ("How many vegetarians," 2003). A 2000 poll showed that about 2.5% of the population was vegetarian ("How many vegetarians," 2003; Sabaté, 2001). A 1994 poll commissioned by the Vegetarian Resource Group had revealed that 1% or less of the population could say that they never ate meat (Stahler, 1994).

Table 1.1, published in 1992, lists the reasons individuals gave for adopting a vegetarian diet (The American vegetarian, 1992). Health has now become a common reason for adopting a vegetarian diet. Also, many North Americans follow a vegetarian diet because of animal welfare concerns.

As the number of vegetarians increases, so too does the number of products marketed to vegetarians. In the past 15 years, more than 2,000 new soy-based meat and dairy substitutes

Table 1.1   Reasons U.S. Individuals Chose a Vegetarian Diet in 1992

Health	46%
Animal rights	15%
Family/Friend influence	12%
Ethics	5%
Environmental	4%
Other/No response	18%

Source: The American Vegetarian: Coming of Age in the 90s—A study of the vegetarian marketplace conducted for *Vegetarian Times* by Yankelovich, Skelly, and White/Clancy, Shulman, Inc., 1992. With kind permission of Taylor and Francis Group, LLC.

have appeared in food markets (V. Messina & M. Messina, 1996). Foods such as meat analogs, nondairy milks, and vegetarian entrees are becoming more and more popular. These products are no longer found only in specialty food stores, but are now commonly appearing on general grocery store shelves. The U.S. market for these foods was estimated to be $1.5 billion in 2002, up from about $310 million in 1996. This market was expected to nearly double by 2006, to $2.8 billion (Mintel International Group Ltd., 2001). Restaurants, schools, and public events are serving more vegetarian items. Vegetarian cookbooks are appearing on best-seller lists.

History of Vegetarian Diets

From ancient Greek times until approximately the end of the seventeenth century, vegetarian diets were advocated primarily on philosophical and religious grounds, rather than scientific principle. Then, during the mid- to late 1700s and early 1800s, a shift occurred: scientifically based arguments in favor of vegetarian diets began emerging. This was in large part due to the fact that about this time science was attaining greater acceptance and authority in European culture (Whorton, 1994).

Beginning in the 1700s, several notable scientists and public figures advocated and advanced the science of meatless diets. In 1739, physician Theophile Lobb presented a treatise on the dissolution of kidney stones and the prevention and cure of gout by means of a flesh-free diet. In the mid-1700s, Antoni Cocchi was advocating a vegetable diet for the preservation of health and the cure of disease (Hardinge & Crooks, 1963b). He claimed that this diet could and should be used to take away pains in the joints, gout, and other rheumatic diseases. In addition, he also suggested that diseases of the nerves, small aneurysms, and scurvy usually responded to this diet. Cocchi's writings stimulated much discussion (Roe, 1986).

In the early 1800s, London physician William Lambe adopted a vegetarian diet to cure himself of gout. He then began advocating a vegetarian diet to others as a cure for illness. He reported his experiences in *Water and Vegetable Diet in Consumption, Scrofula, Cancer, Asthma and Other Chronic Diseases*, a popular medical book that was published in London in 1815 and that later came out in a popular American edition (Roe, 1986). The influence of Lambe's work was widely felt. The poet Shelley, who had been in poor health, adopted a vegetarian diet (Hardinge & Crooks, 1963a). Shelley's 1813 book, *Vindication of Natural Diet*, included not only moral arguments for vegetarianism, but also illustrations of the health benefits of such a diet (Whorton, 1994). In 1833, Harvard University offered a prize for the best thesis on a diet that would "ensure the greatest health and strength to the laborer in the climate of New England." In response, Dr. William Alcott began to collect data on vegetarian diets. He was joined by Dr. Milo North, who published a questionnaire requesting information from those who had adopted

vegetarian diets. The results of these studies, including the reports of a large number of other medical and scientific men, were published in 1838 (Hardinge & Crooks, 1963b). In the late 1800s, London physician Alexander Haig rejected a meat-based diet because of its effect of increasing the body's uric acid (Whorton, 1994).

Throughout the 1800s, several other prominent scientific men also voiced support for a vegetarian diet. Among these were Reuben Mussey (1780–1866), fourth president of the American Medical Association; and Edward Hitchcock (1793–1864), professor of science and then president of Amherst College, whose "Lectures on Diet, Regimen, and Employment" were published in 1831 (Hardinge & Crooks, 1963a).

In 1829, Sylvester Graham, a Presbyterian minister who believed he had regained his own health on a vegetarian diet, began writing and speaking in favor of meatless diets. He launched the popular health movement of the 1830s and 1840s (Whorton, 1994). This movement advocated a vegetarian diet, as well as temperance in many aspects of life. Graham believed that whole-grain flours, which at that time were not considered to be of dietary importance, were more healthful than refined flours. Graham lectured to laypersons as well as to members of the medical profession (Roe, 1986). Many, including members of the educated classes of both America and Europe, were impressed with his arguments and were often persuaded that a vegetarian diet, in which whole-grain breads and cereals held a prominent place, could improve health (Hardinge & Crooks, 1963b; Roe, 1986). Graham's lectures on the "Science of Human Life" raised the standard of the vegetarian literature.

The word *vegetarian* to describe a meatless diet was first used in 1847. In this year, members of the Bible Christian Church in England established the Vegetarian Society of Great Britain. It was at their inaugural meeting that the word *vegetarian* was first used (Whorton, 1994). Most European nations also began forming vegetarian societies during the 1800s. In the United States, Reverend William Metcalf was inspired by the rapid growth of the English vegetarian society, and in 1850 he laid the foundation for the American Vegetarian Society (Hardinge & Crooks, 1963a).

The Seventh-Day Adventist (SDA) Church was founded in the 1840s by Ellen White. She encouraged SDA Church members to eat a vegetarian diet. She advocated the elimination of certain foods and beverages from the diet, feeling that they were unwholesome and a strain on the digestive system, because they were prepared from animals that were carriers of disease, because they were unduly stimulating, or because the use of such foods necessitated taking the lives of God's creatures (Roe, 1986). Today approximately 50% of SDAs are vegetarian. In this country, the SDA Church has had a considerable influence on the acceptance and promotion of vegetarian diets, both by advocating vegetarianism to its members and by being the impetus behind much of the early scientific research into vegetarian diets.

One early SDA was John Kellogg, a physician and vegetarian. In the mid-1870s, Kellogg headed the then-struggling Western Health Reform Institute, a hospital and health education facility operated by the SDA Church. Under his guidance, it became the most famous health institution in the country, preeminent from the 1870s until World War II. Kellogg was an early proponent of dietary fiber and its role in helping to eliminate potentially toxic products from the intestine. Kellogg also believed that the lower protein content of a vegetarian diet was responsible for part of its healthful effects. He and his brother developed products such as meat substitutes and other vegetarian foods, as well as the breakfast cereals that carry their family name (Whorton, 1994). Kellogg was also one of the early enthusiasts of soy milk (Messina & Messina, 1996).

The first two decades of the 1900s also brought an understanding of the crucial role of vitamins and an appreciation for the fact that fruits and vegetables, too often lacking in the general population's diet, are rich in vitamins. At the same time, public awareness was also being raised about the problems caused by lack of dietary fiber (Whorton, 1994).

Inadvertently, some of the first population studies on vegetarian diets emerged from World Wars I and II (Hardinge & Crooks, 1963a). The Allied blockade of 1917 cut off imports into Denmark. The government, fearing acute food shortages, sought aid from its vegetarian society and selected Dr. Mikkel Hindhede to lead its rationing program. Grain-eating meat animals were slaughtered in order to leave all the grain available for humans to eat. On a diet that consisted largely of whole-grain and bran bread, barley porridge, potatoes, greens, and dairy products, the Danish people showed improved health and lowered mortality rates. During World War II, Norway had to make drastic cuts in the consumption of animal foods, leading to increased consumption of fish, cereals, potatoes, and vegetables. These dietary changes led to a decrease in mortality from circulatory disease. After the war, when the nation returned to its prewar diet, these mortality levels returned to prewar levels.

In 1944, the term *vegan* was coined to define a vegetarian who did not eat any animal products, including dairy or eggs. The Vegan Society was founded in that same year (Long, 1981).

Beginning in the 1960s, but especially in the 1970s, scientific research into vegetarian diets began to flourish. Several influential books highlighted the issues involved. In 1971, Frances Moore Lappe's book, *A Diet for a Small Planet*, called attention to the vegetarian cause with special focus on the environmental and world-hunger aspects of diet. *Animal Liberation* (1975), by Peter Singer, focused attention on the animal-cruelty issues associated with the meat, egg, and diary industries and supported vegetarianism as an alternative. John Robbins's book, *Diet for a New America* (1987), drew the public's attention to both the humane and health aspects of a vegetarian diet. Research into vegetarian diets has continued to expand rapidly.

Diets around the World

Today, there is wide variation in the types of diets consumed worldwide. As countries develop economically, consumption of the dominant staple cereals declines. The amount of fats and oils consumed tends to rise sharply. There is a consistent fall in the overall consumption of foods of plant origin and replacement with increasing amounts of foods of animal origin, notably meat and dairy products. Sugar consumption also generally increases rapidly (World Cancer Research Fund, 1997). Such diets are correspondingly lower in fiber and other healthful bioactive compounds found in foods of plant origin. These trends are highlighted in Figure 1.1, which shows regional consumption around the world of major groups of food as a percentage of total energy (World Cancer Research Fund, 1997).

The diets typically consumed in rural areas of Africa, Latin America, Asia, and Oceania often still rely on one or two staple cereal foods. Rice dominates in Asia, wheat in north Africa, corn in Latin America, and corn and starch roots in sub-Saharan Africa (World Cancer Research Fund, 1997).

Average dietary fat content varies widely worldwide, from 8%–15% dietary energy supply (DES) in some parts of Africa and Asia to about 40%–44% in areas of northern and central Europe. In North America, dietary fats provide about 37% DES (World Cancer Research Fund, 1997).

Less (and often much less) than 10% of total energy comes from meat in the less economically developed countries. For example, meat accounts for only about 1% of total energy intake in India, where 25%–30% of the Indian population can be considered completely vegetarian. In more economically developed countries, however, more than 15% of total energy comes from meat, most of which is from domesticated animals (World Cancer Research Fund, 1997).

The reasons for these differences in diet around the world are many. Local conditions, such as food supplies, meat supplies, land conditions, cultural and economic conditions, and environmental factors, all play a role. The degree of industrialization and the availability of transportation play major roles that may supersede local factors: with industry and the ability to transport foods from place to place come the ability to produce many different types of foods and to bring in many foods from distant locations.

History of the "Western" or "Affluent" Diet

In industrialized nations, the "Western" or "affluent" diet has frequently supplanted healthier plant-based diets. The typical Western diet is higher in fat, saturated fat, sugar, and refined grains and lower in fiber and unsaturated fats

Figure 1.1   Consumption of Major Food Groups Worldwide as Percentages of Total Energy

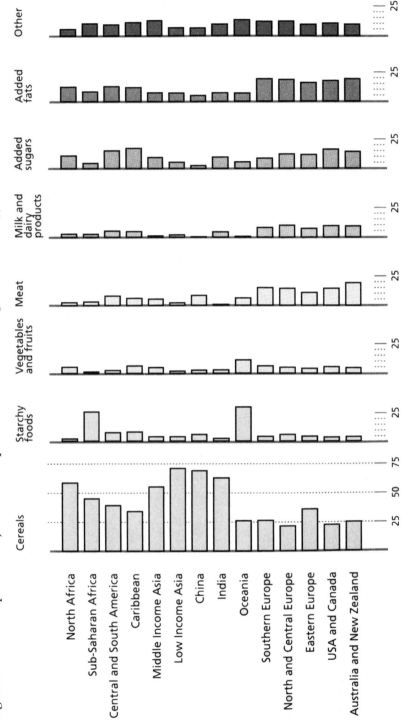

Source: World Cancer Research Fund and American Institute for Cancer Research. *Food, Nutrition and the Prevention of Cancer: A Global Perspective.* Washington, DC: American Institute for Cancer Research, 1997. Reprinted with permission from the American Institute for Cancer Research.

than the more plant-based diets typical of less industrialized nations (Caballero & Popkin, 2002). The reasons why industrialization brings less healthy diets are also many. Understanding these reasons may help society undo some of the dietary problems that exist in the industrialized nations and perhaps prevent the same trend from occurring in less-developed nations as industrialization moves into these countries.

Throughout history, humans have shown themselves capable of subsisting on both mainly meat and mainly plant-based diets (James et al., 1991). Undoubtedly, this versatility enabled survival in times of erratic food supply.

For the first two to three million years, humans were hunters and gatherers. This period represents all but the last 10,000 years since the first appearance of our species. In the hunter-gatherer diet, about 19%–35% of energy came from protein, 22%–40% from carbohydrates, and the rest from fat (Cordain et al., 2000). This is higher in protein and fat, and lower in carbohydrates, than the typical U.S. diet today. Although higher in total fat, there were differences in the types of fats consumed. These early hunter-gatherer diets were lower in saturated fat, higher in the important n-3 fatty acids, and much lower in trans fats (Simopoulos, 1999). The wild animal meat that was consumed had about five times the proportion of polyunsaturated fat as the domestic meat consumed today (Caballero & Popkin, 2002). Among hunter-gatherers, chronic diseases such as heart disease, hypertension, cancer, osteoporosis, and diabetes were relatively unknown. It is felt that the absence of these chronic diseases was due to living patterns rather than a shorter life expectancy (Cordain et al., 2000).

Approximately 10,000 years ago, the cultivation of crops was introduced. Both food production and food storage improved. This provided protection against starvation (James et al., 1991). With this increase in the amount of plant food to eat, protein content in the diet decreased, complex carbohydrates increased to about 69%–75% of DES, and fat decreased to about 10%–15% (Caballero & Popkin, 2002). Anthropological studies show that the diet that fueled most of human evolution was low in fat, very low in sugar, and high in fiber and complex carbohydrates (James et al., 1991).

The arrival of the Industrial Revolution some 200 years ago produced dramatic changes in diet (World Cancer Research Fund, 1997; James et al., 1991). The invention of harvesting machines made grain more readily available to feed to a larger number of animals. With improved transportation, the advent of railways, refrigerated cars, and slaughterhouses, animals raised for meat could be killed in one place and fresh meat could be transported long distances to be sold (World Cancer Research Fund, 1997). As a result, meat became more readily available to more people.

The development of methods to mill grain into refined grain made the more healthful whole-grain products less common (World Cancer Research Fund, 1997; Caballero & Popkin, 2002). Refined sugar made from corn made its appearance (World Cancer Research Fund, 1997). This led to a decrease in dietary fiber and a short-term increase in some deficiency diseases, such as pellagra and beriberi (Caballero & Popkin, 2002).

The ability to hydrogenate fats meant that foods could be made to remain edible for long periods, and thus they could be packaged, transported, and stored without refrigeration (World Cancer Research Fund, 1997). Unfortunately, this hydrogenation process converts the healthier unsaturated vegetable oils into unhealthful fats. The hydrogenation process changes the chemical configuration of the carbon atoms around the double bonds in the fats. These artificially produced hydrogenated fats are known as *trans fats*. In the body, trans fats behave much like saturated fats, in that they increase blood cholesterol levels. Unsaturated fats do not raise blood cholesterol. Saturated fats differ from unsaturated fats in their chemical configuration. Saturated fats have no carbon double bonds, whereas unsaturated fats have one (monounsaturated fats) or more (polyunsaturated fats) double bonds.

These changes during the Industrial Revolution produced another shift in food content. Diets became higher in saturated fat and trans fats and lower in fiber, complex carbohydrates, and unsaturated fats.

In 1917, the USDA began issuing dietary guidelines. There have been many different guidelines, which have shown varying numbers of food groups displayed in different ways. The most recent has been the food pyramid design.

Marion Nestle's recent book, *Food Politics*, outlines the history of and factors behind the changes in the USDA guidelines. These guidelines, unfortunately, often led the public into making poor dietary choices (M. Messina & V. Messina, 1996; Nestle, 2002). The first U.S. government recommendations had five food groups: fruits and vegetables; meats and other protein-rich foods (including milk for children); cereals and other starchy foods; sweets; and fatty foods. From the time of these first guidelines until the late 1960s and early 1970s, the guidelines put no restrictions on any food group. In the 1950s, the USDA invited the food industry to assist in preparation of the dietary guidelines. As a result, throughout the latter part of the history of the USDA guidelines, the powerful influences of parts of the food industry, particularly the meat, dairy, and egg industries, often resulted in weakening of or total absence of any recommendations to decrease or eliminate some foods from the guidelines.

Over the years, the influence of the food industry has also been felt in many other ways. As prepackaged foods, meats, dairy, and eggs became more available, advertising for these products mushroomed. Prepackaged foods with little nutritional value were marketed to the public. The meat, egg, and dairy industries featured prominent and frequent ads for their products, often misrepresenting the nutritional value of those products (Robbins, 1987).

Fast-food restaurants, selling food of poor nutritional value, sprang up rapidly and ubiquitously. Their marketing of "super-size" portions increased not only company profits, but also the caloric contents of their meals ("Cut the fat," 2004).

The food industry has also been influential through its lobbying efforts and financial contributions. Lobbying groups include meat, dairy, and egg associations, such as the National Cattlemen's Association, the National Pork Producers Council, the National Turkey Federation, the United Egg Association, and the International Dairy Foods Association (Nestle, 2002). According to estimates from the Center for Responsive Politics, food and agriculture lobbyists spent $57 million in 2000 on issues other than tobacco (Center for Responsive Politics, 2004). Much of this lobbying money is given to members of the Senate and House agriculture committees (Nestle, 2002).

The food industry has also sought to influence nutrition and health professionals (World Cancer Research Fund, 1997). Food companies and associations donate money to fund nutrition journals, academic conferences, organizations of nutrition professionals, and academic research. Food industry ads have appeared in medical journals. Funds from the food industry also support research about the nutritional value of various industry products. For example, the National Dairy Council has supported research into the role of dairy products on osteoporosis. The egg industry has supported research questioning the effect of eating eggs on elevated blood cholesterol (Robbins, 1987). The objectivity of such research has been questioned.

Increases in industrialization and technology brought not only dietary changes, but also lifestyle changes that can be detrimental to health. Many manual labor jobs were replaced with desk jobs. This, along with increased availability of mass transit, which decreased the necessity to walk as far or as much, led to a more sedentary lifestyle. People began burning fewer calories.

Compared to the diets that fed humans through history, today's diet in the industrialized nations has twice the amount of fat, a much higher ratio of saturated to unsaturated fat, a third of the daily fiber intake, much more sugar and sodium, fewer complex carbohydrates, more foods of animal origin, more processed foods, and a reduced intake of micronutrients (World Cancer Research Fund, 1997; James et al., 1991). Fat intake increased steadily, from about 30% of total energy at the turn of the century to more than 40% in the mid-1980s; this has subsequently declined to around 37%–38% (World Cancer Research Fund, 1997). Diets today also contain more calories.

With these changes have come increased incidence of many chronic diseases, some of which are the major causes of death and disability in the industrialized nations. Diseases such as coronary artery (heart) disease, cancer, stroke, diabetes, vascular diseases, obesity, and gallstones, among others, which are less common in less industrialized societies, have now become common in industrialized nations. Although the etiologies of these diseases are complex, it is clear that diet and lifestyle play important roles.

In the industrialized nations, these changes in diet and lifestyle have appeared gradually over, in some cases, a couple of hundred years. However, in today's developing countries, these changes can come rapidly, even within one to two generations, as industrialization, technology, and transportation move into an area (James et al., 1991). Even people in nations with low per capita income now have access to high-fat and high-added-sugar foods (Caballero & Popkin, 2002). With these changes come rapid increases in the chronic diseases that accompany the westernized diet (James et al., 1991).

Figure 1.2 shows mortality according to per capita gross national product (James et al., 1991).

History of Scientific Research into Diet-Related Diseases

With changes in diet and diet-related illnesses has come a change in nutritional and medical research. Prior to the Industrial Revolution, diets depended primarily on foods grown and produced locally. This was especially true for the poor who did not have access to trading routes. The availability and quality of food were often not reliable. Under such conditions, concerns for nutritional adequacy were paramount. Because of this, nutritional research and concerns centered primarily around problems with dietary inadequacies.

As nations became more industrialized, foods became available from outside the immediate locality. Food supplies became more dependable and abundant, and the classic nutritional inadequacies became less of a problem. Diets, however, became more westernized, and with this came an increase in diet- and lifestyle-related chronic diseases. This led to an increase

Figure 1.2 Mortality from Cardiovascular Disease, Cancer, and Other Diseases According to Per Capita Gross National Product (U.S. $)

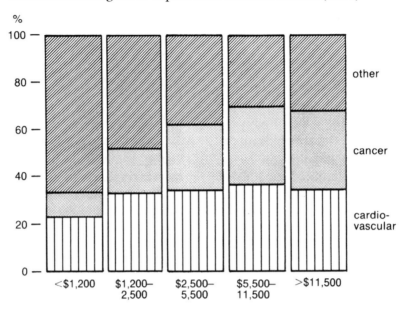

Source: James WP (Chair), Beaton G, Chung-Ming C, et al. for the World Health Organization (excerpted by editors of *Nutrition Review*). Diet, nutrition, and the prevention of chronic diseases: A report of the WHO Study Group on Diet, Nutrition and Prevention of Noncommunicable Diseases. *Nutr Rev.* Oct 1991; 49(10):291–301.

in research related to dietary causes of chronic disease.

Research into vegetarian diets has shown similar changes. Both the amount of research into vegetarian diets, and the emphasis of this research, have changed as the incidence of diet-related diseases has increased. Sabaté, Duk, and Lee (1999) reviewed trends in scientific research from 1966 to 1995. Figure 1.3 shows the average annual publication rate of vegetarian nutrition articles in nutrition journals, non-nutrition journals, and all journals combined.

The focus of research related to vegetarian diets has also changed. Table 1.2 shows the main themes of the vegetarian-related nutrition articles published in the scientific literature from 1966 to 1995 (Sabaté, Duk, & Lee, 1999).

Articles dealing with nutritional adequacy issues, such as nutritional status, deficiency diseases, adequacy of vegetarian diets, and growth indexes prevailed (48%) in the first decade studied, but their overall frequency swiftly decreased over the years. In contrast, articles on disease-preventive or therapeutic applications of vegetarian diets have increased over the years. The major theme in 40% of all vegetarian nutrition articles published in the decade from 1986 to 1995 was the preventive and therapeutic applications of vegetarian diets (Sabaté, Duk, & Lee, 1999).

In addition to frequency, Sabaté et al. also assessed the types of articles dealing with vegetarian diets. In the 1990s, original research articles constituted the largest body of vegetarian

Figure 1.3   Annual Average Publication Rate of Vegetarian Nutrition Articles in Nutrition Journals, Nonnutrition Journals, and Their Combined Total, 1966–1995

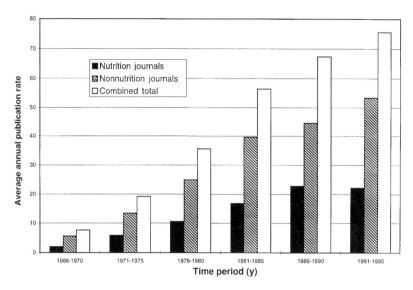

Source: Sabaté J, Duk A, Lee C. Publication trends of vegetarian nutrition articles in biomedical literature, 1966–1995. *Am J Clin Nutr.* 1999;70(3 Suppl): 601S–607S. Reproduced with permission by the *American Journal of Clinical Nutrition,* © Am. J. Clin. Nutr. American Society for Clinical Nutrition.

Table 1.2   Main Themes of Published Vegetarian Nutrition Articles in Biomedical Literature, 1966–1995

	Total	1966–1975	1976–1985	1986–1995	P^1
			n (%)		
Nutritional adequacy issues	162 (29.7)	14 (48.2)	66 (37.2)	82 (24.2)	0.001
Nutritional status	78 (14.3)	9 (31)	29 (16.4)	40 (11.8)	0.006
Deficiency diseases	32 (5.9)	2 (6.9)	16 (9)	14 (4.1)	0.058
Adequacy of vegetarian diets	41 (7.5)	3 (10.3)	16 (9)	22 (6.5)	0.241
Growth and anthropometry	11 (2)	0 (0)	5 (2.8)	6 (1.8)	0.899
Preventive and therapeutic applications	210 (38.6)	7 (24.1)	68 (38.5)	135 (40.0)	0.196
Risk factors	123 (22.6)	3 (10.3)	47 (26.6)	73 (21.6)	0.982
Chronic diseases	38 (7)	2 (6.9)	9 (5.1)	27 (8)	0.333
Medical conditions	49 (9)	2 (6.9)	12 (6.8)	35 (10.4)	0.575
Multiple themes[2]	40 (7.4)	0 (0)	10 (5.6)	30 (8.9)	0.044
Guidelines and recommendations	45 (8.3)	2 (6.9)	12 (6.8)	31 (9.2)	0.193
Other	87 (16)	6 (20.7)	21 (11.9)	60 (17.8)	0.367
Total	544 (100)	29 (100)	177 (100)	338 (100)	

[1]Chi-square test for linear trends (7)
[2]Any combination of 2 of the above-listed themes
Source: Sabaté, Duk, & Lee, 1999. Reproduced with permission by the *American Journal of Clinical Nutrition.* © Am. J. Clin. Nutr. American Society for Clinical Nutrition.

nutrition publications, whereas the opposite was true in the 1960s, when less rigorous publication types, such as anecdotal letters to the editor, were more common.

The original-research studies have also changed over time, in terms of design and, therefore, in strengths and weaknesses. Case-report studies analyze one particular individual's case. Epidemiological studies look at overall risk within specific large groups of people, and can be divided into three main types: observational studies, case-control studies, and prospective (cohort) studies (American Institute for Cancer Research, 2004).

Observational (ecological or correlation) studies look at the incidence of disease and particular factors within a particular population. For instance, this type of study might look at the incidence of heart disease within a large population, such as a country; correlate it with the amount of dietary fat; and then compare this to other large populations and their fat consumption. Although such studies can uncover associations and trends, they cannot prove cause and effect. There may, for instance, be another unrecognized (confounding) factor that occurs in association with the factor under consideration and actually causes the effect under investigation.

Case-control studies begin with a particular endpoint (such as a disease) and look back at the person's history to see what may have affected it. For example, these types of studies might choose two groups, consisting of those who have developed a particular cancer (the study group) and those who have not (the control group), and compare their past diets. Case-control studies are more specific in investigating causes and effects, but must rely on the often-inaccurate memories people have of what they ate in the past. Such studies are also subject to confounding factors.

In contrast, *prospective* (cohort) studies look forward from a particular point in time rather than backward. In cohort studies, a large group of individuals who record their dietary patterns at the start of the study, or who keep records of what they eat at points during the study, is followed for many years to see who develops what diseases. For example, after a set number of years, those in the study group who develop a particular cancer would have their diets analyzed to see if there were identifiable similarities (for instance, lower intake of fruits and vegetables). Although considered more rigorous than case-control studies, cohort studies are still limited by people's estimates of what they are eating. Also, a dietary correlation may be missed if the disease in question was actually affected by dietary choices made years before the study began. The development of certain cancers, for example, might be largely affected by diets consumed many years before the study was initiated. Furthermore, if the participants' diets are recorded only at the start of the study, dietary changes that participants make during the time of the study would not be considered. Finally, cohort studies must be very large to detect a statistically significant number of individuals who develop the disease under study. Like other epidemiological studies, cohort studies may be affected by unrecognized confounding factors.

Whereas all these types of epidemiological studies look at populations of people, *interventional studies* or clinical trials look at changes in some endpoint in an individual person in response to some specific change. For example, such a study might give vitamin E supplements to a group of individuals to see if there is an effect on the incidence of heart disease in that group of individuals. Such studies may be confounded by other factors that might change over the course of the study.

Sabaté, Duke & Lee (1999) concluded that, in terms of study design, intervention studies are becoming more frequent, whereas case-report studies are becoming less common. Similarly, prospective studies are increasing in frequency, while the scientifically weaker observational studies are decreasing.

In summary, the number of research articles on vegetarian diets has ballooned since 1966. Also, the research dealing with vegetarian diets themselves has become more scientific and rigorous. In addition, the research has shifted focus from studies about the nutritional adequacy of vegetarian diets to the disease-prevention and therapeutic aspects of vegetarian diets.

The past few decades have brought an impressive number of studies showing that vegetarian diets can influence the development of several major chronic diseases. Although we often think of this research as a recent development, in fact scientific data suggesting that vegetarian diets can affect health began emerging decades ago. For example, the suggestion that vegetarian diets lower blood pressure dates back at least to 1926 (Beilin, 1986).

It was in 1957 that the American Heart Association proposed modification of dietary fat intake to reduce the incidence of coronary heart disease (CHD) (Krauss et al., 1996). Research dating back 30 years demonstrated a connection between saturated fat intake and serum cholesterol levels and between serum cholesterol levels and CHD. Multiple studies, from as early as the 1960s, have repeatedly reported that vegetarian diets are associated with a relative reduction in cardiovascular risk factors when compared with nonvegetarian diets. More than a decade ago, studies began showing that sufficient reduction of lipids may arrest, and in some cases even reverse, coronary artery disease.

Studies began investigating a link between vegetarian diets and lower cancer incidence as early as the beginning of the 1970s. The National Cancer Act Amendments of 1974 encouraged the National Cancer Program to explore the role of nutrition in the treatment, rehabilitation, and causation of cancer. The first prudent interim dietary principles regarding cancer prevention were issued in a statement by the National Cancer Institute in 1979; they included reduction in dietary fat, generous intake of dietary fiber, moderation in alcohol consumption, avoidance of obesity, and ample fresh fruits and vegetables in the daily diet (Butrum, Clifford, & Lanza, 1988). In 1981, Doll and Peto estimated that 35% of cancer deaths may be related to dietary components, with the possible range of effect being 10%–70% (Doll & Peto, 1981).

Conclusion

From ancient Greek times to the present, there have been proponents of vegetarian diets. In early times, this support was based primarily on philosophical and religious tenets. As scientific methods gained authority, research on vegetarian diets gradually began emerging. Over the past 25 to 35 years, this research has rapidly increased in volume and rigor. During this time there has also been a shift in research emphasis, from the nutritional adequacy of vegetarian diets to their disease-preventive and therapeutic aspects. This book examines the research on both the nutritional and health aspects of vegetarian diets.

References

American Institute for Cancer Research. Available at http://www.aicr.org/information/studies/epidemiological.lasso. Accessed August 15, 2004.

The American vegetarian: Coming of age in the 90s—A study of the vegetarian marketplace conducted for *Vegetarian Times* by Yankelovich, Skelly and White/Clancey, Shulman, Inc.; 1992.

Beilin LJ. Vegetarian approach to hypertension. *Can J Physiol Pharmacol.* 1986;64(6):852-855.

Butrum R, Clifford C, Lanza E. NCI dietary guidelines: Rationale. *Am J Clin Nutr.* 1988;48(3 Suppl): 888-895.

Caballero B, Popkin BM, eds. *The Nutrition Transition: Diet and Disease in the Developing World.* San Diego, CA: Academic Press; 2002.

Center for Responsive Politics. Lobbyist spending. Available at http://www.openseecrets.org. Accessed March 21, 2004.

Cordain L, Miller JB, Eaton SB, et al. Plant-animal subsistence ratios and macronutrient energy estimations in worldwide hunter-gatherer diets. *Am J Clin Nutr.* 2000;71(3):682-692.

Cut the fat. *Consumer Reps.* 2004;69(1):12-16.

Doll R, Peto R. The causes of cancer: Quantitative estimates of avoidable risks of cancer in the United States today. *J Natl Cancer Inst.* 1981; 66(6):1191-1308.

Hardinge MG, Crooks H. Non-flesh dietaries I: Historical background. *J Am Diet Assoc.* 1963a;43: 545-549.

Hardinge MG, Crooks H. Non-flesh dietaries II: Scientific literature. *J Am Diet Assoc.* 1963b;43: 550-558.

How many vegetarians are there? A 2003 national Harris Interactive survey question sponsored by The Vegetarian Resource Group. *Vegetarian J.* 2003;22(3):8-9.

James WP (Chair), Beaton G, Chung-Ming C., et al. for the World Health Organization (excerpted by editors of *Nutrition Review*). Diet, nutrition, and the prevention of chronic diseases: A report of the WHO Study Group on Diet, Nutrition and Prevention of Noncommunicable Diseases. *Nutr Rev.* Oct 1991;49(10):291-301.

Krauss RM (Chair), Deckelbaum RJ, Ernst N, et al. for the American Heart Association. *Dietary Guidelines for Healthy American Adults.* American Heart Association; 1996.

Lappe FM. *A Diet for a Small Planet.* New York: Ballantine Books; 1971.

Long A. The well nourished vegetarian. *New Scientist.* 1981:330-333.

Messina M, Messina V. *The Dietitian's Guide to Vegetarian Diets: Issues and Applications.* Gaithersburg, MD: Aspen Publishers; 1996.

Messina V, Messina M. *The Vegetarian Way.* New York: Crown Trade Paperbacks; 1996.

Mintel International Group Ltd. *The Vegetarian Food Market—U.S. Report.* Chicago: Mintel International Group Ltd.; 2001.

Nestle M. *Food Politics.* Berkeley, CA: University of California Press; 2002.

Robbins J. *Diet for a New America: How Your Food Choices Affect Your Health, Happiness and the Future of Life on Earth.* Walpole, NH: Stillpoint Publishing; 1987.

Roe DA. History of promotion of vegetable cereal diets. *J Nutr.* 1986;116(7):1355-1363.

Sabaté J. *Vegetarian Nutrition.* New York: CRC Press; 2001.

Sabaté J, Duk A, Lee C. Publication trends of vegetarian nutrition articles in biomedical literature, 1966-1995. *Am J Clin Nutr.* 1999;70(3 Suppl): 601S-607S.

Simopoulos AP. Essential fatty acids in health and chronic disease. *Am J Clin Nutr.* 1999;70(3): 560S-569S.

Singer P. *Animal Liberation.* New York: Random House; 1975.

Stahler C. How many vegetarians are there? *Vegetarian J.* 1994;13(4):6-9.

Whorton JC. Historical development of vegetarianism. *Am J Clin Nutr.* 1994;59(Suppl):1103S-1109S.

World Cancer Research Fund/American Institute for Cancer Research. *Food, Nutrition and the Prevention of Cancer: A Global Perspective.* Washington, DC: American Institute for Cancer Research; 1997.

2

Protein

Virginia Messina, MPH, RD

Introduction

The proteins in the foods we eat are digested into individual amino acids. These amino acids are crucial. They are the building blocks the body uses to form its own proteins, such as enzymes used to fuel chemical reactions and tissues such as bone and muscle.

This chapter looks at how plant and animal proteins differ in such aspects as digestibility and amino acid content. We will see that, in spite of the differences, vegetarians can easily meet protein requirements. We then look at *protein complementarity*, which is the concept of mixing plant foods from different sources to ensure that all essential amino acids are consumed daily. We will see that vegetarians should eat protein from different sources each day to ensure adequate intake of all essential amino acids.

Summary of the Scientific Literature

Americans generally consume protein in amounts that significantly exceed recommen-dations; there is little evidence to suggest that such high intakes are beneficial (Metges & Barth, 2000). The protein RDA for adults is 0.8 grams per kilogram of body weight. Protein requirements are met when diets contain about 8%–9% of calories from protein, although the Acceptable Macronutrient Distribution Range for protein has been set at 10%–35% of calories (Food and Nutrition Board, 2002). Data from the third National Health and Nutrition Examination Survey (NHANES-III) indicate that protein intakes in the United States account for nearly 15% of calories (Smit et al., 1999). Individual surveys show that lacto-ovo vegetarian and vegan protein intakes are 12%–14%, and 10%–12%, respectively (Messina, Mangels, & Messina, 2004).

The perceptions that plant protein is vastly inferior in quality to animal protein, and that it is difficult to meet protein needs on plant-based diets, have been largely rejected over the past 10 years. Nevertheless, there is actually considerable debate among scientists over protein and amino acid requirements. Disagreements over protein requirements have arisen for several reasons, including:

- Subtlesigns of protein inadequacy are difficult to detect.
- Humansappear to adapt easily to low protein intakes.
- Energy intake greatly influences protein requirements.
- Theusefulness of nitrogen balance studies for measuring protein needs is unclear.

Protein Quality

The quality of the protein in the diet has some effect on protein needs. Protein quality is determined by two factors: digestibility and amino acid content. The first is of far less importance in Western diets, but does have some bearing on vegetarian requirements.

Digestibility

In North America, protein derived from plant-based diets, consisting largely of whole grains, beans, and vegetables, is about 85% digestible, whereas the protein from mixed diets based on refined grains and meat products, typical of most omnivores, is about 95% digestible (World Health Organization, 1985). Once plant cell-wall constituents are removed, the digestibility of plant proteins is similar to that of animal proteins, which explains why the digestibility of wheat gluten, wheat flour, and soy protein isolate is more than 90%. Beans and some breakfast cereals have lower digestibility, ranging from 50% to 80%.

Differences in digestibility may also arise as a result of inherent differences in the way the amino acids in a protein are linked together; they may also be due to nonprotein factors, such as fiber or polyphenolic compounds. In addition, a variety of processing conditions,

such as heat, oxidation, and the addition of organic solvents and acids, can all adversely affect digestibility. Vegetarian diets in particular may be high in components, such as fiber, that tend to decrease protein digestibility (Acosta, 1988). Overall, however, the digestibility of protein foods in Western vegetarian diets is good.

Still, there are two important methodological considerations regarding the evaluation of protein digestibility that are relevant to both vegetarians and nonvegetarians. One is that individual amino acids may not be as available or digestible as the total protein in a food (Sarwar & Peace, 1986). Consequently, the overall digestibility of a protein may be an overestimate of the actual digestibility of the individual amino acids.

In addition, protein digestibility may typically be overestimated, because the impact of bacterial metabolism in the lower intestines is not considered. Protein is approximately 16% nitrogen on a weight basis. Therefore, protein digestibility is traditionally determined by comparing the amount of nitrogen consumed with the amount of nitrogen excreted in the feces (after correcting for endogenous nitrogen excretion). However, studies have demonstrated that bacteria in the colon metabolize and use some of the nitrogen or amino acids in the intestine, which will decrease the amount of nitrogen excreted and therefore cause overestimation of the amount retained. Although some data suggest that intestinal bacteria can actually contribute indispensable amino acids (IAAs) to the dietary supply (Bingham, 1997; Gibson et al., 1997), other data suggest that amino acid losses due to bacterial metabolism/use may represent 5% or more of the total protein consumed (Millward, 1999). Nevertheless, most tables of protein digestibility do not take this into consideration.

Amino Acid Patterns

A second factor affecting protein quality is the pattern of amino acids in a food. The biologic requirement is not for protein but for amino acids, the building blocks of protein, and for nitrogen. Amino acids from foods are used to synthesize the new proteins needed in the body. Of the 20 amino acids used for protein synthesis, nine are considered indispensable. They must be obtained from food because humans are not able to produce these amino acids.

Proteins are considered "complete" if they supply all the IAAs necessary to meet biologic requirements when consumed at the recommended level of total protein intake. This terminology can be a bit misleading, however, because (with the exception of gelatin) all proteins contain all of the IAAs. Therefore, plant proteins can meet protein and amino acid needs. However, plant proteins tend to be low in one or more IAAs: for example, cereals are low in lysine and threonine, and legumes are low in the sulfur amino acids methionine and cysteine. When these foods are consumed as the sole source of protein at the RDA level (0.8g/kg body weight) for total protein intake, they do not provide the required amount of one or more IAAs. When these lower-quality proteins are eaten, more of the given protein must be consumed to meet amino acid requirements.

Until recently, determination of the protein efficiency ratio (PER) was the official U.S. procedure for evaluating protein quality. It was used for developing the regulations regarding food labeling and the protein recommended daily allowance (RDA). The PER measures the growth of laboratory animals, most often rats, in response to a given amount of protein. Rats grow at a much faster rate than human infants, however, and therefore have much higher protein requirement. Also, rats' requirements for indi-

vidual amino acids differ from humans' needs. For certain amino acids, such as methionine, the rat requirement is a full 50% higher (Sarwar, Peace, & Botting, 1985). Because the limiting amino acid in beans is methionine, the value of legume protein and soy protein, in particular, has been underestimated by use of the PER.

The Food and Agriculture Organization and the World Health Organization (FAO/WHO) and the Food and Drug Administration (FDA) have adopted an alternative method, using the protein digestibility corrected amino acid score (PDCAAS) as an official assay for evaluating protein quality (FAO, 1990; Henley & Kuster, 1994). The PDCAAS is the amino acid score (based on amino acid requirements for two- to five-year-old children) with a correction factor for digestibility. The PDCAAS is calculated by dividing the amount of the IAA in lowest supply in a food (expressed in mg/g of protein) by the requirement for that amino acid for a two- to five-year-old and multiplying the result by the food's digestibility. The PDCAAS has been criticized on several grounds (Sarwar & Peace, 1994; Sarwar & Peace, 1995); nevertheless, it is generally considered to be an improvement over previous methods and is seen as a relatively accurate and quick way to determine protein quality.

Plant Proteins and Nitrogen Balance

The ability of a particular source of protein to meet human needs can be determined by looking at how much of that protein is required to maintain nitrogen balance. When individuals are in nitrogen balance, nitrogen excreted is equal to nitrogen consumed. One study of 16 young men found that to maintain nitrogen balance, twice as much wheat protein as beef protein (178 versus 96 mg of nitrogen/

kg body weight) was required (Young et al., 1975). Similarly, about 35% more rice protein than egg protein was required to achieve nitrogen balance in young men (0.87 versus 0.65 g protein/kg) (Inoue, Fujita, & Niiyama, 1973). Because of the high quality of soybean protein, though, similar amounts of protein from soy and cow's milk (Scrimshaw et al., 1983; Wayler et al., 1983) or beef were required to maintain nitrogen balance.

However, the Michigan State University Bread Study, conducted three decades ago, found that when college students were fed diets for 50 days that provided 70 g of protein per day, 90% to 95% of which was derived from wheat flour, with the remaining protein coming from vegetables, the study subjects were in nitrogen balance (Bolourchi, Friedemann, & Mickelson, 1968). Several other studies (Edwards et al., 1971; Begum, Radhakrishnan, & Pereira, 1970; Hegsted, Trulson, & Stare, 1954; Widdowson & McCance, 1954), though not all (Fujita et al., 1979), have also found that subjects were able to achieve nitrogen balance when fed primarily wheat protein, as well as potato protein (Markakis, 1975; Kon & Kleen, 1928), corn protein (Clark et al., 1967), and rice protein (Lee et al., 1971; Clark, Howe, & Lee, 1971). This may be due to humans' ability to adapt to lower protein intake. It is well known, for example, that in malnourished children, protein catabolism and synthesis are slowed (Young & Scrimshaw, 1977). Short-term studies may fail to allow for this adaptation to low-protein diets and therefore may overestimate protein needs.

Clearly, adaptation occurs, although there is concern that chronic low protein intakes (below the RDA) may result in subtle adverse effects; that is, the level of protein and individual amino acids in these diets may be sufficient for one to survive but not necessarily to thrive (Young & Marchini, 1990).

Protein Complementarity

In the past, vegetarians were advised to compensate for the lower quality of plant proteins by eating plant foods in combination. By combining foods with differing amino acid patterns, "complete" proteins were consumed. According to the American Dietetic Association's 2003 position paper on vegetarian diets, "Research indicates that an assortment of plant foods eaten over the course of a day can provide all essential amino acids and ensure adequate nitrogen retention and use in healthy adults; thus complementary proteins do not need to be consumed at the same time" (Mangels, Messina, & Melina, 2003). Experts in protein nutrition largely concur with this, although recommendations for children may be less flexible (Young & Pellett, 1987; Young & Pellett, 1994). These more flexible guidelines take into consideration the contribution of a pool of extra IAAs that is maintained by the body (Nasset, 1972; Nasset, 1957). This reserve provides free amino acids that can be used to complement dietary proteins. This pool of amino acids comes from as many as four sources (Fuller & Reeds, 1998; Badaloo et al., 1999; Millward et al., 2000):

- Enzymes secreted into the intestine to digest proteins
- Intestinal cells sloughed off into the intestine
- Intracellular spaces of the skeletal musculature
- Synthesis of amino acids by intestinal microflora

Consequently, if one were to consume a meal composed primarily of beans, which are high in lysine, there would be plenty of stored lysine to be used for protein synthesis if a meal comprised primarily of grains was consumed later in the day. The timing of consumption to derive the benefits of complementary amino acid patterns is still not well understood, especially in humans. In children, there is some evidence that combining proteins at a meal can be helpful in meeting protein needs (Young & Pellett, 1994), possibly because of children's higher protein needs on a body-weight basis.

Populations consuming largely plant-based diets tend to eat complementary proteins as part of the normal eating pattern. Some examples include rice and soybean products in Asian countries, chickpeas and sesame tahini in Middle Eastern countries, and pinto beans and corn tortillas in Latin American countries.

Protein Needs of Vegetarians

Although protein needs of vegetarians may be slightly higher due to the somewhat lower digestibility of plant proteins, the Institute of Medicine's Food and Nutrition Board (2002) did not believe there was a need to establish a separate vegetarian RDA for protein. Nevertheless, it may be reasonable to adjust the current RDA somewhat for vegans whose diet consists mainly of beans or harshly processed proteins, or who eat only a limited variety of protein sources. This adjustment would result in a recommendation of about 1.0 g protein/kilogram body weight for adults (Messina, Mangels, & Messina, 2004). This value is consistent with some nitrogen balance studies involving plant-based diets (Agarwal et al., 1984; Yanez et al., 1986; Patwardhan, Mukundan, & Rama Sastri, 1949). This higher level of protein results in a diet that derives approximately 10% of its calories from protein. Both lacto-ovo vegetarians and vegans consume diets that typically contain at least this amount (Messina, Mangels, & Messina, 2004).

The issue of protein adequacy should be of little concern to vegetarians. Protein needs are easily met when the diet includes a variety of plant foods and calorie intake is adequate. The protein intake of vegetarians, even with slightly elevated needs, is adequate. With the exception of fruits, many plant foods are high in protein when expressed on a caloric basis. In fact, because of the high fat content of animal foods, many plant foods are actually higher in percent of calories from protein than animal products such as regular ground beef and 2% whole milk. Furthermore, consuming protein via plant foods will almost certainly result in lower fat, saturated fat, and cholesterol intakes and higher intake of fiber and complex carbohydrates.

Table 2.1 shows the distribution of calories from protein, fat, and carbohydrate in some common foods (Melina, Davis, & Harrison, 1995).

Practical Aspects

Protein requirements are typically met with diets containing about 8%–9% of calories from protein. Vegetarians may need to eat slightly more protein, with vegans having requirements of perhaps 10% of calories as protein. These protein needs are virtually always met by eating a well-balanced vegetarian diet with adequate calories.

Vegetarians should strive to eat protein from a variety of sources (vegetables, legumes, grains) to ensure that all essential amino acids are consumed. One need not combine different sources of protein at each meal; however, different sources should be eaten each day.

Conclusion

Although vegetarians have slightly higher protein needs because plant proteins are less well-

Table 2.1   Distribution of Calories from Protein, Fat, and Carbohydrate in Foods

Percent Calories From:*	Protein	Fat	Carbohydrate
Animal Foods			
Cod	92%	8%	0%
Salmon, sockeye	52%	48%	0%
Beef, lean ground	37%	63%	0%
Beef, regular ground	33%	67%	0%
Eggs	32%	65%	3%
Cow's milk, 2%	27%	35%	38%
Cheddar cheese, medium	25%	74%	1%
Plant Foods			
Legumes and their products			
Tofu, firm	40%	49%	11%
Lentils	30%	3%	67%
Kidney beans	28%	1%	71%
Garbanzo beans (chickpeas)	21%	14%	65%
Vegetables			
Spinach	40%	11%	49%
Broccoli	32%	11%	57%
Carrots	8%	3%	89%
Nuts, seeds, and their products			
Almonds	14%	74%	12%
Sesame butter (tahini)	11%	76%	13%
Grains			
Oatmeal	17%	16%	67%
Wheat	15%	5%	80%
Quinoa	13%	15%	72%
Millet	11%	7%	82%
Rice	9%	5%	86%
Fruits			
Orange	8%	1%	91%
Apples	1%	5%	94%
Recommended Distribution in Diet:	10%–15%	15%–30%	55%–75%

*Percentages were derived using the values 4 calories per gram for protein and carbohydrate and 9 calories per gram for fats.

Source: Melina V, Davis B, Harrison V. *Becoming Vegetarian.* Summertown, TN: Book Publishing Co.; 1995.

digested than animal proteins, these needs are easily met on vegetarian diets that provide adequate calories and a variety of foods. Research shows that lacto-ovo vegetarians and vegans meet protein needs. Vegetarians who consume low-calorie diets may need to make a conscious effort to include high-protein foods, such as soy-based foods, in their diet.

The terms *complete* and *incomplete* exaggerate the differences in quality between animal and plant proteins. By eating a variety of plant foods, all of the indispensable amino acids can be obtained.

Conscious combining of foods at meals is not necessary for adults to meet protein needs, though it is important to eat a variety of plant proteins throughout the day. Young children may benefit from consuming grains and legumes or legumes and nuts at the same meal.

Consuming protein via plant foods will almost certainly result in lower fat, saturated fat, and cholesterol intakes and higher intake of fiber and complex carbohydrates—all aspects of a healthier diet.

References

Acosta PB. Availability of essential amino acids and nitrogen in vegan diets. *Am J Clin Nutr.* 1988; 48:868-874.

Agarwal DK, Agarwal KN, Shankar R, et al. Determination of protein requirements of vegetarian diet in healthy female volunteers. *Indian J Med Res.* 1984;79:60-67.

Badaloo A, Boyne M, Reid M, et al. Dietary protein, growth and urea kinetics in severely malnourished children and during recovery. *J Nutr.* 1999; 129:969-979.

Begum A, Radhakrishnan AN, Pereira SM. Effect of amino acid composition of cereal-based diets on growth of preschool children. *Am J Clin Nutr.* 1970;23:1175-1183.

Bingham SA. Urine nitrogen as an independent validatory measure of protein intake. *Br J Nutr.* 1997;77:144-148.

Bolourchi S, Friedemann CM, Mickelson O. Wheat flour as a source of protein for adult human subjects. *Am J Clin Nutr.* 1968;21:827-835.

Clark HE, Allen PE, Meyers SM, et al. Nitrogen balances of adults consuming opaque-2 maize protein. *Am J Clin Nutr.* 1967;20:825-833.

Clark HE, Howe JM, Lee CJ. Nitrogen retention of adult human subjects fed a high protein rice. *Am J Clin Nutr.* 1971;24:324-328.

Edwards CH, Booker LK, Rumph CH, et al. Utilization of wheat by adult man: Nitrogen metabolism, plasma amino acids and lipids. *Am J Clin Nutr.* 1971;24:181-193.

Food and Agriculture Organization (FAO). *Protein Quality Evaluation.* Rome, Italy: 1990.

Food and Nutrition Board, Institute of Medicine. *Dietary Reference Intakes for Energy, Carbohydrate, Fiber, Fat, Fatty Acids, Cholesterol, Protein and Amino Acids (Macronutrients).* Washington, DC: National Academy Press; 2002.

Fujita Y, Yamamoto T, Rikimaru T, Inoue G. Effect of low protein diets on free amino acids in plasma of young men: Effect of wheat gluten diet. *J Nutr Sci Vitaminol.* 1979;25:427-439.

Fuller MF, Reeds PJ. Nitrogen cycling in the gut. *Ann Rev Nutr.* 1998;18:385-411.

Gibson NR, Ah-Sing E, Badaloo A, et al. Transfer of 15N from urea to the circulating dispensible and indispensible amino acid pool in the human infant. *Proc Nutr Soc.* 1997;56:79A.

Hegsted DM, Trulson MF, Stare FJ. Role of wheat and wheat products in human nutrition. *Physiol Rev.* 1954;34:221-258.

Henley EC, Kuster JM. Protein quality evaluation by protein digestibility-corrected amino acid scoring. *Food Technol.* 1994;48:74-77.

Inoue G, Fujita Y, Niiyama Y. Studies on protein requirements of young men fed egg protein and rice protein with excess and maintenance energy intakes. *J Nutr.* 1973;103:1673-1687.

Kon SK, Kleen A. The value of whole potato protein in human nutrition. *Biochem J.* 1928;22:258.

Lee CJ, Howe JM, Carlson K, Clark HE. Nitrogen retention of young men fed rice with or without supplementary chicken. *Am J Clin Nutr.* 1971; 24:318-323.

Mangels AR, Messina V, Melina V. Position of the American Dietetic Association and Dietitians of Canada: Vegetarian diets. *J Am Diet Assoc.* 2003; 103(6):748-765.

Markakis P. The nutritive quality of potato protein. In: Friedman, M, ed. *Protein Nutritional Quality of Foods and Feeds.* New York: Dekker; 1975.

Melina V, Davis B, Harrison V. *Becoming Vegetarian: The Complete Guide to Adopting a Healthy Vegetarian Diet.* Summertown, TN: Book Publishing; 1995.

Messina V, Mangels R, Messina M. *The Dietitian's Guide to Vegetarian Diets: Issues and Applications.* 2d ed. Sudbury, MA: Jones and Bartlett Publishers; 2004.

Metges CC, Barth CA. Metabolic consequences of a high dietary-protein intake in adulthood: Assessment of the available evidence. *J Nutr.* 2000;130: 886–889.

Millward DJ. The nutritional value of plant-based diets in relation to human amino acid and protein requirements. *Proc Nutr Soc.* 1999;58:249–260.

Millward DJ, Forrester T, Ah-Sing E, et al. The transfer of 15N from urea to lysine in the human infant. *Br J Nutr.* 2000;83:505–512.

Nasset ES. Amino acid homeostasis in the gut lumen and its nutritional significance. *World Rev Nutr Diet.* 1972;14:134–153.

Nasset ES. Role of the digestive tract in the utilization of protein and amino acids. *JAMA.* 1957;164: 172–177.

Patwardhan VN, Mukundan R, Rama Sastri BV. Studies in protein metabolism: The influence of dietary protein on the urinary nitrogen excretion. *Indian J Med Res.* 1949;37:327–346.

Sarwar G, Peace RW. Comparisons between true digestibility of total nitrogen and limiting amino acids in vegetable proteins fed to rats. *J Nutr.* 1986;116:1172–1184.

Sarwar G, Peace RW. Protein quality of enteral nutritionals: A response to Young. *J Nutr.* 1995;125: 1365–1366.

Sarwar G, Peace RW. The protein quality of some enteral products is inferior to that of casein as assessed by rat growth methods and digestibility-corrected amino acid scores [see comments]. *J Nutr.* 1994;124:2223–2232.

Sarwar G, Peace RW, Botting HG. Corrected relative net protein ratio (CRNPR) method based on differences in rat and human requirements for sulfur amino acids. *J Am Oil Chem Soc.* 1985;68: 689–693.

Scrimshaw NS, Wayler AH, Murray E, et al. Nitrogen balance response in young men given one of two isolated soy proteins or milk proteins. *J Nutr.* 1983;113:2492–2497.

Smit E, Nieto FJ, Crespo CJ, Mitchell P. Estimates of animal and plant protein intake in US adults: Results from the Third National Health and Nutrition Examination Survey, 1988–1991. *J Am Diet Assoc.* 1999;99:813–820.

Wayler A, Queiroz E, Scrimshaw NS, et al. Nitrogen balance studies in young men to assess the protein quality of an isolated soy protein in relation to meat proteins. *J Nutr.* 1983;113:2485–2491.

Widdowson EM, McCance RA. *Studies on the Nutritive Value of Bread and on the Effect of Variation in the Extraction Rate of Flour on Growth of Undernourished Children* (Special Report Series 287). London: Medical Research Council; 1954.

World Health Organization. *Joint Food and Agricultural Organization/World Health Organization/United Nations University Expert Consultation.* Geneva: Author; 1985.

Yanez E, Uauy R, Zacarias I, Barrera G. Long-term validation of 1 g of protein per kilogram body weight from a predominantly vegetable mixed diet to meet the requirements of young adult males. *J Nutr.* 1986;116:865–872.

Young VR, Fajardo L, Murray E, et al. Protein requirements of man: Comparative nitrogen balance response within the submaintenance-to-maintenance range of intakes of wheat and beef proteins. *J Nutr.* 1975;105:534–542.

Young VR, Marchini JS. Mechanisms and nutritional significance of metabolic responses to altered intakes of protein and amino acids, with reference to nutritional adaptation in humans. *Am J Clin Nutr.* 1990;51:270–289.

Young VR, Pellett PL. Plant proteins in relation to human protein and amino acid nutrition. *Am J Clin Nutr.* 1994;59(Suppl):1203S–1212S.

Young VR, Pellett PL. Protein intake and requirements with reference to diet and health. *Am J Clin Nutr.* 1987;45:1323–1343.

Young VR, Scrimshaw NS. Human protein and amino acid metabolism and requirements in relation to protein quality. In: Bodwell, CE, ed. *Evaluation of Proteins for Humans.* Westport, CT: AVI; 1977:11–54.

3

Fats

Brenda Davis, RD

Introduction

There is a strong consensus among scientists, health professionals, and the general public that excessive dietary fat is damaging to health. Although we have considerable evidence implicating high-fat diets in chronic diseases such as heart disease, hypertension, type 2 diabetes, certain cancers, and obesity, there is also a solid base of research suggesting that specific fats actually protect against disease. Whether fats support or undermine health depends on several factors, including the quantity and quality of fat consumed.

The dietary fats most consistently linked to negative health consequences are saturated fats, trans fatty acids, and cholesterol. These fats are concentrated in animal products and processed foods. Dietary fats that are generally neutral or beneficial to health are monounsaturated fats (cis- form) and polyunsaturated fats. Polyunsaturated fats include the two essential fatty acids. The intake and balance of these two fatty acids can have profound consequences for health. In addition, methods of processing, storing, and cooking foods can adversely affect the quality of fats and oils.

It is widely recognized that vegetarians enjoy health advantages when compared to omnivores, including lower morbidity and mortality (American Dietetic Association, 1997). It is also generally accepted that these discrepancies are due, at least in part, to the inherent differences in the fat content of these eating patterns. Vegetarian diets are slightly lower in total fat than omnivorous diets: 30%–36% on average for ovo-lacto vegetarians; 28%–33% for vegans, and 34%–38% or more for omnivores (Messina & Messina, 1996). Though the differences in total fat content are not as great as might be expected, the differences in quality of fat are noteworthy. Compared to omnivores, vegetarians consume about one-third less saturated fat (vegans about one-half less), and about half as much cholesterol (vegans consume none) (Draper et al., 1993; Janelle & Barr, 1995; Melby, Foldflies, & Toohey, 1993). Intake of trans fatty acids is highly dependent on the amount of processed foods in the diet. Limited research comparing trans fatty acid intake of omnivores and vegetarians suggests that vegetarians consume slightly smaller amounts, with more pronounced differences found in vegans eating a whole-foods diet (Draper et al., 1993). One study, examining trans fatty acids in subcutaneous fat, found vegetarians to have one-third less trans fatty acids in their tissues than non-vegetarians, with vegans (who eat no refined foods) having no detectable levels (Crane, Zielinski, & Aloia, 1988).

Vegetarian diets appear to offer no advantages over omnivorous eating patterns regarding essential fatty acid balance and intake. Indeed, it has been suggested that vegetarians could be at a disadvantage, as plant sources of omega-3 fatty acids are limited and vegetarian diets are lacking in direct sources of long-chain omega-3 fatty acids (EPA and DHA) (Conquer & Holub, 1997).

This chapter explores current issues and controversies concerning fats in the vegetarian diet, moving us beyond the question of safe and adequate intake to that of optimal intake for vegetarians at every stage of the life cycle. The key issues are examined under four headings:

1. *Defining optimal quantity of fat.* What quantity of fat is recommended in the vegetarian diet?
2. *Achieving recommended essential fatty acid intakes.* How can we ensure that vegetarian diets provide a sufficient quantity and balance of essential fatty acids?
3. *Ensuring highest-quality fat sources.* What sources of fat offer the greatest health advantages?
4. *Practical guidelines for optimal health.* What practical recommendations regarding dietary fat intake can we make to assist vegetarians in making healthful choices?

Summary of the Scientific Literature

Defining Optimal Quantity of Fat

The question of optimal fat intake is among the most hotly debated issues in vegetarian nutrition. On one side of the fence are the proponents of very-low-fat diets (10%–15% fat or less), generally advising against the use of concentrated fats and oils and higher-fat plant foods such as nuts, seeds, avocados, and olives (and often limiting full-fat soy foods). On the other are those advocating much higher-fat (30%–40% fat), "Mediterranean"-style diets with liberal use of olive oil, nuts, seeds, avocados, and olives, in addition to cheese and other dairy products (foods rich in trans fatty acids are avoided). The World Health Organization recommends a total fat intake between 15%–30% of calories. They note that highly active groups with diets rich in vegetables, legumes, fruits, and whole-grain cereals may sustain a total fat intake of up to 35% without the risk of unhealthy weight gain (Report of a Joint FAO/WHO Expert Consultation, 2003). The new *Dietary Reference Intakes for Energy, Carbohydrates, Fiber, Fat, Protein, and Amino Acids* (DRI Macronutrients, 2002) does not set a recommended dietary allowance (RDA), acceptable intake (AI), or upper limit (UL) for total fat (except for during the first year of life), but they do suggest something called the acceptable macronutrient distribution range (AMDR). The AMDR for fat is 20%–35% of calories for everyone four years of age and older, and 30%–40% of calories for children aged one to three years (Food and Nutrition Board, 2002).

The fat debate is generally framed around disease risk reduction and the amount of dietary fat that is most effective in preventing, treating, or reversing chronic diseases. It is often assumed that the diet that best succeeds in this

Box 3.1   A Fatty Acid Primer

Cholesterol   A sterol that is necessary to the structure of every cell. As the human body makes about 800–1,000 mg of cholesterol a day, there is no need of any cholesterol in the diet. Cholesterol comes only from animal foods and is concentrated in eggs and organ meats. High intakes increase the risk for chronic diseases, especially of the heart and blood vessels.

Essential Fatty Acids   Most of the fatty acids that we need for survival can be produced in the body, but there are two that we cannot make and must obtain from food. These are called *essential fatty acids*. One is a parent in the omega-6 family called *linoleic acid*. The other is a parent in the omega-3 family called *alpha-linolenic acid*.

Fatty Acids   Basic components of fats and oils. Fatty acids do not generally roam free in the body; most of them travel in threesomes as part of larger molecules called *triglycerides*. Foods contain three types of fatty acids, in varying amounts: saturated, monounsaturated, and polyunsaturated. Fatty acids are built from a chain of carbon atoms with hydrogen and oxygen molecules attached. The degree of saturation of a fatty acid depends on the amount of hydrogen attached to the carbon atoms.

Highly Unsaturated Fatty Acids (HUFAs)   Larger polyunsaturated fatty acid molecules. These fatty acids originate from either of two places. We can convert "parent" fatty acids to these longer-chain fatty acids in the body, or we can consume these long-chain fatty acids directly from food. In the omega-6 family, we may either convert linoleic acid to arachidonic acid (AA) or AA can be consumed directly from animal products, such as meat and dairy products. In the omega-3 family, we may convert alpha-linolenic acid to eicosapentaenoic acid (EPA) and docosahexaenoic acid (DHA), or they can be consumed directly from fish (both EPA and DHA), eggs (small amounts of DHA), seaweed (small amounts of EPA), and microalgae (single-celled organisms that provide EPA and DHA; varieties currently available in North America provide only DHA). See Table 3.1 for the metabolism of essential fatty acids.

Lipids   A family of compounds that do not dissolve in water. They include fats and oils (made up of fatty acids), sterols (such as cholesterol), and phospholipids (such as lecithin). Although fats are only one type of lipid, the words *fat* and *lipid* are commonly used interchangeably. The main feature that distinguishes fats from oils is that fats are hard at room temperature, whereas oils are liquid. Fats are generally found in animal products, such as meat, poultry, and dairy; oils are commonly derived from plant seeds, such as olive, canola, corn, and sunflower.

Monounsaturated Fats   Fatty acids having one spot in the carbon chain where hydrogen is missing (one point of unsaturation). Monounsaturated fat has been shown to have neutral or slightly beneficial effects on health, with modest effects on blood cholesterol levels. When monounsaturated fat replaces saturated, trans fatty acids, or refined carbohydrates, it decreases total and LDL cholesterol, and slightly increases HDL cholesterol. There is some evidence that monounsaturated fat may slightly reduce blood pressure and enhance blood flow. Oils rich in monounsaturated fat are generally liquid at room temperature, but become cloudy and thick when refrigerated, as does olive oil. The richest dietary sources of

continued

Box 3.1 *Continued*

monounsaturated fat are olives, olive oil, canola oil, avocados, most nuts (except for walnuts and butter-nuts), high-oleic sunflower oil, and high-oleic safflower oil (sunflower and safflower oils are usually mainly omega-6 oils, but the high-oleic varieties are bred to have a high monounsaturated fat content).

Phytosterols   Sterols naturally present in plants and in the body. We absorb far less plant sterols, and they also help to block cholesterol absorption from the gut. All whole-plant foods contain small amounts of these compounds. Some new products on the market have added sterols. Vegetarian diets are naturally higher in phytosterols than nonvegetarian diets.

Polyunsaturated Fats   Fatty acids having more than one spot in the carbon chain where hydrogen is missing (more than one point of unsaturation). Fats high in polyunsaturates are liquid at room temperature and when refrigerated. There are two distinct families of polyunsaturated fats, the omega-6 and the omega-3 families. The family names describe the first point of unsaturation on the carbon chain. In the omega-6 family, the first double bond occurs at the sixth carbon from the methyl end, and in the omega-3 family it occurs at the third carbon from the methyl end. The effects of polyunsaturated fats on health are generally favorable, and certain polyunsaturated fats are absolutely necessary for human survival. When they replace saturated fats, trans fatty acids, or refined carbohydrates in the diet, total and LDL cholesterol levels decrease, and HDL levels may slightly increase. Their impact on other risk factors for cardiovascular disease is varied. Their impact on cancer risk appears to be mixed: some studies show a beneficial effect, and others show a negative effect. Their effect on other diseases seems no less contradictory. Some of the discrepancy can be explained by inherent differences in the two distinct families of polyunsaturated fatty acids, and the balance in quantities of each. The main dietary sources of polyunsaturated fats are vegetable oils, seeds, nuts, grains, legumes, and other plant foods.

Saturated Fats   Fatty acids completely packed or "saturated" with hydrogen. Fats containing primarily saturated fatty acids are generally hard at room temperature. Excessive intakes of saturated fats have consistently been linked to an increased risk of chronic diseases, including coronary artery disease, type 2 diabetes, kidney disease, gallstones, and some forms of cancer. Animal products are the main sources of saturated fats in Western diets. Approximately 20%–30% of the fat in fish, 33% of the fat in poultry, 40%–44% of the fat in red meat, and 62% of the fat in dairy is saturated. Most high-fat plant foods contain much less fat, with about 5%–20% of fat being saturated. The one exception is tropical oils. Coconut fat is more than 85% saturated; palm kernel oil more than 80%, and palm oil about 50%. These foods are rarely a major part of any North American diet, in most cases accounting for less than 2% of the fat. Most governments and health authorities recommend that saturated fat should not exceed 10% of energy. The World Health Organization (WHO), in Technical Report 916, *Diet, Nutrition and the Prevention of Chronic Diseases* (2003), suggests saturated fat intakes of less than 10% of energy in healthy populations and less than 7% of energy in high-risk populations.

Trans Fatty Acids   Unsaturated fatty acids with two hydrogen atoms on opposite sides of the double bond. In nature, most unsaturated fatty acids are cis fatty acids. This means that the hydrogen atoms are on the same side of the double carbon bond, giving the molecule a curved shape. In trans fatty acids, a hydrogen atom flips to the other side of the double bond, changing the cis configuration to a trans con-

Box 3.1 *Continued*

figuration. This changes the curved, flexible molecule to a straight, rigid molecule. The vast majority of trans fatty acids are formed during the process of hydrogenation—a process that turns liquid oils into solid, stable fats. Trans double bonds can also occur in nature as the result of fermentation in grazing animals. Hydrogenated fats were developed to improve the shelf life of foods, increase the melting point of fat (good for deep-frying), and permit high-temperature cooking. Trans fatty acids have been demonstrated to have highly negative consequences for human health, though naturally formed trans fatty acids may be less damaging than those formed by artificial hydrogenation. Gram for gram, trans fatty acids appear to be two to four times more damaging than saturated fats. Trans fatty acids increase the risk of heart disease, interfere with liver function, increase insulin resistance, contribute to low-birth-weight babies, and interfere with essential fatty acid metabolism. Our most concentrated sources are margarine, shortening, crackers, cookies, granola bars, chips, snack foods, baked goods, and deep-fried fast foods.

endeavor would be the diet of choice for the entire vegetarian population. However, although disease risk reduction is a vital consideration in the pursuit of optimal health, it is not the sole consideration. Other important factors are ensuring adequate growth and development, meeting nutrient needs (including essential fatty acids, vitamins, and minerals), and maximizing the absorption of nutrients and protective phytochemicals.

Very-Low-Fat Vegetarian Diets

Very-low-fat vegetarian diets have enjoyed considerable popularity among Western vegetarian populations. The attraction is ascribed to research studies demonstrating the phenomenal success of such diets (often in combination with other lifestyle changes) in treating patients with severe coronary artery disease. In 1990, Dr. Dean Ornish proved that diet and lifestyle changes (<10% fat vegetarian diet, stress management, aerobic exercise, and group therapy) could not only slow the progression of atherosclerosis, but also significantly reverse it. In the first phase of this randomized, controlled clinical trial, 48 patients were followed

for one year. Eighty-two percent of the experimental group participants experienced regression of their disease, while in the control group the disease continued to progress (control group participants followed a 30% fat, <200-mg-cholesterol diet). Total and LDL cholesterol dropped an average 24% and 37%, respectively, in the experimental group, and 5% and 6%, respectively, in the control group. Patients in the experimental group reported a 91% reduction in the frequency of angina, while patients in the control group reported a 165% rise in frequency (Ornish et al., 1990). The second phase of this research took place over the next four years, during which time more regression of atherosclerosis occurred in the experimental group, and more progression in the control group. In addition, the control group experienced twice as many cardiac events as the experimental group (Ornish et al., 1998). The powerful cholesterol-reducing effects of very-low-fat vegetarian or near-vegetarian diets have been further supported by the work of Esselstyn (1999), Barnard (1991), and McDougall et al. (1995).

Although Ornish and others have provided valuable contributions to science and medicine, the evidence for health benefits of a very-low-fat vegetarian diet lies primarily in treating patients with severe coronary artery disease. It is important to recognize that the dietary goals for a healthy vegetarian population, and particularly for growing children, are different than they are for individuals with severe cardiovascular disease. There are no scientific studies to indicate that healthy vegetarians would benefit from eliminating nuts, seeds, and other high-fat, whole-plant foods from their diet. Indeed, eliminating such foods may prove to be a disadvantage for this population. The concerns associated with the use of very-low-fat diets among healthy vegetarians include:

- Very-low-fat diets may provide insufficient energy, particularly for infants and children.

Among the most common reasons a vegetarian diet would fail to adequately nourish an infant or child is that it provides insufficient energy. Studies of malnutrition in vegetarian/vegan populations have consistently demonstrated that overly restrictive diets (with little or no added fat) do not adequately support growth and development (Dagnelie & van Staveren, 1994; Shinwell & Gorodischer, 1982), and thus are not advised for this age group (Kaplan & Toshima, 1992; Jarvis & Millre, 1996; Zlotkin, 1996). Individuals with high energy needs, such as pregnant and lactating women or competitive athletes, may also have difficulty achieving energy requirements when consuming very-low-fat diets.

- Very-low-fat diets may not provide sufficient essential fatty acids (especially omega-3 fatty acids).

Diets providing less than 10% of calories from fat may compromise essential fatty acid intakes. These nutrients are necessary for the formation of healthy cell membranes, the proper development and functioning of the brain and nervous system, the absorption of vital nutrients, and the production of hormone-like substances called *eicosanoids*. Very-low-fat vegetarian diets (no added fat, limited fat-rich plant foods) generally provide sufficient omega-6 fatty acids when liberal amounts of grains are consumed. In contrast, such diets provide only about 25%–30% of omega-3 fatty acid needs, unless omega-3-rich foods are included (e.g., flaxseeds or flaxseed oil). Diets supplying less than 10% of energy from fat generally do not supply sufficient essential fatty acids during pregnancy and lactation (Hachey, 1994).

- The absorption of fat-soluble vitamins, minerals, and phytochemicals may be compromised when very-low-fat diets are consumed.

Studies indicate that the absorption of fat-soluble vitamins, minerals (including iron, zinc, manganese, and calcium), and phytochemicals is enhanced with moderate levels of dietary fat as compared to very-low-fat diets (Siguel & Lerman, 1994; Kies, 1988; Gartner, Stahl, & Sies, 1997). The absorption of certain nutrients (iron and zinc in particular) is lower in vegetarian diets; thus, further reduction could potentially compromise nutritional status, especially in children. Phytochemicals play an important role in reducing disease processes; hence, maximizing their absorption would be well advised.

- The overall nutritional value of the diet may be reduced when consumers make total fat content their highest priority for food selection.

Many individuals following very-low-fat diets become "fat phobic," avoiding all foods that contain fat. In so doing, they may shun nutritious, whole-plant foods in favor of much less nourishing fat-free processed foods. A bag of non-fat potato chips or fat-free cookies may be selected over a handful of almonds or edamame (green soybeans) or a loaf of white bread over whole-grain bread containing flax and pumpkin seeds. Higher-fat plant foods (e.g., tofu, full-fat soy milk and other soy products, nuts, seeds, wheat germ, avocados, and olives) provide valuable nutrients, including antioxidants such as vitamin E, selenium, other trace minerals, and a host of protective phytochemicals.

- Very-low-fat, high-carbohydrate diets can cause a drop in HDL cholesterol and a rise in triglycerides.

High-carbohydrate, low-fat eating patterns have been associated with a drop in HDL cholesterol and a rise in triglycerides. These changes in blood lipids are most significant when diets are low in fiber, such as when the carbohydrates are derived predominately from refined grains (e.g., "white flour" products such as bread, bagels, pasta, crackers, pretzels, etc.). Preliminary research suggests that when whole-plant foods are used, changes in triglycerides are favorable (Anderson et al., 1991; Turley et al., 1998; Nicholson et al., 1999). It is important to note that a drop in HDL is a natural consequence of total cholesterol reduction, as the primary function of HDL is the removal of excess cholesterol from the bloodstream (when there is less cholesterol to remove, there is less need for HDL cholesterol). Thus, although some decrease in HDL levels may occur with high-carbohydrate, low-fat diets, it is not necessarily detrimental to health. Indeed, low HDL levels are seen in many societies that eat plant-based diets, and these social groups are at very low risk for coronary artery disease (CAD).

Mediterranean-Style Diets

Although the evidence supporting a very-low-fat diet in the reversal of coronary artery disease is strong, epidemiological evidence suggests that certain high-fat diets can be protective against chronic disease. Key's classic "Seven Countries" study demonstrated a positive connection between saturated animal fats and coronary artery disease. The lowest mortality rate was not, however, in the country with the lowest total fat intake, but rather in Crete, where people consumed high amounts of fat but relatively small amounts of damaging saturated fats, trans fatty acids, and cholesterol (Keys, Menotti, & Toshima, 1986). These findings made the experts question whether the *types* of fats consumed could actually be a greater predictor of disease than the *amount* of fat consumed.

In the Lyon heart study, 605 post-heart-attack patients were assigned to either a "prudent Western-type diet" (AHA) or a modified version of the Crete diet. The Crete diet was based on grains, vegetables, fruits, legumes, and fish, with liberal use of olive and canola oil. (Actual intake based on final visit: Total fat—30% for Crete diet, 34% for prudent diet; saturated fat—8% for Crete diet, 12% for prudent diet; omega-6:omega-3 ratio—4:1 for Crete diet, 18:1 for prudent diet.) Within four months of the start of the trial, preliminary results indicated that participants on the Crete diet had significantly fewer deaths than participants on the AHA diet. By the end of two years, patients on the Crete diet had an unprecedented 76% lower risk of dying of a heart attack or stroke (de Lorgeril, Salen, & Delaye, 1996).

Mediterranean diets provide a compelling argument for higher fat intakes being perfectly compatible with optimal coronary health. However, the advantages experienced by consumers may be related more to other beneficial components of the diet than its high fat content. A strong message provided by the Mediterranean diet is that it is not nuts, seeds, avocados, olives, or soybeans that are responsible for the epidemic of chronic disease that plagues us.

Diets containing more than 35% of calories from fat are not recommended. Potential problems associated with high-fat diets include the following.

- High-fatdiets can dilute nutrient density, making it a challenge to meet recommended intakes for nutrients.

This is of particular concern when the main sources of fat are concentrated fats and oils, such as vegetable oils, margarine, mayonnaise-type spreads, coconut oil, and foods prepared or manufactured with these fats (as opposed to nuts, seeds, soy, avocados, etc.). Concentrated fats and oils, such as commercial lards, shortenings, and vegetable oils, contribute very few nutrients (vitamins and minerals) and other protective components (phytochemicals and fiber) to the diet. Thus, when these fats and oils are abundant in the diet, it can be difficult to meet needs for nutrients that are sometimes marginal (e.g., trace minerals such as zinc).

- High-fatdiets can lead to excessive caloric intake, thereby contributing to obesity in some individuals.

Ounce for ounce, fat provides more than double the calories of protein or carbohydrate. It also has less bulk and a lower satiety value than carbohydrates or protein, making overconsumption more likely. In addition, dietary fat is stored as body fat more readily than carbohydrate or protein. Generally, where populations consume high levels of fat, the incidence of obesity is greater (especially where that population also tends to be sedentary). Obesity in and of itself increases risk of several chronic diseases.

- High-fat diets may be linked to other chronic diseases.

A great deal of research has been conducted on the association between total fat and the risk of chronic disease. Evidence shows that diets high in saturated fat increase the risk for cardiovascular diseases, and possibly diabetes and stroke. High-fat diets may also be linked to some cancers.

- High-fatdiets may result in increased oxidative damage to body tissues.

Free radicals are reactive oxygen molecules containing one or more unpaired electrons (most molecules are stable, containing only paired electrons) that react quickly with other molecules, turning them into free radicals too, and thereby setting off a destructive chain of oxidative damage to tissues. Free radicals preferentially react with polyunsaturated fats (unstable molecules); thus, people consuming large amounts of these fats could be more susceptible to oxidative damage. Oxidative stress has been linked to numerous disease processes, including heart disease, cancer, diabetes, arthritis, age-related diseases, and neurological disorders.

Making Sense of the Dichotomy

While it may appear that this debate is between diametrically opposed eating patterns, very-low-fat vegetarian diets have more in common with the Mediterranean-style diets than not. Both are plant-centered diets based on vegetables, legumes, fruits, and whole grains, providing abundant plant protein, fiber, phytochemicals, vitamins, and minerals—all dietary components that are protective to health. Neither eating pattern is high in saturated fat, trans fatty acids, cholesterol, animal protein, or refined carbohydrates—dietary components that contribute to chronic disease. Nor does either diet contain excessive omega-6 fatty acids, and when sources of omega-3 fatty acids are included in very-low-fat eating patterns, both provide a reasonable quantity and balance of these essential nutrients.

In making dietary recommendations appropriate for the entire vegetarian population, it is important to recognize that requirements for fat vary substantially throughout the life cycle and among individuals. It is recommended that fat not be restricted during the first two years of life (human breast milk provides 50% of its energy from fat) (Jarvis & Millre, 1996; Zlotkin, 1996). After the age of two years, until the end of linear growth, dietary fat gradually declines, from 40%–50% of calories during infancy, to about 30%–40% during early childhood, then closer to 30% or less by the teen years. Healthy vegetarian adults should aim for a total of 15%–30% of energy from fat. Less than 15% of energy from fat could jeopardize essential fatty acid intake and absorption of important nutrients and phytochemicals, although fat intakes closer to 10% of energy may be advantageous for the reversal of atherosclerosis. For most people, there appears to be no advantage to consuming diets providing in excess of 30% of calories from fat. Such diets are often energy dense (potentially contributing to excessive energy intake and obesity) (IOM/FNB, 2002), with poor nutrient density (especially when the fat comes from oil, as opposed to more nutrient-dense foods such as nuts or seeds). In addition, diets high in fat (saturated fat, in particular) have been linked to other chronic diseases, including cardiovascular disease, and possibly diabetes, stroke, and some cancers (World Cancer Research Fund, 1997).

Although total fat intake has received a great deal of attention from scientists and consumers, there is mounting evidence that the amount of fat consumed may be less important than the source of fat. Fats derived from animal foods and processed vegetable oils (saturated fats and trans fatty acids) are more strongly associated with chronic disease, whereas fats from whole-plant foods are generally benign or, in some cases, protective (especially foods rich in monounsaturated fat and/or omega-3 fatty acids).

Achieving Recommended Essential Fatty Acid Intakes

Within the two families of polyunsaturated fats (PUFAs), there is one essential fatty acid (EFA) or "parent" fatty acid. Linoleic acid (LA) is the EFA in the omega-6 family and alpha-linolenic acid (ALA) is the EFA in the omega-3 family. These fatty acids cannot be made by the body and must be obtained through diet. There are several other very important fats in each family, called highly unsaturated fatty acids (HUFAs). Humans have the ability to convert LA and ALA to HUFAs through a series of elongation and desaturation reactions. These fatty acids are critical to health; however, because they can be made in the body from parent fatty acids, they are not generally "essential" in our diets. Highly unsaturated fatty acids are even more physiologically active in the body than essential fatty acids, and have powerful impacts on health. These fats are needed for the formation of healthy cell membranes; they help cells keep their shape and flexibility, and allow substances to flow in and out. They are critical to the development and functioning of the brain and nervous system, and are involved in the production of hormone-like substances called *eicosanoids* (thromboxanes, leucotrienes, prostaglandins, and prostacyclins), which regulate many organ systems. In the omega-6 family, the most important HUFAs are arachidonic acid (AA) and dihommogamma-linolenic acid (DGLA). In the omega-3 family, the most important HUFAs are eicosapentaenoic acid (EPA) and docosahexaenoic acid (DHA). All of these HUFAs, except for DHA, serve as raw materials for making eicosanoids. The eicosanoids formed from AA have very potent effects, such as increasing blood pressure, inflammation, and thrombosis, all of which can increase the risk of cardiovascular disease. Those formed from EPA and DGLA are less potent, and tend to have the opposite effects. Although we need the eicosanoids formed from AA for fight-or-flight reactions (such as running from danger), chronic disease risk increases when they are overexpressed in the human body.

Docosahexaenoic acid is not a precursor of eicosanoids, but is an important structural component of the gray matter of the brain, the retina of the eye, and specific cell membranes, and is found in high levels in the testes and sperm. Low levels of DHA have been associated with several neurological and behavioral disorders, such as depression, schizophrenia, Alzheimer's disease, and attention deficit hyperactivity disorder (ADHD) (Conquer & Holub, 1997). In addition, low levels of DHA are also linked to suboptimal visual acuity and reduced brain development in infants (Uauy et al., 2001). Thus, although these long-chain fatty acids are not technically "essential" nutrients, it is important to ensure sufficient levels, whether by relying on conversion from parent fatty acids or by direct consumption.

Essential Fatty Acid Conversion

Vegetarians have few direct sources of EPA and DHA (highly unsaturated omega-3 fatty acids) in the diet, and thus must convert alpha-linolenic acid to EPA and DHA in the body. Although conversion of essential fatty acids to longer-chain fatty acids is, at least in part, dependent on genetics, age, and overall health, several dietary factors also have a significant impact on the conversion process. First, it is important to ensure that the diet is nutritionally adequate, as poorly designed diets can impair the conversion process. Insufficient energy or protein decreases the activity of conversion enzymes, as can deficiencies of pyridoxine, biotin, calcium, copper, magnesium, and zinc (Siguel & Lerman, 1994; Horrobin, 1992). Trans fatty acids can also depress conversion enzymes, and com-

petitively inhibit the incorporation of essential fatty acids into cell membranes. In addition, alcohol inhibits the activity of delta-5 and delta-6 desaturase and depletes tissues of long-chain omega-3 fatty acids (Nervi, Peluffo, & Brenner, 1980). High intakes of omega-6 fatty acids can have a profound effect on omega-3 fatty acid conversion, reducing it as much as 40% (Emken, Adlof, & Gulley, 1994). Conversion enzymes may also be compromised in people with diabetes or certain metabolic disorders, and those who inherit a limited ability to produce these enzymes (possibly in populations where fish has been a major component of the diet for generations) (Simopoulos, 1999).

Conversion of linoleic acid to AA is typically efficient; conversion of alpha-linolenic acid to EPA and DHA tends to be less efficient. In healthy individuals, an estimated 5%–10% of alpha-linolenic acid is converted to EPA, but less than 2%–5% is converted to DHA (Emken, Adlof, & Gulley, 1994; Ghafoorunissa, 1998; Gerster, 1998). There is some evidence that the conversion may be significantly better in women than men. Two recent UK studies found that young men converted alpha-linolenic acid at a rate of approximately 8% to EPA and 0% to DHA, whereas young women converted 21% to EPA and 9% to DHA (Burge, Jones, & Wootton, 2002; Burge & Wootton, 2002).

Although conversion is slow and incomplete, it appears to be sufficient to meet the needs of most healthy people, if intake of alpha-linolenic acid is sufficient (Conquer & Holub, 1997). It is important to note that there is a rapidly expanding database that demonstrates significant effects of omega-3 fatty acids on primary and secondary prevention of chronic diseases, particularly cardiovascular disease. Both epidemiologic and randomized controlled clinical studies have evaluated the effects of both marine and plant sources of omega-3 fatty acids—from food sources as well as supplements. These studies have established that both forms of omega-3 fatty acids have protective effects (Davis & Kris-Etherton, 2003).

EFA Intake and Status of Vegetarians

Total omega-3 fatty acid intakes are similar for vegans, vegetarians, and omnivores: approximately 1–3 g/day, with the current average being about 1.0–1.8 g/day (IOM/FNB, 2002; Messina, Mangels, & Messina, 2004). However, the intakes of very-long-chain omega-3 fatty acids (EPA and DHA) vary appreciably. Vegans consume negligible amounts of EPA and DHA, whereas vegetarians consume minimal EPA (less than 5 mg/day) and varying amounts of DHA depending on egg consumption (a source of DHA, averaging approximately 33 mg/day) (Ferrier et al., 1995). Consumption of EPA and DHA in omnivores varies according to fish and egg intake, with average intakes in the 100–150 mg/day range. Omega-6 intakes are significantly higher in vegan and vegetarian populations than in omnivorous populations, ranging from a low of about 5%–7% of calories in omnivores to a high of about 10%–12% of calories in vegans. As a result, the omega-6:omega-3 ratio is generally considered to be elevated in vegans (approximately 14:1–20:1) and ovo-lacto vegetarians (approximately 10:1–16:1) compared with omnivores (approximately 10:1).

Reports to date suggest that the low consumption of EPA and DHA, and generous intakes of linoleic acid, have resulted in reduced levels of EPA and DHA in body fluids and tissues of vegetarians, and especially vegans. In 1978, Sanders et al. first noted that the plasma and total erythrocyte lipid levels of vegans were significantly decreased. In vegans, EPA levels were only 12%–15% those of nonvegetarians, and DHA levels were 32%–35% those of nonvegetarians (Sanders, Ellis, & Dickerson, 1978). Melchert et al. (1987) examined the fatty acid levels in the serum of vegetarians and nonvegetarians and found that DHA levels were approximately 40% lower in vegetarians than nonvegetarians. Sanders and Roshanai (1992) found that vegan EPA plasma levels were only 22% that of omnivores and DHA levels were 38% of omnivores, although AA levels were similar. In 1994, Reddy et al. again demonstrated that vegetarians (who appeared to be vegan, based on a zero intake of EPA and DHA) had reduced EPA in plasma phospholipids (37% of nonvegetarians), and DHA (52% of nonvegetarians) (Reddy, Sanders, & Obeid, 1994). Krajcovicova-Kudlackova et al. (1997) compared the fatty acid status of vegans, ovo-lacto vegetarians, semi-vegetarians, and omnivores between the ages of 11 and 15 years. Though the levels of EPA and DHA were similar in vegetarians and nonvegetarians, they were significantly lower in vegans (62%–65% of nonvegetarians). Interestingly, while long-chain omega-3 fatty acids were reduced in vegan children, they were not as severely decreased as reported in vegan adults. The higher EPA and DHA levels in vegan children may be the result of reserves from extended breastfeeding, or from better conversion in this age group. Ågren et al. (1995) compared serum lipid levels of vegans eating uncooked food with that of nonvegetarians. The proportions of EPA and DHA in vegans were only 29%–36% and 49%–52%, respectively, those of nonvegetarian controls, and the levels of AA were similar, indicating no difficulty with the n-6 conversion. Sanders and Reddy (1992) compared the LA, ALA, and DHA content of vegan, vegetarian, and omnivorous human milk. The mean percent of linoleic acid was 23.8%, 19.7%, and 10.9%, respectively; alpha-linolenic acid was 1.36%, 1.25%, and 0.49%, respectively; and DHA was 0.14%, 0.30%, and 0.37%, respectively. Milk from vegan mothers had more than double the linoleic and alpha-linolenic acid of the nonvegetarian mothers, but less than half of the DHA. The EPA status of the infants (as determined by erythrocyte lipids) reflected the levels in the milk they received. Vegan infants had less than 30% of the EPA and DHA of omnivorous infants.

Two other groups comparing EPA and DHA status of vegetarians and nonvegetarians found little difference in their levels (Kirkeby & Bjerkedal, 1968; Holub & Conquer, 1997). Holub and Conquer suggest that it is possible that Canadian vegetarians have elevated alpha-linolenic acid intakes due to the high consumption of canola oil in their diets and, thus, better DHA status. These studies did not assess EPA status in vegans.

Recommended Intakes for EFA

The Institute of Medicine recently established adequate intake (AI) values for essential fatty acids, based on current average intakes. The adequate intakes for linoleic acid are 12 g/day for women and 17 g/day for men. The adequate intakes for alpha-linolenic acid are 1.1 g/day for women and 1.6 g/day for men (IOM/FNB, 2002). This provides a ratio of omega-6 fatty acids relative to omega-3 fatty acids of approximately 10:1 or 11:1. The World Health Organization recommends 5%–8% of calories from omega-6 fatty acids and 1%–2% of calories from omega-3 fatty acids (Report of a Joint FAO/WHO Expert Consultation, 2003). This provides a ratio of omega-6 fatty acids relative to omega-3 fatty acids (or a ratio of omega-6 to omega-3) of 2.5:1 to 8:1. Both sets of recommendations are meant for the general population, and assume some direct intake of EPA and DHA. For vegetarians and vegans, who consume little if any direct sources of EPA and DHA, smaller ratios have been suggested to help maximize conversion. Indu and Ghafoorunissa (1992) found significant increases in both EPA and DHA with an omega-6:omega-3

ratio of 4:1. Masters (1996) suggested that maximum conversion occurs with an omega-6: omega-3 ratio of 2.3:1. Experts generally recommend a ratio of omega-6 to omega-3 fatty acids ranging from 2:1 to 4:1 as being optimal for vegetarians and vegans to enhance conversion of alpha-linolenic acid to EPA and DHA (Davis & Kris-Etherton, 2003).

For those with increased needs for EPA and/or DHA (e.g., pregnant and lactating women), or who are at greater risk for poor conversion (people with diabetes or hypertension, those with neurological disorders, premature infants, and the elderly), it may be prudent to ensure a direct source of EPA and/or DHA. Though not common, it is possible to overconsume omega-3 fatty acids. If a person minimizes omega-6 fatty acids and uses large amounts of omega-3 fatty acids, resulting in a ratio of omega-6 to omega-3 of less than 1:1, insufficient linoleic acid conversion to AA can occur. Elongase and desaturase enzymes preferentially convert omega-3 fatty acids, when compared to omega-6 fatty acids. (See Table 3.1 for a chart of how essential fatty acids are metabolized.)

Achieving Optimal EFA Intake and Status in Vegetarians

The primary challenge for vegetarians is to improve their omega-3 fatty acid status. In short, that means adjusting dietary intake to ensure optimal conversion of alpha-linolenic acid to EPA and DHA, and, in some cases, taking a direct source of DHA. Most vegetarians consume insufficient omega-3 fatty acids while consuming adequate, and sometimes excessive, amounts of omega-6 fatty acids. To achieve the recommended ratio of omega-6 to omega-3 (2:1 to 4:1), vegetarians are well advised to aim for approximately 5%–8% of energy from omega-6 fatty acids and at least 1.5%–2% from omega-3

Table 3.1 Metabolism of Essential Fatty Acids

Omega-6 Family	Enzyme	Omega-3 Family
Linoleic acid 18:2 n-6		Alpha-linolenic acid 18:3 n-3
↓	*Delta 6 desaturase* *(add a double bond)*	↓
Gamma-linolenic acid (GLA) 18:3 n-6		Stearidonic acid (SDA) 18:4 n-3
↓	*Elongase* *(add a carbon)*	↓
Dihommogamma-linolenic acid $20:3\text{ n-}6 \rightarrow PG_1^*$		Eicosatetraenoic acid 20:4 n-3
↓	*Delta 5 desaturase* *(add a double bond)*	↓
Arachidonic acid (AA) $20:4\text{ n-}6 \rightarrow PG_2; TXA_2; LTB_4^*$		Eicosapentaenoic acid (EPA) $20:5\text{ n-}3 \rightarrow PG_3; TXA_3; LTB_5^*$
↓	*Elongase* *(add a carbon)*	↓
Adrenic acid 22:4 n-6		Docosapentaenoic acid 22:5 n-3
↓	*Elongase* *(add a carbon)*	↓
Tetracosatetraenoic acid 24:4 n-6		Tetracosapentaenoic acid 24:5 n-6
↓	*Delta 6 desaturase* *(add a double bond)*	↓
Tetracosapentaenoic acid 24:5 n-6		Tetrahexaenoic acid 24:6 n-3
↓	*Retroconversion* β-*oxidation*	↓
Docosapentaenoic acid 22:5 n-6		Docosahexaenoic acid (DHA) 22:6 n-3

*Abbreviations for eicosanoids:
PG_1 = series 1 prostaglandins   LTB4 = series 4 leukotrienes
PG_2 = series 2 prostaglandins   LTB5 = series 5 leukotrienes
PG_3 = series 3 prostaglandins   TXA2 = series 2 thromboxanes
                                      TXA3 = series 3 thromboxanes

Table 3.2 EFA Content of Selected Plant Foods

Food/serving size	ALA %	LA %	n-6:n-3 Ratio	ALA g/serving
Flaxseed oil, 1 tbsp.	57	16	0.28:1	8.0
Flaxseed, whole, 2 tbsp.	57	16	0.28:1	5.2
Flaxseed, ground, 2 tbsp.	57	16	0.28:1	3.8
Greens (mixed), 1 cup	56	11	0.19:1	0.1
Hempseed oil, 1 tbsp.	19	57	3:1	2.7
Hempseeds, 2 tbsp.	19	57	3:1	1.0
Walnuts, 1 oz. (¼ c)	14	58	4:1	2.6
Canola oil, 1 tbsp.	11	21	2:1	1.6
Soybean oil, 1 tbsp.	7	51	7:1	0.9
Soybeans, 1 cup cooked	7	50	7:1	1.0
Tofu, firm, ½ cup (4.5 oz.)	7	50	7:1	0.7

fatty acids. Individuals with increased needs or decreased capacity for conversion may need to increase intake of omega-3 fatty acids to 2%–2.5% of energy. In practical terms, a healthy vegetarian consuming a 2,000-kcal-per-day diet should aim for approximately 11–18 grams of omega-6 fatty acids and 3–5 grams of omega-3 fatty acids. There are four simple steps that will help improve omega-3 fatty acid status:

1. *Include good sources of alpha-linolenic acid (the plant omega-3 fatty acid) in the daily diet.* The very best sources of alpha-linolenic acid are flaxseeds, flaxseed oil, hempseeds, hempseed oil, canola oil, walnuts, and green leafy vegetables. Aim for 3–5 grams per day for most adults. Flaxseeds are by far the richest source of alpha-linolenic acid (57% of the fat is ALA). One teaspoon of flaxseed oil or 1.5 tablespoons of ground flaxseed, plus the usual intake of vegetables, walnuts, and other foods, provides plenty of omega-3 fatty acids for most people. (See Table 3.2 for the EFA content of selected plant foods.)

2. *Moderate the use of oils rich in omega-6 fatty acids, and high-fat processed foods rich in these oils.* Although increasing omega-3 fatty acids is an important first step in correcting EFA imbalance, vegetarians with especially high omega-6 intakes would be well advised to moderate their omega-6 intake. The best way of doing this, without compromising nutrient intake, is to reduce use of omega-6-rich/omega-3-poor oils and processed foods containing large amounts of these oils. Sunflower, safflower, corn, grapeseed, soybean, and cottonseed oils contain the greatest amounts of omega-6 fatty acids, relative to omega-3 fatty acids. Hempseed and walnut oils are rich in omega-6 fatty acids, but are beautifully balanced with omega-3 fatty acids, so these are good options. Omega-6-rich whole foods, such as sunflower seeds, pumpkin seeds, sesame tahini, soybeans, and wheat germ, are highly nutritious, whole-plant foods, and can be enjoyed as part of a varied plant-based diet.

3. *Make the primary dietary fat monounsaturated, if consuming more than 15% of calories from fat.* When dietary fat is less than 15% of total calories, polyunsaturated fats should predominate. If fat in-

take is higher, generally monounsaturated fatty acids will be highest. When mono-unsaturated fats (cis- configuration) become the primary dietary fat, saturated fats, trans fatty acids, and omega-6 fatty acids are kept in check, and the balance of omega-6 to omega-3 fatty acids improves. Fats in the following foods contain primarily monounsaturated fatty acids: nuts (except for walnuts and butternuts), peanuts, olive oil, olives, avocados, canola oil, and high-oleic sunflower and high-oleic safflower oils. Whole foods, rather than oils, are the preferred sources of monounsaturated fat, because they contribute many other nutrients to the diet as well.

4. *Consider including a direct source of EPA and/or DHA in the diet.* Individuals at risk for poor conversion of EPA to DHA, and those with increased needs for long-chain omega-3 fatty acids, may benefit from direct sources of EPA and DHA. The primary sources of EPA and DHA are fish and seafood. Thus, for vegetarians, increasing consumption of these long-chain omega-3 fatty acids can be a challenge. For ovo-lacto vegetarians, eggs provide a reasonable amount of DHA (approximately 50 mg/egg), though very little EPA. Most supermarkets also sell DHA-rich eggs, providing two to three times the DHA of conventional eggs. Eggs from chickens fed flax generally provide 60–100 mg DHA per egg, whereas those from chickens fed microalgae contain 100–150 mg DHA per egg. The only plant sources of long-chain omega-3 fatty acids are plants of the sea: microalgae and seaweed. Macroalgae, otherwise known as seaweed, is even lower in fat than most vegetables (less than 1%–14% of calories from fat), although it does contain small amounts of long-chain omega-3 fatty acids. A 100-gram serving provides, on average, about 100 mg of EPA, but little DHA. Seaweeds do not contribute significantly to EPA intakes in the Western world, but are sources where people use large quantities of seaweed on a daily basis (e.g., Japan and other parts of Asia). Very large intakes of seaweeds are not recommended, as they may contain excessive quantities of iodine. For example, just one gram of dried kelp contains about 3,000 mcg of iodine. The upper limit to avoid toxicity is 1,100 mcg. Microalgae is the most promising source of long-chain omega-3 fatty acids for people who do not consume fish. One variety, which provides 10%–40% DHA by dry weight, is currently available in supplement form. When supplementing with a direct DHA source, 100–300 mg/day is recommended (look for veg caps). EPA-rich microalgae exists, but is not currently being cultured in North America. Blue-green algae (spirulina and aphanizomenon flos aquae) are low in long-chain omega-3 fatty acids. Spirulina is rich in gamma-linolenic acid (GLA), an omega-6 fatty acid, and aphanizomenon flos aquae (AFA) is more concentrated in ALA. Although blue-green algae is not a significant source of EPA or DHA, some research indicates that it has a very high conversion rate in comparison to other plants (Kushak et al., 1999). Thus, although vegetarians can rely on eggs and/or microalgae supplements for DHA, most consume little if any EPA. However, approximately 10%–11% of DHA is retroconverted back to EPA; thus, if sufficient alpha-linolenic acid and DHA are consumed, total EPA production would be expected to be adequate (Conquer & Holub, 1996).

Box 3.2   Why Not Just Eat Fish?

Fish is loaded with omega-3 fatty acids. High-fat, cold-water fish contains up to 1,600 mg DHA and 1,000 mg EPA per 100-gram (3.5-oz.) serving. So why not just eat fish?

There are plenty of sound reasons to forgo fish. For starters, increased fish consumption does not appear to protect against coronary heart disease in individuals at low risk who enjoy healthy lifestyles (Marckmann & Gronbaek, 1999). Perhaps more importantly, fish is the most concentrated source of two types of contaminants: heavy metals (such as lead, mercury, and cadmium) and industrial pollutants (such as PCBs, DDT, and dioxin). The potential human health effects of these compounds include increased risk of certain cancers, damage to the immune system, infertility, birth defects, and altered levels of sex hormones.

Of course, being an animal food, fish is a source of cholesterol and saturated fat, and provides no fiber or phytochemicals. Fish is also a primary source of foodborne illness, poisoning hundreds and perhaps thousands of people in North America each day.

There are also compelling ecological and ethical arguments for avoiding fish. Large commercial fishing operations are leaving the vast majority of the world's fish stocks in jeopardy. The Natural Resources Defense Council (NRDC) estimates that about 70% of the world's fish populations are now fully fished, overexploited, depleted, or slowly recovering. From an ethical perspective, eating fish requires taking a life, or several lives. Indeed, commercial fishing operations generally have huge bycatches (fish and other sea life that is unintentionally caught). These creatures generally do not survive, and are simply tossed back into the water.

Practical Aspects

Ensuring Highest-Quality Fat Sources: Whole Foods as the Optimal Source of Dietary Fat

The highest quality of fat is naturally present in fresh nuts, seeds, soybeans, avocados, olives, and other plant foods. These plant foods come packaged by nature to protect them from damaging light, heat, and oxygen. There is simply no contest between the fats found in these foods and the chemically altered fats found in margarine, shortening, and other hydrogenated vegetable oils, or the highly saturated fats found in animal products. Even vegetable oils that are thought of as being very healthful pale in comparison to the whole foods from which they were extracted. Whole-plant foods are brimming with valuable vitamins, minerals, phytochemicals, plant protein, plant sterols, essential fatty acids, and fiber. Seeds are also good sources of vitamins, trace minerals, essential fatty acids, phytochemicals, and fiber. Consider what we know about the health benefits of nuts and seeds:

- *Nuts.* The studies looking at the health effects of eating nuts annihilate the myth that "all fat is bad fat."

During the last decade, studies have consistently confirmed the health benefits of these foods. In four large epidemiological studies, those eating nuts most frequently had a 50% reduction in risk of dying from heart disease, on average, compared with those eating nuts the most infrequently (Albert et al., 2002; Fraser et al., 1992; Kushi et al., 1996; Hu et al., 1998).

Numerous smaller studies looking at the effects of individual nuts, including peanuts (not technically a tree nut, but a legume), have provided further evidence that nuts are extremely protective of health. The Adventist Health Study, a prospective study with more than 31,000 participants, found that when contrasted with 65 other foods, nuts had one of the strongest inverse relationships to coronary artery disease (Fraser et al., 1992). Clinical research by Sabaté and coworkers examined the effects of two cholesterol-lowering American Heart Association Step 1 diets—the only difference in the diets was that one provided 20% of its calories in the form of walnuts (replacing other visible fats in the diet). Study participants were assigned to one of the two diets, then after four weeks were switched to the other. When compared to the control diet, those on the walnut diet experienced a total cholesterol reduction of 12% and LDL reduction of 16% (Sabaté et al., 1993).

In addition to the cardioprotective effects of nuts, they also appear to reduce the risk of stroke (Yochum, Folsom, & Kushi, 2000), type 2 diabetes (Jiang et al., 2002), dementia (Zhang et al., 2002), advanced macular degeneration (Seddon, Cote, & Rosner, 2003), and gallstones (Tsai et al., 2004). Calculations suggest that daily nut eaters gain an extra five to six years of life free of coronary disease (Hu & Stampfer, 1999), and that regular nut eating appears to increase longevity by about two years (Fraser & Shavik, 2001). The frequency of nut consumption has been found to be inversely related to all-cause mortality in several population groups (Sabaté, 1999). Maximum benefits appear to occur with intakes of 1–2 ounces per day (30–60 g). Moderate intakes are recommended, as nuts are high in energy (approximately 800 kcal per cup).

Although nuts are loaded with protective dietary components, the relative impact of these components has not been well quantified. They are rich in antioxidants, including selenium and vitamin E (possibly reducing LDL oxidation), plant protein, and fiber. They contain significant levels of arginine, a dietary precursor of nitric oxide, a potent endogenous vasodilator. In addition, their folic acid levels may help reduce levels of homocysteine (a possible risk factor for CAD). Nuts are important sources of copper and magnesium, both shown to protect against heart disease. In addition to these beneficial nutrients, nuts and seeds are rich in inositol hexaphosphate (phytic acid), ellagic acid, lignans, phytosterols, and other phytochemicals shown to have anticarcinogenic potential (Rainey & Nyquist, 1997). Nuts are warehouses of healthful fats, mainly monounsaturated fat (except for walnuts, which are high in polyunsaturated fats and are an excellent source of essential fatty acids), are low in saturated fat, and are free of trans fatty acids and cholesterol.

- *Seeds.* Seeds are the life-giving part of a plant, responsible for the survival of their species. The value of seeds in human nutrition is sorely underestimated. These concentrated foods are our most plentiful sources of essential fatty acids.

Pumpkin seeds, sunflower seeds, poppy seeds, hemp seeds, and sesame seeds are all rich in linoleic acid, the omega-6 fatty acid. Flax seeds, chia seeds (grown in the deserts of Mexico), canola seeds, and hemp seeds (hemp contains plentiful amounts of both essential fatty acids) are all rich in alpha-linolenic acid, the omega-3 fatty acid. Seeds vary in their protein content, ranging from about 12% of calories to more than 30% of calories. They are among our richest sources of vitamin E, and provide an impressive array of other vitamins, minerals, phytochemicals, and fiber.

Flaxseeds offer a significant advantage for vegetarians because they have the greatest omega-3 content of any food, averaging about

57% alpha-linolenic acid. Thus, flax can go a long way toward helping correct the imbalance in essential fatty acids. Flax is very high in soluble fiber (the type of fiber that lowers cholesterol), and is one of the richest known sources of boron (a mineral important to bone health). Studies show that flaxseeds can help to reduce blood cholesterol levels (Cunnane et al., 1995), and improve a number of other markers of coronary artery disease (Caughey et al., 1996; Lucas et al., 2002; Jenkins et al., 1999; Nestel et al., 1997). They also improve blood sugar response in people with diabetes (Cunnane et al., 1993), and may improve immune/inflammatory disorders (Ingram et al., 1995). Flaxseeds are the richest known source of lignans, and preliminary evidence suggests that they may help to reduce growth of human cancer cells (Thompson et al., 2000; Sung, Lautens, & Thompson, 1998).

- *Do flaxseeds and flaxseed oil increase risk of prostate cancer?*

At least eight studies since 1993 have found a positive connection between blood levels of alpha-linolenic acid (the type of omega-3 fatty acid found in plants and animals, excluding fish) and prostate cancer (De Stéfani et al., 2000; Gann et al., 1994; Harvei et al., 1997; Newcomer et al., 2001; Ramon et al., 2000; Yang et al., 1999; Brouwer, Katan, & Zock, 2004; Leitzmann et al., 2004). As a result, prostate cancer experts often warn men to limit their use of foods rich in alpha-linolenic acid. Flaxseed and flaxseed oil, with their exceptionally high alpha-linolenic acid content, have been singled out as foods to be cautiously avoided, especially by those with prostate cancer or at high risk for the disease. Many experts suggest that men stick to fish as their primary source of omega-3 fatty acids.

Although it certainly makes sense to assume that flaxseed would be a problem if high alpha-

linolenic acid increases prostate cancer risk, close examination of the literature, particularly the studies in question, suggest that flaxseed may not be the culprit. To begin, flaxseed and flaxseed oil were not the source of the alpha-linolenic acid in any of these studies. Indeed, the primary sources of alpha-linolenic acid in most of these reports were animal products, such as butter, red meat, and bacon. In addition, the actual differences in the alpha-linolenic acid intakes of the study participants (from the highest to lowest intakes) were small. However, in one recent study both plant and animal sources of alpha-linolenic acid, significantly increased risk (Attar-Bashi, Frydenberg, Li, & Sinclair, 2004). Still, at least three other studies have found that high alpha-linolenic acid does not increase prostate cancer risk (Shuurman et al., 1999; Bairati et al., 1998; Godley et al., 1996).

In 2001, a research team decided to look specifically at the effects of flaxseed use on men with prostate cancer (Demark-Wahnefried et al., 2001). Although this was a small, short-term pilot study with only 25 participants, the results were encouraging. The participants were given a low-fat diet (20% or less of calories from fat) and about 30 grams (3 heaping tablespoons) of finely ground flaxseed per day for an average of 34 days. There were favorable changes in prostate cancer biology and associated biomarkers, including a reduction in tumor cell division and greater rate of tumor cell death in the entire group. Another study conducted by the same researchers in 2004 looked at the potential effect of a low-fat, flaxseed-supplemented diet on prostatic growth and disease in 15 subjects. This trial also suggested favorable changes in prostate cell biology and associated biomarkers (Demark-Wahnefried et al., 2004). Larger studies will be needed before conclusions can be made about flaxseed, flaxseed oil, and prostate cancer.

Why would an essential nutrient appear to be a marker for prostate cancer? It is possible that the unstable nature of alpha-linolenic acid is to blame. Alpha-linolenic acid is very easily damaged during commercial processing, storage, and food preparation, especially barbequing and frying. Without the necessary antioxidants to prevent such reactions, products of oxidation may be formed that have negative health consequences. From a practical perspective, this means being conscious about how omega-3-rich foods are used. Until more research is completed, it would be prudent for vegetarian men to be especially cautious with omega-3-rich oils. A reasonable option is to stick with ground flaxseed rather than flaxseed oil. Flaxseeds are loaded with antioxidants, and based on the evidence to date, they do not appear to increase the risk of prostate cancer; rather, preliminary research suggests that they may actually offer protection.

Practical Guidelines for Optimal Health: Fats in the Vegetarian Diet

The following guidelines help to translate science into practical recommendations for vegetarian consumers—an important step in ensuring optimal health in this population.

Total Dietary Fat

- Aim for 15%–30% of calories from fat for healthy vegetarian adults.
- Do not restrict fat in the diets of infants under the age of two years.
- Fat should gradually drop from about 40%–50% of calories during infancy to 30%–40% of calories during early childhood; thereafter it should gradually decline to the recommended 15%–30% of calories when full height is attained.

If the primary source of fat is whole-plant foods (nuts, seeds, soy, avocados, and olives), one can expect to maintain excellent health eating a relatively high proportion of total calories as fat (i.e., 30% of calories). In contrast, when fat is derived from animal sources and processed fats (e.g., hydrogenated oils), adverse health consequences could occur even with relatively moderate total fat intakes. Those who are inactive, overweight, or have chronic disease are generally well advised to aim for the lower end of this 15%–30% range, whereas children, athletes, and those who are lean and active may do best aiming for the higher end of this range. It is best not to exceed 35% of calories from fat. How much fat is 15% to 30% of calories? For a person eating 2,000 calories a day, it would allow 2.5–5 tablespoons of fat, including fat naturally present in whole foods and concentrated fats and oils. The following foods provide approximately 1 tablespoon of fat each:

> 1 oz. nuts or seeds
> 250 mL (1 cup) medium tofu or 125 mL (1/2 cup) of firm tofu or tempeh
> 500 mL (2 cups) regular soy milk
> 185 mL (3/4 cup) boiled soybeans
> 1/2 avocado
> 20 large olives
> 125 mL (1/2 cup) shredded coconut

Thus, an individual consuming 2,000 kcal/day and aiming for approximately 25% of calories from fat could include 1 oz. nuts, 1 oz. seeds, 1 cup soy milk, and half an avocado in the daily diet, in addition to the usual intakes of vegetables, fruits, legumes, and whole grains.

The best way to ensure that an infant receives the necessary fat to support growth and development is to provide the child with the appropriate milk. The best choice is breast milk, and it is recommended that breastfeeding continue for a full two years and beyond. If breastfeeding is not possible or not chosen, commercial infant formula is the only safe alternative during the first 12 months of life. From 12 to 24 months of age, ovo-lacto vegetarian children can be switched to whole-fat cow's milk (lower-fat milk can be used after this time), and vegan children can continue on soy formula or switch to full-fat, fortified soy milk.

Intake of Saturated Fat and Trans Fatty Acids

Limit intake of saturated fat to less than 7% of calories. Avoid trans fatty acids.

Saturated Fat. Vegetarian diets are naturally lower in saturated fat than nonvegetarian diets. Ovo-lacto vegetarian intakes average between 8% and 10% of calories from saturated fat. Vegans eat even less, averaging 4% to 7% of calories from saturated fat. To keep saturated fat under 7% of calories, 16 grams would be the maximum allowable intake. Vegetarians who eat a lot of full-fat dairy products and eggs could find themselves over the top almost as quickly as nonvegetarians. Two ounces of cheddar cheese contain 12 grams of saturated fat, and one cup of whole milk has more than 5 grams. In contrast, a person could eat 10 servings of fruits and vegetables, 8 servings of whole grains, 2 servings of beans, a serving of tofu, 2 ounces of nuts, and 2 ounces of seeds, and still come in at less than 10 grams of saturated fat.

To reduce saturated fat in the vegetarian diet:

- Replace high-fat dairy products with low-fat or skim products or soy milk and soy products.
- Replace butter with nut or seed butters, liquid vegetable oils, or nonhydrogenated soft margarine.
- Replace scrambled eggs with scrambled tofu, and substitute ground flaxseeds for eggs in baking (1 tbsp. ground flaxseeds plus 3 tbsp. water = 1 egg).
- If using concentrated fats and oils, use primarily liquid oils rather than tropical oils.

Trans Fatty Acids. Trans fatty acids should be avoided, with an absolute maximum intake less than 1% of calories. For someone eating 2,000 calories a day, that amounts to no more than 2.2 grams of trans fatty acids. The main sources of trans fatty acids are processed foods containing hydrogenated or partially hydrogenated oils, shortening, margarine, and deep-fried fast foods. Table 3.3 shows the trans fatty acid content of selected foods.

To minimize consumption of trans fatty acids:

- Use whole foods as the foundation of the diet.
- Become a label reader. When using processed foods, avoid those containing shortening and/or hydrogenated or partially hydrogenated oils.
- Avoid deep-fried foods.
- Avoid hydrogenated margarine. Use nut or seed butters or vegetable oils instead. If you do use margarine, select a nonhydrogenated variety.

Intake of Essential Fatty Acids

- Aim for a minimum of 1.5% omega-3 fatty acids (2% omega-3 fatty acids during pregnancy and lactation).
- Aim for an omega-6:omega-3 fatty acid ratio between 2:1 and 4:1.
- Consider a direct source of DHA in your diet.

Aim for a Minimum of 1.5% Omega-3 Fatty Acids (2% Omega-3 Fatty Acids during Pregnancy and Lactation). It is easy to achieve sufficient omega-6 fatty acids on almost any

Table 3.3   Trans Fatty Acid Content of Selected Foods*

Food	Total fat, g	Trans fatty acids, g
Microwave popcorn, 3.5 oz.	25	7.5
French fries, medium	23.7	5
Cookies, chocolate chip, 4	12	5
Donut, honey-glazed, 1	15	3.8
Shortening, 1 tbsp.	14	3.7
Cake, yellow with frosting, 1 piece	12.8	3.2
Margarine, hard, 1 tbsp.	12	3.1
Crackers, snack, 8	7	2.6
Margarine, soft, 1 tbsp.	12	1.4
Potato chips, 2 oz.	19.6	1.1

*From the USDA Nutrient Database.

vegetarian diet, even one that is fairly low in fat. Omega-6 fatty acids are abundant in many plant foods, including grains, sunflower, safflower, soy, sesame, cottonseed, walnut, and corn oil. It is considerably more difficult to achieve sufficient omega-3 fatty acids, as they are less prevalent in today's food supply. The richest sources of omega-3 fatty acids are flaxseeds and flaxseed oil, hempseed and hempseed oil, dark green leafy vegetables (especially purslane), canola oil, and walnuts. The richest plant source of alpha-linolenic acid is flaxseed oil. Other omega-3-rich plant foods are much less concentrated sources of this nutrient, often coming packaged with higher amounts of linoleic acid (for example, soy is approximately 7% omega-3 fatty acids and 54% omega-6 fatty acids). On a 2,000-calorie-per-day diet, one would require approximately 3 to 4.5 grams of alpha-linolenic acid. This amount of omega-3s could be supplied by 2 to 3 servings of the following (each contains about 1.5 grams of alpha-linolenic acid):

½ tsp. flaxseed oil
2 tsp. flaxseeds (ground)
2 tsp. hempseed oil
3 tbsp. hempseeds

15 cups dark greens (measured raw)
1 tbsp. canola oil
2 heaping tbsp. walnuts (0.5 oz.)

Aim for an Omega-6:Omega-3 Fatty Acid Ratio of Approximately 2:1–4:1.   To ensure good balance between linoleic and alpha-linolenic acid, vegetarians are advised to:

- Limit concentrated sources of omega-6 fatty acids, if excessive in diet. If using concentrated oils, do not use omega-6-rich oils in daily food preparation (e.g., corn, safflower, sunflower, grapeseed, soy, sesame, and cottonseed oils). Commercial products such as margarine, salad dressing, and mayonnaise that are made with these oils should also be used in moderation.
- Do not use excessive flaxseed oil (more than a tablespoon per day). If flaxseed oil is the primary oil used, and the diet is otherwise low in fat, it is possible to have a balance of omega-6 to omega-3 that is less than 1:1. Although most people get too little omega-3 fatty acid, it is possible to get too much. Omega-6 fatty acids are also essential to health, so balance is the key.

- Monounsaturated fats should make up the largest portion of fat in the diet, unless the diet is very low in fat (<15% of calories). Emphasizing monounsaturated fats will help to keep saturated fats, trans fatty acids, and omega-6 fatty acids in check. Whole foods rich in monounsaturated fat include most nuts (hazelnuts, pistachios, almonds, macadamia nuts, peanuts, and pecans), avocados, and olives. If using concentrated oils, select those rich in monounsaturated fats (e.g., extra-virgin olive oil) and/or omega-3 fatty acids (e.g., flaxseed oil, organic canola oil, balanced EFA oils).

Consider a Direct Source of DHA in Your Diet.   The best source for vegetarians is DHA from a special type of microalgae that is being cultured and sold in veg caps. When using these supplements, 100–300 mg/day DHA is generally recommended (the higher end of the range is recommended for pregnant and lactating women). For ovo-lacto vegetarians, omega-3-rich eggs are also an option. Most contain approximately 100 mg DHA per egg.

Quality of Dietary Fats

- Whole foods should be the primary source of dietary fat.
- If using concentrated fats and oils, select them wisely.
- Store high-fat plant foods and oils with care.
- Do not expose highly unsaturated oils to excessive or prolonged heating.

Whole Foods Should Be the Primary Source of Dietary Fat.   To shift from a diet of poor-quality fats to one with the highest-quality fats available:

- Cook or sprout whole grains for breakfast (kamut berries, oat groats, triticale, millet, barley, quinoa, etc.) and top with soy milk or other nondairy milk; seeds, including ground flaxseeds; nuts, including walnuts; and fresh fruit, such as blueberries.
- Use nut or seed butters in place of other spreads.
- Use toasted nuts, seeds, avocados, and/or marinated tofu in salad.
- Add legumes, tofu, nuts, seeds, or olives to casseroles, stews, or stir-fries.
- Make spreads, dips, and dressings using avocados, tofu, or nut/seed butters instead of sour cream, cream cheese, or mayonnaise.

Allow time for meal preparation; make it a priority. Make bread, granola, crackers, muffins, cookies, and other baked goods from scratch. Use whole grains with added ground flax, seeds, nuts, and/or wheat germ.

Select Fats and Oils Wisely.   Is it acceptable to use some concentrated fats and oils? There is no question that the best-quality fat comes from whole-plant foods, and this is where most of our fat should come from. However, moderate amounts of concentrated fats and oils can fit into the diet of healthy vegetarians. High-quality oils can make meals more enjoyable, add extra calories (without adding bulk), and help to improve the absorption of certain vitamins and protective phytochemicals.

Although refined oils (e.g., commercial vegetable oils) offer important advantages over hydrogenated oils (e.g., shortening), they provide little nutritional value other than fat calories. If using concentrated oils, select unrefined, mechanically pressed oils whenever possible. Extra-virgin olive oil is often the only unrefined oil available on supermarket shelves. The monounsaturated fat content makes it a good choice. Other high-quality, fresh-pressed oils are available in natural food stores or natural foods sections of supermarkets (those with high omega-3 content will be kept refrigerated). Among the best choices are flaxseed, hempseed, canola, walnut, almond, and hazelnut oil. Nonorganic canola oil is often produced from genetically engineered crops, so if you want to be sure to avoid these products, buy organic.

Can we get sufficient fat without using any concentrated fats and oils? Absolutely! Just as you can get all the carbohydrates your body needs from whole foods, without any added refined starches or sugars, so you can get all the fat your body needs without using any concentrated fats and oils. However, it is best to include a wise selection of fresh, whole-plant foods that are naturally high in fat. Nuts, seeds and their butters, avocados, olives, and soybeans and soy products are all excellent sources of good-quality fats.

Store Fats and Oils with Care.   High-fat plant foods can easily become rancid if not properly stored. This could well be nature's way of letting us know that a food has lost its freshness and is no longer wholesome. Nuts and seeds are naturally protected: nuts by their shells and seeds by their hard outer coats. Once the shell is broken or the seeds ground, they are much more susceptible to oxidative damage. Naturally occurring antioxidants help to slow this process; however, proper storage is very important. Nuts in the shell or unbroken seeds are best stored in a cool, dry place. When stored properly, unshelled nuts and whole seeds will last up to a year. Shelled nuts and ground seeds can be stored in the refrigerator for up to four months or in an airtight container in the freezer for up to one year.

The storage requirements for oils depend on the relative amounts of saturated, monounsaturated, and polyunsaturated fatty acids in the product and the method of processing used. The more highly unsaturated oils will go rancid more quickly than oils with a higher monounsaturated and saturated fat content. Refining oil also increases the shelf life, so these oils can last many months in the pantry. Fresh-pressed oils (other than olive oil) should be refrigerated and used within two months. Olive oil is more resistant than many other oils to oxidative damage, because of its high monounsaturated fat content. The more refined the oil, the less highly unsaturated fats it will contain. Extra-virgin olive oil (first pressing) should be kept for no more than three to four months (best used within two months after opening).

Do Not Expose Highly Unsaturated Oils to Excessive or Prolonged Heating.   When oils are subjected to high-temperature cooking, a number of toxic products are formed, including peroxides, hydroperoxides, polymers, cyclic monomers, and hydrocarbons. These substances can be toxic to the liver, cardiocirculatory system, immune system, and the kidneys (Viola, 1997; Aw, 1999). For optimal health, it is best to avoid exposing oils to direct heat. Although high-temperature heating of oils is not recommended, some fats are more resistant to destruction than others. The oils that survive best under "heat" are those richest in saturated and monounsaturated fats, such as coconut oil, palm oil, palm kernel oil, peanut oil, and high-oleic sunflower or safflower oil (those made from plants grown to have a high mono content). Oils rich in omega-3 fatty acids, particularly flax and hempseed oils, should not be used in cooking at all.

Boiling and baking are less destructive to oils. The temperature in baked goods generally goes up only to about 240°F, a temperature that most oils can withstand without damage.

Ground flaxseeds are recommended as a source of omega-3 fatty acids. These seeds can be used raw or in baking. A study assessing level of peroxidation products in muffins containing ground flaxseed found no significant increases of peroxidation products with normal cooking time and temperatures (Cunnane et al., 1993). Although flax is a rich source of alpha-linolenic acid, it has been shown to be stable when baked at usual baking temperatures. Raw flaxseed contains cyanogenic glycosides that could, under certain circumstances, contribute to iodine deficiency and goiter. This problem is not a concern where iodine intake is sufficient; however, some vegan populations have reported low iodine intakes. Cyanogenic glycosides are destroyed by heat, even fairly low baking temperatures (Vaisey-Genser, 1997). Some experts suggest that intake of raw flax be limited to not more than 3–4 tablespoons per day.

Conclusion

Vegetarians enjoy many health advantages, and these benefits are related, at least in part, to a more favorable intake of fats and oils. Vegetarians eat less fat overall, and consume less damaging saturated fats, cholesterol, and trans fatty acids.

Within Western vegetarian populations, there has been substantial emphasis on the use of very-low-fat diets as means of preventing and treating disease. Although such diets have proved valuable in the treatment of coronary artery disease, they may not be optimal for healthy vegetarian/vegan populations, particularly children. Fat intakes for vegetarians of all ages (and health states) must take into account not only disease risk reduction, but also growth and development, nutrient needs (including essential fatty acids, vitamins, and minerals), and absorption of nutrients and protective phytochemicals. For healthy vegetarian adults, a total fat intake of 15%–30% of calories is recommended.

Vegetarian food choices could be significantly improved where dietary fat is concerned. The primary challenges for this population are:

- To improve the quantity and balance of essential fatty acids in the diet by increasing intake of omega-3 fatty acids, moderating intake of omega-6 fatty acids, and making monounsaturated fats the primary dietary fat if fat intake is above 15% of calories.
- To eliminate trans fatty acids by decreasing reliance on processed foods containing shortening and other hydrogenated or partially hydrogenated fats, and deep-fried fast foods.
- To select whole foods, such as nuts, seeds, avocados, olives, and soybeans, as the main source of dietary fat.

The questions and challenges that remain for scientists center around the essentiality of preformed, long-chain omega-3 fatty acids and how best to supply these fatty acids to vegetarian consumers. There is also still a question about the optimal intake of alpha-linolenic acid in the vegetarian diet in light of its relatively poor conversion to EPA and DHA.

References

Ågren J, Törmälä M, Nenonen M, Hänninen O. Fatty acid composition of erythrocyte, platelet, and serum lipids in strict vegans. *Lipids.* 1995;30: 365–369.

Albert CM, Gaziano JM, Willett WC, Manson JE. Nut consumption and decreased risk of sudden cardiac death in the Physicians' Health Study. *Arch Intern Med.* 2002;162(12):1382–1387.

American Dietetic Association. Position of the American Dietetic Association: Vegetarian diets. *J Am Diet Assoc.* 1997;97(11):1317–1321.

Anderson JW, Zeigler JA, Deakins DA, et al. Metabolic effects of high-carbohydrate, high-fiber diets for insulin-dependent diabetic individuals. *Am J Clin Nutr.* 1991;54(5):936–943.

Attar-Bashi NM, Frydenberg M, Li D, Sinclair AJ. Lack of correlation between plasma and prostate tissue alpha-linolenic acid levels. *Asia Pac J Clin Nutr.* 2004;13(Suppl):S78.

Aw TY. Molecular and cellular responses to oxidative stress and changes in oxidation-reduction imbalance in the intestine. *Am J Clin Nutr.* 1999; 70(4):557–565.

Bairati I, Meyer F, Fradet Y, Moore L. Dietary fat and advanced prostate cancer. *J Urology.* 1998;159: 1271–1275.

Barnard RJ. Effects of life-style modification on serum lipids. *Arch Intern Med.* 1991;151:1389–1394.

Brouwer IA, Katan MB, Zock PL. Dietary alpha-linolenic acid is associated with reduced risk of fatal coronary heart disease, but increased prostate cancer risk: A meta-analysis. *J Nutr.* April 2004;134(4):919–922.

Burge GC, Jones AE, Wootton SA. Eicosapentaenoic and docosapentaenoic acids are the principal products of alpha-linolenic acid metabolism in young men. *Br J Nutr.* 2002;88(4):355–363.

Burge GC, Wootton SA. Conversion of alpha-linolenic acid to eicosapentaenoic, docosapentaenoic and docosahexaenoic acids in young women. *Br J Nutr.* 2002;88(4):411–420.

Caughey GE, Mantzioris E, Gibson RA, et al. The effect on human tumor necrosis factor α and interleukin 1β production of diets enriched in n-3 fatty acids from vegetable oil or fish oil. *Am J Clin Nutr.* 1996;63:116–122.

Conquer JA, Holub BJ. Docosahexaenoic acid (omega-3) and vegetarian nutrition. *Vegetarian Nutr: An Intl J.* 1997;1/2:42–49.

Conquer JA, Holub BJ. Supplementation with an algae source of docosahexaenoic acid increases (n-3) fatty acid status and alters selected risk factors for heart disease in vegetarian subjects. *J Nutr.* 1996;126:3032–3039.

Crane MG, Zielinski R, Aloia R. Cis and trans fats in omnivores, ovo-lacto vegetarians and vegans. *Am J Clin Nutr.* 1988;48:920.

Cunnane SC, Ganguli S, Menard C, et al. High alpha-linolenic acid flaxseed: Some nutritional properties in humans. *Br J Nutr.* 1993;69:443–453.

Cunnane SC, Hamadeh MJ, Liede AC, et al. Nutritional attributes of traditional flaxseed in healthy young adults. *Am J Clin Nutr.* 1995;61:62–68.

Dagnelie PC, van Staveren W. Macrobiotic nutrition and child health: Results of a population-based, mixed-longitudinal cohort study in the Netherlands. *Am J Clin Nutr.* 1994;59(Suppl):1187S–1196S.

Davis B, Kris-Etherton PM. Achieving optimal essential fatty acid status in vegetarians: Current knowledge and practical implications. *Am J Clin Nutr.* 2003:78(3, Suppl);640S–646S.

de Lorgeril M, Salen MP, Delaye J. Effect of a Mediterranean type of diet on the rate of cardiovascular complications in patients with coronary artery disease. *J Am Coll Cardiology.* 1996;28(5): 1103–1108.

Demark-Wahnefried W, Price DT, Polascik TJ, et al. Pilot study of dietary fat restriction and flaxseed supplementation in men with prostate cancer before surgery: Exploring the effects on hormonal levels, prostate-specific antigen, and histopathologic features. *Urology.* 2001;58:47–52.

Demark-Wahnefried W, Robertson CN, Walther PJ, Polascik TJ, Paulson DF, Vollmer RT. Pilot study to explore effects of low-fat, flaxseed-supplemented diet on proliferation of benign prostatic epithelium and prostate-specific antigen. *Urology.* 2004; 63(5):900–904.

De Stéfani E, Deneo-Pellegrini H, Boffetta P, et al. α-Linolenic acid and risk of prostate cancer: A case-control study in Uruguay. *Cancer Epidemiol Biomarkers Prev.* 2000;9:335–338.

Draper A, Lewis J, Malhotra N, Wheeler E. The energy and nutrient intakes of different types of vegetarian: A case for supplements? *Br J Nutr.* 1993;69(1):3–19 [published erratum appears in *Br J Nutr.* 1993;70(3):812].

Emken EA, Adlof RO, Gulley RM. Dietary linoleic acid influences desaturation and acylation of deuterium-labeled linoleic and ALAs in young adult males. *Biochim Biophys Acta.* 1994;1213: 277–288.

Esselstyn CB Jr. Updating a 12-year experience with arrest and reversal therapy of coronary heart disease (an overdue requiem for palliative cardiology). *Am J Cardiol.* 1999;84(3):339-341.

Ferrier LK, Caston LJ, Leeson S, Squires J, Weaver BJ, Holub BJ. Alpha-linolenic acid and docosahexaenoic acid-enriched eggs from hens fed flaxseed: Influence on blood lipids and platelet phospholipids fatty acids in humans. *Am J Clin Nutr.* 1995;62(1):81-86.

Food and Nutrition Board, Institute of Medicine. *Dietary Reference Intakes for Energy, Carbohydrate, Fiber, Fat, Fatty Acids, Cholesterol, Protein, and Amino Acids (Macronutrients).* Washington, DC: National Academy Press; 2002.

Fraser GE, Sabaté J, Beeson WL, Strahan TM. A possible protective effect of nut consumption on risk of coronary heart disease: The Adventist health study. *Arch Intern Med.* 1992;152(7):1416-1424.

Fraser GE, Shavik DJ. Ten years of life: Is it a matter of choice? *Arch Intern Med.* 2001;161:1645-1652.

Gann PH, Hennekens CH, Sacks FM, et al. Prospective study of plasma fatty acids and risk of prostate cancer. *J Natl Cancer Inst.* 1994;86:281-286.

Gartner C, Stahl W, Sies H. Lycopene is more bioavailable from tomato paste than from fresh tomatoes. *Am J Clin Nutr.* 1997;66:116-122.

Gerster H. Can adults adequately convert α-linolenic acid (18:3 n-3) to eicosapentaenoic acid (20:5n-3) and docosahexaenoic acid (22:6 n-3)? *Intl J Vit Nutr Res.* 1998;68:159-173.

Ghafoorunissa SA. Requirements of dietary fats to meet nutritional needs and prevent the risk of atherosclerosis—An Indian perspective. *Indian J Med Res.* 1998;108:191-202.

Godley PA, Campbell MK, Gallagher P, et al. Biomarkers of essential fatty acid consumption and risk of prostatic carcinoma. *Cancer Epidemiol Biomarkers Prev.* 1996;5:889-895.

Hachey DL. Benefits and risks of modifying maternal fat intake in pregnancy and lactation. *Am J Clin Nutr.* 1994; 59(Suppl):454S-464S.

Harvei S, Bjerve KS, Tretli S, et al. Prediagnostic level of fatty acids in serum phospholipids: Ω-3 and Ω-6 fatty acids and the risk of prostate cancer. *Intl J Cancer* 1997;71:545-551.

Holub BJ, Conquer JA. Dietary docosahexaenoic acid as a source of eicosapentaenoic acid in vegetarians and omnivores. *Lipids.* 1997;21:341-345.

Horrobin DF. Nutritional and medical importance of gamma-linolenic acid. *Prog Lipid Res.* 1992; 31(2):163-194.

Hu FB, Stampfer, MJ. Nut consumption and risk of coronary heart disease: A review of the epidemiologic evidence. *Curr Atherosclerosis Reps.* 1999; 1:204-209.

Hu FB, Stampfer MJ, Manson JE, et al. Frequent nut consumption and risk of coronary heart disease in women: Prospective cohort study. *BMJ.* 1998; 317(7169):1341-1345.

Indu M, Ghafoorunissa SA. N-3 fatty acids in Indian diets—Comparison of the effects of precursor (alpha-linolenic acid) vs. product (long-chain n-3 polyunsaturated fatty acids). *Nutr Res.* 1992;12: 569-582.

Ingram AJ, Parbtani A, Clark WF, et al. Effects of flaxseed and flax oil diets in a rat-5/6 renal ablation model. *Am J Kidney Dis.* 1995;25:320-329.

Janelle KC, Barr SI. Nutrient intakes and eating behavior scores of vegetarian and nonvegetarian women. *J Am Diet Assoc.* 1995;95:180-189.

Jarvis K, Millre G. Fat in infant diets. *Nutr Today.* 1996;31(5):182-191.

Jenkins DJA, Kendall CWC, Vidgen E, et al. Health aspects of partially defatted flaxseed, including effects on serum lipids, oxidative measures, and ex vivo androgen and progestin activity: A controlled crossover trial. *Am J Clin Nutr.* 1999;69: 395-402.

Jiang R, Manson JE, Stampfer MJ, Liu S, Willet WC, Hu FB. Nut and peanut butter consumption and risk of type 2 diabetes in women. *JAMA.* 2002; 288:2554-2560.

Kaplan R, Toshima M. Does a reduced fat diet cause retardation in child growth? *Prev Med.* 1992;21: 33-52.

Keys A, Menotti A, Toshima H. The diet and 15-year death rate in the Seven Countries study. *Am J Epidemiol.* 1986;124(6):903-915.

Kies CV. Mineral utilization of vegetarians: Impact of variation in fat intake. *Am J Clin Nutr.* 1988; 48:884-887.

Kirkeby K, Bjerkedal I. The fatty acid composition in serum of Norwegian vegetarians. *Acta Med Scand.* 1968;183:143–148.

Krajcovicova-Kudlackova M, Simoncic R, Bederova A, Klvanova J. Plasma fatty acid profile and alternative nutrition. *Ann Nutr Metab.* 1997;41(6): 365–370.

Kushak R, Drapeau C, van Corr E, Winter H. Blue-green algae Aphanizomenon flos-aquae as a source of dietary polyunsaturated fatty acids and a hypocholesterolemic agent. *Ann Meeting of Am Chem Soc.* March, 1999.

Kushi LH, Folsom AR, Prineas RJ, Mink PJ, Bosick RM. Dietary antioxidant vitamins and death from coronary heart disease in postmenopausal women. *N Engl J Med.* 1996;334:1156–1162.

Leitzmann MF, Stampfer MJ, Michaud DS, et al. Dietary intake of n-3 and n-6 fatty acids and the risk of prostate cancer. *Am J Clin Nutr.* 2004; 80(1):204–216.

Lucas EA, Wild RD, Hammond LJ, et al. Flaxseed improves lipid profile without altering biomarkers of bone metabolism in postmenopausal women. *J Clin Endocrinol Metab.* 2002;87:1527–1532.

Marckmann P, Gronbaek M. Fish consumption and coronary heart disease mortality. A systematic review of prospective cohort studies. *Eur J Clin Nutr.* 1999;53(8):585–590.

Masters C. Omega-3 fatty acids and the peroxisome. *Mol Cell Biochem.* 1996;165(2):83–93.

McDougall J, Litzau K, Haver E, Saunders V, Spiller GA. Rapid reduction of serum cholesterol and blood pressure by a twelve-day, very low fat, strictly vegetarian diet. *J Am Coll Nutr.* 1995;14(5):491–496.

Melby CL, Foldflies DG, Toohey ML. Blood pressure differences in older black and white long-term vegetarians and nonvegetarians. *J Am Coll Nutr.* 1993;3:262–269 [published erratum appears in *J Am Coll Nutr.* 1993;12(6):following table of contents].

Melchert HU, Limsathayourat N, Mibajlovic H, Eichber J, Thefeld W, Rottkea H. Fatty acid patterns in triglycerides, diglycerides, free fatty acids, cholesterol esters and phosphatidylcholine in serum from vegetarians and nonvegetarians. *Atherosclerosis* 1987;65:159–166.

Messina M, Messina V. *The Dietitian's Guide to Vegetarian Diets: Issues and Applications.* Gaithersburg, MD:Aspen Publishers; 1996.

Messina V, Mangels R, Messina M. *The Dietitian's Guide to Vegetarian Diets: Issues and Applications.* 2d ed. Sudbury, MA: Jones and Bartlett Publishers; 2004.

Nervi AM, Peluffo RO, Brenner RR. Effects of ethanol administration on fatty acid desaturation. *Lipids.* 1980;15:263–268.

Nestel PJ, Pomeroy SE, Sasahara T, et al. Arterial compliance in obese subjects is improved with dietary plant n-3 fatty acid from flaxseed oil despite increased LDL oxidizability. *Arterioscler Thromb Vasc Biol.* 1997;17:1163–1170.

Newcomer LM, King IB, Wicklund KG, Stanford JL. The association of fatty acids with prostate cancer risk. *Prostate.* 2001;47:262–268.

Nicholson AS, Sklar M, Barnard ND, Gore S, Sullivan R, Browning S. Toward improved management of NIDDM: A randomized, controlled, pilot intervention using a lowfat, vegetarian diet. *Preven Med.* 1999;29(2):87–91.

Ornish D, Brown SE, Scherwitz LW, et al. Can lifestyle changes reverse coronary heart disease? The Lifestyle Heart Trial. *Lancet.* 1990;336(8708): 129–133.

Ornish D, Scherwitz LW, Billings JH, et al. Intensive lifestyle changes for reversal of coronary heart disease. *JAMA.* 1998;280(23):2001–2007.

Rainey C, Nyquist L. Nuts—Nutrition and health benefits of daily use. *Nutr Today.* 1997;32(4): 157–163.

Ramon JM, Bou R, Romea S, et al. Dietary fat intake and prostate cancer risk: A case-control study in Spain. *Cancer Causes Control.* 2000;11:679–685.

Reddy S, Sanders TAB, Obeid O. The influence of maternal vegetarian diet on the essential fatty acid status of the newborn. *Eur J Clin Nutr.* 1994; 48:358–368.

Report of a Joint FAO/WHO Expert Consultation. *Diet, Nutrition and the Prevention of Chronic Diseases.* Technical Report Series No. 916. Geneva, Switzerland: World Health Organization; 2003.

Sabaté J. Nut consumption, vegetarian diets, ischemic heart disease risk, and all-cause mortality:

Evidence from epidemiologic studies. *Am J Clin Nutr.* 1999;70(3 Suppl):500S–503S.

Sabaté J, Fraser GE, Burke K, Knutsen S, Bennett H, Lindsted KD. Effects of walnuts on serum lipid levels and blood pressure in normal men. *N Engl J Med.* 1993;328:603–607.

Sanders TAB, Ellis FR, Dickerson JWT. Studies of vegans: The fatty acid composition of plasma choline phosphoglycerides and some indicators of susceptibility to ischemic heart disease in vegan and omnivore control. *Am J Clin Nutr.* 1978;31:805–813.

Sanders TAB, Reddy S. The influence of a vegetarian diet on the fatty acid composition of human milk and the essential fatty acid status of the infant. *J Pediatr.* 1992;120(4, Pt 2):S71–S77.

Sanders TAB, Roshanai F. Platelet phospholipid fatty acid composition and function in vegan compared with age- and sex-matched omnivore controls. *Eur J Clin Nutr.* 1992;46(11):823–831.

Schuurman AG, van den Brandt PA, Dorant E, Brants HA, Goldbohm RA. Association of energy and fat intake with prostate carcinoma risk: Results from The Netherlands Cohort Study. *Cancer.* 1999; 86(6):1019–1027.

Seddon JM, Cote J, Rosner B. Progression of age-related macular degeneration: Association with dietary fat, transunsaturated fat, nuts and fish intake. *Arch Ophthalmology.* 2003;121:1728–1737.

Shinwell ED, Gorodischer R. Totally vegetarian diets and infant nutrition. *Pediatrics.* 1982;4:582–586.

Siguel EN, Lerman RH. Altered fatty acid metabolism in patients with angiographically documented coronary artery disease. *Metabolism.* 1994;43: 982–993.

Simopoulos AP. Essential fatty acids in health and chronic disease. *Am J Clin Nutr.* 1999;70(3): 560S–569S.

Sung MK, Lautens M, Thompson LU. Mammalian lignans inhibit the growth of estrogen-independent human colon tumor cells. *Anticancer Res.* 1998; 18:1405–1408.

Thompson LU, Li T, Chen J, Goss PE. Biological effects of dietary flaxseed in patients with breast cancer [abstract]. *Breast Cancer Res. Treatment* 2000;64:50.

Tsai CJ, Leitzmann MF, Hu FB, Willett WC, Giovannucci EL. Frequent nut consumption and decreased risk of cholecystectomy in women. *Am J Clin Nutr.* 2004;80:76–81.

Turley ML, Skeaff CM, Mann JI, Cox B. The effect of a low-fat, high-carbohydrate diet on serum high-density lipoprotein cholesterol and triglyceride. *Eur J Clin Nutr.* 1998;52(10):728–732.

Uauy R, Hoffman DR, Peirano P, Birch DG, Birch EE. Essential fatty acids in visual and brain development. *Lipids.* 2001;36(9):885–895.

Vaisey-Genser M. *Flaxseed: Health, Nutrition and Functionality.* Winnipeg, Canada: Flax Council of Canada; 1997.

Viola P. *Olive Oil and Health.* Spain: International Olive Oil Council; 1997.

World Cancer Research Fund and American Institute for Cancer Research. *Food, Nutrition and the Prevention of Cancer: A Global Perspective.* Washington, DC: American Institute for Cancer Research; 1997.

Yang YJ, Lee SH, Hong SJ, Chung BC. Comparison of fatty acid profiles in the serum of patients with prostate cancer and benign prostatic hyperplasia. *Clin Biochem.* 1999;32:405–409.

Yochum LA, Folsom AR, Kushi LH. Intake of antioxidant vitamins and risk of death from stroke in postmenopausal women. *Am J Clin Nutr.* 2000; 72(2):476–483.

Zhang SM, Hernan MA, Chen H, Spiegelman D, Willett WC, Ascherio A. Intakes of vitamins E and C, carotenoids, vitamin supplements, and PD risk. *Neurology.* 2002;59:1161–1169.

Zlotkin SH. A review of the Canadian "Nutrition Recommendations Update: Dietary Fat and Children." *J Nutr.* 1996;126:1022S–1027S.

4

Fiber

Peggy Carlson, MD

Introduction

Dietary fiber is crucial for maintaining good health. Vegetarians typically consume much more fiber than omnivores. This increased fiber intake is responsible for many of the health benefits of a vegetarian diet.

This chapter starts by describing what fiber is, where it is found in the diet, and how it is used by the body. We then look at the effects of fiber on health. Lastly, we discuss some practical ways to ensure that a diet contains adequate fiber.

Summary of the Scientific Literature

Facts about Fiber

Definition of Fiber

Dietary fiber is the portion of consumed plant material that is resistant to degradation by the enzymes of the small intestine. There are different types of fiber, but they are all nonstarch polysaccharides, with the exception of lignin, which is an alcohol derivative. No animal products, including meat, dairy, and eggs, contain fiber.

Fiber can be classified into soluble and insoluble types based on the extent to which it is soluble in water or forms a gel. Cellulose, lignin, and some hemicelluloses are considered insoluble forms of fiber, whereas pectins, gums, mucilages, and the remaining hemicelluloses are soluble in water. Although indigestible by intestinal enzymes, most soluble and some insoluble fiber is fermented by intestinal bacteria.

Fiber Content of Foods

All unprocessed plant foods are high in dietary fiber. Different plant foods also contain different proportions of soluble and insoluble fiber. Wheat, rye, rice, and most other grains contain primarily insoluble fiber. Oats have a greater proportion of soluble fiber than any other grain. Legumes, beans, and peas are excellent sources of both soluble and insoluble fiber. Among fruits and vegetables, some are better sources

Table 4.1   Food Sources of Dietary Fiber

Food	Grams of fiber per 100 g dry weight			Grams of fiber according to dietary food portions				
	Dietary Fiber	Soluble	**Insoluble**	Portion	Weight (g)	Dietary Fiber	Soluble	**Insoluble**
Fruits								
Apple	13	4	**9**	1 medium	138	2.9	0.9	**2.0**
Orange	11	7	**4**	1 medium	140	2.0	1.3	**0.7**
Banana	7	2	**5**	1 medium	114	2.0	0.6	**1.4**
Vegetables								
Broccoli	30	14	**16**	1 stalk	100	2.7	1.3	**1.4**
Carrots	24	11	**13**	1 large	100	2.9	1.3	**1.6**
Tomato	13	2	**11**	1 small	100	0.8	0.1	**0.7**
Potato	9	5	**4**	1 medium	100	1.8	1.0	**0.8**
Corn	9	1	**8**	2/3 cup	100	1.6	0.2	**1.4**
Grains								
All-Bran	32	5	**27**	1/2 cup	28	9.0	1.4	**7.6**
Oat bran	16	8	**8**	1/2 cup	28	4.4	2.2	**2.2**
Rolled oats	11	5	**6**	3/4 cup, cooked	175	3.0	1.3	**1.7**
Whole-wheat bread	9	2	**7**	1 slice	25	1.4	0.3	**1.1**
White bread	3	2	**1**	1 slice	24	0.4	0.3	**0.1**
Macaroni	3	2	**1**	1 cup, cooked	90	0.8	0.5	**0.3**
Cornflakes	2	0	**2**	1 cup	28	0.5	0	**0.5**
Legumes								
Green peas	21	3	**18**	2/3 cup, cooked	100	3.9	0.6	**3.3**
Kidney beans	21	5	**16**	1/2 cup, cooked	100	6.5	1.6	**4.9**
Pinto beans	19	4	**15**	1/2 cup, cooked	100	5.9	1.2	**4.7**
Lentils	16	2	**14**	2/3 cup, cooked	100	4.5	0.6	**3.9**

Source: Gray, 1995.

of soluble and insoluble fiber than others (Van Horn, 1997). Table 4.1 lists the fiber content and distribution of some common foods.

Fiber Intake

The United States has one of the lowest per-capita daily fiber intakes of any country. The typical American omnivorous diet contains only about 10–20 grams of fiber per day. Lacto-ovo vegetarians typically consume 20–35 grams of fiber per day, whereas most vegans consume 25–50 grams per day (Messina & Messina, 1996). A plant-based diet can contain 60 grams or more of fiber. Current U.S. dietary recommendations call for 14 grams of fiber per 1,000 kilo-

Figure 4.1   Dietary Fiber Intakes in Different Populations

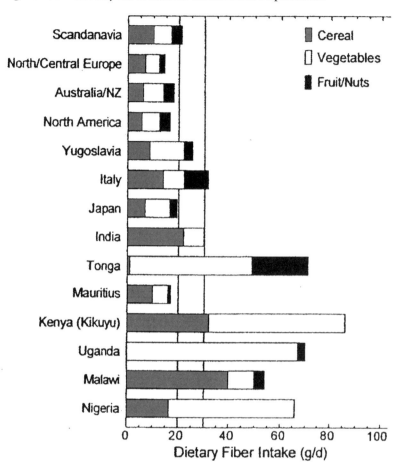

Source: Wolever TM, Jenkins DJ. What is a high fiber diet?. *Adv Expl Med Biol.* 1997;427:35–42. With kind permission of Springer Science and Business Media.

calories, or about 38 grams for the average man and 25 grams for the average woman (Food and Nutrition Board [FNB], 2002). As Figure 4.1 shows, the intakes of dietary fiber in different populations worldwide vary widely, from less than 20 grams to more than 80 grams per day. Although there is no standard, accepted definition of what constitutes a high-fiber diet, Figure 4.1 shows that, internationally, high-fiber intakes range from 55–90 grams per day (Wolever & Jenkins, 1997).

Dwyer (1995) reported that dietary fiber in-

takes of most American children are lower than current American Academy of Pediatrics recommendations. Studies show that fiber intakes of vegetarian children come closer to recommended amounts (Dwyer, 1995; Sanders & Manning, 1992; Williams & Bollella, 1995). Adequate guidelines for daily fiber intake by children are 19 grams per day for 1- to 3-year-olds, 25 grams per day for 4- to 8-year-olds, 31 grams per day for 9- to 13-year-old boys, 38 grams per day for 14- to 18-year-old boys, and 26 grams per day for 9- to 18-year-old girls (FNB, 2002).

Physiological Effects of Fiber

The physiological effects of soluble and insoluble fiber differ. Insoluble fiber has greater water-holding capacity, which increases stool bulk, accelerates intestinal transit time, and increases stool frequency. Soluble fiber increases stool bulk by stimulating intestinal bacterial growth; these bacteria may constitute up to one-half of the entire stool mass. Soluble fiber also tends to form viscous solutions that delay gastric (stomach) emptying and nutrient absorption from the small intestine. More soluble than insoluble fiber is fermented by intestinal bacterial. This fermentation process produces short-chain fatty acids (SCFAs) and the gases hydrogen, carbon dioxide, and methane. SCFAs play an important functional role in the metabolism of cells in the colon, and may have other functions as well.

Health Effects of Fiber

Constipation

Dietary fiber is a mainstay for the prevention and treatment of constipation. Insoluble fiber is the most effective treatment for constipation, because of its ability to increase stool bulk through increased water retention and its ability to speed transit time through the intestine. However, soluble fiber is also effective, because it increases stool bulk by increasing bacterial mass.

Hemorrhoids

Hemorrhoids result from the straining necessary to pass hard stools. Because fiber intake results in softer stools, it also reduces the incidence of hemorrhoids.

Cholesterol Levels and Coronary Artery Disease

Several studies, including several large prospective studies, have reported significant inverse associations between cereal fiber/whole-grain intake and coronary artery disease (CAD) (Pereira & Pins, 2000; Truswell, 2002; Steffen et al., 2003). A meta-analysis of 10 prospective studies concluded that each 10-gram-per-day increase in dietary fiber is associated with a 14% decrease in the risk of coronary events (Pereira et al., 2004).

Part of fiber's role in decreasing the risk of coronary artery disease is its effect on serum lipids. Fiber has an independent effect of lowering total cholesterol and low-density lipoprotein (LDL) cholesterol, thereby lowering the risk of CAD (Van Horn, 1997; Pereira & Pins, 2000). The soluble fraction of fiber results in the greatest reduction in total cholesterol and LDL cholesterol (Glore et al., 1994).

Several mechanisms have been proposed to explain how fiber decreases serum cholesterol (Van Horn, 1997; Pereira & Pins, 2000). Soluble fiber binds bile acids, which in turn leads to increased LDL cholesterol uptake from circulation to synthesize further bile acids. There is evidence that soluble fiber also decreases the absorption of cholesterol and its precursors. The fermentation of fiber produces SCFAs, which inhibit hepatic cholesterol synthesis. Fiber may also affect the concentration of enzymes that are involved in cholesterol synthesis. In addition, specific compounds or amino acids found in fiber-containing foods may produce a cholesterol-lowering effect.

Higher-fiber diets may also afford protection from CAD in ways other than by their effects on lipids. The increased satiety that accompanies a diet higher in fiber may lead to decreased consumption of food—including fat and cholesterol. Fiber can improve blood sugar control in persons with diabetes and may play a role in lowering blood pressure and reducing obesity, all of which can decrease the risk of CAD. High-fiber foods also are often high in phytoestrogens, antioxidants, vitamins, and unsaturated fats, which themselves may be cardioprotective. Fiber may also affect blood-clotting mechanisms in ways that favor a lower CAD risk (Reddy, 1999).

Diverticular Disease

Diverticula are small pouches that project from the intestine. These pouches can become obstructed, leading to infection, perforation, or bleeding. Diverticular disease affects 30%–40% of Americans over the age of 50, but is rare in societies that consume high-fiber, plant-based diets (Kennedy & Zarling, 1998). Numerous studies have consistently found that patients with diverticular disease consume less fiber (Aldoori, 1997). Increased dietary fiber is also used in the treatment of diverticular disease. It is theorized that the bulkier, softer stools attributable to a higher-fiber diet result in lower pressures in the colon when the stool is passed and, therefore, reduce the formation of outpouchings (diverticula) from the intestinal wall.

Cancer

Colon Cancer. Many case-control and observational studies suggest that greater fiber consumption lowers the risk of colon cancer:

- In a combined analysis of 13 case-control studies, Howe et al. (1992) showed that the risk of colon cancer decreased as fiber intake increased; those in the highest quintile of intake (median, 31.2 grams of fiber per day) had about half the risk of colon cancer as those in the lowest quintile (median, 10.1 grams of fiber per day). Of the 13 studies, all but one showed a decrease in risk of at least 26% per 27 grams of fiber per day. Howe et al. also estimated that if the U.S. population increased fiber intake to at least 39 grams per day, the corresponding reduction in risk in colon cancer would be about 31%.
- Shankar and Lanza (1991) reviewed 15 observational studies of colon cancer and found that 13 showed a protective effect of fiber. They also summarized 17 case-control studies and found that 12 showed an inverse association between fiber and colon cancer, 3 showed no association, and 2 showed a positive association.
- Trock and associates (Trock, Lanza, & Greenwald, 1990) analyzed 37 observational studies and 16 case-control studies and found that the majority of both types of studies indicated a protective effect of high-fiber diets.
- Another meta-analysis of 13 case-control studies (Friedenreich, Brant, & Riboli, 1994) showed that high intake of fiber-rich food reduces the risk of colon cancer by one-half.
- More recently, Kim (2000) concluded that of 28 observational studies, 82% showed a strong or moderate protective effect of dietary fiber or "fiber-rich foods," or yielded results that were consistent with a positive effect of fiber. Kim also concluded that most of the published case-control studies showed a significant inverse relationship between dietary fiber and colorectal cancer.
- In a review of the case-control studies published from 1986 to 2000, Sengupta, Tjandra, and Gibson (2001) found that 13 of 24 case-control studies found a positive

association between dietary fiber and colorectal cancer.

In contrast to these observational and case-control studies, more recent prospective studies have been, at best, only weakly supportive, with some studies finding no association and others finding some protection. Kim summarized the results from six large prospective studies and concluded that the relationship between fiber intake and colon cancer was equivocal, but noted that in a recent large prospective study, involving more than 1 million people, there was a significant 30% reduction in colorectal cancer in the group with the highest fiber intake (Kim, 2000). Sengupta reviewed 13 prospective studies, published from 1988 to 2000, which looked at the risk of colorectal cancer in relation to fiber intake. Of the 12 that reported on dietary fiber specifically, only 3 found a protective effect of dietary fiber. Four of eight found a protective effect of vegetables or vegetable fiber and two of five found a protective effect of cereal or cereal fiber. The studies included the U.S. Health Professionals Study of 47,949 men, the Iowa Women's Study of 41,837 participants, and the Nurses' Health Study of 88,757 women (Sengupta, Tjandra, & Gibson, 2001).

Interventional studies to investigate the relationship of cancer with diet would be very difficult to conduct. Cancer may take years to develop to a detectable stage; therefore, the study participants would have to be on a particular diet for many years. In addition, because the incidence of cancer in the study participants would be low, many thousands of people would have to be studied. As an alternative, several studies have focused on the rate of recurrence of colon polyps (frequent precursors to cancer) among those on different diets. Very few of the interventional studies looking at the rate of polyp recurrence have found

a relationship with dietary fiber (Ferguson, Chavan, & Harris, 2001). Of five such trials that Sengupta reviewed, none showed any significant protective effect of fiber (Sengupta, Tjandra, & Gibson, 2001). It is not known if these interventional studies of polyps mimic the effect of diet on colon cancer.

Several hypotheses have been proposed to explain how fiber might protect against colon cancer (Reddy, 1999; Kim, 2000; Sengupta, Tjandra, & Gibson, 2001; Andoh, Tsujikawa, & Fujiyama, 2003; Klurfield, 1997). Fiber-rich diets are typically lower in fat, which may be a risk factor for colon cancer. Fiber may bind potential carcinogens (secondary bile acids), thereby removing them from the body. Because transit times through the colon are faster with a higher-fiber diet, potential carcinogens have less contact time with the colon. Fiber, because it increases stool bulk, may dilute potential carcinogens. The SCFAs produced by fiber fermentation may themselves inhibit the growth of cancer cells. SCFAs may also be anticarcinogenic because, by lowering intestinal pH, they may reduce the solubility of fecal bile acids and affect their conversion to carcinogenic secondary bile acids. The lower risk may also be due to anticarcinogenic properties of the phytochemicals associated with fiber. Fiber may also promote changes in the colonic bacterial population, which can influence the presence of carcinogens in the colon. It has further been proposed that softer stools may reduce the amount of mechanical abrasion in the colon, thereby reducing tumor promotion. Lastly, fiber may affect gene expression and enzyme and hormone functions.

Breast Cancer. Although a considerable number of studies suggest that higher fiber intakes are associated with a decreased risk of breast cancer, several other studies have not supported this relationship. Shankar reported that, of seven case-control studies evaluating the relationship between a fiber-rich diet and breast cancer, six demonstrated a decreased risk with increased fiber consumption (Shankar & Lanza, 1991). In a 1990 report, Howe et al. pooled data from 12 case-control studies and reported that dietary fiber appeared protective among postmenopausal women, but not among premenopausal women (Howe et al., 1990). In 1997, Clavel-Chapelon analyzed nine case-control studies and three cohort studies and found a slight decrease in breast cancer risk with higher fiber consumption, but also reported a fair amount of discrepancy among the studies (Clavel-Chapelon, Niravong, & Joseph, 1997). A 1998 review by Gerber summarized 10 case-control studies and noted that of these, 8 found a decreased risk of breast cancer with increased fiber intake; however, in only 5 was the change statistically significant (Gerber, 1998). Included in this review were case-control studies from Australia and Uruguay, which reported that total dietary fiber reduced breast cancer risk by 54% and 49%, respectively, among those with the highest levels of fiber intake (Baghurst & Rohan, 1994; De Stefani et al., 1997). A 1997 Italian study comparing 2,569 women with breast cancer and 2,588 controls found a trend toward a negative association of fiber with breast cancer risk that was significant for cellulose, but not other types of fiber (La Vecchia et al., 1997). A 1999 study comparing 568 women with breast cancer with 1,451 controls reported minimal, if any, protective effects with high intake of cereals and grains, vegetables, and beans (Potischman et al., 1999).

Prospective studies have been less supportive of any effect by fiber on breast cancer. Gerber (1998) summarized four prospective studies, of which two found no change and two found a nonsignificant decrease in risk of breast cancer with fiber intake. Gerber also noted that when data indicate a reduction in risk, the reduction appears to be dependent on the level of intake, indicating a possible reason for the discrepancy among studies. Included in this review were the Nurses' Health Study of 89,494 women (Willet et al., 1992), which found no association of breast cancer with fiber, and the Netherlands Cohort Study of 62,573 women (Verhoeven et al., 1997), which also found no significant association. Gerber's study also included the Canadian National Breast Screening Study of 56,837 women, which found a nearly significant 30% reduction in breast cancer risk in those at the highest versus the lowest quintiles of fiber intake (Rohan et al., 1993). A 2002 Canadian study, which followed 49,536 women for 16.2 years, found no association between breast cancer risk and the amount or type of dietary fiber, including soluble and insoluble fiber, cereal fiber, fruit and vegetables, lignin, and cellulose (Terry et al., 2002).

Several plausible mechanisms could explain a possible link between greater fiber intake and lower breast cancer risk (Gerber, 1998; Gorbach & Goldin, 1987; Duncan, 2004). Fiber-rich diets are usually lower in fat, which has itself been hypothesized to be a risk factor for breast cancer. However, several studies have suggested an independent effect of fiber beyond that which could be accounted for by lower fat intake (Bennett & Cerda, 1996). There is general agreement that hormones such as estrogen are involved in the development of breast cancer, and many studies have shown that increased fiber intake is associated with decreased estrogen levels. Fiber may decrease estrogen levels by binding or preventing reabsorption of it, thereby increasing the excretion of estrogen in the stool. Fiber may also promote the growth of bacteria that can inhibit intestinal reabsorption of estrogen. The effect of fiber may be due to the ability of some of its associated phytoestrogens to act as estrogen antagonists. Fiber may also act indirectly by reducing obesity, which itself may be a risk factor for breast cancer.

Other Cancers.   Five of six case-control studies have shown a decreased risk of pancreatic cancer with increasing consumption of fiber (World Cancer Research Fund/American Institute for Cancer Research, 1997). Although there are studies linking increased fiber intake to lower risks of other cancers, the data are limited and inconclusive (Gerber, 1998; World Cancer Research Fund/American Institute for Cancer Research, 1997).

Appendicitis

Many studies have either supported or been consistent with the hypothesis that appendicitis is less common in those on a fiber-rich diet (Westlake, St. Leger, & Burr, 1980; Walker et al., 1973; Appleby et al., 1995; Brender et al., 1985; Arnbjornsson, 1983; Jones et al., 1985). Appendicitis is generally recognized to be caused by the obstruction and subsequent inflammation of the appendix. Protection against appendicitis may be afforded by fiber because of the associated softer stools and more rapid gastrointestinal transit time, which would make obstruction of the small opening of the appendix less likely.

High Blood Pressure

Although low-fat, high-fiber vegetarian diets do appear to reduce blood pressure in hypertensive individuals, there is no conclusive evidence that it is specifically the fiber content that is responsible for this effect. Some studies have shown that increasing fiber intake does lower blood pressure, but other studies have not been able to duplicate this finding (Van Horn, 1997; Keenan, Huang, & McDonald, 1997; Beilin, 1994).

The mechanism by which fiber might lower blood pressure is not well understood.

Diabetes

Higher-fiber diets can probably produce modest improvement in the blood glucose control of persons with diabetes (Messina & Messina, 1996; Anderson, Smith, & Gustafson, 1994; Vessby, 1994; Anderson & Akanji, 1991; Chandalia et al., 2000; Jenkins et al., 2003; Liu et al., 2000). A review of 53 studies that examined the effects of a high-fiber diet in diabetic patients reported that 62% showed improved glucose control, 15% reported no change, and 4% noted worsening of glucose control (Anderson & Akanji, 1993).

Generally, studies show that it takes an increase in fiber consumption to two to three times the average American intake to produce this positive effect (Messina & Messina, 1996). This level of intake is more consistent with an average vegetarian diet than with an omnivorous diet. It is the soluble, as opposed to insoluble, fiber that yields the beneficial effect on glucose control.

Proposed mechanisms for this effect of fiber on blood glucose control include the longer time it takes to eat a higher-fiber diet; slower gastric emptying and intestinal absorption, which can blunt the rise in glucose after meals; decreased absorption of glucose; changes in the actions of gastrointestinal hormones; and the effects of SCFAs on liver and muscle metabolism (Pereira et al., 2002; Ha & Lean, 1998). Several recent studies have also shown that higher intakes of whole grains are associated with increased insulin sensitivity (Pereira et al., 2002; McKeown et al., 2002; Liese et al., 2003). Increased dietary fiber may also contribute to weight loss, which itself improves glucose control. In addition, other factors associated with dietary fiber, such as antioxidants, phytochemicals, and magnesium, may contribute to improved glucose control (Liu et al., 2000; Liese et al., 2003).

In addition to helping with glucose control in diabetics, dietary fiber, especially cereal fiber, appears to help prevent the onset of diabetes. Most prospective epidemiologic studies (Parillo & Riccardi, 2004), including the Nurses' Health Study (Schulze et al., 2004), the Health Professionals Follow-up Study (Fung et al., 2002), and the Iowa's Women's Study (Meyer et al., 2000), indicate that low fiber intake correlates with a higher prevalence of diabetes.

Obesity

Fiber has long been touted as a beneficial part of a healthy diet for preventing or correcting obesity. Many studies have shown that increasing fiber intake can lead to better weight management; however, the evidence is not conclusive (Van Horn, 1997; Gray, 1995; Bennett & Cerda, 1996; Hamilton & Anderson, 1992; Rolls, 1995; Pereira & Ludwig, 2001; Howarth, Saltzman, & Roberts, 2001). There are many proposed mechanisms by which fiber could help with weight control (Pereira & Ludwig, 2001; Howarth, Saltzman, & Roberts, 2001). Fiber is relatively calorie-free. Because of its bulkiness and effect on slowing gastric emptying, it may lead to an earlier feeling of satiety. Fiber may provide a mechanical barrier to enzymatic digestion of food in the small intestine. In addition, fiber can be fermented by bacteria, thereby producing intestinal gas and a resultant sensation of bloating and fullness. Food intake may also be modulated by SCFAs formed by fiber fermentation, by fiber-stimulated release of gastrointestinal hormones, and by the longer time needed to chew a higher-fiber diet. Fiber also decreases insulin secretion, thereby decreasing appetite.

Other Gastrointestinal Disorders

Gallstones. It has been theorized that increasing one's fiber intake may decrease the occurrence of gallstones. Fiber decreases the intestinal absorption of cholesterol (the primary component of gallstones) and bile acids (a minor component of gallstones). In addition, fiber-mediated decreases in intestinal transit time may also affect gallstone formation by decreasing the time available for bile acid absorption (VanBerge-Henegouwen, Portincasa, & van Erpecum, 1997). Despite these theoretical considerations, and despite the fact that vegetarians seem less predisposed to gallstones, there is currently no clinical evidence that fiber itself decreases the occurrence of gallstone disease (Bennett & Cerda, 1996; VanBerge-Henegouwen, Portincasa, & van Erpecum, 1997). One study that looked at the reformation of gallstones in patients who had undergone previous medical dissolution of gallstones found that patients in the placebo and fiber groups had similar (30%) rates of recurrence (Hood et al., 1993).

Irritable Bowel Syndrome, Inflammatory Bowel Disease, Ulcer Disease. A few studies have looked at the effect of fiber on irritable bowel syndrome, inflammatory bowel disease, and ulcer disease. In the case of irritable bowel disease, the results of a handful of studies have been mixed, with some showing improvement and others showing no effect (Bennett & Cerda, 1996).

Nair and Mayberry (1994) reviewed studies that investigated the role of fiber in the development and treatment of inflammatory bowel disease (Crohn's disease and ulcerative colitis). The studies are too few in number to be conclusive.

The relationship of fiber to peptic ulcer disease is also not clear. A study by Katschinski

et al. (1990) found that fiber intake was not related to peptic ulcer disease. However, Rydning
et al. (1982) reported a 45% rate of recurrence
of duodenal ulcers in those on a higher-fiber
diet, compared with an 80% rate of recurrence
in those on a lower-fiber diet. The Health Professionals Follow-up Study of 43,881 men found
that fiber, particularly fiber from legumes, fruits,
and vegetables, was associated with a significant decreased risk of duodenal ulcer (Aldoori
et al., 1995).

Side Effects of Increased Fiber Intake

Increased fiber consumption can sometimes
cause flatulence, diarrhea, abdominal discomfort, and/or a sensation of bloating. It may be
possible to decrease these symptoms by increasing fiber intake gradually.

Fiber does bind minerals, including zinc,
iron, and calcium. This does not, however, appear to be clinically significant. There is no evidence of deficiencies of these minerals among
people with higher fiber intake if adequate mineral intake is maintained (Anderson & Akanji,
1991; Rattan et al., 1981).

Practical Aspects

It is generally recommended that adults consume 14 grams of fiber per 1,000 kilocalories
per day. In practice, this is much easier to do
when consuming a plant-based diet that emphasizes whole, unprocessed foods. Vegetarians generally have fiber intakes equal to or
greater than the recommended 25–38 grams
per day.

Table 4.1 lists the fiber content of common
foods.

Conclusion

Fiber is an important dietary component for
maintaining optimal health. Fiber is found only
in plant foods, and thus typically is consumed
in greater amounts in a vegetarian diet. Although most Americans consuming a meat-
based diet fall short of the recommended daily
intake of fiber, those consuming a vegetarian
diet likely meet the recommendations easily.

Scientific studies have fairly conclusively
linked a fiber-rich diet with decreased incidences of constipation and hemorrhoids, lower
cholesterol levels, decreased risk of coronary
artery disease, and a lower occurrence of diverticular disease. Many, but not all, studies suggest that a higher-fiber diet is protective against
colon cancer. Evidence also suggests that
greater fiber intake leads to lower rates of appendicitis, and also to small or modest improvements in the control of blood glucose levels in
persons with diabetes.

Despite a number of studies, the jury is still
out as to whether fiber has a protective role
against breast cancer and whether fiber intake
has an important role in the treatment of obesity or hypertension. There are far too few
studies to draw any conclusions about the possible role of fiber in other cancers, gallstone
disease, irritable bowel syndrome, inflammatory bowel disease, and ulcer disease.

An excellent way to meet recommendations
for fiber intake is to consume a plant-based diet
built around unprocessed foods. The higher
fiber content of a vegetarian diet is at least
partly responsible for many of the health benefits enjoyed by vegetarians.

References

Aldoori WH. The protective role of dietary fiber in diverticular disease. *Adv Expl Med Biol.* 1997; 427:291–308.

Aldoori WH, Giovannucci E, Stampfer M, et al. A prospective study of diet and the risk of duodenal ulcer in men. *Am J Clin Nutr.* 1995;61:897 [abstract].

Anderson J, Akanji A. Treatment of diabetes with high fiber diets. In: Spiller GA, ed. *Handbook of Dietary Fiber in Human Nutrition.* Boca Raton, FL: CRC Press; 1993.

Anderson JW, Akanji AO. Dietary fiber—An overview. *Diabetes Care.* 1991;14(12):1126–1231.

Anderson JW, Smith BM, Gustafson NJ. Health benefits and practical aspects of high-fiber diets. *Am J Clin Nutr.* 1994;59(5, Suppl):1242S–1247S.

Andoh A, Tsujikawa T, Fujiyama Y. Role of dietary fiber and short-chain fatty acids in the colon. *Curr Pharm Des.* 2003;9(4):347–358.

Appleby P, Thorogood M, McPherson K, Mann J. Emergency appendicectomy and meat consumption in the U.K. *J Epidemiol & Community Health.* 1995;49(6):594–596.

Arnbjornsson E. Acute appendicitis and dietary fiber. *Arch Surg.* 1983;118(7):868–870.

Baghurst PA, Rohan TA. High-fiber diets and reduced risk of breast cancer. *Intl J Cancer.* 1994; 56(2):173–176.

Beilin L. Vegetarian and other complex diets, fats, fiber, and hypertension. *Am J Clin Nutr.* 1994; 59(Suppl):1130S–1135S.

Bennett WG, Cerda JJ. Dietary fiber: Fact and fiction. *Dig Discuss.* 1996;14(1):43–58.

Brender JD, Weiss NS, Koepsell TD, Marcuse EF. Fiber intake and childhood appendicitis. *Am J Public Health.* 1985;75(4):399–400.

Chandalia M, Garg A, Lutjohann D, et al. Beneficial effects of high dietary fiber intake in patients with type 2 diabetes mellitus. *N Eng J Med.* 2000;342(19):1392–1398.

Clavel-Chapelon F, Niravong M, Joseph RR. Diet and breast cancer: Review of the epidemiologic literature. *Cancer Detect Preven.* 1997;21(5):426–440.

De Stefani E, Correa P, Ronco A, et al. Dietary fiber and risk of breast cancer: A case-control study in Uruguay. *Nutr Cancer.* 1997;28(1):14–19.

Duncan AM. The role of nutrition in the prevention of breast cancer. *AACN Clin Issues.* 2004;15(1): 119–135.

Dwyer JT. Dietary fiber for children: How much? *Pediatrics.* 1995;96(5, Pt. 2):1019–1022.

Ferguson LR, Chavan RR, Harris PJ. Changing concepts of dietary fiber: Implications for carcinogenesis. *Nutr Cancer.* 2001;39(2):155–169.

Food and Nutrition Board, Institute of Medicine. *Dietary Reference Intakes for Energy, Carbohydrate, Fiber, Fat, Fatty Acids, Cholesterol, Protein, and Amino Acids (Macronutrients).* Washington, DC: National Academy Press; 2002.

Friedenreich CM, Brant RF, Riboli E. Influence of methodologic factors in a pooled analysis of 13 case-control studies of colorectal cancer and dietary fiber. *Epidemiology.* 1994;5(1):66–79.

Fung TT, Hu FB, Pereira MA, et al. Whole-grain intake and the risk of type 2 diabetes: A prospective study in men. *Am J Clin Nutr.* 2002;76(3):535–540.

Gerber M. Fibre and breast cancer. *Eur J Cancer Preven.* 1998;7(Suppl 2):S63–S67.

Glore SR, Van Treeck D, Knehans AW, Guild M. Soluble fiber and serum lipids: Literature review. *J Am Dietetic Assoc.* 1994;94(4):425–436.

Gorbach SL, Goldin B. Diet and the excretion and enterohepatic cycling of estrogens. *Preven Med.* 1987;16(4):525–531.

Gray D. The clinical uses of dietary fiber. *Am Fam Physician.* 1995;51(2):419–426.

Ha TK, Lean ME. Recommendations for the nutritional management of patients with diabetes mellitus. *Eur J Clin Nutr.* 1998;52(7):467–481.

Hamilton CC, Anderson JW. Fiber and weight management. *J Fla Med Assoc.* 1992;79(6):379–381.

Hood KA, Gleeson D, Ruppin DC, Dowling RH. Gall stone recurrence and its prevention: The British/ Belgian Gall Stone Study Group's post-dissolution trial. *Gut.* 1993;34(9):1277–1288.

Howarth NR, Saltzman E, Roberts SB. Dietary fiber and weight regulation. *Nutr Rev.* 2001;59(5): 129–139.

Howe GR, Benito E, Castelleto R, et al. Dietary intake of fiber and decreased risk of cancers of the colon and rectum: Evidence from the combined analysis of 13 case-control studies. *J Natl Cancer Inst.* 1992;84(24):1887–1896.

Howe GR, Hirohata T, Hislop TG, et al. Dietary factors and risk of breast cancer: Combined analysis of 12 case-control studies. *J Natl Cancer Inst.* 1990;82(7):561–569.

Jenkins DJ, Kendall CW, Marchie A, et al. Type 2 diabetes and the vegetarian diet. *Am J Clin Nutr.* 2003;78(3, Suppl):610S–616S.

Jones BA, Demetriades D, Segal I, Burkitt DP. The prevalence of appendiceal fecaliths in patients with and without appendicitis: A comparative study from Canada and South Africa. *Ann Surg.* 1985;202(1):80–82.

Katschinski B, Logan RF, Edmond M, Langman MJ. Duodenal ulcer and refined carbohydrate intake: A case-controlled study assessing dietary fibre and refined sugar intake. *Gut.* 1990;31(9):993–996.

Keenan JM, Huang Z, McDonald A. Soluble fiber and hypertension. *Adv Expl Biol.* 1997;427:79–87.

Kennedy MV, Zarling EJ. Answers to 10 key questions on diverticular disease of the colon. *Comp Ther.* 1998;24(8):364–369.

Kim YI. AGA technical review: Impact of dietary fiber on colon cancer occurrence. *Gastroenterology.* 2000;118(6):1235–1257.

Klurfield DM. Fiber and cancer protection—mechanism. *Adv Expl Biol.* 1997;427:249–257.

La Vecchia C, Ferraroni M, Franceschi S, et al. Fibers and breast cancer risk. *Nutr Cancer.* 1997;28(3):264–269.

Liese AD, Roach AK, Sparks KC, et al. Whole-grain intake and insulin sensitivity: The Insulin Resistance Atherosclerosis Study. *Am J Clin Nutr.* 2003;78(5):965–971.

Liu S, Manson JE, Stampfer MJ, et al. A prospective study of whole-grain intake and risk of type 2 diabetes mellitus in US women. *Am J Public Health* 2000;90(9):1409–1415.

McKeown NM, Meigs J, Liu S, et al. Whole-grain intake is favorably associated with metabolic risk factors for type 2 diabetes and cardiovascular disease in the Framingham Offspring Study. *Am J Clin Nutr.* 2002;76(2):390–398.

Messina M, Messina V. *The Dietitian's Guide to Vegetarian Diets: Issues and Applications.* Gaithersburg, MD: Aspen Publishers; 1996.

Meyer KA, Kushi LH, Jacobs DR, et al. Carbohydrates, dietary fiber, and incident type 2 diabetes in older women. *Am J Clin Nutr.* 2000;71(4):921–930.

Nair P, Mayberry JF. Vegetarianism, dietary fibre and gastro-intestinal disease. *Dig Dis.* 1994;12(3):177–185.

Parillo M, Riccardi G. Diet composition and the risk of type 2 diabetes: Epidemiological and clinical evidence. *Br J Nutr.* 2004;92(1):7–19.

Pereira MA, Jacobs DR, Pins JJ, et al. Effect of whole grains on insulin sensitivity in overweight hyperinsulinemic adults. *Am J Clin Nutr.* 2002;75(5):848–855.

Pereira MA, Ludwig DS. Dietary fiber and bodyweight regulation. *Pediatr Clin N Am.* 2001;48(4):969–980.

Pereira MA, O'Reilly E, Augustsson K, et al. Dietary fiber and risk of coronary heart disease: A pooled analysis of cohort studies. *Arch Intern Med.* 2004;164(4):370–376.

Pereira MA, Pins JJ. Dietary fiber and cardiovascular disease: Experimental and epidemiologic advances. *Curr Atheroscler Reps.* 2000;2(6):494–502.

Potischman N, Swanson CA, Coates RJ, et al. Intake of food groups and associated micronutrients in relation to risk of early-stage breast cancer. *Intl J Cancer.* 1999;82(3):315–321.

Rattan J, Levin N, Graff E, et al. A high-fiber diet does not cause mineral and nutrient deficiencies. *J Clin Gastroenterol.* 1981;3(4):389–393.

Reddy BS. Role of dietary fiber in colon cancer: An overview. *Am J Med.* 1999;106(1A):16S–19S.

Rohan TE, Howe GR, Friedenreich CM, et al. Dietary fiber, vitamins A, C, and E, and the risk of breast cancer: A cohort study. *Cancer Causes Control.* 1993;4(1):29–37.

Rolls BJ. Carbohydrates, fats and satiety. *Am J Clin Nutr.* 1995;61(4, Suppl):960S–967S.

Rydning A, Berstad A, Aaland E, Odegaard B. Prophylactic effect of dietary fibre in duodenal ulcer disease. *Lancet.* 1982;2(8301):736–739.

Sanders TAB, Manning J. The growth and development of vegan children. *J Hum Nutr Diet.* 1992; 5:11–21.

Schulze MB, Liu S, Rimm EB, et al. Glycemic index, glycemic load, and dietary fiber intake and incidence of type 2 diabetes in younger and middle-aged women. *Am J Clin Nutr.* 2004;80(2): 348–356.

Sengupta S, Tjandra JJ, Gibson PR. Dietary fiber and colorectal neoplasia. *Dis Colon Rectum.* 2001; 44(7):1016–1033.

Shankar S, Lanza E. Dietary fiber and cancer prevention. *Hematol Oncol Clin N Am.* 1991;5(1): 25–41.

Steffen LM, Jacobs DR, Stevens J, et al. Associations of whole-grain, refined-grain, and fruit and vegetable consumption with risks of all-cause mortality and incident coronary artery disease and ischemic stroke: The Atherosclerosis Risk in Communities (ARIC) study. *Am J Clin Nutr.* 2003; 78(3):383–390.

Terry P, Jain M, Miller AB, et al. No association among total dietary fiber, fiber fractions, and risk of breast cancer. *Cancer Epidemiol Biomarkers Preven.* 2002;11(11):1507–1508.

Trock B, Lanza E, Greenwald P. Dietary fiber, vegetables, and colon cancer: Critical review and meta-analyses of the epidemiologic evidence. *J Natl Cancer Inst.* 1990;82(8):650–661.

Truswell AS. Cereal grains and coronary heart disease. *Eur J Clin Nutr.* 2002;56(1):1–14.

VanBerge-Henegouwen GP, Portincasa P, van Erpecum KJ. Effect of lactulose and fiber-rich diets on bile in relation to gallstone disease: An update. *Scand J Gastroenterol.* 1997;222(Suppl):68–71.

Van Horn L. Fiber, lipids, and coronary heart disease: A statement for healthcare professionals from the Nutrition Committee, American Heart Association. *Circulation.* 1997;95(12):2701–2704.

Verhoeven DT, Assen N, Goldbohm RA, et al. Vitamins C and E, retinol, beta-carotene and dietary fiber in relation to breast cancer risk: A prospective cohort study. *Br J Cancer.* 1997;75(1):149–155.

Vessby B. Dietary carbohydrates in diabetes. *Am J Clin Nutr.* 1994;59(3, Suppl):742S–746S.

Walker AR, Richardson BD, Walker BF, Woolford A. Appendicitis, fibre intake and bowel behaviour in ethnic groups in South Africa. *Postgrad Med J.* 1973;49(570):243–249.

Westlake CA, St. Leger AS, Burr ML. Appendectomy and dietary fiber. *J Hum Nutr.* 1980;34(4): 267–272.

Willet WC, Hunter DJ, Stampfer MJ, et al. Dietary fat and fiber in relation to risk of breast cancer. An 8-year follow-up. *JAMA.* 1992;268(15):2037–2044.

Williams CL, Bollella M. Is a high-fiber diet safe for children? *Pediatrics.* 1995;96(5 Pt. 2):1014–1019.

Wolever TM, Jenkins DJ. What is a high fiber diet?. *Adv Expl Med Biol.* 1997;427:35–42.

World Cancer Research Fund/American Institute for Cancer Research. *Food, Nutrition and the Prevention of Cancer: A Global Perspective.* Washington, DC: American Institute for Cancer Research; 1997.

5

Iron

Dina Aronson, MS, RD

Introduction

Iron is one of the most controversial nutrients in the vegetarian diet. Measurements of overall iron intake from foods and supplements are not sufficient to assess adequacy in the diet, because of a wide range of factors affecting absorption of iron from the small intestine. Iron from plant foods is not as well absorbed as iron from animal foods; indeed, this issue is so significant that the recommended iron intake value (Food and Nutrition Board [FNB], 2001) for vegetarians is actually higher than for the rest of the population.

Iron is a relatively well-understood mineral; knowledge of the relationship between blood and iron dates back to the 16th century. Its use as a treatment for anemia began in the 1830s, and it was one of the first nutrients to be used for fortification. (Iron was added to milk in the 1920s in England.)

Summary of the Scientific Literature

Functions of Iron in the Body

The best-known function of iron is as an essential component of the protein hemoglobin, the component of red blood cells that carries oxygen in the blood. Two-thirds to three-quarters of the body's iron is found in hemoglobin. Iron is also a part of myoglobin, a protein similar in structure to hemoglobin, that stores oxygen in muscle tissue. Iron provides a building block for the production of enzymes involved in synthesizing new amino acids, tissues, hormones, and neurotransmitters. As a component of metabolic enzymes, iron is needed for cellular oxidation processes. Iron is necessary for normal brain development in children and for learning. Over and above these main functions, research has shown that iron is also a major factor in heart health, cell-mediated immunity, and bone health.

Iron in Food

Heme iron is found in the flesh of animals; this iron is in the form of hemoglobin and myoglobin in that animal. Non-heme iron is found in meat, as well as plants, eggs, and dairy foods. The vast majority of iron found in the diet is non-heme; even the iron in meat is only up to 40% heme.

Metabolism and Absorption of Iron

Iron is recycled very efficiently by the body; that which is broken down is reused over and over again. Only a small fraction of iron is lost from the body pool each day. Iron balance differs from that of other trace elements in that it is regulated primarily by absorption, not excretion. The body's ability to excrete iron is very limited; to maintain iron balance, adult men absorb (and excrete) about 1 mg per day, and menstruating women absorb (and excrete) an average of 1.5 mg per day. Only about 10%–15% of the iron consumed is absorbed (FNB, 2001; Sabaté, 2001).

Iron is absorbed in the proximal small intestine (mostly the duodenum), and is absorbed in the ferrous form (2+). Ferric salts (3+) are reduced to ferrous salts prior to absorption. Iron is readily absorbed directly into the bloodstream, where it is transported by ferritin. Absorbed iron goes to the bone marrow for red blood cell synthesis; to tissues for cellular oxidation processes; and to the liver, spleen, and bone marrow for storage.

Heme iron is better absorbed than non-heme iron. This is thought to be due to the presence of specific heme-binding sites in the intestinal tract that facilitate absorption (Sabaté, 2001). Oxidized (ferric, 3+) iron is less readily absorbed than reduced (ferrous, 2+) iron. Most of the iron in the diet is non-heme, even for those who consume meat regularly.

The absorption of non-heme iron is particularly vulnerable to other factors in the diet, as well as an individual's iron status. The body is a superb regulator of absorption rate; iron status itself will determine the absorption of iron at the gut level. Non-heme iron absorption adapts to maintain body iron stores (Hunt & Roughead, 2000). The mechanism for this regulation is thought to take place within the mucosal cells; it appears that intestinal cells are programmed to contain ferritin in larger amounts when iron stores are high and in lower amounts when stores are low (FNB, 2001; Monsen, 1999). Table 5.1 lists factors that affect (reduce or enhance) iron absorption.

Overcoming Iron Absorption Inhibitors

It is difficult to accurately assess the degree to which absorption inhibitors affect overall iron absorption and status. Because there are so many competing factors, and because the body is such a good regulator of absorption, it is always best to assess iron intake and status on an individual basis. Given the dietary inhibitors listed in Table 5.1, however, it is useful to identify ways to overcome inhibitory effects of certain plant foods, especially with regard to vegetarian diets.

Phytates. Found mainly associated with fiber in whole grains and legumes, phytates are the most potent inhibitors of iron absorption. Refining grains is one way to reduce phytate, but refining also removes iron. (This is why iron-fortified refined grains are recommended for infants.) Refining also removes the fiber and other protective nutrients that are important components of whole grains, so refinement for the purpose of removing phytate is

Table 5.1   Factors Affecting Iron Absorption

Factors That Reduce Absorption of Iron	Examples and Notes
Phytic acid	Legumes, rice, grains
Polyphenols	Tannins (in tea and coffee), flavonoids (in red wine)
Vegetable protein	Whole soybeans, soy flour, nonfermented soybean products, beans, nuts
Whey and casein	Dairy products
Eggs	Also, egg albumin added to foods
Fiber	Wheat bran, fiber supplements
Antacids	Calcium carbonate, magnesium hydroxide; decrease stomach acidity
Zinc	Zinc supplements are of concern, not zinc from foods
High calcium intakes	Calcium supplements or meals with high calcium loads may interfere with degradation of phytic acid; may block absorption in intestinal mucosa

Factors That Enhance Absorption of Iron	Examples and Notes
Ascorbic acid (vitamin C)	Citrus fruits, bell peppers, potatoes, leafy green vegetables are good sources. Ferric iron is reduced to ferrous iron, which is more easily absorbed.
Other organic acids, such as citric, lactic, and malic acids	Fruits (especially citrus fruits), vegetables, condiments with organic acids added for flavor and preservation
Heme iron	Meat, poultry, fish
Low iron intakes	Regulation at gut level
Low iron status	Regulation at gut level
Pregnancy	Regulation at gut level

not recommended in general. Instead, using foods rich in vitamin C and other organic acids is recommended as a strategy to overcome the effects of phytate. In addition, soaking, sprouting, leavening, and fermenting whole grains render the iron more bioavailable by degrading the phytates (Meerschaert, Sullivan, & Aronson, 2002).

Soy.   In the vegetarian diet, soy is commonly eaten in many forms, such as tofu, tempeh, isolated soy protein, soy milk, and soy flour. Some studies have shown soy to have an inhibitory effect on iron absorption, although a few, including a study that investigated human iron absorption from soybeans, have shown

soybeans to be a good source of absorbable iron, particularly for marginally iron-deficient women (Murray-Kolb et al., 2003). Fermented soy products—tempeh, nato, and miso—have been shown to have higher iron bioavailability because the phytate is hydrolyzed during the fermentation process (Meerschaert, Sullivan, & Aronson, 2002). Thus, increasing the variety of soy products to include such fermented products is one strategy that may help some individuals improve their iron status. Another is to consume vitamin C-rich foods with meals.

Polyphenols.   Phenolic acids, flavonoids, and tannins are all examples of polyphenols that, when consumed in high amounts, may lead to decreased iron absorption. Tea, coffee, cocoa, red wine, and some herbal teas are common foods that are rich in polyphenols. As with phytates, some of the inhibitory effects of these polyphenols can be overcome, at least partially, by consuming them with enhancers of iron absorption.

Vitamin C Enhances Absorption

As indicated in Table 5.1, the presence of ascorbic acid (vitamin C) in a meal increases iron absorption by reducing iron to a more bioavailable state. Thus, inclusion of more vitamin C-rich foods with foods containing inhibitors (e.g., orange juice with a meal of whole grains and beans) helps increase iron absorption. Other organic acids help too; these are found in fruits and vegetables and some processed foods. Malic acid, for example, is found in apples, and citric acid is often added to sauces and dressings to add or enhance a sour flavor.

Mineral Interactions

Iron absorption is affected by the presence of other minerals, such as zinc. With zinc, the effect goes both ways: too much zinc may inhibit iron absorption, and too much iron may inhibit zinc absorption. Zinc-containing supplements, which give a bigger one-time dose of zinc than typical meals, have been shown to decrease iron absorption. Thus, it is recommended to avoid zinc-only supplements, at least at mealtime, if iron status is compromised. The effect of calcium on iron absorption is unclear; studies demonstrate that calcium interferes with iron absorption in the short term, but long-term effects and mechanisms are unknown. Because of the many competing inhibitory and enhancing effects on iron absorption, it is difficult to isolate the influence of calcium (Meerschaert, Sullivan, & Aronson, 2002).

The World's Primary Nutrient Deficiency

Iron deficiency is extremely common, affecting between 500 million and 600 million people worldwide (Bothwell, 1995). Fortunately, deficiency is preventable and readily reversible with supplementation and/or the addition of iron-rich foods to the diet.

Iron-deficiency anemia is, by far, the most common cause of anemia. It is most common in children and women of childbearing age. This anemia is characterized by red blood cells that are small and pale because of low amounts of hemoglobin. The main symptom of iron deficiency is fatigue; indeed, the lowered capacity to provide oxygen to the tissues is largely responsible for the fatigue and apathy characteristic of iron-deficiency anemia (Tver & Russel, 1989). Other signs and symptoms of iron deficiency include skin pallor, dizziness, rapid pulse, weakness, shortness of breath, and impaired immune function (e.g., increased susceptibility to infection) (FNB, 2001). Anemia appears only after the body's iron stores have been depleted; thus, blood tests for anemia (such as the hemoglobin or hematocrit tests) are not satisfactory measures for detecting early iron depletion (Liberman & Bruning, 2003).

Iron deficiency, sometimes leading to anemia, is also a problem seen in infants fed cow's milk or formula based on cow's milk. Human babies' digestive systems are designed for the milk of a human, not that of a cow. The cow's-milk protein may cause micro-tears in the lining of the small intestine, causing bleeding (FNB, 2001). The blood loss via the stools, over time, may lead to iron deficiency and possibly anemia (Udall & Suskind, 1999).

Table 5.2   Recommended Dietary Allowances for Iron (and Other DRIs)

Life Stage		RDA (mg/d)	RDA for vegetarians (mg/d)**	Upper Limit (mg/d)
Infants	0–6 months	0.27*	0.27*	40
	7–12 months	11	19.8	40
Children	1–3 years	7	12.6	40
	4–8 years	10	18	40
Males	9–13 years	8	14.4	40
	14–18 years	11	19.8	45
	19+ years	8	14.4	45
Females	9–13 years	8	14.4	45
	14–18 years	15	27	45
	19–50 years	18	32.4	45
	51+ years	8	14.4	45
Pregnancy	all ages	27	48.6	45
Lactation	≤18 years	10	18	45
	19–30 years	9	16.2	45
	31–50 years	9	16.2	45

Source: Food and Nutrition Board, Institute of Medicine. *Dietary Reference Intakes for Vitamin A, Vitamin K, Arsenic, Boron, Chromium, Copper, Iodine, Iron, Manganese, Molybdenum, Nickel, Silicon, Vanadium, and Zinc.* Washington, DC: National Academy of Sciences; 2001. Courtesy of the National Academies Press.
*This value is the "Adequate Intake" value based on the amount of iron present in human breast milk.
**The RDA for vegetarians is calculated by multiplying the RDA by 1.8.

Iron Requirements

Most people need about eight milligrams of iron per day to keep up normal stores (FNB, 2001). The blood demands of pregnancy, menstruation, blood donation, gastrointestinal bleeds, growth, and increased metabolism (e.g., exercise, lactation, disease states) all increase iron requirements. In addition, according to the National Academy of Sciences, high intakes of plant foods increase iron needs almost twofold (FNB, 2001); hence the recommendation for vegetarians to consume more iron (1.8 times more) than the RDA for people following a mixed diet (see Table 5.2). Whether this rather high intake of iron has been shown to be truly necessary in cross-cultural studies of vegetari-

ans is a matter of debate. Given that the RDA for vegetarians during pregnancy (48.6 mg/d) actually exceeds the upper limit for safety (45 mg/d) set by the same organization, it is important to assess vegetarians' iron needs on an individual basis.

Iron Throughout the Lifespan

Children

Full-Term Infants.   Infants are born with large iron stores. Breast milk provides all the iron necessary for proper growth and development until approximately six months of age (Messina, Mangels, & Messina, 2004). Babies who are not fed human milk should be given an iron-fortified infant formula (FNB, 2001). When babies begin eating solids, iron-fortified cereals and iron-rich fruits and vegetables are recommended (Messina, Mangels, & Messina, 2004).

Children and Adolescents. Children and adolescents need enough iron, especially during rapid growth periods, for normal growth and brain development. The RDA is set to cover these needs. A study looking at risk factors for low iron intake in British children and young adults aged 4 to 18 years found that girls aged 11 to 18 years had the poorest iron intakes and status; this group may be at higher risk of poor iron status due to menstruation, lower socio-economic conditions, and poor diet. In this study, vegetarianism was not identified as a risk factor for low iron intake or poor iron status (Thane, Bates, & Prentice, 2003).

Men

Healthy adult men have no regular iron losses, so this population has the lowest adult RDA. As with other RDA values, the eight milligrams recommended should cover both normal losses and absorption challenge issues.

Women

Menstruating Women. Menstruating women lose about 50% more iron than men, hence the much higher RDA. Absorption rates of iron among this population are typically higher because of higher demand. Women taking oral contraceptives lose less blood during menstruation, so require a bit less per day: 10.9 milligrams (11.4 mg for adolescent girls). Women who use birth control injections menstruate very little or not at all, and thus may require less iron. Women who use IUDs may have higher-than-average blood loss and thus may need more than 18 mg per day.

Pregnant Women. Pregnant women have the highest need for iron of all populations, despite the fact that menstruation ceases during pregnancy. The demand for iron during pregnancy is substantial due to increased blood volume, fetal development, and any blood loss during delivery. Iron needs increase as pregnancy progresses, and pregnancy's strong positive effect on iron absorption is an important physiological adjustment. Maternal iron stores typically meet the needs of the fetus, so that even infants who are born to iron-deficient mothers are unlikely to be anemic unless the mother's anemia is severe. This is not to say that iron deficiency will not put the fetus at risk; adequate iron intakes and good iron status during pregnancy are important to minimize outcome risks of both mother and fetus (Messina, Mangels, & Messina, 2004).

Supplements are generally recommended to meet the iron needs of pregnancy. The Institute of Medicine recommends 30 mg per day starting at week 12 of gestation (Institute of Medicine [IOM], 1990). However, some health practitioners argue that the recommendation for iron supplements should not be generalized to all pregnant women (Cogswell, Kettel-Khan, & Ramakrishnan, 2003), and that supplements should be prescribed only to those who show the need for them. Although it would be extremely challenging to meet the iron intake needs of the pregnant vegetarian without supplements, it is possible that a carefully planned, iron-rich diet will provide adequate iron to the growing fetus, as well as keep maternal iron stores optimal throughout pregnancy. Pregnant women who do not take iron supplements should be carefully monitored throughout pregnancy; often the need for extra iron is not evident until the second or third trimester (IOM, 1990).

Iron supplements often cause gastrointestinal discomfort and/or constipation. A liquid supplement (Meerschaert, Sullivan, & Aronson, 2002) or form other than iron sulfate (such as glycinate, fumarate, and gluconate) may be better tolerated (Liberman & Bruning, 2003). It has been shown that intermittent (weekly) iron supplementation may be just as effective as daily supplementation (Mukhopadhyay et al., 2004); this may be an acceptable compromise for women who need the extra iron but experience adverse side effects. Another option might be a lower iron dose in a daily multivitamin-mineral supplement (Ahn, Nava-Ocampo, & Koren, 2004).

Seniors

Seniors often develop iron deficiency, a condition usually secondary to illness, chronic blood loss, and poor nutrient intakes. Seniors should be screened for iron deficiency and prescribed supplements as needed.

Iron Toxicity

Because of the effect of mixed foods on absorption, as well as the precise regulation of absorption at the gut level, iron toxicity from foods (in healthy people) is typically not a concern. (However, iron overload from foods—especially heme iron—may increase the risk of some chronic diseases; see the following section on "Iron and Its Relationship to Disease.") Iron toxicity most often results from overconsumption of iron-containing supplements, and is quite serious. In fact, accidental iron overdose is the most common cause of poisoning deaths in children under six years of age in the United States (FNB, 2001). For this reason, supplements containing more than 250 mg per package must have a child safety cap. Symptoms

of an acute iron overdose include vomiting and diarrhea, and advanced intoxication will lead to compromised function of the cardiovascular and central nervous systems, as well as the kidneys and liver (FNB, 2001).

Iron in the Vegetarian Diet

Because liver and other organ meats, beef, and other meats are the richest sources of heme iron, it is widely believed that those following a meatless eating pattern are automatically at risk for iron deficiency. The scientific literature suggests otherwise; well-nourished vegetarians and vegans can get plenty of absorbable iron as long as they consume a well-balanced, varied diet based on healthful plant foods. In fact, many plant foods contain more iron per calorie than red meat. For example, 96 calories of spinach provide 15 milligrams of iron. To get that much iron from steak, one would have to consume 850 calories worth (Meerschaert, Sullivan, & Aronson, 2002). Indeed, many studies have shown that vegetarians consume more iron than nonvegetarians (with vegans consuming even more than ovo-lacto vegetarians) (Messina, Mangels, & Messina, 2004; Mangels, Messina, & Melina, 2003). The EPIC-Oxford study, one of the largest studies on vegetarians in the world (Davey et al., 2003), reported that vegans have the highest iron intake of the four groups studied (vegans, ovo-lacto vegetarians, fish eaters, and meat eaters). However, the concern for vegetarians is not so much the amount of iron in the diet as the absorption of iron from the diet. Though it is true that more iron will be absorbed from beef, this comparison ignores the important contribution of plant foods as good iron sources.

Well-planned vegetarian diets are perfectly adequate to provide enough bioavailable iron. A diet high in vitamin C-rich fruits and vegetables, combined with adequate amounts of iron derived from a variety of grains, legumes, nuts, and seeds, can meet all the nutritional requirements. The richest plant sources of iron are tofu, dried beans, vegetables (especially leafy greens), dried fruits, nuts, and whole grains. Fortification of cereals, flours, and processed foods such as energy bars has contributed significantly to iron consumption across the board. Bran flakes, cream of wheat, oatmeal, tofu, soybeans, and lentils are the richest sources of iron among grains and legumes. Vegetables such as green beans, peas, mushrooms, and broccoli are good sources of iron; large amounts of iron are found especially in sea vegetables such as kelp. Prunes, apricots, dates, and raisins rank high among iron-containing fruits, and pine nuts, sunflower seeds, and pumpkin seeds among nuts and seeds.

It is important to maximize the absorption of iron in the diets of children; fortified cereals and enriched bread, rice, or pasta are good choices, especially when combined with vitamin C-rich food. Good meal combinations include pasta with tomato sauce, cereal with orange juice, or soy milk and strawberry shakes/smoothies. See Table 5.3 for iron content of selected foods.

Iron Status among Vegetarians

Vegetarians have no more incidence of iron-deficiency anemia than nonvegetarians (Messina, Mangels, & Messina, 2004; Mangels, Messina, & Melina, 2003; Hunt & Roughead, 1999; Hunt, 2003; Ball & Bartlett, 1999). Studies have shown that although vegetarians have lower iron stores than nonvegetarians, these stores are still in the normal range (Messina, Mangels, & Messina, 2004; Mangels, Messina, & Melina, 2003; Hunt & Roughead, 1999). Although iron levels of vegetarians are typically low-normal, several studies do indicate that more vegetarians are likely to have iron stores considered to be deficient or very low in comparison to nonvegetarians (Messina, Mangels, & Messina, 2004). The most recent study on iron intake and iron status is the German Vegan Study, which looked at the iron intake and status of 75 vegan women. This study showed that the average iron intake was actually above the recommended 18 mg/day, but that several of the study participants were iron deficient at a rate of twice the general population (Waldmann et al., 2004). (It is important to note that this study did not have a non-vegan control group.) In spite of the lower iron stores seen in this and other studies, adverse health effects from lower iron absorption have not been demonstrated in persons following varied vegetarian diets; indeed, such moderately lower iron stores have even been hypothesized to reduce the risk of some chronic diseases (Hunt, 2003). Because dairy products are not good sources of iron (and tend to inhibit iron absorption), and the bioavailability of iron from eggs is poor, a lacto-ovo vegetarian would have no advantage (perhaps even a disadvantage) over a vegan as far as iron intake or status is concerned (Sabaté, 2001).

A study on female athletes showed that antioxidant supplementation (vitamins E and C, and beta-carotene) prevented the drop in serum iron and iron saturation index that was seen in the placebo group after both groups were subjected to the same exercise routine over three months (Aguilo et al., 2004). In another study, vegetarians given vitamin C supplements showed significant improvement in all measurements of iron status (Sharma & Mathur, 1995). These and other research studies show a possible protective effect of high antioxidant intake regarding iron status. Vegetarians consume significantly more antioxidants than nonvegetarians; perhaps this is one reason vegetarians tend to have normal iron status, despite the bioavailability challenges inherent in a plant-based diet.

Table 5.3 Food Sources of Iron

Food	Serving Size	Iron content (mg)
Vegetables		
Spinach	½ cup cooked	3.2
Carrots	½ cup cooked	0.5
Green beans	½ cup cooked	0.8
Potato with skin, baked	1 medium	2.3
Bok choy	½ cup cooked	0.9
Mushrooms	½ cup cooked	1.4
Tomato	1 medium	0.8
Fruits		
Watermelon	1 slice	1.5
Strawberries	10 large	1.0
Prune juice	½ cup	1.5
Dried apricots	1/4 cup	1.5
Raisins	1/4 cup	0.9
Avocado	½ each	1.0
Legumes		
Navy (white) beans	½ cup	2.3
Peas	½ cup	1.5
Firm tofu	3 ounces	8.8
Soy milk	8 fluid ounces	1.0–1.8 (depends on brand)
Tahini (sesame butter)	2 tablespoons	2.7
Chick peas	½ cup	2.4
Kidney beans	½ cup	1.8
Pumpkin seeds	2 tablespoons	2.5
Soybeans	½ cup	2.7
Cashew nuts	1 ounce	1.7
Lentils	½ cup	1.6
Grains		
Pasta, enriched	½ cup	1.0
Cream of Wheat	½ cup	6.0
Fortified breakfast cereal	1 serving according to package	up to 18 (check label)
Instant oatmeal	1 packet	4.0
Whole-wheat bread	1 slice	0.8
Brown rice	½ cup	0.4
Quinoa	½ cup	3.1
Other		
Blackstrap molasses	1 tablespoon	3.5
Animal foods (as comparison)		
Beef sirloin	3 ounces	2.3
Chicken breast	3 ounces	0.9
Tuna fish	3 ounces	1.3
Whole milk	8 fluid ounces	0.1
Egg	1 large	0.6

Source: USDA National Nutrient Database for Standard Reference, Release 20. Accessed May 12, 2005 at http://www.ars.usda.gov/nutrientdata.

Hemochromatosis

Hemochromatosis is characterized by excessive absorption of food iron, associated with failure to store the additional iron properly. Even though iron intake is normal, people with this disease accumulate iron at a rate of about 2 mg/day, resulting in eventual organ damage between the fourth and sixth decade of life. Untreated, this condition can lead to skin hyperpigmentation, cirrhosis of the liver, liver cancer, heart failure, and damage to the pancreas (typically leading to diabetes) and pituitary gland. Between 1 in 200 and 1 in 400 individuals of northern European descent are affected by hereditary hemochromatosis, which is an autosomal, recessive disorder (Bacon et al., 1999). Treatment for this condition is phlebotomy, to remove the excess iron (Meerschaert, Sullivan, & Aronson, 2002). Those diagnosed early and treated properly can live normal, healthy lives. The mechanism for increased iron absorption in hemochromatosis is not understood; however, it appears that there is some normal regulation of absorption of non-heme (plant-based) iron, but little or no regulation of heme (meat-based) iron (Fairbanks, 1999). It is important to note that the determination of the upper limit values as part of the Dietary Reference Intakes (DRIs) was not influenced by this disorder; only people without hemochromatosis were considered when these levels were being established (FNB, 2001).

Iron and Its Relationship to Disease

Abnormally high or low levels of iron may contribute to disease states by affecting the immune system, damaging cells, or compromising oxygen transport (Meerschaert, Sullivan, & Aronson, 2002). The exact mechanisms by which iron contributes to disease or disease risk are not clear and are still being studied. Low iron status may result in anemia, which can be treated by diet therapy and/or supplementation. However, iron overload is more controversial and has been studied quite extensively. Excess iron intake, usually in the form of supplements but possibly from diet alone (particularly meat-centered), can lead to diarrhea, constipation, abdominal pain, and other gastrointestinal problems. Its relationship to some chronic diseases is hypothesized to be due to iron's role as an oxidative agent, leading to free radical formation (Sabaté, 2001; Meerschaert, Sullivan, & Aronson, 2002).

Heart Disease

Several studies have looked at the relationship between iron intake/status and heart disease risk. The studies focused on different measures of iron status (such as serum ferritin concentration and total iron-binding capacity), as well as different disease outcomes (coronary artery disease, myocardial infarction, ischemic heart disease, or mortality from coronary heart disease). A review of the scientific literature suggests that iron levels (over and above a certain level) may be positively correlated with heart disease risk, but the body of evidence is not conclusive (FNB, 2001). One proposed mechanism for this relationship is the pro-oxidant effect of iron (Meerschaert, Sullivan, & Aronson, 2002).

Cancer

The increased risk of liver cancer among people with hemochromatosis is well established (FNB, 2001), but studies on the relationship between iron status and cancer among the general population are not as clear. Studies that have shown correlations have looked at colon cancer, but not all studies showed a positive relationship between iron intake and colon cancer risk. Those that have show a correlation with heme iron specifically (Sesink et al., 1999). Other cancers that may be related to iron overload include liver, stomach, lung, esophagus, and bladder. There is currently not enough evidence to pinpoint iron status as a risk factor for cancer except among people with hemochromatosis (FNB, 2001). The mechanisms by which iron overload may increase cancer risk is still unclear, but, as with heart disease, the pro-oxidant effect of iron may play a role, as may iron's role in cellular proliferation and differentiation (Meerschaert, Sullivan, & Aronson, 2002).

Insulin Resistance and Diabetes

Studies of serum ferritin levels and insulin resistance have shown that those with low-normal ferritin levels (commonly seen in vegetarians) have significantly improved insulin sensitivity over those with higher ferritin levels. This suggests an advantage for vegetarians with regard to insulin sensitivity (Messina, Mangels, & Messina, 2004).

Because most patients with hemochromatosis develop type 2 diabetes, researchers in one study tested the hypothesis that accumulation of iron predicts the development of type 2 diabetes. The researchers followed 1,038 men for 4 years and found that men with high iron stores were 2.4 times more likely to develop diabetes than those with lower stores (Salonen et al., 1998). More research is needed to describe a definitive relationship, however.

Bone Health

A 2003 study demonstrated a positive relationship between dietary iron intake and bone mineral density among postmenopausal women (Harris et al., 2003). However, relationships between iron status and bone mineral density have not been studied as of the writing of this chapter. Such a comparison could provide valuable understanding of the relationship between iron intake, iron status, and bone health.

Parkinson's Disease

People with Parkinson's disease have more iron in their brains (observed postmortem) than people without the disease (Gotz et al., 2004). Some studies have found a high iron intake to be a risk factor for Parkinson's disease (Powers et al., 2003), but these findings are not conclusive.

Practical Aspects

Measurements of Iron Status

Hemoglobin and hematocrit (measures of the red blood cells in the body) are nonspecific and crude tests of iron status. They are lower in more advanced stages of iron deficiency and in many conditions other than iron deficiency. Alone, they are not sufficient for a determination of iron status, particularly among those who are borderline iron deficient. For a full workup, other values should be measured, such as serum iron, plasma ferritin (iron stores), total iron-binding capacity, and cell morphology (to help determine type of anemia).

Iron Supplementation

Iron supplements sometimes lead to gastrointestinal effects, notably constipation, but sometimes also nausea, vomiting, and diarrhea (FNB, 2001). Iron is available as an individual supplement or as part of a multiformula. The most common form is iron sulfate, but some manufacturers sell iron glycinate, iron fumarate, and iron gluconate, which are reportedly less irritating to the digestive tract than iron sulfate (Liberman & Bruning, 2003).

Iron supplements have proven beneficial when used as a therapeutic aid among persons with compromised iron status. The decision to supplement should be based not on iron intake but on iron status as measured by blood tests. Those with compromised iron status—either iron deficiency or iron-deficiency anemia—may benefit from supplements, despite what the diet currently supplies. Of course, more is not better; when iron stores return to normal, supplementation should be lowered or discontinued, and iron status closely monitored before, during, and after supplementation. Among persons with normal iron status, iron intake over and above the RDA (via supplements and/or food) has not been shown to be beneficial.

There seems to be controversy about whether to recommend iron supplements to all vegans and vegetarians (more specifically, to all female vegans/vegetarians or all pregnant vegans/vegetarians). Clearly, there is a risk-benefit issue with regard to optimal iron status versus health risks resulting from overintake of iron. For this reason, there is no generalized recommendation for iron supplementation in the absence of a blood test for iron status. Experts agree, however, that when iron supplements are used, iron status should be monitored before, during, and after supplementation.

For those taking iron supplements, it is recommended to:

- Take the supplement between meals for better absorption (Waldman et al., 2004), but with meals if there are gastrointestinal side effects.
- Take the supplement with water or juice rather than with tea, coffee, or milk (Waldman et al., 2004).

- Get regular blood tests to monitor iron status.
- Eat plenty of antioxidant-rich foods (fruits, vegetables, and legumes), as iron is a pro-oxidant and should be balanced with an antioxidant-rich diet.

Maximizing Iron Status in Vegetarians

Maximizing iron absorption from plant foods is the number-one strategy to optimize iron status among vegetarians. Indeed, enhancers and inhibitors can vary iron absorption up to 20-fold (Messina, Mangels, & Messina, 2004), so choosing foods wisely makes a tremendous difference. Basing the diet on an abundance of fruits and vegetables (both of which are rich sources of organic acids that enhance iron absorption), whole grains, and legumes; selecting a wide variety of foods at each meal; and avoiding the overconsumption of iron absorption inhibitors (e.g., several cups of tea at every meal or adding wheat bran to everything) should work together to maximize iron absorption. In addition, using cast-iron cookware, consuming iron-fortified foods (grain products such as cereals and pasta, meat substitutes, energy bars), and choosing foods that have undergone processes that increase the bioavailability of iron (leavened whole grain breads, fermented soy products, sprouted grains, seeds, and legumes) are all good strategies. In addition, it is important to get regular blood tests to check iron status.

Conclusion—Vegetarians: At Risk, or Having an Edge?

Despite the unquestionable health benefits of vegetarian diets, health experts still question the adequacy of a vegetarian or vegan diet when it comes to iron. However, there is absolutely no requirement to eat animal foods to have optimal iron intake and iron status. The fact that iron from plant foods is more influenced by absorption inhibitors and enhancers may actually be advantageous. As discussed in this chapter, high body stores of iron are not healthy, and may even be harmful due to the pro-oxidant quality of iron and its relationship to heart disease and cancer. The human body protects itself from excess iron by controlling absorption, and vegetarian diets are far more likely to protect against excess iron than are meat-containing diets. In addition, the very factors that inhibit iron absorption—phytates and polyphenols (which are antioxidants) and vegetable protein—are those that also contribute to reduced chronic disease risk ("The Iron Balancing Act," 2001). Iron-rich plant foods are also rich in components that protect against chronic disease. The bottom line is that no human needs red meat to provide adequate iron. Plant foods provide plenty of iron; it is our job to consume a balanced diet with plenty of iron-rich foods and plenty of fruits and vegetables to help that iron get absorbed.

References

Aguilo A, Tauler P, Fuentespina E, et al. Antioxidant diet supplementation influences blood iron status in endurance athletes. *Intl J Sport Nutr Exer Metab.* Apr 2004;14(2):147–160.

Ahn E, Nava-Ocampo AA, Koren G. Multivitamin supplements for pregnant women: New insights. *Can Fam Physician.* May 2004;50:705–706.

Bacon BR, Olynyk JK, Brunt EM, Britton RS, Wollf RK. HFE genotype in patients with hemochromatosis and other liver diseases. *Ann Intern Med.* 1999;130(12):953–962.

Ball MJ, Bartlett MA. Dietary intake and iron status of Australian vegetarian women. *Am J Clin Nutr.* 1999;70:353–358.

Bothwell TH. Overview and mechanisms of iron regulation. *Nutr Rev.* Sept 1995;53(9):237–245.

Cogswell ME, Kettel-Khan L, Ramakrishnan U. Iron supplement use among women in the United States: Science, policy, and practice. *J Nutr.* 2003; 133:1974S–1977S.

Davey GK, Spencer EA, Appleby PN, Allen NE, Knox KH, Key TJ. EPIC-Oxford: Lifestyle characteristics and nutrient intakes in a cohort of 33,883 meat-eaters and 31,546 non meat-eaters in the UK. *Public Health Nutr.* 2003;6(3):259–268.

Fairbanks VF. Iron in medicine and nutrition. In: Shils ME, Olson JA, Shike, M, Ross, AC, eds. *Modern Nutrition in Health and Disease.* 9th ed. Baltimore, MD: Williams & Wilkins; 1999:193–221.

Food and Nutrition Board, Institute of Medicine. *Dietary Reference Intakes for Vitamin A, Vitamin K, Arsenic, Boron, Chromium, Copper, Iodine, Iron, Manganese, Molybdenum, Nickel, Silicon, Vanadium, and Zinc.* Washington, DC: National Academy of Sciences; 2001.

Gotz ME, Double K, Gerlach M, Youdim MB, Riederer P. The relevance of iron in the pathogenesis of Parkinson's disease. *Ann NY Acad Sci.* Mar 2004;1012:193–208.

Harris MM, Houtkooper LB, Stanford VA, et al. Dietary iron is associated with bone mineral density in healthy postmenopausal women. *J Nutr.* 2003;133:3598–3602.

Hunt JR. Bioavailability of iron, zinc, and other trace minerals from vegetarian diets. *Am J Clin Nutr.* 2003;78(3, Suppl):633S–639S.

Hunt JR, Roughead ZK. Adaptation of iron absorption in men consuming diets with high or low iron bioavailability. *Am J Clin Nutr.* 2000;71: 94–102.

Hunt JR, Roughead ZK. Nonheme-iron absorption, fecal ferritin excretion, and blood indexes of iron status in women consuming controlled lacto-ovovegetarian diets for 8 wks. *Am J Clin Nutr.* 1999;69:944–952.

Institute of Medicine. *Nutrition during Pregnancy.* Washington, DC: National Academy Press; 1990.

The iron balancing act: Vegetarians may have the edge. *Loma Linda University Nutrition & Health Letter.* Aug 2001.

Liberman S, Bruning N. *The Real Vitamin and Mineral Book.* 2d ed. New York: Avery; 2003.

Mangels AR, Messina V, Melina V. Position of the American Dietetic Association and Dietitians of Canada: Vegetarian Diets. *J Am Diet Assoc.* 2003; 103(6):748-765.

Meerschaert C, Sullivan CL, Aronson DL. *Minerals from Plant Foods: Strategies for Maximizing Nutrition.* Chicago: American Dietetic Association; 2002.

Messina V, Mangels R, Messina M. *The Dietitian's Guide to Vegetarian Diets: Issues and Applications.* 2d ed. Sudbury, MA: Jones and Bartlett Publishers; 2004.

Monsen ER. The ironies of iron. *Am J Clin Nutr.* 1999;69:831-832.

Mukhopadhyay A, Bhatla N, Kriplani A, Agarwal N, Saxena R. Erythrocyte indices in pregnancy: Effect of intermittent iron supplementation. *Natl Med J India.* 2004;17(3):135-137.

Murray-Kolb LE, Welch R, Theil EC, Beard JL. Women with low iron stores absorb iron from soybeans. *Am J Clin Nutr.* 2003;77:180-184.

Powers KM, Smith-Weller T, Franklin GM, Longstreth WT Jr, Swanson PD, Checkoway H. Parkinson's disease risks associated with dietary iron, manganese, and other nutrient intakes. *Neurology.* Jun 10, 2003;60(11):1761-1766.

Sabaté J, ed. *Vegetarian Nutrition.* CRC Series in Modern Nutrition. Boca Raton, FL: CRC Press; 2001.

Salonen JT, Tuomainen TP, Nyyssonen K, Lakka HM, Punnonen K. Relation between iron stores and non-insulin dependent diabetes in men: Case-control study. *BMJ.* 1998;317:727-728.

Sesink AL, Termont DS, Kleibeuker JH, Van der Meer R. Red meat and colon cancer: The cytotoxic and hyperproliferative effects of dietary heme. *Cancer Res.* 1999;59:5704-5709.

Sharma DC, Mathur R. Correction of anemia and iron deficiency in vegetarians by administration of ascorbic acid. *Indian J Physiol Pharmacol.* Oct 1995;39(4):403-406.

Thane CW, Bates CJ, Prentice A. Risk factors for low iron intake and poor iron status in a national sample of British young people aged 4-18 years. *Public Health Nutr.* 2003;6(5):485-496.

Tver DF, Russel P. *The Nutrition and Health Encyclopedia.* 2d ed. New York: Van Nostrand Reinhold; 1989.

Udall JN Jr, Suskind RM. Cow's milk versus formula in older infants: Consequences for human nutrition. *Acta Paediatrica Suppl.* 1999;88(430): 61-67.

Waldmann A, Koschizke JW, Leitzmann C, Hahn A. Dietary iron intake and iron status of German female vegans: Results of the German Vegan Study. *Ann Nutr Metab.* 2004;48(2):103-108.

6

Calcium and Vitamin D

Suzanne Havala Hobbs, DrPH, MS, RD
John J. B. Anderson, PhD

Introduction

Calcium and vitamin D are of keen interest in discussions about vegetarian diets because of their roles in bone health and concerns that arise when vegetarians limit or exclude from the diet animal products that are rich sources of these nutrients. Dairy products such as milk, cheese, and yogurt are the foods most commonly associated with dietary calcium by North Americans. The use of dairy products as an integral part of the diet has been reinforced for more than 50 years by food guides such as the Basic Four Food Groups and, more recently, the Food Guide Pyramid, which graphically and narratively depict dairy products as being important—or even essential—components of a balanced diet. In comparison, plant sources of calcium, though often superior in terms of absorbability, are seldom viewed by consumers as being as desirable or realistic a source of dietary calcium.

Inclusion of dairy products in the diet is an ethnocentricity not shared by most people in the world. The majority of Asians, for instance, have no tradition of including dairy products in the diet. This topic is likely to receive increased attention in coming years, as anticipated changes in American demographics due to immigration, as documented by Census 2000, lead to a greater number of individuals living in the United States who are lactose intolerant or for whom no tradition exists for consumption of dairy products (Office of Minority Health, 2001; Institute for the Future, 2000). Health professionals need to adapt national dietary recommendations to accommodate cultural food preferences that differ from traditional North American eating patterns.

Lacto-ovo and lacto vegetarians—all of whom to some extent include dairy products in the diet—have calcium intakes equal to or greater than those of nonvegetarians (Slattery et al., 1991; Tesar et al., 1992) but vegan diets typically contain less calcium than any of these other groups and may fall below current recommended intakes (Tesar et al., 1992; Janelle & Barr, 1995; Larsson & Johansson, 2002; Weaver, Proulx, & Heaney, 1999). Calcium is widely available in plant foods and some fortified foods (American Dietetic Association, 2003), and the bioavailability of calcium varies depending on the source and the presence of factors that may inhibit or enhance intestinal absorption.

Questions about the vitamin D status of vegetarians are equally important. Among its functions, vitamin D is largely responsible for regulating intestinal absorption of calcium. Few foods are natural sources of vitamin D. Instead, vitamin D is primarily produced by the skin in response to exposure to ultraviolet (UV) radiation in sunlight. Vitamin D production is generally high in the summer months and low in late fall and winter. Insufficient vitamin D and calcium may result in rickets, a disease in children characterized by bow legs, swollen joints, pigeon breast, and other deformities of the bones. In adults, vitamin D deficiency results in osteomalacia (softening of the bones) or widened osteoid seams (areas of unmineralized young bone) that do not mineralize because of insufficient calcium availability.

When exposure to sunlight is inadequate, supplemental vitamin D is needed to prevent deficiency. In the United States, dairy products have been fortified with vitamin D since the 1930s, serving as an alternate source for those who might otherwise be deficient. The primary dietary source of vitamin D in the United States is fortified cow's milk. However, the labeling of vitamin D-fortified dairy products throughout this country may be highly inaccurate: some milk samples contain greatly more or less vitamin D than stated on the label (Anderson & Toverud, 1993). Because vegans do not use dairy products, they need supplemental vitamin D to meet requirements if they do not have sufficient exposure to sunlight.

Summary of the Scientific Literature

Calcium status is determined as much by factors that affect calcium absorption and retention as by calcium intake. Diets with a high ratio of sulfur-containing amino acids to calcium result in increased losses of calcium from bone, due to production of sulfuric acid, which requires buffering with calcium from the skeleton (American Dietetic Association, 2003). Foods high in sulfur-containing amino acids include meat, fish, eggs, dairy products, nuts, and grains. In a typical North American diet, which is high in sulfur-containing amino acids, total protein intakes above 75 grams per day produce substantial calcium losses (Heaney, 1994). Vegetarian diets that exclude or limit animal sources of protein may favor bone health (Anderson, 1991).

Other studies indicate that a high ratio of calcium to protein in the diet is predictive of bone health. The relevance of this balance, however, is greatest when calcium intakes are low and the body is already maximizing its absorption. At that point, a low intake of calcium relative to protein intake is likely to result in the greatest net loss of calcium. Messina, Mangels, & Messina (2004, pp. 104-105) have written a comprehensive review of the clinical data supporting the relationship between protein intake and calcium balance. Lacto-ovo vegetarian diets generally have favorable calcium-to-protein ratios, whereas vegan and nonvegetarian diets have less favorable profiles (Weaver, Proulx, & Heaney, 1999; Remer, 2000).

High levels of dietary sodium can also increase urinary loss of calcium (Nordin et al., 1993). Foods high in sodium in both vegetarian and nonvegetarian diets include numerous processed foods, such as pizza, frozen entrees, processed cheese, instant pudding and cake mixes, condiments, fast food, and soups.

Dietary calcium is provided by a wide range of foods from a variety of food groups, though bioavailability varies (Remer, 2000; American Dietetic Association, 2003). Low-oxalate greens—which exclude spinach, beet greens, Swiss chard, and rhubarb—provide calcium with the highest bioavailability. (The oxalic acid in spinach, beet greens, Swiss chard, and rhubarb binds with calcium and prevents absorption.) Examples include kale, collards, broccoli, bok choy, Chinese or Napa cabbage, and turnip and mustard greens. Other foods with relatively high calcium bioavailability include tofu processed with calcium, fortified fruit juices and cow's milk, fortified soy milk, sesame seeds, almonds, and red and white beans (Weaver, Proulx, & Heaney, 1999; American Dietetic Association, 2003; Heaney et al., 2000; Weaver & Plawecki, 1994). Negative effects of such food constituents as phytates, dietary fiber, and phosphorus on calcium bioavailability are negligible in healthy individuals, and thus are not considered a significant issue for individuals consuming vegetarian diets (Anderson, 1991).

In contrast to calcium, for which there are food sources, the primary natural source of vitamin D is the body's own production. Biosynthesis of vitamin D is affected by several factors, including location (latitude), exposure to UV rays, clothing (the amount of the body covered), color of the skin, environmental conditions such as smog, and the time of year (Anderson & Toverud, 1993). Light-skinned individuals are likely to have adequate vitamin D production if hands, arms, and face are exposed to sunlight for about 15 minutes per day during the summer, assuming a latitude equivalent to that of Boston, Massachusetts (Anderson & Toverud, 1993; Holick, 1996). The body's capacity to produce vitamin D varies with age; infants, children, and older adults produce vitamin D less efficiently than do middle-aged individuals (Holick, 1996; Food and Nutrition Board [FNB], 1997; Lee, Drake, & Kendler, 2002). Limited data document vitamin D deficiencies in unsupplemented individuals consuming vegan diets and living in northern latitudes (Parsons et al., 1997; Dagnelie et al., 1990).

Practical Aspects

Dietary calcium needs of vegetarians likely differ from those of nonvegetarians. Vegetarians and nonvegetarians differ from one another in diet and, likely, lifestyle (exercise and use of tobacco, caffeine, and alcohol), both of which may have implications for calcium absorption and retention. Defining precise recommendations for vegetarian groups is also difficult because of a lack of sufficient data, particularly for vegans living in the United States. For that reason, vegetarians should err on the side of caution and strive to meet recommendations set by the Institute of Medicine for the nonvegetarian general public (FNB, 1997). The amounts of calcium and vitamin D recommended per day are listed in Table 6.1. Although these levels are relatively high, they can be met by choosing plenty of calcium-rich plant foods and limiting foods with low nutritional value, such as cakes, cookies, candy, soft drinks, snack chips, and other junk foods. A vegetarian food guide developed by Messina, Melina, and Mangels (2003) lists food sources of calcium appropriate for all types of vegetarians, including vegans, with recommended numbers of servings and portion sizes. (See Chapter 22.)

Most adult vegetarians can meet recommended intakes of calcium by including at least eight servings of calcium-rich foods in the diet daily. Calcium supplements or fortified foods are an option if recommendations cannot be met through diet. However, it is preferable to meet calcium needs via whole foods rather than supplements, because whole foods contribute other essential nutrients as well. In addition to calcium, plant sources of calcium often contain substantial amounts of other nutrients that support health, including vitamins A, C, and E, folacin and B vitamins, iron, and dietary fiber. They are also low in saturated fat,

Table 6.1 Amounts of Vitamin D and Calcium Recommended per Day

Age Group	Calcium (mg)	Vitamin D (μg)[a,b]
Infants		
0–6 months	210	5
7–12 months	270	5
Children		
1–3 years	500	5
4–8 years	800	5
Males		
9–13 years	1,300	5
14–18 years	1,300	5
19–30 years	1,000	5
31–50 years	1,000	5
51–70 years	1,200	10
>70 years	1,200	15
Females		
9–13 years	1,300	5
14–18 years	1,300	5
19–30 years	1,000	5
31–50 years	1,000	—
51–70 years	1,200	10
>70 years	1,200	15
Pregnancy		
14–18 years	1,300	5
19–30 years	1,000	5
31–50 years	1,000	5
Lactation		
14–18 years	1,300	5
19–30 years	1,000	5
31–50 years	1,000	5

[a]Listed as cholecalciferol. One microgram (μg) cholecalciferol = 40 International Units (IU) vitamin D
[b]Recommended only in the absence of adequate exposure to sunlight
Source: Food and Nutrition Board, Institute of Medicine. *Dietary Reference Intakes for Calcium, Phosphorus, Magnesium, Vitamin D and Fluoride.* Washington, DC: National Academy Press; 1997.

which is present in excess in the traditional U.S. diet and to which dairy products are a major contributor.

Vegetarians who suspect that they may be at risk for vitamin D deficiency should seek an assessment from a qualified health professional. Blood vitamin D levels can be measured. Individuals who are housebound, live in smog-filled cities, use sunblock regularly, or have dark skin and live in northern latitudes are among those most likely to be at risk. If exposure to sunlight is inadequate and dairy products are not consumed, other vitamin D-fortified foods or a daily supplement are indicated. In addition to dairy products, many commercial breakfast cereals, orange juice, and some brands of soy milk and other nondairy milks are fortified with vitamin D. These products are now widely available in mainstream supermarkets.

Conclusion

Vegans and other vegetarians who consume adequate but moderate amounts of protein and limit their intakes of sodium and junk foods may have calcium needs lower than those of the general, nonvegetarian population. Because of the complexity of estimating needs for disparate groups, and until more data are available for American vegetarians and vegans, it is suggested that all vegetarians strive to meet age-specific recommendations for calcium and vitamin D intakes set forth by the Institute of Medicine report (FNB, 1997).

The recommended amount of calcium can be consumed if vegetarians include several servings of calcium-rich plant foods or nonfat or low-fat dairy products in the diet daily, and limit junk foods that may otherwise displace calcium. Consuming calcium-rich foods not only assists in meeting calcium needs, but also helps to ensure adequate intakes of other essential nutrients commonly found in the same foods. Vegetarians who include dairy products in the diet should choose nonfat or low-fat varieties to minimize intake of saturated fat.

Vegans who have inadequate exposure to sunlight should take a vitamin D supplement or add vitamin D-fortified foods to their diets. Those who suspect they may be deficient in vitamin D should consult a qualified health care professional for an assessment.

References

American Dietetic Association. Position of the American Dietetic Association: Vegetarian diets. *J Am Diet Assoc.* 2003;103(6):748-765.

Anderson JJB. Nutritional biochemistry of calcium and phosphorus. *J Nutr Biochem.* 1991;2:300-307.

Anderson JJB, Toverud SU. Diet and vitamin D: A review with an emphasis on human function. *J Nutr Biochem.* 1993;5:58-65.

Dagnelie PC, Vergote FJ, van Staveren WA, van den Berg H, Dingjan PG, Hautvast JG. High prevalence of rickets in infants on macrobiotic diets. *Am J Clin Nutr.* 1990;51:202-208.

Food and Nutrition Board (FNB), Institute of Medicine. *Dietary Reference Intakes for Calcium, Phosphorus, Magnesium, Vitamin D, and Fluoride.* Washington, DC: National Academy Press; 1997.

Heaney RP. Nutrient interactions and the calcium economy. *J Lab Clin Med.* 1994;124:15-16.

Heaney RP, Dowell MS, Rafferty K, Bierman J. Bioavailability of the calcium in fortified soy imitation milk, with some observations on method. *Am J Clin Nutr.* 2000;71(5):1166-1169.

Holick, MF. Vitamin D and bone health. *J Nutr.* 1996; 126(Suppl):1159S-1164S.

Institute for the Future. *Health & Health Care 2010: The Forecast, The Challenge.* San Francisco: Jossey-Bass; 2000:3.

Janelle KC, Barr, SI. Nutrient intakes and eating behavior scores of vegetarian and nonvegetarian women. *J Am Diet Assoc.* 1995;95:180-189.

Larsson CL, Johansson GK. Dietary intake and nutritional status of young vegans and omnivores in Sweden. *Am J Clin Nutr.* 2002;76:100-106.

Lee LT, Drake WM, Kendler DL. Intake of calcium and vitamin D in 3 Canadian long term care facilities. *J Am Diet Assoc.* 2002;102:244-247.

Messina V, Mangels R, Messina M. *The Dietitian's Guide to Vegetarian Diets: Issues and Applications.* 2d ed. Sudbury, MA: Jones and Bartlett Publishers; 2004.

Messina V, Melina V, Mangels AR. A new food guide for North American vegetarians. *J Am Diet Assoc.* 2003;103(6):771-775.

Nordin BEC, Need AG, Morris HA, Horowitz M. The nature and significance of the relationship between urinary sodium and urinary calcium in women. *J Nutr.* 1993;123:1615-1623.

Office of Minority Health, U.S. Department of Health and Human Services. *National Standards for Culturally and Linguistically Appropriate Services: Final Report.* March 2001;25.

Parsons TJ, van Dusseldorp MV, van der Vliet M., et al. Reduced bone mass in Dutch adolescents fed a macrobiotic diet in early life. *J Bone Miner Res.* 1997;12:1486-1494.

Remer T. Influence of diet on acid-base balance. *Semin Dial.* 2000;13:221-226.

Slattery ML, Jacobs DR, Hilner JE Jr, et al. Meat consumption and its association with other diet and health factors in young adults: The CARDIA study. *Am J Clin Nutr.* 1991;54:930-935.

Tesar R, Notelovitz M, Shim E, Dauwell G, Brown J. Axial and peripheral bone density and nutrient intakes of postmenopausal vegetarian and omnivorous women. *Am J Clin Nutr.* 1992;56:699-704.

Weaver C, Plawecki K. Dietary calcium: Adequacy of a vegetarian diet. *Am J Clin Nutr.* 1994;59(Suppl): 1238S-1241S.

Weaver CM, Proulx WR, Heaney R. Choices for achieving adequate dietary calcium with a vegetarian diet. *Am J Clin Nutr.* 1999;70(3, Suppl): 543S-548S.

7

Vitamin B12

Michael A. Klaper, MD

Introduction

Vitamin B12 is needed by the body in only very small amounts—but needed it is. A deficiency of B12 can cause serious health problems. Fortunately, it is easy to ensure that one is getting enough.

This chapter first looks at the many roles B12 plays in the human body, where the vitamin occurs naturally, who is at risk for developing B12 deficiency, and what tests can be done to determine if one is getting enough B12. Lastly, the chapter provides a number of ways to ensure that B12 intake is adequate. Once you know where it is found, it is easy to make sure that you are getting enough vitamin B12.

Summary of the Scientific Literature

Why the Body Needs Vitamin B12

Vitamin B12 is a large and beautifully complex molecule with a structure similar to the hemoglobin molecules in our red blood cells. In contrast to hemoglobin, which contains an atom of iron in its center, the vitamin B12 molecule is constructed around an atom of cobalt, making the vitamin a "cobalt-amine"—from which comes its common name, *cobalamin*. Crystalline cobalamin, which is red, also contains the elements carbon, oxygen, phosphorus, and nitrogen.

Needed for utilization of proteins, fats, and carbohydrates, cobalamin is also essential for synthesis of the double helix of DNA. Thus, it plays an especially key role in fast-growing cells that synthesize DNA rapidly, such as the cells in bone marrow that produce new blood cells. Chronic insufficiency of vitamin B12 in the diet—or an inability to absorb sufficient cobalamin into the bloodstream from food—can result in anemia as well as abnormally shaped red and white blood cells.

Vitamin B12 is also required for the functioning of the cells of the nervous system, including the brain, spinal cord, and peripheral nerves. If the brain tissue is deprived of adequate vitamin B12, confusion, depression, irritability, and inability to concentrate can result. When the spinal cord and peripheral nerves are injured by B12 deficiency, the person can experience numbness and tingling in the arms and legs. Left untreated, this condition can progress to "subacute combined degeneration" of the spinal cord, eventually leading to paralysis and even death.

Vitamin B12 may help to sustain healthy arteries; cobalamin is required for the degradation and elimination of homocysteine, a sulfur-containing byproduct of protein metabolism. Insufficient vitamin B12 can contribute to elevated homocysteine levels in the blood, which some studies suggest may, in turn, lead to injury of the delicate inner lining of the arteries. The injured blood vessel lining invites deposition of atherosclerotic plaques, which can foster clogging of the arteries, heart attacks, and strokes (Ubbink, 1994; Selhub et al., 1995).

Vitamin B12 deficiency is also suspected to play a causative role in other serious degenerative diseases (especially in the elderly) (Pennypacker et al., 1992; Yao, 1992), and in some of the neurological and psychological disorders seen in AIDS (Herbert, 1988a). Vitamin B12 is also needed for synthesis of the vitamin choline and the amino acid methionine. Fortunately, vitamin B12 deficiency can often be reversed if cobalamin supplementation is provided before severe tissue injury is sustained.

The body is very efficient in recycling and conserving vitamin B12. Consequently, the amount of cobalamin required to meet the body's daily B12 needs is extremely tiny: The current recommended daily allowance for nonpregnant adults—the amount that will exceed all known requirements for dietary cobalamin—is two millionths of a gram (2 micrograms), about the weight of a period on a piece of paper. Pregnant women are advised to consume 2.6 micrograms daily.

Vitamin B12 Sources

Omnivorous humans obtain most of their dietary vitamin B12 from animal-based sources, namely, the muscles and organ meats of various animals and the milk of cows and goats. It is not widely appreciated that vitamin B12 is not produced by the animals themselves. With the possible exception of *Crithidia fasciculata*, a microscopic protozoan that lives in the intestines of mosquitoes (and technically is part of the animal kingdom), the earth's cobalamin is created by nonanimals: common, single-celled bacteria and fungi that populate the planet's healthy soils, fresh water, and ocean environments. Some cobalamin-producing organisms are carried on the winds. These master chemists produce cobalamin—one of the most complex molecules in the universe—as a natural byproduct of their normal metabolism.

Vitamin B12-producing organisms—with musical-sounding names like *Streptomyces aureofaciens*, *Propionibacterium shermanii*, *Pseudomonas denitrificans*, *Clostridium stricklandii*, and *Streptomyces griseus*—also populate the digestive tracts of animals that live in the soils. These include earthworms, beetles, gophers, moles, rabbits, and related creatures—as well as all their predators that ingest the vitamin B12-containing contents of their prey's digestive tracts.

Grazing animals regularly consume particles of soils that cling to the roots of the plants they eat, and to the surfaces of the grains they are fed. As a result, vitamin B12-producing bacteria predictably dwell in the intestines of cattle, chickens, and pigs. Their cobalamin is absorbed into the animal's bloodstream and is deposited in the liver, muscles, and other organs. Thus, the cobalamin that makes flesh and milk products "good sources of vitamin B12" is produced by microbes.

Humans who consume root vegetables freshly pulled from the earth, or apples picked from trees, will also ingest naturally occurring vitamin B12, as well as the organisms that produce it. People living rural existences commonly consume vitamin B12 as they draw their drinking water from dug wells or from rivers or streams running through the forest. The ubiquitous, cobalamin-producing bacteria, and the animals that carry them, assure that vitamin B12 finds its way into these waters. In healthy ecosystems, there is even vitamin B12 in the rainwater (Parker, 1968).

People living traditional, "earth-connected" lifestyles, utilizing the food sources and drinking water supplies just described, will continually have their digestive tracts "seeded" with cobalamin-generating organisms. As a result, it is theoretically possible for a resident population of vitamin B12-producing bacteria to establish themselves in the healthy human mouth and intestines (Albert, 1980). Whether humans can absorb and utilize the vitamin B12 produced in their own intestines is still uncertain.

Cobalamin can enter the human food supply during the traditional preparation of fermented foods, such as sauerkraut. Airborne vitamin B12-producing bacteria naturally alight on the freshly shredded cabbage and generate cobalamin while the vegetables mature in the jar or crock over several days. Foods prepared in traditional manners, like tempeh made from fermented soybeans aged in porcelain crocks, can contain substantial quantities of vitamin B12. (Unfortunately, modern methods of tempeh production—sterilized, stainless-steel vats, shorter maturing times, and so on—reduce the time of production and hence the number of organisms required to create cobalamin. Thus, commercially produced tempeh and similar products should not be relied upon as

a sole source of vitamin B12, unless one receives proof of cobalamin content from the producer.)

There are many bacteria in the human intestine that synthesize vitamins, such as vitamin K and biotin. We know that human fecal material is rich in vitamin B12. However, there is debate as to whether the bacterially produced cobalamin synthesized in the human colon is actually absorbed or is produced too far down in the colon for absorption to occur. Until it is proven that persons with a healthy population of B12-producing organisms in their digestive systems can meet their vitamin B12 requirements entirely through vitamin synthesis within their own bodies, consuming an assured vitamin B12 source in the diet is advised for everyone—especially vegetarians who consume no animal products.

Although the naturally occurring form of vitamin B12 is cobalamin, the most widely available commercial preparation is cyanocobalamin, in which a molecule of cyanide (carbon and nitrogen) is attached to the B12 molecule during production. Additional forms of vitamin B12 are hydroxycobalamin (known technically as vitamin B12a), aquacobalamin (with a molecule of water attached, known as vitamin B12b), and nitrocobalamin (known as vitamin B12c). Vitamin B12 requires hydrochloric acid in the stomach for absorption, as well as adequate levels of thyroid hormone, calcium, and a "helper protein" made in the lining of the stomach known as *intrinsic factor*. This protein allows the vitamin to be absorbed at its main site of uptake, at the end segment of the small intestine, the terminal ileum. Here, vitamin B12 enters the bloodstream, is separated from the intrinsic factor molecule, and rides on another carrier protein (transcobalamin) as it is distributed to tissues throughout the body.

Bye, Bye, B12

Since 1900, food and water supplies in Western-style societies have become ever more processed. As a result, traditional vitamin B12 sources are disappearing from the diets of vegetarians and nonvegetarians alike. Few people spend their days working their hands in the black soils of an organic garden. Rather, most people eat commercially grown fruits and vegetables, produced in soils that are repeatedly saturated with hydrocarbon pesticides and herbicides. These potent chemicals eradicate many of the B12-producing microbes that normally live in healthy soils. Years of repeated overuse of pesticides have, in many places, transformed nutrient-rich soils into lifeless sands and clays. Consequently, the surfaces of carrots, beets, radishes, and other vegetables can no longer be depended on as cobalamin sources.

Similarly, modern sanitary methods of water treatment—especially adding chlorine to kill dysentery-producing microbes—also destroy cobalamin-producing bacteria. Ironically, rather than being a healthy sign of our connection with nature, cobalamin in the municipal drinking supplies today often signals sewage contamination leaking into the water system. As more people turn to bottled or other purified water sources completely devoid of vitamin B12, our daily drinking supply is no longer a friendly source of cobalamin.

Today, even people who consume meat and other animal products may not be protected from vitamin B12 deficiency (Gray, 1990). Cobalamin supplies in omnivore diets may be insufficient due to:

- Destruction of vitamin B12 by the heat of cooking. (Up to 25% of B12 in stew meat is lost during cooking.)
- Reduced consumption by North Americans of beef and lamb and other vitamin B12-dense meats; these meats are being replaced with relatively B12-poor poultry, fish, and pork.
- Inhibition of absorption of vitamin B12 by other foods. Egg whites and egg yolks, for example, contain substances that inhibit vitamin B12 absorption (Doscherholmen, McMahon, & Ripley, 1976).
- Hypothyroidism or lack of sufficient secretion of hydrochloric acid by the stomach.
- Inadequate pancreatic enzyme secretion (common after years of pancreatic damage due to alcohol ingestion).
- Inflammation of the small intestine from Crohn's disease, intestinal inflammation from anti-arthritis drugs, and other inflammation problems.
- Bacterial overgrowth due to unbalanced diet or antibiotic therapy.
- Surgical resection of the stomach (which produces the intrinsic factor protein) and/or the last 12 inches of small intestine (where most B12 absorption occurs).
- Intestinal infestation with fish tapeworms.
- Nitrous oxide anesthesia (Amess et al., 1978), cigarette smoke, and birth control pills.
- Rarer medical causes such as Zollinger-Ellison syndrome, celiac sprue, strictures and anastomoses, biguanidine therapy for diabetes, and inborn errors of cobalamin metabolism, which are known to and investigated by medical science.

If any of these conditions exist, it is important to work with a physician, nutritionist, or other practitioner to choose an appropriate vitamin B12 source that ensures effective cobalamin levels in the tissues.

Vitamin B12 deficiency caused by lack of cobalamin consumption in the diet is not to be confused with the far more common disease known as *pernicious anemia*. This disease state results when adequate cobalamin is ingested in the food, but the body is unable to absorb the vitamin from the intestine into the bloodstream due to the lack of the transport protein, intrinsic factor (IF). As discussed previously, IF is secreted by the stomach; it is needed to ferry cobalamin molecules from the food, across the intestinal lining membranes, and into the blood. Pernicious anemia, which is caused by gastric lining failure rather than lack of vitamin B12 in the diet, is common in the elderly and far more frequent in the meat-eating population than among vegetarians. Treatment for this particular type of anemia usually requires intramuscular injection or oral administration of large quantities of vitamin B12 (approximately 1,000 mcg per day), under the supervision of a physician. Recent experience has suggested that mega-doses of oral vitamin B12—daily consumption of 1,000–5,000 mcg of B12 sublingually or by nasal spray administration—can overcome the "block" produced by lack of intrinsic factor. If this method of treatment is chosen, blood B12 levels and clinical response must still be monitored by a physician.

Blood Testing for Vitamin B12 Levels

Any adult who has followed a vegan diet for more than three years, and who has not been regularly consuming cobalamin-fortified foods or supplements (or who has any concern at all about vitamin B12 status) should have his or her blood tested. The blood test should include total serum levels of cobalamin as well as a complete blood count (CBC) with red blood cell indices and morphology (a test that describes the size, shape, and density of the red cells).

Optimal levels of cobalamin have not been established. The range of normal values, from 200 to 900 pg/ml, are based on blood samples drawn from the general American, meat-consuming population. Vegans frequently have lower levels in general, but amounts below 250 pg/ml in anyone should prompt consideration of supplementation.

Blood tests that measure cobalamin levels only can be falsely reassuring. The pitfall lurks in conventional laboratory testing, which measures cobalamin levels in the circulating blood but not in vital tissues, such as the brain and peripheral nerves, where cobalamin actually functions. Thus, the laboratory tests for total B12 circulating in the blood may yield normal-range results even when the actual cobalamin levels in the brain and other tissues are critically low, resulting in injury to these vital organs.

A more accurate picture of the body's true vitamin B12 status is generated by measuring the levels of the carrier form of the vitamin, holotranscobalamin II (HTC II). Because HTC II levels decrease significantly before the total vitamin B12 level falls, decreasing HTC II values can sound the alarm of impending cobalamin deficiency before actual tissue damage occurs (Herzlich & Herbert, 1988; Herbert, 1988b; Herbert, 1986). Blood tests for HTC II will soon be widely available through medical testing laboratories. Until then, if vitamin B12 deficiency is suspected, blood or urine tests for methylmalonic acid (MMA), a metabolic product that accumulates with deficiencies of vitamin B12, should be done along with blood cobalamin levels. MMA levels may rise significantly before the total vitamin B12 level falls, and thus elevated MMA in the blood or urine should always prompt consideration of supplementation with B12. Fortunately, the adverse effects of vitamin B12 deficiency can usually be reversed if cobalamin supplementation is provided before significant tissue damage is done.

Practical Aspects

Strategies for Assuring Cobalamin Sufficiency

The adult human liver can store a three- to seven-year supply of vitamin B12, and thus acts as a B12 sponge or buffer. For this reason, vegetarians who eliminate all sources of vitamin B12 from their diet may take up to seven years to display clinical evidence of cobalamin deficiency. However, the body tissues may begin functioning at suboptimal levels, or even suffer damage, long before noticeable symptoms appear. Fortunately, this B12 buffer effect also makes it unnecessary for an adult to consume cobalamin daily. Most adults require vitamin B12-containing foods or supplements only a few times per week; for some people who have very efficient reutilization of the vitamin, ingestion of a few micrograms of cobalamin a few times per month will be enough to keep them in positive vitamin B12 balance.

In adult vegans with insufficient vitamin B12 sources in the diet, cobalamin stored in the liver will be steadily depleted through small but steady daily losses in the feces. The threat of "creeping" vitamin B12 deficiency in vegans is real, and should be taken seriously (Herbert, 1994; Herbert, 1987). Anemia and numbness in the hands and feet (due to nerve damage) are all signs of advanced vitamin B12 deficiency; such conditions should be diagnosed and treated —or better, prevented—before they progress to the stage of tissue injury. Most people, including vegans past the age of adolescence, can meet their needs for cobalamin with a vitamin B12 top-off of 5 to 10 micrograms two or three times weekly.

The developing fetus and the newborn infant are totally dependent upon the mother for their cobalamin supplies (Sanders & Roshanai, 1992). The vitamin B12 stored in the mother's liver is not available to the fetus, who must rely upon the cobalamin circulating in the mother's bloodstream. Consequently, for the health of their babies, pregnant women and nursing mothers are wise to consume at least 3 to 5 mcg of vitamin B12 daily (Sanders & Reddy, 1992; Rana & Sanders, 1986).

Children require 1–2 mcg of vitamin B12 daily to maintain normal growth. Studies show that children who consume a broad-based vegan diet, with adequate vitamin B12, grow steadily and healthfully into full-sized, normally functioning adults (Sanders, 1988; O'Connell et al., 1989) with normal intellectual development (Dwyer et al., 1980).

The medical literature contains reports of severe cases of vitamin B12 deficiency in children. In almost every instance, the patient was an infant or child whose well-intentioned but nutritionally naive parents provided a diet based on diluted soy milks or similar formulas that were deficient not only in vitamin B12, but also in calories, protein, and other essential nutrients (Wighton et al., 1979; Higginbottom, Sweetman, & Nyhan, 1978). The deficiency of all these necessary substances conspires to cause malnutrition in these children, including cobalamin deficiency. Fortunately, most of the clinical problems resolved promptly when adequate nutrition, including vitamin B12, was provided.

Concern has been expressed about children raised as macrobiotic vegetarians, who rely only on sea vegetables for their vitamin B12. A few such children were found to suffer from cobalamin deficiency and resulting slowed growth (Dagnelie, 1994). Fortunately, most of these children experienced catch-up growth when sufficient, active vitamin B12 was supplied. Such problems in children are completely preventable through use of fortified foods or vitamin supplements. The lesson from the macrobiotic example should be that sea vegetables cannot be relied on as the sole source of vitamin B12, and that it is wise to include several, varied cobalamin sources in the diet (Dagnelie, 1991).

The advice to utilize vitamin B12-fortified foods should not be taken as evidence of the inherent dietary deficiency of a vegan diet. Rather, it is a commentary on the price we have all paid for convenience, commercialization, and sterilization of our food supply.

In summary, it would seem prudent for all vegans—as well as lacto vegetarians, lacto-ovo vegetarians, and even omnivores who are not certain of the vitamin B12 adequacy of their diets—to take steps to ensure that they get sufficient dietary cobalamin. For vegans, the most practical method is to include vitamin B12-fortified cereals, soy milks, and other foods in the daily diet, and vitamin supplements if deemed necessary. Ideally, cobalamin from several sources will be consumed.

Great Britain has an established history of B12-fortified food products, including soy milk (Plamil), and a yeast-derived paste (Marmite) that is commonly used as a soup base or as a spread for breads. Canada has recently decided to permit production and importation of B12-fortified food products.

In the United States, vitamin B12-containing foods include breakfast cereals, soy milks, rice milks, and cobalamin-fortified nutritional yeast (a pleasant-tasting and highly nutritious ingredient, available in both powder and flake form). Nutritional yeast can be blended into salad dressings, and is a savory topping to sprinkle over steamed vegetables, pastas, and popcorn! As stated on the label, one tablespoon of Red Star Nutritional Yeast (Model T-6635) powder contains 3 mcg of cobalamin (Red Star, 2007). Twin Lab nutritional yeast and other brands all supply significant amounts of cobalamin per serving. These and other vitamin B12-fortified products (see Table 7.1) are appearing in increasing numbers at natural food stores and supermarkets everywhere. Consumed regularly, these products can conveniently and deliciously ensure vitamin B12 adequacy.

In addition, anyone can fortify foods by simply crushing a vitamin B12 tablet and adding the powder to common dishes such as salad dressings and sauces. For children, parents can add a few drops of B12-containing liquid multivitamins to a daily fruit smoothie or glass of juice.

The Supplement Question

Until recently, commercially produced vitamin B12 was extracted from beef liver and other slaughterhouse sources. Currently, most cobalamin is produced for commercial use by large-scale culture of a B12-synthesizing organism, *Streptomyces griseus*. The cobalamin is then separated from the culture broth, purified, and concentrated for use in processed foods and vitamin supplements.

People who consume a standard multivitamin one or more times per week can expect to meet their B12 requirements easily. Almost every standard multivitamin tablet contains cobalamin in amounts that usually exceed the body's actual requirement, as well as the (higher) U.S. Recommended Dietary Intake (RDI) values. However, if oral vitamin supplements are the *sole* source of cobalamin in the diet—and especially if blood tests reveal low vitamin B12 levels (< 250 pg/ml)—the label of the vitamin preparation should be examined to assure that the U.S. RDA of at least 2–4 mcg of cobalamin is present. This amount should be ingested at least two to three times weekly. If levels stay depressed on this regimen, it may be that the vitamin tablet is dissolving beyond the stomach

Table 7.1   Vitamin B12 in Foods Used by Vegetarians

Vegan Food	Volume	Mcg B12
Nutritional yeast powder	1 tsp.	1.0
Red Star T-6635, large flakes	1 Tbsp.	2.0
Kellogg's Nutri-Grain Post Grape Nuts	½ cup	1.5
Ralston Muesli	1 serving	2.0
Western Family Nutritional Nuggets	1 serving	2.4
Ralston Graham Chex	1 serving	2.7
Eden Soy Extra Soy Beverage, Original	1 cup	3.0
Healthy Choice, Just Right Cereals	1 serving	6.0
Fortified infant formula	(see product label)	
For Comparison Purposes Only:		
Egg, cooked	1	0.4–0.6
Milk, whole, 2% or skim	1 cup	0.9
Yogurt	6 oz.	0.2–1.2
Cheese	1 oz.	0.2

Source: Melina V, Davis B, Harrison V. *Becoming Vegetarian.* Summertown, TN: Book Publishing Co.; 1995.

and the cobalamin is thus unable to combine with the intrinsic factor required for absorption into the bloodstream. In this case, an alternative form of vitamin B12 should be considered, such as sublingual "dots" that are absorbed through the mouth tissues, or intranasal gels and sprays.

Vitamin B12 is essentially nontoxic, even in amounts hundreds of times the RDI. Dosages from 5 mcg up to 1,000 mcg are widely available for use several times weekly. (As the dosage increases, the fraction that is absorbed decreases. Thus, from a 1,000-mcg microdot, only approximately 5 to 10 mcg are absorbed.) Cobalamin supplement tablets taken in the evening have a longer time to be absorbed, and thus result in higher blood levels than those taken in the morning.

In some vitamin B12-containing preparations, including many algae and sprout-based food supplements (e.g., spirulina [Dagnelie, 1991; Herbert & Drivas 1982]), molecules called *cobalamin analogues* are supplied. Analogues can occupy the B12 receptor sites on cell surfaces. These molecules are similar to cobalamin, but are chemically inert and thus block active cobalamin from performing its metabolic functions. In this way, vitamin B12 analogues can act as "anti-B12" molecules, and the supplement ingested to prevent vitamin B12 deficiency can actually contribute to that very condition (Herbert et al., 1982). Obviously, the vitamin B12 supplement upon which one is relying should be as free from cobalamin analogues as possible. If the B12 analogue content is of concern, write or call the quality control officer at the vitamin company, supplement producer, or food processor. They should provide upon request confirmation that the vitamin B12 in their product is present in adequate amounts and is relatively free from analogues.

Experience among vegans who use standard supplements—tablets, sprays, sublingual dots, etc.— indicates that analogues are not a significant problem in these preparations. Algae and sprout-based supplements are of greater concern. The issue of analogues is yet another reason for including more than one vitamin B12 source in the diet.

Conclusion

In summary, vitamin B12 deficiency due to lack of dietary intake of cobalamin is completely preventable. Dietary cobalamin sources are widely available, even to pure vegetarians (vegans), so vitamin B12-containing foods can and should be part of every vegan diet. Concern over vitamin B12 adequacy should not be a deterrent to people who choose to nourish themselves on exclusively plant-based diets.

References

Albert MJ. Vitamin B12 synthesis by human small intestinal bacteria. *Nature.* 1980;283:781–782.

Amess J, Burman JF, Rees GM, Nancekievill DG, Mollin DL. Megaloblastic haemopoiesis in patients receiving nitrous oxide. *Lancet.* 1978;2(8085): 339–342.

Dagnelie PC, van Staveren W. Macrobiotic nutrition and child health: Results of a population-based, mixed-longitudinal cohort study in the Netherlands. *Am J Clin Nutr.* 1994;59(Suppl):1187S–1196S.

Dagnelie PC. Vitamin B12 from algae appears not to be bioavailable. *Am J Clin Nutr.* 1991;53: 695–697.

Doscherholmen A, McMahon J, Ripley D. Inhibitory effect of eggs on vitamin B12 absorption: Description of a simple ovalbumin co-vitamin B12 absorption test. *Br J Haematol.* 1976;33: 261–272.

Dwyer JT, Miller LG, Arduino, NL, et al. Mental age and I.Q. of predominantly vegetarian children. *J Am Diet Assoc.* 1980;76:142–147.

Gray SR. Where's the B12? *Solstice.* February, 1990; 39:10–15.

Herbert V. Staging vitamin B12 (cobalamin) status in vegetarians. *Am J Clin Nutr.* 1994;59(Suppl): 1213S–1222S.

Herbert V. B12 deficiency in AIDS [letter]. *JAMA.* 1988a;260:2837.

Herbert V. Don't ignore low serum cobalamin (vitamin B12) levels. *Arch Intern Med.* 1988b;148: 1705–1707.

Herbert V. Recommended dietary intakes (RDI) of vitamin B12. *Am J Clin Nutr.* 1987;45:671–678.

Herbert V. What is normal? Variation from the individual's norm for granulocyte "lobe average" and holo-transcobalamin II (Holo-TC II) diagnoses vitamin B12 deficiency before variation from the laboratory norm. *Clin Res.* 1986;342:718A [abstract].

Herbert V, Drivas G. Spirulina and vitamin B12. *JAMA.* 1982;248(23):1096–1097.

Herbert V, Drivas G, Foscaldi R, et al. Multi-vitamin/ mineral food supplements containing vitamin B12 may also contain analogues of vitamin B12. *N Engl J Med.* 1982;307:255–256.

Herzlich B, Herbert V. Depletion of serum holo-transcobalamin II: An early sign of negative vitamin B12 balance. *Lab Invest.* 1988;58:332–337.

Higginbottom MC, Sweetman L, Nyhan WL. A syndrome of methylmalonic aciduria, homocystinuria, megaloblastic anemia and neurologic abnormalities in a vitamin B12-deficient breast-fed infant of a strict vegetarian. *N Engl J Med.* 1978;299: 317–323.

O'Connell JM, Dibley MJ, Sierra J, Wallace B, Marks JS, Yip R. Growth of vegetarian children: The Farm study. *Pediatrics.* 1989;84:475–481.

Parker BC. Rain as a source of vitamin B12. *Nature.* 1968;219:617.

Pennypacker LC, Allen RH, Kelly JP, et al. High prevalence of cobalamin deficiency in elderly outpatients. *J Am Geriatr Soc.* 1992;40:1197–1204.

Rana SK, Sanders TA. Taurine concentrations in the diet, plasma, urine and breast milk of vegans compared with omnivores. *Br J Nutr.* 1986;56(1): 17–27.

Red Star Nutritional Yeast, Model T-6635+ [package label]. Midland, MI: Universal Foods; 2007.

Sanders TAB. Growth and development of British vegan children. *Am J Clin Nutr.* 1988;48:822–825.

Sanders TAB, Reddy S. The influence of a vegetarian diet on the fatty acid composition of human milk and the essential fatty acid status of the infant. *J Pediatr.* 1992;120(4, Pt 2):S71–S77.

Sanders TAB, Roshanai F. Platelet phospholipid fatty acid composition and function in vegans compared with age- and sex-matched omnivore controls. *Eur J Clin Nutr.* 1992;46(11):823–831.

Selhub J, Jacques PF, Bostom AG, et al. Association between plasma homocysteine concentrations and extracranial carotid-artery stenosis. *N Engl J Med.* 1995;332(5):286–291.

Ubbink JB. Vitamin nutrition status and homocysteine: An atherogenic risk factor. *Nutr Rev.* 1994; 52(11):383–387.

Wighton MC, Manson JL, Speed I, Robertson E, Chapman E. Brain damage in infancy and dietary vitamin B12 deficiency. *Med J Australia.* 1979;2(1):1–3.

Yao Y. Low serum vitamin B12 in seniors. *J Fam Pract.* 1992;35:524–529.

8

Zinc

Virginia Messina, MPH, RD
Reed Mangels, PhD, RD, FADA

Introduction

Zinc status among vegetarians is poorly understood. The existing disagreement among experts about zinc requirements is further complicated by the fact that zinc status is not easily assessed and signs of marginal zinc deficiency are not well defined. This chapter reviews zinc recommendations and the bioavailability of zinc from plant foods. The zinc status of vegetarians is then discussed. We conclude with discussion of the dietary sources of zinc and ways to ensure adequate zinc intake.

Summary of the Scientific Literature

Functions of Zinc

Zinc plays extensive biochemical roles via catalytic, structural, and regulatory functions. Zinc is a co-factor of many enzymes and is involved in DNA synthesis, protein synthesis, blood formation, reproductive function, and maintenance of a healthy immune system. Overt signs of zinc deficiency include severe growth reduc-

tion, and sexual immaturity in children and adolescents. In some parts of the world where low-income populations consume plant-based diets, zinc deficiency is common. Researchers estimated that as many as 30% of children in China could suffer stunted growth due to zinc deficiency (Chen et al., 1985). However, diet is only one factor affecting zinc status in these populations: parasitic infections and pica—the practice of eating clay—also appear to contribute to zinc deficiency. Although zinc intake appears to be low among many low-income American children, overt deficiency is still rare in Western populations.

Zinc Bioavailability and Recommendations

Many factors affect zinc bioavailability. Zinc absorption increases when zinc status is poor and losses decrease when zinc intakes are low (Johnson et al., 1993). As a result, it is relatively easy to maintain zinc balance at marginal levels; however, it is not clear whether this marginal status supports optimal health. Foods can also affect zinc absorption and bioavailability. Zinc absorption can vary as much as fourfold, from as little as 8% absorbed from a meal to as much as 38% of the zinc in a meal being absorbed (Sandstrom et al., 1980; Sandstrom & Cederblad, 1980). Two factors that appear to be important in determining the amount of zinc absorbed are the phytate and protein content of the diet.

Phytate, a phosphorus-containing compound found largely in whole grains, legumes, nuts, and seeds, is a potent inhibitor of zinc absorption (Larsson et al., 1996; Reinhold et al., 1973). Zinc absorption from high-phytate meals has been shown to be only about 5%–15% (Navert, Sandstrom, & Cederblad, 1985; Fordyce et al., 1987). However, foods high in phytate should not be dismissed as poor sources of zinc, as their total zinc content can be high compared to low-phytate plant foods. Although zinc is more efficiently absorbed from white bread than from whole-wheat bread, more total zinc is absorbed from the latter (Sandstrom et al., 1980; van Dokkum, Wesstra, & Schippers, 1982).

Food processing or preparation techniques that result in fermentation can decrease the phytate content of foods, resulting in as much as a fourfold increase in zinc absorption. For example, fermentation in yeast-leavened bread breaks down phytate, so zinc is better absorbed from whole-wheat bread than from unleavened wheat products (Sandstrom et al., 1980). Zinc is also more bioavailable from fermented soy products like tempeh and miso (Ikeda & Murakamai, 1995). Organic acids, such as citric, lactic, and acetic acid, also improve zinc absorption, and foods that contain these acids (such as sourdough products, sauerkraut, fruits, cheeses, and yogurt) can improve the total zinc absorption from a meal (Tabekhia & Luh, 1980). Sprouting of legumes also increases zinc bioavailability, although eating sprouts may not be a common practice among many vegetarians (Ellis et al., 1982).

Though all these factors mitigate some effects of phytate, it is likely that the high phytate content of vegetarian diets does adversely affect zinc absorption to some extent. Vegetarian diets may contain as much as two to three times more phytate than omnivore diets (Rosado et al., 1992). Because vegetarian diets are also frequently lower in zinc, the potential effects of phytate cannot be ignored. A number of studies have shown zinc to be less available in vegetarian diets (Campbell-Brown et al., 1985; Pecoud, Donzel, & Schelling, 1975; Sandstrom, 1989). Research suggests that Western vegetarians absorb about 15% to 20% of zinc from their diet, compared to 30% from omnivore diets (Hunt, Matthys, & Johnson, 1998). A short-term study of lacto-ovo vegetarian women showed average zinc intake and absorption to be 14% and 21% lower, respectively, than in omnivores (Sandstead, 1982).

The amount and type of protein in the diet also may affect zinc needs, although findings on this point conflict. Some studies suggest that high protein diets increase zinc needs—which would suggest that vegetarians have lower needs (Hunt et al., 1995). Other studies suggest that protein decreases the need for zinc (Wood & Zheng, 1997). Protein from beef, eggs, and cheese have been shown to enhance zinc absorption (Sandstrom & Cederblad, 1980), but casein in milk inhibits zinc absorption.

Calcium also inhibits zinc absorption and may also increase the effects of phytates (Fordyce et al., 1987). This suggests that lacto-ovo vegetarians are at greater risk for poor zinc status (because of their higher calcium intake) than vegans, who often have zinc intakes similar to those of lacto-ovo vegetarians. In one study, when diets with identical zinc content were either low in calcium, supplemented with calcium phosphate, or supplemented with milk, zinc absorption was 35%, 6%, and 2.6%, respectively (O'Brien et al., 2000). This suggests that diets with generous amounts of milk, as are typical with some lacto-ovo vegetarians, can interfere with zinc absorption. The potentially higher phytate content of a lacto-ovo vegetarian diet compared to a nonvegetarian diet, as well as the higher calcium level seen in some lacto-ovo vegetarian diets, raise concerns about the effects of these factors on zinc absorption in lacto-ovo vegetarians.

Zinc absorption of lacto-ovo vegetarians may not be markedly lower than in people eating nonvegetarian diets, however. United States Department of Agriculture (USDA) researchers (Sandstead, 1982) found that zinc absorption was only 20% lower in lacto-ovo vegetarians than in nonvegetarians, suggesting a smaller effect of calcium and phytate interactions than was seen in the study using low calcium, calcium-supplemented, or milk-supplemented diets (O'Brien et al., 2000).

Iron supplements also appear to impair zinc absorption (O'Brien et al., 2000; Chung et al., 2002; Solomons, 1986), especially supplements containing 30 mg or more of iron. If iron supplements are used, taking them between meals may reduce their effect on zinc absorption (Ruz et al., 2001).

The RDA for zinc is 11 mg/day for adult men and 8 mg/day for adult women (Food and Nutrition Board [FNB], 2001). Although there is no specific RDA for vegetarians, low zinc absorption from foods like grains and dried beans, which are often staples of a vegetarian diet, has prompted the suggestion that vegetarians may need as much as 50 percent more zinc than the current RDA (FNB, 2001). This would yield a suggested intake of 16.5 mg/day for men and 12 mg/day for women. The World Health Organization (WHO) bases zinc recommendations on the zinc bioavailability of different diets (WHO/FAO, 2004). WHO recommendations for those on diets with the lowest zinc bioavailability (many vegan diets fall into this category) are 14 mg/day for adult men and 9.8 mg/day for adult women, somewhat higher than the RDA.

Vegetarian Zinc Status

Studies show that zinc intakes of vegetarians are often comparable to those of omnivores, although some have reported low zinc intakes among vegetarians (Messina, Mangels, & Messina, 2004). Sensitive measures for assessing zinc status are unknown at this time. Although zinc levels in serum, hair, and saliva are often measured, and frequently found to be low in cases of severe zinc deficiency, other conditions unrelated to zinc status could also affect these measurements (WHO/FAO, 2004). Despite the limitations of these measures, it is noteworthy that vegetarians have been shown to have serum zinc levels similar to those of nonvegetarians (Ball & Ackland, 2000). Similarly, levels of zinc in the hair and saliva of vegetarians were in the normal range, although these levels were lower than those seen in nonvegetarians (Morris et al., 1986; Kies, Young, & McEndree, 1983; Freeland-Graves, Bodzy, & Epright, 1980; Srikumar, Ockerman, & Akesson, 1992). However, other studies have found that vegetarians are more likely than nonvegetarians to have very low blood zinc levels (Srikumar, Ockerman, & Akesson, 1992; Latta & Liebman, 1984). Although stunted growth that may be linked, in part, to zinc deficiency has been seen in some children on macrobiotic diets, frank zinc deficiency has not been observed in Western vegetarian populations.

There are legitimate questions about the problem of marginal zinc deficiency in some vegetarians. Symptoms of chronic marginal nutrient deficiencies are much harder to identify and define than overt zinc deficiency. Some studies suggest that low blood levels of zinc, in the absence of overt deficiency, could be linked to suboptimal health. Increased zinc intake caused improvements in children with marginal intakes who experienced poor appetite, impaired taste acuity, and suboptimal growth but were otherwise healthy (Gibson et al., 1989; Vanderkooy & Gibson, 1987). Males with mild zinc deficiency have been shown to have low testosterone levels (Prasad et al., 1996).

Also of interest is the effect of zinc on conditions—such as cancer—that are related to a complex interaction of many factors and therefore difficult to link to any single nutrient deficiency. Because zinc is a co-factor in enzymes involved in carcinogen detoxification, it is reasonable to speculate that inadequate zinc intake could raise the risks for cancer.

Thus, though it is clear that zinc balance and normal blood levels can be maintained on low zinc intakes, it is not clear that these marginal intakes are enough to prevent more subtle symptoms or consequences of poor zinc nutrition. The ubiquitous nature of zinc in metabolism suggests that marginal deficiency could have important effects. Whether or not this has consequences for vegetarians is not known. Presumably, however, this is not a concern unique to vegetarians, as large segments of the American population in general do not meet zinc recommendations. However, it is clear that meeting zinc needs is a somewhat greater challenge on plant-based diets and therefore is one that deserves some attention in vegetarian diets.

Practical Aspects

Steps to ensure optimal zinc status include the following:

- Choose good sources of zinc daily, such as bran flakes, fortified cereals such as Wheat Chex, wheat germ, corn, beans, nuts, and seeds.
- Include daily servings of both legumes and nuts/seeds in the diet. These foods are sometimes underutilized in vegetarian diets.
- Choose whole grains over refined foods. Although they are high in phytates, the total zinc absorbed from these foods is greater than from refined foods.
- Choose yeast-raised breads over crackers and flatbreads, as zinc is better absorbed from these foods.
- Choose fermented soy foods, such as tempeh and miso, more often than unfermented soy products such as tofu and soy milk.
- Include foods high in organic acids, such as sauerkraut, sourdough bread, lemon juice, citrus fruits, vinegar, and fruits.
- Include sprouted legumes in meals.
- Avoid taking calcium supplements with meals, as this may inhibit zinc absorption.

Conclusion

Vegetarians consume either comparable amounts of or less zinc than omnivores, and zinc is at least somewhat less bioavailable from plant foods than from animal-source foods. However, it is possible that, over the long term, the body compensates for this by conserving zinc more efficiently. Overt zinc deficiency is not common among vegetarians. However, it is difficult to accurately assess zinc status and even harder to pinpoint signs of marginal zinc deficiency. Concerns about the effects of marginal zinc deficiency on health suggest that it is prudent to maximize zinc intake and absorption on all diets. Vegetarians can improve zinc nutrition with relatively moderate adjustments to the diet. Although dairy foods are the best sources of well-absorbed zinc in vegetarian diets, well-planned vegan diets can provide adequate zinc (WHO/FAO, 2004).

References

Ball MJ, Ackland ML. Zinc intake and status in Australian vegetarians. *Br J Nutr.* 2000; 83:27–33.

Campbell-Brown M, Ward RJ, Haines AP, et al. Zinc and copper in Asian pregnancies—Is there evidence for a nutritional deficiency? *Br J Obstet Gyn.* 1985;92:875–885.

Chen XC, Yin TA, He JS, et al. Low levels of zinc in hair and blood, pica, anorexia and poor growth in Chinese preschool children. *Am J Clin Nutr.* 1985;42:694–700.

Chung CS, Nagey DA, Veillon C, et al. A single 60-mg iron dose decreases zinc absorption in lactating women. *J Nutr.* 2002;132:1903–1905.

Ellis R, Morris ER, Hill AD, Smith JC. Phytate:zinc molar ratio, mineral and fiber content of three hospital diets. *J Am Diet Assoc.* 1982;81:26–29.

Food and Nutrition Board, Institute of Medicine. *Dietary Reference Intakes for Vitamin A, Vitamin K, Arsenic, Boron, Chromium, Copper, Iodine, Iron, Manganese, Molybdenum, Nickel, Silicon, Vanadium, and Zinc.* Washington, DC: National Academy Press; 2001.

Fordyce EJ, Forbes RM, Robbins KR, Erdman JW Jr. Phytate calcium/zinc molar ratios: Are they predictive of zinc bioavailability? *J Food Sci.* 1987; 52:440–444.

Freeland-Graves JH, Bodzy PW, Epright MA. Zinc status of vegetarians. *J Am Diet Assoc.* 1980;77: 655–661.

Gibson RS, Vanderkooy PD, MacDonald AC, et al. A growth-limiting, mild zinc-deficiency syndrome in some southern Ontario boys with low height percentiles. *Am J Clin Nutr.* 1989;49: 1266–1273.

Hunt JR, Gallagher SK, Johnson LK, et al. High-versus low-meat diets: Effects on zinc absorption, iron status, and calcium, copper, iron, magnesium, manganese, nitrogen, phosphorus, and zinc balance in postmenopausal women. *Am J Clin Nutr.* 1995;62:621–632.

Hunt JR, Matthys LA, Johnson LK. Zinc absorption, mineral balance, and blood lipids in women consuming controlled lacto-ovo-vegetarian and omnivorous diets for 8 wks. *Am J Clin Nutr.* 1998; 67:421–430.

Ikeda S, Murakamai T. Zinc chemical form in some traditional soy foods. *J Food Sci.* 1995;60:1151–1155.

Johnson PE, Hunt CD, Milne DB, Mullen LK. Homeostatic control of zinc metabolism in men: Zinc excretion in men fed diets low in zinc. *Am J Clin Nutr.* 1993;57:557–565.

Kies C, Young E, McEndree L. Zinc bioavailability from vegetarian diets: Influence of dietary fiber, ascorbic acid, and past dietary practices. In: Inglett GE, ed. *Nutritional Bioavailability of Zinc* (American Chemical Society Symposium Series 210B). Washington, DC: American Chemical Society; 1983:115–126.

Larsson M, Hulten LR, Sandstrom B, Sandberg A. Improved zinc and iron absorption from breakfast meals containing malted oats with reduced phytate content. *Br J Nutr.* 1996;76:677–688.

Latta D, Liebman M. Iron and zinc status of nonvegetarian males. *Nutr Reps Intl.* 1984;30:141–149.

Messina V, Mangels R, Messina M. *The Dietitian's Guide to Vegetarian Diets: Issues and Applications.* 2d ed. Sudbury, MA: Jones and Bartlett Publishers; 2004.

Morris ER, Ellis R, Hill AD, et al. Apparent zinc and iron balance of adult men consuming three levels of phytate. *Fed Proc.* 1986;45:819.

Navert B, Sandstrom B, Cederblad A. Reduction of the phytate content of bran by leavening in bread and its effect on zinc absorption in man. *Br J Nutr.* 1985;53:47–53.

O'Brien KO, Zavaleta N, Caulfield LE, et al. Prenatal iron supplements impair zinc absorption in pregnant Peruvian women. *J Nutr.* 2000;130: 2251–2255.

Pecoud A, Donzel P, Schelling JL. Effect of foodstuffs on the absorption of zinc sulfate. *Clin Pharmacol Ther.* 1975;17:469–473.

Prasad AS, Mantzoros CS, Beck FW, et al. Zinc status and serum testosterone levels of healthy adults. *Nutrition.* 1996;12:344–348.

Reinhold JG, Nast K, Lahimgarzadeh A, Hedayati H. Effects of purified phytate and phytate-rich bread upon metabolism of zinc, calcium, phosphorus, and nitrogen in man. *Lancet.* 1973;1:283–288.

Rosado JL, Lopez P, Morales M, et al. Bioavailability of energy, nitrogen, fat, zinc, iron, and calcium from rural and urban Mexican diets. *Br J Nutr.* 1992;68:45–58.

Ruz M, Codeceo J, Rebolledo A, et al. Effects of iron supplementation on zinc absorption in Chilean women. *Ann Nutr Metab.* 2001;45(Suppl):363 [abstract].

Sandstead HH. Availability of zinc and its requirement in human subjects. In: Prasad AS, ed. *Clinical, Biochemical, and Nutritional Aspects of Trace Elements.* New York: Liss;1982:83–101.

Sandstrom B. Dietary pattern and zinc supply. In: Mills CF, ed. *Zinc in Human Biology.* New York: Springer-Verlag; 1989:351–363.

Sandstrom B, Arvidsson B, Cederblad A, Bjorn-Rasmussen E. Zinc absorption from composite meals. I. The significance of wheat extraction rate, zinc, calcium, and protein content in meals based on bread. *Am J Clin Nutr.* 1980;33: 739–745.

Sandstrom B, Cederblad A. Zinc absorption from composite meals. II. Influence of the main protein source. *Am J Clin Nutr.* 1980;33:1778–1783.

Solomons NW. Competitive interaction of iron and zinc in the diet: Consequences for human nutrition. *J Nutr.* 1986;116:927–935.

Srikumar TS, Ockerman PA, Akesson B. Trace element status in vegetarians from southern India. *Nutr Res.* 1992;12:187–198.

Tabekhia MM, Luh BS. Effect of germination, cooking, and canning on phosphorus and phytate retention in dried beans. *J Food Sci.* 1980;45: 406–408.

van Dokkum W, Wesstra A, Schippers FA. Physiological effects of fibre-rich types of bread. *Br J Nutr.* 1982;47:451–460.

Vanderkooy PD, Gibson RS. Food consumption patterns of Canadian preschool children in relation to zinc and growth status. *Am J Clin Nutr.* 1987; 45:609–616.

WHO/FAO. *Vitamin and Mineral Requirements in Human Nutrition,* 2d ed. Rome:WHO/FAO; 2004.

Wood RJ, Zheng JJ. High dietary calcium intakes reduce zinc absorption and balance in humans. *Am J Clin Nutr.* 1997;65:1803–1809.

9

Other Vitamins and Minerals

Reed Mangels, PhD, RD, FADA

Introduction

A number of other vitamins and minerals, in addition to iron, calcium, vitamin D, vitamin B12, and zinc, play important roles in human health. Issues germane to these nutrients include their function, how much is needed on a daily basis, adequacy of a vegetarian diet to supply them, and sources of the nutrients in question. Nutrients discussed are thiamin, riboflavin, niacin, vitamin B6, folate, biotin, pantothenic acid, vitamin C, vitamin A, vitamin E, vitamin K, phosphorus, magnesium, iodine, selenium, copper, chromium, and molybdenum.

Summary of the Scientific Literature

Thiamin

Thiamin, also called *vitamin B1*, is needed for the metabolism of carbohydrates. It plays an important role in nerve and muscle function. In the United States, thiamin deficiency is observed most commonly among alcoholics, due to their low intake and absorption of thiamin and increased need for thiamin.

The recommended intake level of thiamin is 1.2 milligram (mg) per day for adult males and 1.1 mg per day for adult females (Food and Nutrition Board [FNB], 1998). The average daily thiamin intake of U.S. adults is nearly 2.0 mg for men and 1.2 mg for women (FNB, 1998). Major sources of thiamin for U.S. adults are yeast breads, ready-to-eat cereals, pasta, ham, and cow's milk (Cotton et al., 2004).

There is no evidence that vegetarians eating a varied diet are at risk of thiamin deficiency. Most recent studies indicate that vegetarians consume adequate thiamin (Messina, Mangels, & Messina, 2004).

Riboflavin

Riboflavin, also called *vitamin B2*, is also important in energy metabolism, as well as for supporting normal vision and skin health. A deficiency of riboflavin is quite uncommon in the United States.

The recommended intake level of riboflavin is 1.3 mg per day for adult males and 1.1 mg per day for adult females (FNB, 1998). Cow's milk, ready-to-eat cereals, yeast breads, and beef account for close to half of the riboflavin intake of U.S. adults (Cotton et al., 2004).

Lacto-ovo vegetarians generally consume adequate levels of riboflavin if they have two to three servings of cow's milk daily (Messina, Mangels, & Messina, 2004). However, riboflavin has been mentioned as a potential problem for vegans. Vegan diets do not contain what are considered major sources of riboflavin, such as cow's milk, meat, and eggs. In reality, other good sources of riboflavin are found in vegan diets, such as wheat germ, soybeans, leafy green vegetables, sea vegetables, fortified soy milk, nutritional yeast, and whole-grain or enriched breads and cereals. Thus, vegan diets can easily provide sufficient riboflavin. The few extant studies of vegans' riboflavin intake indicate that intakes are generally at or above the recommended level (Messina, Mangels, & Messina, 2004).

Niacin

Niacin, also called *vitamin B3*, is produced to some extent from an amino acid, tryptophan. Niacin plays an important role in energy metabolism and is needed for the nervous and digestive systems to function properly.

The recommended intake level for niacin is 16 mg per day for adult males and 14 mg per day for adult females (FNB, 1998). Major food sources for U.S. adults are poultry, yeast breads, beef, and ready-to-eat cereals (Cotton et al., 2004).

Niacin from cereal grains is not well absorbed because the niacin is bound to other substances (Carter & Carpenter, 1982). Absorption from corn is especially low unless the corn is treated with lime (Goldsmith et al., 1956). Niacin that is added to refined grains as a part of the enrichment process is well absorbed.

Despite lower absorption of niacin from grains, vegetarian diets can easily supply adequate niacin. Both lacto-ovo vegetarians and vegans appear to have adequate intakes of niacin (Messina, Mangels, & Messina, 2004).

Vitamin B6

Vitamin B6 functions as a coenzyme for more than 60 enzymes used in amino-acid and fatty-acid metabolism. Vitamin B6 also is important for nervous system function and for the immune system.

The intake level recommended for vitamin B6 is 1.3 mg per day for adults aged 19 to 50 years, 1.7 mg per day for older males, and 1.5 mg per day for older females (FNB, 1998). Major food sources for adults in the United States are ready-to-eat cereals, poultry, beef, potatoes, bananas, and cow's milk (Cotton et al., 2004).

A deficiency of vitamin B6 is rarely seen, but can produce convulsions, dermatitis, and anemia. Several popular articles have implied that vegetarians might be at risk of vitamin B6 deficiency. The concern for vegetarians is based on reports that high-fiber diets may reduce absorption of vitamin B6 (Leklem et al., 1980). Fiber appears to have only a minor effect on vitamin B6 absorption (Lindberg, Leklem, & Miller, 1983), however, and many fiber-rich foods are also rich in vitamin B6.

Vegetarians who consume a variety of foods do not appear to be at risk for vitamin B6 deficiency. Vitamin B6 intakes and blood levels of Seventh-Day Adventist vegetarian women have been shown to be similar to those of nonvegetarians (Shultz & Leklem, 1987). Other studies of intakes of vegans have shown that vitamin B6 intakes meet recommendations

(Draper et al., 1993; Janelle & Barr, 1995; Davey et al., 2003; Larsson & Johansson, 2002). Vegetarians may actually be at lower risk of vitamin B6 deficiency than nonvegetarians, because particularly good sources of vitamin B6 include many of the foods commonly eaten in vegetarian diets.

Folate

Folate, also called *folic acid* or *folacin*, is a water-soluble vitamin that functions as a coenzyme in amino acid metabolism and nucleic acid production. A deficiency of folate can lead to anemia, depression, confusion, and immune suppression. Folate and vitamin B12 work together to synthesize DNA. Large amounts of folate can take the place of vitamin B12 in some functions and prevent vitamin B12 deficiency anemia. Even large amounts of folate, however, cannot fulfill the role of vitamin B12 in the nervous system. Some studies have suggested that elevated blood homocysteine levels may be a risk factor for heart disease. If so, folate may be protective against heart disease, because it lowers homocysteine levels (Kang, Wong, & Malinow, 1992; Graham et al., 1997).

Folate appears to play an important role in prevention of neural tube defects (FNB, 1998). Neural tube defects, also called *spina bifida* and *anencephaly*, occur in about 2,500 infants born each year in the United States. Studies have shown that women who have infants with neural tube defects have lower intakes of folate and lower blood folate levels than other women. Folate is needed early in pregnancy (before many women know they are pregnant) for normal neural tube development.

The recommended intake level for folate is 400 micrograms (mcg) per day for adults (FNB, 1998). The National Academy of Sciences recommends that all women capable of becoming pregnant consume 400 mcg of synthetic folic acid from fortified foods or supplements, in addition to food folate from a varied diet (FNB, 1998). Major food sources of folate for U.S. adults are ready-to-eat cereals, yeast breads, dried beans and lentils, orange or grapefruit juice, lettuce, and cow's milk (Cotton et al., 2004).

Folate intakes and folate status of vegetarians appear to be similar to or better than those of nonvegetarians (Messina, Mangels, & Messina, 2004); however, vegetarians who eat few fruits, vegetables, and enriched breads and cereals may not meet folate needs.

Beginning in 1998, flour and grain products were enriched with folic acid to increase the folate intake of women in their childbearing years. Although there is some concern that the amount of folic acid added to grains could mask vitamin B12 deficiency, at least one study did not find any increase in the number of people with vitamin B12 deficiency but without anemia following fortification of grains with folic acid (Mills et al., 2003).

Biotin

Biotin is a sulfur-containing vitamin that is essential for humans. It is involved in energy metabolism, fat synthesis, and amino acid metabolism. Biotin deficiency is very rare, but can be produced by ingestion of large amounts of raw egg whites, because of a biotin-binding protein found in raw egg white (FNB, 1998).

An adequate intake (AI) for biotin is 30 mcg per day for adults (FNB, 1998). Biotin is found in a number of foods, including egg yolk, soy flour, cereals, and yeast. The bioavailability of biotin is quite variable.

Little information is available on biotin intakes or status of vegetarians. Seventh-Day Adventist vegetarians were found to have higher blood levels of biotin than nonvegetarians, and

vegans had higher levels than lacto-ovo vegetarians (Lombard & Mock, 1989).

Pantothenic Acid

Pantothenic acid is part of a coenzyme used
in energy metabolism. Evidence of dietary deficiency has not been recognized in humans.

The AI for pantothenic acid is 5 mg per day
for adults (FNB, 1998). Pantothenic acid is found
in many foods and is especially abundant in
animal flesh, whole-grain cereals, and legumes.
Because both whole-grain cereals and legumes
play an important role in the diet of many vegetarians, pantothenic acid status of vegetarians
should be adequate.

Vitamin C

Vitamin C, also called *ascorbic acid*, has many
important functions, including collagen synthesis, thyroxine synthesis, amino acid metabolism, immune system function, and promotion
of iron absorption. Vitamin C, which serves as
an antioxidant, may also play a role in cancer
prevention (Block, 1991).

The Recommended Dietary Allowance (RDA)
for vitamin C is 90 mg per day for adult men
and 75 mg per day for adult women (Jacob,
1999). Approximately 90% of the vitamin C in
Western diets comes from fruits and vegetables.
Grains, legumes, and dairy products contain almost no vitamin C. Orange and grapefruit juices,
fruit drinks, tomatoes, peppers, potatoes, and
broccoli account for more than 60% of the intake of vitamin C among U.S. adults (Cotton
et al., 2004).

Vegetarians commonly consume more vitamin C than do nonvegetarians, and vegans tend
to consume more than lacto-ovo vegetarians
(Messina, Mangels, & Messina, 2004), possibly
because of increased use of fruits and vegetables. Consumption of five servings per day
of fruits and vegetables can provide more than
200 mg per day of vitamin C (Jacob, 1999).

Vitamin A

Beta-carotene is a substance found in plants
that the human body converts to retinol (*vitamin A*). Retinol is also found in foods, but only
in those from animals, so beta-carotene is an
important source of vitamin A for many vegetarians. Vegans get all their vitamin A from
carotenoids.

Vitamin A is essential for vision and appears
to play a role in immune function. In addition
to their roles as vitamin A precursors, beta-
carotene and alpha-carotene also function as
antioxidants. Lutein and lycopene, neither of
which are vitamin A precursors, are among
the other carotenoids that are found most commonly in our diets. Dietary carotenoids appear
to play an important role in disease prevention.
They may help to protect against cardiovascular disease and cancer (Osganaian et al., 2003,
McCann et al., 2003). Carotenoids also reduce
the risk of developing macular degeneration, the
leading cause of irreversible blindness among
persons older than 65 years (Beatty et al., 2000;
Mares-Perlman et al., 2002). Increasing dietary
alpha-carotene and beta-carotene intake can
provide both protection from several common
diseases and a way to meet the requirement
for vitamin A.

The RDA for vitamin A is 900 mcg retinol
for males and 700 mcg retinol for females.
This can be obtained from foods containing
beta-carotene: 12 mcg of dietary beta-carotene
provides 1 mcg of retinol. Alpha-carotene and
beta-cryptoxanthin (other carotenoids) can also

be used to form vitamin A; 24 mcg of these carotenoids is equivalent to 1 mcg of retinol (FNB, 2001). Foods that are especially high in beta-carotene include sweet potatoes, carrots, spinach, cantaloupes, pumpkins, kale, and winter squash (Mangels et al., 1993).

Vegetarians appear to have both higher carotenoid intakes and serum carotenoid levels than do nonvegetarians (Messina, Mangels, & Messina, 2004). Vegetarians can easily meet the requirement for vitamin A.

Vitamin E

Vitamin E functions as one of the body's main defenses against oxidative damage and free radical attack. Although several early studies suggested a role for vitamin E in reducing risk of heart disease (Kushi et al., 1996; Stampfer et al., 1993; Rimm et al., 1993) and cancer (Bostick et al., 1993), more recent studies are inconsistent (The Heart Outcomes Prevention Evaluation Study Investigators, 2000; Wu, 2002).

Because vitamin E can protect polyunsaturated fats from oxidation, the requirement for vitamin E is based on the amount of polyunsaturated fats in the diet (FNB, 2000). When the main polyunsaturated fat in the diet is linoleic acid, as in most U.S. diets, 0.4 mg of RRR-alpha-tocopherol is needed for every gram of polyunsaturated fat (Witting & Lee, 1975). We would expect vegetarians to consume more unsaturated fat than saturated fat, because of their avoidance of meat, a significant source of saturated fat. Vegetarians tend to have intakes of polyunsaturated fat that are similar to the intakes of nonvegetarians, although the overall fat intake of vegetarians is lower (Messina, Mangels, & Messina, 2004). In this case, the requirement for vitamin E would be similar to that of nonvegetarians. In some cases, however, vege-

tarians have much higher intakes of polyunsaturated fat than do nonvegetarians (Messina, Mangels, & Messina, 2004), and thus may need additional vitamin E.

Foods that are high in polyunsaturated fats, such as oils, also tend to be high in vitamin E. Although sunflower oil contains vitamin E mainly in its most biologically active form, alpha-tocopherol, corn or soybean oils and other oils do not have high levels of alpha-tocopherol and may more likely be oxidized (Gey, 1995). Major food sources of vitamin E among U.S. adults include salad dressings and mayonnaise, oils, ready-to-eat cereals, margarine, and baked goods (Cotton et al., 2004). Other good sources are unprocessed cereal grains and nuts.

Several studies of vegetarians have shown that their blood levels of vitamin E were similar to or higher than those of nonvegetarians (Messina, Mangels, & Messina, 2004).

Vitamin K

Vitamin K is important for blood clotting. It is also required for normal bone and kidney function.

The AI for vitamin K for adult men is 120 mcg per day; for adult women, it is 90 mcg per day (FNB, 2001). Vitamin K deficiency is quite rare because vitamin K is found in a wide variety of foods, the body conserves it, and bacteria in the human colon synthesize some vitamin K.

Primary sources of vitamin K are vegetables. For both men and women in the United States, the top four sources of vitamin K are spinach, collard greens, iceberg lettuce, and broccoli (Booth, Pennington, & Sadowski, 1996). Other good sources include cabbage, French dressing, peas, and margarine. In one study (Lloyd et al., 1991), vegetarians were found to consume more vitamin K than did nonvegetarians. Vegetarians should be able to meet their vitamin K needs easily, especially if foods that have been shown to be important contributors to vitamin K intake (Kohlmeier, Garris, & Anderson, 1997), such as broccoli, lettuce, cabbage, asparagus, or greens, are consumed regularly.

Phosphorus

Phosphorus is one of the minerals that, along with calcium, make up bone and teeth. It also plays an important role in many processes in the body, including energy metabolism, maintenance of acid-base balance, and growth and replacement of tissue. Because almost all foods contain phosphorus, dietary phosphorus deficiency does not usually occur (FNB, 1997).

The recommended intake of phosphorus is 700 mg per day for adults (FNB, 1997). U.S. adults typically consume much more phosphorus than this. Mean intake of U.S. males was 1,495 mg and of females was 1,024 mg (FNB, 1997). Phosphate salts are commonly used as food additives, and nutrient databases may not include phosphorus salts when the phosphorus content of foods is calculated (Calvo & Park, 1996). Thus, phosphorus intakes may be even higher among those who use lots of heavily processed foods. Major food sources of phosphorus among U.S. adults are cow's milk, cheese, beef, yeast breads, and poultry (Cotton et al., 2004).

Phosphorus intakes of vegetarians are similar to those of nonvegetarians (Messina, Mangels, & Messina, 2004). Although vegetarians do not use animal protein, which is quite high in phosphorus, they do use cereals and beans, which are also high in phosphorus. The phosphorus in plant seeds, such as legumes, cereals, and nuts, is in the form of phytic acid. This form of phosphorus is not as well absorbed as

phosphorus from animal foods. Despite this, when young women were placed on a lacto-ovo vegetarian diet for eight weeks, their phosphorus balance was no different from when they were on a nonvegetarian diet for eight weeks (Hunt, Matthys, & Johnson, 1998).

Magnesium

Magnesium is needed for hundreds of enzymes to function properly and is involved in the metabolism of potassium, calcium, and vitamin D. It plays a role in muscle function and promotes resistance to tooth decay. Magnesium deficiency symptoms in normal, healthy people are rare (FNB, 1997). Deficiency can occur due to prolonged vomiting or diarrhea and alcoholism. Low intakes of magnesium have also been associated with an increased incidence of hypertension (Ma et al., 1995; Joffres, Reed, & Yano, 1987) and osteoporosis (Sojka & Weaver, 1995; Tucker et al., 1995), although these associations are controversial and are not supported by all studies.

The recommended intake of magnesium is 400 mg per day for males aged 19–30 years, 420 mg per day for older males, 310 mg per day for females aged 19–30 years, and 320 mg per day for older females (FNB, 1997). Major food sources of magnesium among U.S. adults are cow's milk, yeast breads, coffee, ready-to-eat cereals, potatoes, and beef (Cotton et al., 2004). Drinking water is a variable source of magnesium intake.

Vegetarian diets are frequently much higher in magnesium than are nonvegetarian diets (Messina, Mangels, & Messina, 2004). This is partially because of the use of whole grains, unrefined cereals, vegetables, dried beans, and nuts, all of which are good sources of magnesium. Although the high levels of phytate and fiber that are typically found in vegetarian diets decrease magnesium absorption (Kelsay, Behall, & Prather, 1979; Siener & Hesse, 1995; Wisker et al., 1991), this does not seem to affect magnesium balance (Hunt, Matthys, & Johnson, 1998), and the higher magnesium content of vegetarian diets should compensate for any reduction in absorption (Messina, Mangels, & Messina, 2004).

Iodine

Iodine is a part of the thyroid hormones. Iodine deficiency leads to a variety of problems ranging from mental retardation to a slight enlargement of the thyroid gland. Table salt is fortified with iodine, and this is a major source for most Americans. In other parts of the world, iodine deficiency is a major problem because low levels of iodine in the soil result in low dietary iodine intakes.

The RDA for iodine for adults is 150 mcg (FNB, 2001). Food sources include seafood and sea vegetables, and plants. Water from near the ocean is also frequently high in iodine. Iodine content in plants is quite variable depending on soil content and other factors. Iodine is also found in commercially produced breads, because iodates are used as a dough oxidizer.

Although there are a limited number of studies of iodine status of vegetarians, there is some evidence that vegetarians may be at risk for iodine deficiency. Iodine intake was found to be very low in a study of Swedish vegans (Abdulla et al., 1981), although it should be noted that Sweden has low soil iodine levels. Consumption of plant foods grown on soil that is low in iodine can lead to a very low iodine intake. In another study, iodine intake of vegans was below the British recommendations (Draper et al., 1993); use of iodized salt was not considered. Another study found that 25% of the vegetarians and 80% of the vegans studied suffered from iodine deficiency, compared to 9% of those on a mixed diet (Krajcovicova-Kudlackova et al., 2003). Vegetarians using iodized salt on a daily basis should have adequate intakes of iodine; those not using iodized salt should use other reliable sources of iodine. The most reliable source of iodine, besides iodized salt, is a small daily iodine supplement. Sea vegetables such as kombu or hijiki can serve as alternative iodine sources, but it is easy to get too much iodine from some sea vegetables (Teas, Pino, Critchley, & Braveman, 2004).

Selenium

Selenium is a *trace element*, a substance that is needed in very small amounts by humans. The food content of selenium and other trace elements, including copper and manganese, is quite variable. Such factors as the amount and availability of the metal in the soil in which a plant is grown, food preparation and processing, type and amount of fertilizer, and the containers used for storage and processing can affect the level of a trace element in a plant-based food (Yang et al., 1988).

Selenium functions as an antioxidant along with vitamin E. It also plays a role in thyroid function. Dietary deficiency has been reported in areas of China where soil selenium is low (Yang et al., 1983); toxicity has been reported in areas of China where soil selenium is high (Pennington, Young, & Wilson, 1989).

The adult RDA for selenium is 55 mcg per day for adults (FNB, 2000). Typical North American diets appear to provide ample selenium (Ganapathy & Dhandra, 1980). Seafoods, liver, and kidney are consistently good sources of selenium; plant foods have a variable content depending on where they were grown.

Studies of North American vegetarians find little difference in selenium status between vegetarian and nonvegetarians (Messina, Mangels,

& Messina, 2004; Yang et al., 1988). When diets were planned to represent typical vegan, lacto-ovo vegetarian, and nonvegetarian diets in the United States, the selenium content of all diets was similar and above the minimum recommended intake (Sandstead, 1982). Gibson (1994) concluded that vegetarians are unlikely to be at risk of selenium deficiency.

Copper

Copper is needed for many copper-containing proteins and enzymes, and is used to help form hemoglobin and collagen. Under normal circumstances, dietary copper deficiency is not known to occur in adults.

The RDA for copper is 900 mcg per day for adults (FNB, 2001). Major food sources of copper for U.S. adults are potatoes, yeast breads, tomatoes, beef, ready-to-eat cereals, and dried beans (Cotton et al., 2004).

Vegetarians' diets tend to have more copper than nonvegetarian diets, with vegan diets containing the highest levels of copper (Messina, Mangels, & Messina, 2004; Yang et al., 1988). There has been some concern about the bioavailability of copper from vegetarian diets because of the high fiber and high phytate content of vegetarian diets (Turnlund et al., 1984; Turnlund et al., 1985); in reality, though, phytate and dietary fiber have little adverse effect on copper absorption (Anderson et al., 1983). Copper balance was not different in women on lacto-ovo vegetarian or nonvegetarian diets for eight weeks (Hunt, Matthys, & Johnson, 1998).

High intakes of zinc have been shown to reduce copper bioavailability (Yang et al., 1988). This is unlikely to be problematic for vegetarians, because zinc intakes are typically low. High-protein diets appear to enhance the bioavailability of copper (Yang et al., 1988). Vegetarian diets are typically lower in protein than nonvegetarian diets (Messina, Mangels, & Messina, 2004). The effect of protein may be counterbalanced by the effect of zinc. The copper status of most adult vegetarians in North America appears adequate (Yang et al., 1988).

Chromium

Chromium is needed for proper insulin action to regulate blood glucose levels. Many adults in the United States do not appear to consume adequate chromium. In the case of inadequate intake, chromium supplements can improve impaired glucose tolerance (Anderson et al., 1983).

The AI for adults for chromium is 35 mcg for adult men and 25 mcg for adult women (FNB, 2001). Good sources of chromium include whole-grain products, spices, and nuts. The effect of processing on food levels is variable. Chromium is lost when grains are refined, but chromium can also be added to food during processing and preparation (Anderson, Bryden, & Polansky, 1992; Kumpulainen, 1992; Khan et al., 1990).

The chromium intake of Western vegetarians has not been assessed.

Molybdenum

Molybdenum plays a role in several enzymes. Naturally occurring deficiency is not known.

Molybdenum concentration in foods varies depending on where the food is grown. Important sources of molybdenum for U.S. adults include cow's milk, legumes, breads, and cereals (Tsongas et al., 1980). As these foods play an important role in vegetarian diets, the molybdenum intake of most vegetarians would be expected to be adequate.

The RDA for adults for molybdenum is 45 mcg per day (FNB, 2001).

Table 9.1 Vegetarian Sources of Vitamins and Minerals

Nutrient	Food Sources
Thiamin	Whole grains, legumes, nuts and seeds, orange juice, nutritional yeast, enriched and fortified grains and baked goods. Not found in fats, oils, and refined sugars. Dairy products, vegetables, and most fruits are not good sources.
Riboflavin	Wheat germ, soybeans, mushrooms, leafy green vegetables, sea vegetables, fortified soy milk, avocados, nutritional yeast, whole-grain or enriched breads and cereals, cow's milk, eggs.
Niacin	Fortified cereals and grains, legumes, mushrooms, potatoes, peanuts, peanut butter.
Vitamin B6	Legumes (including soybeans and tempeh), potatoes, walnuts, ready-to-eat cereals, and bananas.
Folate	Leafy vegetables (such as spinach, collard greens, and mustard greens), asparagus, orange juice, legumes, enriched flour, bread, cereals, rolls, buns, corn grits, corn meal, farina, rice, macaroni, and noodles.
Biotin	Egg yolk, soy flour, cereals, yeast.
Pantothenic Acid	Whole-grain cereals, legumes.
Vitamin C	Many fruits and vegetables, especially citrus fruits and juices; tomatoes, potatoes, cabbage, broccoli, and green leafy vegetables.
Vitamin A	Carrots, sweet potatoes, spinach, cantaloupe, pumpkin, kale, winter squash. (These sources provide vitamin A in the form of beta-carotene.)
Vitamin E	Salad dressings and mayonnaise, margarine, ready-to-eat cereals, vegetable oils, unprocessed cereal grains, nuts.
Vitamin K	Broccoli, lettuce, cabbage, asparagus, greens.
Phosphorus	Cereals, beans.
Magnesium	Whole grains, unrefined cereals, vegetables, dried beans, nuts.
Iodine	Vegetarians using iodized salt should have adequate intakes of iodine; those not using iodized salt should use a low-dose iodine supplement.
Selenium	Plant foods grown on selenium-rich soil.
Copper	Yeast breads, potatoes, tomatoes, ready-to-eat cereals, dried beans.
Chromium	Whole-grain products, spices, nuts.
Molybdenum	Legumes, breads, cereals, cow's milk.

Practical Aspects

A vegetarian diet can easily supply all essential nutrients. Table 9.1 gives examples of vegetarian sources of many vitamins and minerals.

Conclusion

Vegetarian diets can provide adequate amounts of thiamin, riboflavin, niacin, vitamin B6, folate, biotin, pantothenic acid, vitamin C, vitamin A, vitamin E, vitamin K, phosphorus, magnesium, iodine, selenium, copper, chromium, and molybdenum. Although some nutrients are less bioavailable from the sources usually found in vegetarian diets, the higher absolute content of those nutrients often compensates for the lower bioavailability. As with almost all food-source nutrients, eating a wide variety of plant foods helps ensure adequate supplies.

References

Abdulla M, Andersson I, Asp NG, et al. Nutrient intake and health status of vegans: Chemical analyses of diets using the duplicate portion sampling technique. *Am J Clin Nutr.* 1981;34:2464-2477.

Anderson RA, Bryden NA, Polansky MM. Dietary chromium intake: Freely chosen diets, institutional diets, and individual foods. *Biol Trace Elem Res.* 1992;32:117-121.

Anderson RA, Polansky MM, Bryden NA, Roginski EE, Mertz W, Glinsmann WH. Chromium supplementation of human subjects: Effects on glucose, insulin, and lipid variables. *Metabolism.* 1983;32: 894-899.

Beatty S, Koh H, Phil M, Henson D, Boulton M. The role of oxidative stress in the pathogenesis of age-related macular degeneration. *Surv Ophthalmol.* 2000;45:115-134.

Block G. Vitamin C and cancer prevention: The epidemiologic evidence. *Am J Clin Nutr.* 1991;53: 270S-283S.

Booth SL, Pennington JAT, Sadowski JA. Food sources and dietary intakes of vitamin K-1 (phylloquinone) in the American diet: Data from the FDA Total Diet Study. *J Am Diet Assoc.* 1996;96:149-154.

Bostick RM, Potter JD, McKenzie DR, Sellers TA, Kushi LH, Steinmetz KA, et. al. Reduced risk of colon cancer with high intakes of vitamin E: The Iowa Women's Health Study. *Cancer Res.* 1993; 15:4230-4237.

Calvo MS, Park YK. Changing phosphorus content of the US diet: Potential for adverse effects on bone. *J Nutr.* 1996;126:1168S-1180S.

Carter EGA, Carpenter KJ. The bioavailability for humans of bound niacin from wheat bran. *Am J Clin Nutr.* 1982;36:855-861.

Cotton PA, Subar AF, Friday JE, Cook A. Dietary sources of nutrients among US adults, 1994-1996. *J Am Diet Assoc.* 2004;104:921-930.

Davey GK, Spencer EA, Appleby PN, Allen NE, Knox KH, Key TJ. EPIC-Oxford: Lifestyle characteristics and nutrient intakes in a cohort of 33,883 meat-eaters and 31,546 non-meat-eaters in the UK. *Public Health Nutr.* 2003;6(3):259-268.

Draper A, Lewis J, Malhotra N, Wheeler E. The energy and nutrient intakes of different types of vegetarians: A case for supplements? *Br J Nutr.* 1993;69(1):3-19 [published erratum appears in *Br J Nutr.* 1993;70(3):812].

Food and Nutrition Board, Institute of Medicine. *Dietary Reference Intakes for Calcium, Phosphorus, Magnesium, Vitamin D, and Fluoride.* Washington, DC: National Academy Press; 1997.

Food and Nutrition Board, Institute of Medicine. *Dietary Reference Intakes for Thiamin, Riboflavin, Niacin, Vitamin B6, Folate, Vitamin B12, Pantothenic Acid, Biotin, and Choline.* Washington, DC: National Academy Press; 1998.

Food and Nutrition Board, Institute of Medicine. *Dietary Reference Intakes for Vitamin A, Vitamin K, Arsenic, Boron, Chromium, Copper, Iodine, Iron, Manganese, Molybdenum, Nickel, Silicon, Vanadium, and Zinc.* Washington, DC: National Academy Press; 2001.

Food and Nutrition Board, Institute of Medicine. *Dietary Reference Intakes for Vitamin C, Vitamin E, Selenium, and Carotenoids.* Washington, DC: National Academy Press; 2000.

Ganapathy SN, Dhandra R. Selenium content of omnivorous and vegetarian diets. *Indian J Nutr Diet.* 1980;17:53-59.

Gey KF. Extra vitamin E beyond PUFA-dependent vitamin E requirement is supplied by olive oil and sunflower oil but not by soybean oil and other oils with insufficient a-tocopherol/PUFA ratio. *Intl J Vitamin Nutr Res.* 1995;65:61-64.

Gibson RS. Content and bioavailability of trace elements in vegetarian diets. *Am J Clin Nutr.* 1994; 59:1223-1232.

Goldsmith GA, Gibbens J, Unglaub WG, Miller ON. Studies on niacin requirements in man. III. Comparative effects of diets containing lime-treated and untreated corn in the production of experimental pellagra. *Am J Clin Nutr.* 1956;4: 151-160.

Graham IM, Daly LE, Refsum HM, et al. Plasma homocysteine as a risk factor for vascular disease: The European Concerted Action Project. *JAMA.* 1997;277:1775-1781.

The Heart Outcomes Prevention Evaluation Study Investigators. Vitamin E supplementation and cardiovascular events in high-risk patients. *N Engl J Med.* 2000;342:154–160.

Hunt JR, Matthys LA, Johnson LK. Zinc absorption, mineral balance, and blood lipids in women consuming controlled lacto-ovo-vegetarian and omnivorous diets for 8 wks. *Am J Clin Nutr.* 1998;67:421–430.

Jacob RA. Vitamin C. In Shils ME, Olson JA, Shike M, Ross AC. eds. *Modern Nutrition in Health and Disease.* 9th ed. Baltimore, MD: Williams & Wilkins; 1999:467–483.

Janelle KC, Barr SI. Nutrient intakes and eating behavior scores of vegetarian and nonvegetarian women. *J Am Diet Assoc.* 1995;95:180–189.

Joffres MR, Reed DM, Yano, K. Relationship of magnesium intake and other dietary factors to blood pressure: The Honolulu heart study. *Am J Clin Nutr.* 1987;45:469–475.

Kang SS, Wong PWK, Malinow MR. Hyperhomocyst(e)inemia as a risk factor for occlusive vascular disease. *Ann Rev Nutr.* 1992;12:279–298.

Kelsay JL, Behall KM, Prather ES. Effect of fiber from fruits and vegetables on metabolic responses of human subjects. II. Calcium, magnesium, iron, and silicon balances. *Am J Clin Nutr.* 1979;32:1876–1880.

Khan A, Bryden NA, Polansky MM, Anderson RA. Insulin potentiating factor and chromium content of selected foods and spices. *Biol Trace Elem Res.* 1990;24:183–188.

Kohlmeier M, Garris S, Anderson JJB. Vitamin K: A vegetarian promoter of bone health. *Vitamin Nutr Intl J.* 1997;1/2:53–57.

Krajcovicova-Kudlackova M, Buckova K, Klimes I, Sebokova E. Iodine deficiency in vegetarians and vegans. *Ann Nutr Metab.* 2003;47(5):183–185.

Kumpulainen JT. Chromium content of foods and diets. *Biol Trace Elem Res.* 1992;32:9–18.

Kushi LH, Folsom AR, Prineas RJ, Mink PJ, Bosick RM. Dietary antioxidant vitamins and death from coronary heart disease in postmenopausal women. *N Engl J Med.* 1996;334:1156–1162.

Larsson CL, Johansson GK. Dietary intake and nutritional status of young vegans and omnivores in Sweden. *Am J Clin Nutr.* 2002;76:100–106.

Leklem JE, Miller LT, Perera AD, Prefers DE. Bioavailability of vitamin B-6 from wheat bread in humans. *J Nutr.* 1980;110:1819–1828.

Lindberg AS, Leklem JE, Miller LT. The effect of wheat bran on the bioavailability of vitamin B-6 in young men. *J Nutr.* 1983;113:2578–2586.

Lloyd T, Schaeffer JM, Walder MA, Demers L. Urinary hormonal concentrations and spinal bone densities of premenopausal vegetarian and nonvegetarian women. *Am J Clin Nutr.* 1991;54:1005–1010.

Lombard KA, Mock DM. Biotin nutritional status of vegans, lactoovovegetarians, and nonvegetarians. *Am J Clin Nutr.* 1989;50:486–490.

Ma J, Folsom AR, Melnick SL, et al. Associations of serum and dietary magnesium with cardiovascular disease, hypertension, diabetes, insulin, and carotid arterial wall thickness: The ARIC study. *J Clin Epidemiol.* 1995;48:927–940.

Mangels AR, Holden JM, Beecher GR, Forman MR, Lanza E. Carotenoid content of fruits and vegetables: An evaluation of analytic data. *J Am Diet Assoc.* 1993;93:284–296.

Mares-Perlman JA, Millen AE, Ficek TL, et al. The body of evidence to support a protective role for lutein and zeaxanthin in delaying chronic disease: Overview. *J Nutr.* 2002;132:518S–524S.

McCann SE, Freudenheim JL, Marshall JR, Graham S. Risk of human ovarian cancer is related to dietary intake of selected nutrients, phytochemicals and food groups. *J Nutr.* 2003;133:1937–1942.

Messina V, Mangels R, Messina M. *The Dietitian's Guide to Vegetarian Diets: Issues and Applications.* 2d ed. Sudbury, MA: Jones and Bartlett Publishers; 2004.

Mills JL, VonKohorn I, Conley, MR, et al. Low vitamin B-12 concentrations in patients without anemia: The effect of folic acid fortification of grain. *Am J Clin Nutr.* 2003;77:1474–1477.

Osganaian SK, Stampfer MF, Rimm E, et al. Dietary carotenoids and the risk of coronary artery disease in women. *Am J Clin Nutr.* 2003;77:1390–1399.

Pennington JAT, Young BE, Wilson DB. Nutritional elements in US diets: Results from the Total Diet Study, 1982-1986. *J Am Diet Assoc.* 1989;89: 659-664.

Rimm EB, Stampfer MJ, Ascherio A, Giovannucci E, Colditz GA, Willett WC. Vitamin E consumption and the risk of coronary heart disease in men. *N Engl J Med.* 1993;328:1450-1456.

Sandstead HH. Copper bioavailability and requirements. *Am J Clin Nutr.* 1982;35:809-814.

Shultz TD, Leklem JE. Vitamin B-6 status and bioavailability in vegetarian women. *Am J Clin Nutr.* 1987;46:647-651.

Siener R, Hesse A. Influence of a mixed and a vegetarian diet on urinary magnesium excretion and concentrations. *Br J Nutr.* 1995;73:783-790.

Sojka JE, Weaver CM. Magnesium supplementation and osteoporosis. *Nutr Rev.* 1995;53:71.

Stampfer MJ, Hennekens CH, Manson JE, Colditz GA, Rosner B, Willett WC. Vitamin E consumption and the risk of coronary disease in women. *N Engl J Med.* 1993;328:1444-1449.

Teas J, Pino S, Critchley A, Braverman LE. Variability of iodine content in common commercially available edible seaweeds. *Thyroid.* 2004;14(10): 836-841.

Tsongas TA, Meglen RR, Walravens PA, Chappell WR. Molybdenum in the diet: An estimate of average daily intake in the United States. *Am J Clin Nutr.* 1980;33:1103-1107.

Tucker K, Kiel DP, Hannan MT, Felson DT. Magnesium intake is associated with bone-mineral density in elderly women. *J Bone Miner Res.* 1995;10:S466.

Turnlund JR, King JC, Gong B, Keyes WR, Michel MC. A stable isotope study of copper absorption in young men: Effect of phytate and alpha-cellulose. *Am J Clin Nutr.* 1985;42:18-23.

Turnlund JR, Michel MC, Keyes WR, Schultz Y, Margen S. Copper absorption in elderly men determined by using stable 65-Cu. *Am J Clin Nutr.* 1984;36:587-591.

Wisker E, Nagel R, Tanudjaja TK, Feldheim W. Calcium, magnesium, zinc, and iron balances in young women: Effects of a low-phytate barley-fiber concentrate. *Am J Clin Nutr.* 1991;54:553-559.

Witting LA, Lee I. Dietary levels of vitamin E and polyunsaturated fatty acids and plasma vitamin E. *Am J Clin Nutr.* 1975;28:571-576.

Wu K, Willett WC, Chan JM, Fuchs CS, Colditz GA, Rimm EB, et al. A prospective study on supplemental vitamin E intake and risk of colon cancer in women and men. *Cancer Epidemiol Biomarkers Prev.* 2002;11:1298-1304.

Yang G, Ge K, Chen J, Chen X. Selenium-related endemic diseases and the daily selenium requirement of humans. *World Rev Nutr Diet.* 1988;55: 98-152.

Yang GQ, Wang S, Zhou R, Sun S. Endemic selenium intoxication of humans in China. *Am J Clin Nutr.* 1983;37:872-881.

10

Heart Disease

Peggy Carlson, MD

Introduction

Heart disease is the leading cause of death in America. An estimated 13 million people in the United States have coronary artery disease (CAD). Each year, 1.5 million people with CAD suffer heart attacks, and half a million people die from CAD (Schaefer, 2002).

Heart attacks are caused by decreased blood flow through the vessels that supply the heart muscle—the coronary arteries. This decreased flow is most typically caused by a narrowing of the vessels due to a buildup of atherosclerotic plaque consisting of cholesterol, cellular debris, clotting material, and calcium. Coronary atherosclerotic changes often begin to appear in Americans in young adulthood and even childhood (Enos, Holmes, & Beyer, 1986; McNamara et al., 1971; Berenson et al., 1992; McGill & Mc-Mahan, 1998).

A vegetarian diet provides protection from coronary artery disease because of many factors. Compared with a nonvegetarian diet, it has a lower saturated fat and cholesterol content and a higher content of fiber and unsaturated fat. Lower rates of hypertension and obesity among vegetarians may also serve as protective factors. Science has also begun focusing attention on other factors that may decrease the risk of CAD, such as antioxidants, soy protein, and phytochemicals. Although the evidence is much less clear, blood-clotting parameters and the iron status of vegetarians may also be protective.

This chapter first looks at the studies linking a vegetarian diet to lower rates of CAD. We then examine each of the protective factors individually, and conclude with a discussion on the use of vegetarian diets for treating CAD.

Summary of the Scientific Literature

Vegetarianism and Risk of Coronary Artery Disease

Although CAD is very common in the United States, in rural societies of China and Japan, where diets are still largely plant-based, CAD is quite rare (Ryde, 1996; Campbell, Parpia, & Chen, 1998; Esselstyn, 1999). A study of 1,001 men from Ireland and Boston also demonstrated decreased mortality from CAD among those whose diet contained more vegetable protein, fiber, and starches; that is, who followed more of a plant-based diet (Kushi et al., 1985).

Several studies that have demonstrated lower rates of CAD among vegetarians have focused on Seventh-Day Adventists (SDAs), who offer a unique opportunity to study vegetarian diets. As a group, they share a similar lifestyle, in that most SDAs abstain from alcohol and tobacco and emphasize family and religious life. However, they differ in that approximately 50% are vegetarian, thus providing researchers an opportunity to examine the effect of a vegetarian diet compared to a nonvegetarian diet in an already health-conscious population.

- In one study (California Adventist Health Study), 25,000 SDAs were examined at baseline and then at 6 and 20 years later. At six years, the risk of fatal CAD among nonvegetarian SDA males, aged 35 to 64 years, was three times greater than that of vegetarian SDA males of comparable age. Vegans had an even lower risk of CAD than lacto-ovo vegetarians. The authors of the study felt that although the difference in risk might be partially accounted for by other risk factors, such as smoking, hypertension, diabetes, obesity, exercise, and use of coffee and dairy products, which are more frequent among nonvegetarians, a significant differential persisted after adjustment for these risk factors. In this study, vegetarian/nonvegetarian status showed little or no relationship to risk of CAD death in males over the age of 65 nor in females of any age (Phillips et al., 1978). This same group was studied again at 20 years. Again, for 45- to 64-year-old men there was approximately a threefold difference in risk of fatal CAD between men who ate meat daily and those who did not

eat meat. The researchers also found that those who had been vegetarian longest were at the least risk. Also, the risk of CAD rose steadily with the frequency of meat consumption. The study found that meat consumption was unrelated to risk in premenopausal women; however, in postmenopausal women the relationship between meat consumption and risk was modest but statistically significant. Once again, similar results were found after correcting for the potential confounding effects of marital status, smoking history, weight, and dairy and coffee consumption (Snowdon, Phillips, & Fraser, 1984).

- A 1997 study of SDAs from California who were more than 84 years old found that beef consumption increased the risk of CAD in men. This was evident even among men who ate beef less than three times per week. Consumption of beef four or more times per week was associated with a twofold relative risk. The study found no association, however, between CAD and beef consumption in the women (Fraser & Shavlik, 1997).
- Data from SDA groups in other countries have shown similar results. In a Dutch study, SDAs had only 43% as many deaths from CAD as did non-SDAs. Because this difference was greater than could be accounted for by the lower prevalence of cigarette smoking among SDAs, the authors concluded that the vegetarian diet played a role in the lower CAD risk (Berkel & de Waard, 1983). In a Norwegian study, the standardized mortality ratio (observed/expected deaths) for CAD was 64% for the SDA vegetarian men. For the SDA vegetarian women, it was 94% (Waaler & Hjort, 1981). In Japan, a 16-year follow-up study of 122,261 men found that those who followed an SDA-like lifestyle (no

smoking, no drinking, no meat consumption, and daily consumption of vegetables) had less than one-half the risk of heart disease as compared with Japanese with opposite lifestyles. The researchers found that even among those who did not smoke or drink, eating meat raised the risk of CAD (Hirayama, 1985). In another study from Japan, where the death rates from CAD in about 7,700 SDAs were compared with CAD death rates in the general Japanese population, no difference was found for the men; however, among women the CAD death rate was significantly less for the SDAs (Kuratsune, Ikeda, & Hayashi, 1986).

Several studies have also looked at the risk of CAD among vegetarians in non-SDA populations:

- Non-SDA vegetarians were compared in a British study of about 5,000 vegetarians and 6,000 nonvegetarians. Approximately 60% of the participants were female. At seven years into the study, the researchers found that vegetarians had a statistically significant decreased risk of mortality from CAD, and that this decreased risk occurred mainly in men. These results did not seem to be due to a confounding effect of smoking (Burr & Sweetnam, 1982). The results were confirmed in a follow-up analysis five years later (Burr & Butland, 1988).

- Another British study compared 4,555 vegetarians with 4,898 meat eaters. In this study, both vegetarian and meat-eating participants ate diets with less saturated fat and more fiber than the average for the British population. The study found a 17% reduction in CAD in vegetarians after adjusting for age, smoking, and social class. The results were not reported by sex. Although not statistically significant, the difference was suggestive. When those with preexisting heart disease were studied, it was found that CAD mortality was significantly lower in the vegetarian/vegan group (Mann et al., 1997).

- A third British Study (the EPIC-Oxford Study) looked at 55,041 participants, of whom 32% were vegetarian. Preliminary results, after approximately a six-year follow-up, showed that the vegetarians had a nonsignificant reduced mortality from all circulatory diseases and CAD (Key et al., 2003).

- The risk for cardiovascular disease was evaluated in an 11-year follow-up of a group of 1,904 "strict" and "moderate" vegetarians in Germany. The strict vegetarians avoided meat and fish completely; the moderate vegetarians ate fish or meat occasionally. For the moderate vegetarians, mortality for CAD was reduced by half when compared to the general German population. For the strict vegetarians, mortality from CAD was only one-quarter that of the general population. Results were not corrected for such factors as socioeconomic status, smoking, and body weight (Chang-Claude, Frentzel-Beyme, & Eilber, 1992).

- A 1998 meta-analysis of 5 prospective studies (including studies mentioned earlier in this list), with a combined total of 76,000 male and female participants and a mean of 10.6 years of follow-up, showed that consuming a vegetarian diet was associated with a 24% reduction in mortality from CAD (Key et al., 1998). This reduction in mortality among vegetarians varied significantly with age: mortality ratios for vegetarians compared to nonvegetarians were 0.55 at less than 65 years of age, 0.69 at 65 to 79 years of age, and 0.92 at 80 to 89 years of age. When the reference group was restricted to those who ate meat at least one time per week, the vegetarians showed a 34% reduction in mortality from CAD.

- Vegetarian diets were also found to have a protective effect against CAD in a study from India, which evaluated 200 patients who were admitted to the hospital with a first heart attack and compared them with 200 age- and sex-matched controls chosen from patients in the hospital's outpatient and elective surgery departments. This protective effect of a vegetarian diet persisted after adjustment for smoking (Pais et al., 1996).

- A study of Chinese women compared 90 vegetarian women who were more than 70 years old with 90 nonvegetarian women of similar age. A vegetarian diet was found to be an independent protective factor for probable ischemic heart disease, as defined by questionnaire, history, and EKG (Kwok et al., 2000).

- One study reported no reduction in mortality from "circulatory diseases" among vegetarians (Kinlen, Hermon, & Smith, 1983). This study looked at the causes of death for 759 members of a vegetarian society and compared them with mortality rates for the general population. In this study the term "circulatory disease" was not defined.

In general, nearly every study has shown a decrease in CAD risk among those consuming a vegetarian diet. A few studies suggest that the protective effect may be greater for men than for women.

Aspects of a Vegetarian Diet That Protect Against Coronary Artery Disease

Many aspects of a vegetarian diet could contribute to the decreased risk in CAD seen with these diets:

- Fats and cholesterol
- Fiber
- Antioxidants
- Soy products
- Iron
- Phytochemicals
- Fruits and vegetables
- Blood clotting
- Hypertension
- Homocysteine
- Body weight

This section investigates these potentially protective aspects.

Fats and Cholesterol

The average American diet contains about 300 mg of cholesterol each day and derives about 32%–34% of its calories from fat, of which about one-third (11%–12% of total calories) is saturated fat. The remainder of fat calories comes from unsaturated (polyunsaturated and monounsaturated) fats and hydrogenated oils (trans fats). The average serum cholesterol in the United States is slightly over 200 mg/dl (Ford et al., 2003).

Many years of research have shown that elevated serum cholesterol is associated with an increased risk for CAD. For every 1% rise in serum cholesterol, the risk of CAD increases by 2%–4%. Therefore, small changes in serum cholesterol can translate into big changes in CAD risk. Studies have also confirmed that lowering total cholesterol is associated with a significant decrease in CAD risk (Schaefer, 2002). International epidemiological studies have shown a near-absence of CAD in populations with serum cholesterols of less than 150 mg/dl (Esselstyn, 1999; Roberts, 1995; Leaf, 1989). Evidence suggests that an elevated cholesterol level must be present before other risk factors become important (Roberts, 1995; Glueck, 1979). For example, it was seen that in Japan, where blood pressure levels are high and smoking is common, CAD was rare because dietary fat intake and serum cholesterol levels were so low (Roberts, 1995; Castelli, 1984).

The greatest determinant of serum cholesterol is the amount of saturated fat and trans fat (partially hydrogenated vegetable fats) in the diet. Dietary cholesterol can also contribute to an elevated serum cholesterol, although the effect is less than that of saturated fats and trans fats. Meat, dairy products, oils, shortening, and eggs are the chief dietary sources of saturated fat in the American diet. Saturated fat can also be found in coconut oil, palm oil, and palm kernel oil. Cholesterol, however, is found only in foods of animal origin. Trans fats can be found in such products as packaged baked goods and margarine.

Saturated fats, trans fats, and cholesterol are not essential nutrients and need not be included in the diet. The human body produces all the cholesterol it needs. Walter Willett, MD, one of the world's experts on nutrition, writes that the optimal intake of cholesterol is probably zero; this, of course, would mean avoiding all animal products (Willett & Sacks, 1991). The scientists who develop the Recommended Dietary Allowances (RDAs) concluded that any amount of saturated fat, trans fat, or cholesterol in the diet increases LDL cholesterol levels and heart disease risk (Food and Nutrition Board, 2002; Glueck, 1979).

Many ecological studies (studies of large populations) and studies of people who have migrated from one culture to another have shown a positive correlation between saturated fat consumption and CAD (Shrapnel et al., 1992; Hu & Willett, 2002; Renaud & Lanzmann-Petithory, 2001). Some, but not all, prospective studies have also found an increased risk of CAD with increased dietary saturated fat (Hu & Willett, 2002; Renaud & Lanzmann-Petithory, 2001; Wolfram, 2003).

Vegetarians eat considerably less saturated fat and less cholesterol than nonvegetarians. Veg-

ans consume less saturated fat than lacto-ovo vegetarians (Messina & Messina, 1996; Resnicow et al., 1991). Vegans, because they eat no animal products, consume no cholesterol.

Studies have shown that vegetarians have lower serum cholesterol levels than nonvegetarians, with vegans having lower values than lacto-ovo vegetarians (Messina & Messina, 1996; Resnicow et al., 1991). Vegans have average cholesterol levels of about 150–158 mg/dl (Resnicow et al., 1991). It is at this level—about 150 mg/dl—that coronary artery atherosclerotic plaques do not form and at which those present shrink. As the level increases above the 150 mg/dl mark, the risk of CAD increases roughly proportionally to the cholesterol level and to the amount of time that the elevated cholesterol level has been present (Roberts, 1995).

Cholesterol is carried in the blood in several lipoproteins, including low-density lipoprotein (LDL) and high-density lipoprotein (HDL). When attached to LDL, cholesterol builds up on the insides of arteries, increasing plaque formation. When attached to HDL, cholesterol is removed from the body.

It is the LDL form of cholesterol (specifically, the oxidized form of LDL cholesterol) that is most correlated with an increased risk of CAD. Lowering LDL cholesterol decreases the risk of CAD (Schaefer, 2002). Compared with meat eaters, vegetarians on average have lower levels of serum LDL cholesterol (Resnicow et al., 1991; Sacks et al., 1985; Barnard, Scherwitz, & Ornish, 1992; Fisher et al., 1986).

HDL cholesterol offers protection from CAD, especially in those at high risk of CAD. The protective effect of HDL cholesterol may, at least in part, be due to the fact that in the HDL form cholesterol is transported out of the body (Lichtenstein, 1996). In addition, some researchers propose that HDL cholesterol may attenuate the atherogenicity of LDL cholesterol (Grundy et al., 1998); therefore, it may be that a low HDL cholesterol level is an additional risk factor for CAD only if LDL and total cholesterol levels are elevated (Roberts, 1995).

Although most studies have not, some studies have suggested that HDL cholesterol levels are lower in vegetarians than in nonvegetarians (Messina & Messina, 1996; Fisher et al., 1986; Masarei et al., 1984). This drop in HDL cholesterol, which can be seen in some individuals consuming vegetarian and low-fat, high-carbohydrate diets, may be attenuated by the presence of fiber or unsaturated fats in the diet (Stone & Van Horn, 2002; Coulston, 1999). The significance of lower levels of HDL cholesterol in those who have low overall cholesterol levels is not known. Some evidence suggests that low HDL cholesterol may not have the same significance in those with low total cholesterol as in those with high total cholesterol. When the total cholesterol level is low, there is less cholesterol to be transported out of the body; therefore, the HDL cholesterol level is low. In countries where very low-fat diets are the norm, the incidence of CAD is much lower than in the United States, despite significantly lower HDL cholesterol. Also, regression of atherosclerosis has been reported in those consuming very-low-fat diets, despite the fact that such diets also lower HDL cholesterol levels (Kenney, Barnard, & Inkeles, 1999).

Despite having possibly lower levels of HDL cholesterol, vegetarians still have a favorable ratio of HDL cholesterol to total cholesterol. The ratio of total cholesterol to HDL cholesterol should, ideally, be less than 4.0 (Castelli, 1998). In a comparison of vegetarians, marathon runners, and males and females with and without CAD, Castelli (1984) found that vegetarians have the best ratio of total cholesterol to HDL cholesterol, averaging about 2.9. He reported that the average American male without CAD has a ratio of 5.1; for females, the ratio is 4.4. The averages for those with CAD were 5.8 and 5.3, respectively.

Both polyunsaturated (safflower, corn, sunflower, cottonseed, sesame, soybean, and fish oils) and monounsaturated (olive and canola oil, peanuts) fats lower total serum cholesterol and LDL cholesterol when they replace saturated fat in the diet (Schaefer, 2002; Lada & Rudel, 2003). Although the effect of the unsaturated fatty acids on HDL cholesterol appear less clear, saturated and monounsaturated fats, and possibly polyunsaturated fats, may elevate HDL cholesterol when they replace carbohydrates in the diet (Hu & Willett, 2002; Lada & Rudel, 2003; Perez-Jimenez, Lopez-Miranda, & Mata, 2002).

A few studies have suggested that monounsaturated fats may decrease the risk of CAD (Perez-Jimenez, Lopez-Miranda, & Mata, 2002; Hu, 2003). It has been hypothesized that monounsaturated fats are the reason for low cholesterol levels and low rates of CAD in southern Italy and Greece, where diets are relatively high in total fat, low in saturated fat, and high in olive oil, which is 70% monounsaturated fat (Kris-Etherton et al., 1988). The Nurses' Health Study, which followed 80,082 women for 14 years, also found that dietary monounsaturated fats were associated with decreased risk of CAD (Kark et al., 2003). Similarly, a Finnish study that followed 21,930 individuals for about 6 years suggested an inverse association of monounsaturated fat and CAD (Pietinen et al., 1997). Early evidence suggests that monounsaturated fats may have a beneficial effect on blood pressure, blood vessels, and blood-clotting mechanisms (Perez-Jimenez, Lopez-Miranda, & Mata, 2002). There is also some evidence that monounsaturated fats may reduce the susceptibility of LDL cholesterol to oxidation (Garg, 1998).

The n-3 long-chain polyunsaturated fatty acids EPA and DHA, and probably their parent compound (the n-3 polyunsaturated fatty acid alpha-linolenic acid), appear to protect against CAD (Lada & Rudel, 2003; Lopez & Ortega, 2003;

von Schacky, 2003; Erikkila et al., 2003; Baylin et al., 2003).This may be due to their effects of decreasing clotting tendencies, lowering blood pressure, and decreasing serum triglycerides, as well as their protective effects on blood vessels themselves, or to their role in preventing heart rhythm irregularities (Lopez & Ortega, 2003, von Schacky, 2003).

The n-6 long-chain polyunsaturated fatty acids have effects opposite those of the n-3 fatty acids. They can cause an increase in blood clotting and inflammatory responses and a constriction of arteries. Studies investigating any association between linoleic acid (the parent fatty acid of the n-6 long-chain polyunsaturated fatty acids) and CAD have been few in number and have yielded conflicting findings (Kark et al., 2003; Vos & Cunnane, 2003).

Epidemiological and dietary intervention studies have shown that substituting unsaturated fats for saturated fats in the diet is more effective in lowering the risk of CAD than simply reducing the total amount of fat (Hu & Willett, 2002). It has been estimated that replacement of 5% energy from saturated fat by unsaturated fat would reduce risk of CAD by 42% (Hu, 2003).

The higher unsaturated fat content of vegetarian diets (Draper et al., 1993) in comparison with meat-based diets may contribute to the low CAD rate in vegetarians. With respect to the n-3 long-chain polyunsaturated fatty acids specifically, vegetarian diets do not appear to offer any advantage over omnivorous diets. Vegans, in particular, appear to have lower levels of EPA and DHA when compared to nonvegetarians. This is because, although alpha-linolenic acid (ALA) is obtained primarily from plant sources, there is limited conversion of ALA to EPA and DHA; the primary sources of dietary EPA and DHA are foods not included in a vegan diet, such as fish and seafood, with eggs also providing a reasonable amount of DHA.

Although unsaturated fats do have beneficial cardioprotective effects, one should not use excessive amounts of unsaturated fat in the diet. All fats are high in calories and, therefore, should be used in moderation when obesity and its resultant health risks (including increased CAD risk) are concerns. In addition, the long-term health consequences of diets high in polyunsaturated fats (more than 10% of total calories) are unknown. Concerns have been voiced about a possible increased risk of cancer and decreased immune function in those with diets high in polyunsaturated fats; however, evidence for this is inconclusive (Dwyer, 1995).

Fiber

Dietary fiber is another factor that may contribute to the low rate of CAD among vegetarians. Vegetarians consume between 50%–100% more fiber than nonvegetarians (Messina & Messina, 1996, Resnicow et al., 1991). Several large prospective epidemiological studies have found significant inverse associations between consumption of cereal fiber or whole grains and coronary artery disease (Truswell, 2002; Pereira & Pins, 2000; Steffen et al., 2003). These studies include the Health Professionals Follow-up Study (43,757 participants), the Iowa Women's Health Study (38,740 women), the U.S. Nurses' Health Study (75,521 nurses), and the Atherosclerosis Risk in Communities (ARIC) Study (11,940 people). A 2004 study analyzed the data from 10 prospective studies and found that each 10-gram-per-day increment of dietary fiber was associated with a 14% decrease in risk of all coronary events and a 27% decrease in coronary-related deaths (Pereira et al., 2004).

Several mechanisms have been proposed to explain the correlation between high cereal fiber and whole-grain intakes and low CAD risk. Soluble fiber, particularly oat fiber, in the diet lowers total blood cholesterol and LDL cholesterol (Glore et al., 1994; Fernandez, 2001). The majority of more than 40 human trials of the effect of oatmeal or oat bran on plasma lipids have found modest reductions (0%–18%) in total and LDL cholesterol (Truswell, 2002). Another explanation may be an increased feeling of fullness due to dietary fiber, which may lead to decreased consumption of food, including total fat, saturated fat, and cholesterol (Dwyer, 1995; Van Horn, 1997). Other factors proposed to explain the protection afforded by fiber include lower blood pressure, better glucose control in diabetics, lower body weight, and favorable effects on blood-clotting factors (Pereira & Pins, 2000).

Evidence also suggests that the protective effects of cereals and whole grains on CAD go beyond the protection afforded by fiber alone (Pereira & Pins, 2000). Other factors in cereals and whole grains that have the potential to affect the risk of CAD include phytoestrogens, antioxidants, unsaturated fats, and vitamins such as folate.

Antioxidants

Considerable evidence now suggests that oxidative chemical reactions, especially the oxidation of LDL cholesterol, play a key role in the development of CAD. When LDL cholesterol is oxidized, it can more readily lead to atherosclerosis in the coronary arteries (Tribble, 1999). Dietary antioxidants appear to decrease the oxidation of LDL cholesterol (Tribble, 1999; Czernichow & Hercberg, 2001).

In studies of antioxidants, particular attention has been given to vitamin E, beta-carotene (β-carotene), and vitamin C, all known to be powerful antioxidants. They are in abundant supply in fruits, vegetables, and grains.

Epidemiological studies, including ecological studies, case-control studies, and prospective studies, indicate that greater antioxidant intake is associated with lower risk of CAD (Tribble, 1999; Czernichow & Hercberg, 2001; Asplund, 2002). Some case-control studies have found lower risk of CAD among those with higher blood concentrations of antioxidant vitamins, although the data have been inconsistent (Marchioli et al., 2001). Interventional trials, however, have generally not substantiated any cardioprotective effects of antioxidants (Czernichow & Hercberg, 2001; Asplund, 2002; Marchioli et al., 2001). One reaon for this difference may be that the interventional studies have looked at dietary supplements, rather than antioxidants from foods. This may be an important difference, because supplements may contain forms of vitamins different from those in foods. In addition, the interventional studies have generally studied only one, or possibly two, antioxidants at a time; such protocols might miss effects due to combinations of antioxidants found in foods.

Vegetarians have higher dietary intakes of both vitamins E and C and beta-carotene. In addition, vegetarians have a higher intake of many phytochemicals, such as flavonoids and polyphenols, which are potent antioxidants (Messina & Messina, 1996). Although the protective effect of these vitamins are attributed primarily to their antioxidant abilities, they may also have other cardioprotective properties, such as effects on blood vessels and blood clotting (Pandya, 2002).

As mentioned previously, there are low rates of CAD in southern Italy and Greece, where diets are low in saturated fat and high in monounsaturated fat. Although one explanation may be the high monounsaturated-fat content in the Mediterranean diet, another explanation may be the increased amounts of antioxidants in the diet, both from the olive oil and from the many fruits and vegetables prevalent in this diet (Jones & Kubow, 1999).

Soy Products

Numerous studies over the past three decades have shown that soy consumption reduces total and LDL cholesterol in hypercholesterolemic individuals (Merz-Demlow et al., 2000; Hermansen et al., 2003); there may also be a cholesterol-lowering effect in individuals with normal cholesterol (Merz-Demlow et al., 2000; Setchell, 2001). These studies have involved both the addition of soy to the diet and the substitution of soy protein for animal protein (Merz-Demlow et al., 2000). The decreases in LDL cholesterol ranged from 4%–21% depending on the individual's initial cholesterol level (Hermansen et al., 2003). A 1995 meta-analysis of 38 studies concluded that consumption of soy protein rather than animal protein significantly decreased serum concentration of total cholesterol and LDL cholesterol in people with hypercholesterolemia, and that these effects were independent of total fat, saturated fat, and cholesterol in the diet (Anderson, Johnstone, & Cook-Newell, 1995). Because decreases in cholesterol are directly related to decreases in CAD, soy protein may be a contributing factor to the lower risk of CAD in vegetarians who eat soy products.

Soy may also decrease CAD risk by means other than its cholesterol-lowering effect (Stone et al., 1996; Clarkson, 2002). Soy protein contains phytochemicals that may reduce the clumping of platelets and the formation of blood clots (Marckmann, Sandstrom, & Jespersen, 1993; Rajaram, 2003). Soy flavonoids also have anti-inflammatory and antioxidant effects and may prevent the oxidation of LDL, thereby reducing CAD risk (Setchell, 2001; Clarkson, 2002; Wiseman et al., 2000). These flavonoids may also have beneficial effects on blood vessels themselves (Clarkson, 2002; Steinberg et al., 2003; Kannel, D'Agostino, & Belanger, 1987; Anthony, 2002). Soy is also a rich source of isoflavonoids, which are phytoestrogens, and which may decrease the risk of coronary artery disease.

Iron

It has been hypothesized that higher body iron stores may increase the risk of CAD. This has theoretical support in that it is the oxidized form of LDL cholesterol, rather than the native form, that is most atherogenic—and iron serves as a catalyst in the formation of free radicals that oxidize LDL cholesterol. Although a few studies have shown that higher iron stores are associated with an increased CAD risk, most studies have not found such a relationship (deValk & Marx, 1999; Haidari et al., 2001). There have, likewise, been conflicting results regarding total dietary iron intake and risk of CAD, with some studies showing a positive association and others showing a negative or no association (deValk & Marx, 1999; Heath & Fairweather-Tait, 2003). In their study, Ascherio et al. (1994) found no association between total iron intake and risk of CAD; however, they further subdivided dietary iron intake into heme iron (found mainly in red meats) and non-heme iron. Having done this, they found that dietary intake of heme iron, though not significantly associated with risk of CAD, was associated with an increased incidence of fatal CAD or nonfatal myocardial infarction. They, as well as others, have hypothesized that high iron stores may worsen heart damage caused by a lack of blood flow to the heart muscles, rather than by promoting atherosclerosis (Ascherio et al., 1994). Although data regarding iron supplements are very limited, there is no evidence that such supplements increase the risk of CAD (deValk & Marx, 1999).

If iron is a risk factor for CAD, then the iron status of vegetarians may decrease their risk. Vegetarians, though they have adequate iron stores, generally have lower stores than omnivores (Messina & Messina, 1996). Also, because they consume no meat, vegetarians consume only non-heme iron.

Phytochemicals

Plant foods contain many chemicals. At least 8,000 of these *phytochemicals*, as they are called, have been identified. Many of these have actions that may protect against CAD.

The flavonoids are some of the most common and most well-studied phytochemicals. More than 4,000 types of flavonoid compounds have been isolated from various plants. Several, but not all, prospective studies have documented an inverse association between flavonoid intake and coronary artery disease (Hu & Willett, 2002; Mojzisova & Kuchta, 2001). Several mechanisms could account for this. Flavonoids, as well as some other phytochemicals (Visioli, Borsani, & Galli, 2000), are antioxidants (Mojzisova & Kuchta, 2001; Visioli, Borsani, & Galli, 2000; Prior, 2003), have anti-platelet activity (Rajaram, 2003; Murphy et al., 2003; Mojzisova & Kuchta, 2001), and may decrease LDL cholesterol (Merz-Demlow et al., 2000; Clarkson, 2002; Wangen et al., 2001; Nestel, 2002). They may also have protective effects on blood vessels themselves (Steinberg et al., 2003; Mojzisova & Kuchta, 2001). Their anti-inflammatory properties may also protect against the development of atherosclerosis (Murphy et al., 2003).

It has long been felt that estrogen protects premenopausal women from CAD. *Phytoestrogens* are plant compounds that are structurally similar to estrogen. They are found in many plant foods, including soy products, cereals, legumes, and vegetables. It has been suggested that phytoestrogens, because of their similarities to estrogen, may protect against heart disease (Cassidy, 2003). In addition, the isoflavone phytoestrogens have been shown to lower LDL cholesterol.

A number of studies have also indicated that *phytosterols* (phytochemicals that are structurally related to cholesterol) reduce serum cholesterol (Jones et al., 1997). An intake of 2 g/day of sterols and stanols (saturated sterols) reduces LDL cholesterol by about 10% (Katan et al., 2003). The mechanism for the cholesterol-lowering effect of phytosterols appears to be a decrease in intestinal cholesterol absorption, which in turn leads to an increase in excretion (St. Onge & Jones, 2003). No trials have been done to determine the effects of phytosterols on the risk of coronary artery disease (Katan et al., 2003).

Fruits and Vegetables

Several studies have found fruit and vegetable intake to be inversely related to the risk of CAD (Hu, 2003; Rastogi et al., 2004; Ness & Powles, 1997), including many recent large prospective studies such as the Nurses' Health Study (Joshipura et al., 2001), the Health Professionals Follow-up Study (Joshipura et al., 2001), the Women's Health Study (Liu et al., 2000), the first National Health and Nutrition Examination Survey Epidemiologic Follow-up Study (Bazzano et al., 2002), and the Physicians' Health Study (Liu et al., 2001). In another large prospective study, the Atherosclerosis Risk in Communities (ARIC) study, fruit and vegetable intake was inversely associated with CAD in African Americans, but not Caucasians (Steffen et al., 2003). Not all epidemiologic studies, however, have found an association between fruit and vegetable intake and risk of heart disease (Ness & Powles, 1997). No interventional studies examining the effects of increased consumption of fruits and vegetables on CAD endpoints (i.e., heart attacks, angina, etc.) have been conducted (Hu, 2003).

Many factors could account for the protective effect of fruits and vegetables. Fruits and vegetables are excellent sources of fiber, phytochemicals, antioxidants, potassium (which has blood-pressure-lowering effects), and vitamins, including folate. Also, diets high in fruits and vegetables may be lower in saturated fat.

Blood Clotting

Another possible factor in the reduced CAD risk of vegetarians is decreased blood clotting. There is a small amount of emerging data in this area. Heart attacks, which are due to blockage of coronary arteries, can be precipitated by blood clots in narrowed arteries; therefore, dietary effects on the blood-clotting mechanism can affect CAD risk.

Some studies have shown a decreased tendency toward blood clotting in individuals on a low-fat, high-fiber diet (Marckmann, Sandstrom, & Jespersen, 1993). Also, a review of five studies that looked at the effect of vegetarian diets on different aspects of blood clotting found indications of a favorable impact of vegetarian diets, although there are not enough data to draw any definitive conclusions (Rajaram, 2003). Although the mechanisms behind any differences in blood clotting between vegetarians and nonvegetarians remain speculative, several possibilities have been proposed.

Many things play a role in the blood-clotting mechanism. These include platelets (blood-clotting cells in the blood), coagulation factors (substances that work together to cause blood to clot), and fibrinolysis (dissolution of fibrin clots). The Framingham study (Kannel, D'Agostino, & Belanger, 1987) and the Northwick Park Heart study (Meade et al., 1980) indicate that elevated factor VII, factor VIII, and fibrinogen (factor I) levels are risk factors for CAD.

Differences in the cholesterol or fatty acid composition of platelets between vegetarians and nonvegetarians may contribute to changes in platelet function (Rajaram, 2003; Fraser, 1994;

Renaud et al., 1986; Sanders & Roshanai, 1992; Ågren et al., 1995). Saturated fat causes platelets to aggregate (Renaud & Lanzmann-Petithory, 2002). The n-6 long-chain polyunsaturated fatty acids have an effect of increasing platelet clumping, whereas the n-3 long-chain polyunsaturated fatty acids produce the opposite effect (Rajaram, 2003; Dutta-Roy, 2002). A vegetarian diet, with its lower saturated fat content, would yield the more beneficial anti-clumping effect. There is also evidence that phytochemicals such as isoflavonoids may reduce the clumping of platelets and perhaps the formation of clots (Rajaram, 2003; Murphy et al., 2003). Two studies that investigated platelet function in vegetarians found increased platelet aggregation compared with nonvegetarians (Rajaram, 2003).

There may also be differences in the individual blood-clotting factors that would make the blood of vegetarians less likely to clot. Several studies have reported lower factor VII levels in vegetarians (Rajaram, 2003; Meade, 1983). Increased fiber levels were shown in one study to decrease factor VII levels. This may account for a difference in factor VII levels in vegetarians (Rajaram, 2003). Some, but not all, studies have shown decreased fibrinogen levels in vegetarians (Rajaram, 2003; Haines et al., 1980; Hostmark et al., 1993). It has also been reported that vegetarians may have less viscous blood (Sanders & Roshanai, 1992; Ernst et al., 1986). The few studies that have looked at factor VIII have found no differences between vegetarians and omnivores (Haines et al., 1980; Mezzano et al., 1999; Pan et al., 1993). The breakdown of blood clots (fibrinolysis) has also been reported to be greater in vegetarians than in nonvegetarians (Rajaram, 2003).

A blockage of the coronary arteries can be caused not only by atherosclerosis and blood clots, but also by constriction of the vessels. Dilation of the vessels would decrease the impediments caused by blockages. There may be differences between vegetarians and omnivores in the ability of blood vessels to dilate. A small study that compared 20 vegetarians with 20 omnivores found better vasodilatory responses among the vegetarians (Lin, Fang, & Gueng, 2001). Along similar lines, very early evidence suggests that folic acid, which is higher in vegetarian diets, may also improve vasodilation (Wilmink et al., 2000).

Hypertension

Vegetarians tend to have lower blood pressures and a lower incidence of hypertension than nonvegetarians (Beilin, 1993). Because hypertension is a risk factor for CAD, this decreased prevalence of hypertension may contribute to the decreased amount of CAD seen among vegetarians.

Homocysteine

Cross-sectional and retrospective studies have found evidence that elevated homocysteine levels are associated with an increased risk of CAD, although several more recent prospective studies have not been as supportive of this conclusion (Pasceri & Willerson, 1999; Falk, Zhou, & Moller, 2001; Taylor, Oudit, & Evans, 2000). It is unclear whether there is a cause-and-effect relationship between homocysteine and CAD, or whether they merely occur together for other reasons. It has also been theorized that homocysteine may play a detrimental role only in persons with established CAD disease, rather than being involved in the development of CAD (Falk, Zhou, & Moller, 2001).

Several factors, including vitamin deficiencies (folic acid, vitamin B12, vitamin B6), smoking, genetics, and some systemic diseases and drugs, can increase plasma homocysteine levels (Guthikonda & Haynes, 1999). Of these, vitamin deficiencies (particularly in folic acid) seem to be strong predictors of elevated homocysteine levels (Pasceri & Willerson, 1999; Guthikonda & Haynes, 1999). Homocysteine levels can be reduced by increasing intake of folic acid and, to a lesser degree, vitamin B12.

Although it has been demonstrated that homocysteine levels can be reduced by increasing intake of folic acid and vitamin B12, it is not known whether a reduction of plasma homocysteine levels by diet and/or vitamin therapy will reduce cardiovascular risk (Taylor, Oudit, & Evans, 2000; Guthikonda & Haynes, 1999; Andreotti et al., 2000). The data from some epidemiologic studies, though not entirely consistent, have shown an inverse association between folate, vitamin B6, and occasionally vitamin B12 intake and risk of CAD (Hu & Willett, 2002; Taylor, Oudit, & Evans, 2000). In addition, two controlled trials found evidence of decreased atherosclerosis in those receiving folate supplementation (Hu & Willett, 2002). Irrefutable proof that homocysteine actually causes CAD will come only if interventions to lower plasma homocysteine also are shown to decrease CAD (Andreotti et al., 2000).

Plasma homocysteine levels are lower in those with higher folate intake. Because vegetarians consume considerably more folate than nonvegetarians, there has been speculation that this increased folate consumption may be another protective mechanism of a vegetarian diet. To a lesser degree, homocysteine levels are higher in those with lower vitamin B12 and vitamin B6 levels. Vegetarians appear to have adequate vitamin B6 intake, although vitamin B12 intakes tend to be lower in vegetarians, particularly in vegans. Therefore, the higher folate levels found in vegetarian diets would tend to lower homocysteine levels, while lower vitamin B12 levels would tend to raise homocysteine levels.

A few studies have compared homocysteine levels between vegetarians and omnivores. In 1999, two population studies were published that compared homocysteine levels in meat eaters, lacto-ovo vegetarians, and vegans (Mezzano et al., 1999; Mann et al., 1999). Both studies found higher homocysteine levels in the vegetarians than in the nonvegetarians. Because in both studies serum vitamin B12 levels were lower in the vegetarians, and serum folate levels were either the same or higher in the vegetarians, the authors concluded that the increase in homocysteine levels in the vegetarians could be attributed to their lower vitamin B12 levels. A 2001 study that compared 44 high meat eaters, 19 low meat eaters, 34 lacto-ovo vegetarians, and 7 vegans found elevated homocysteine levels in the lacto-ovo vegetarians and even higher levels in the vegans (Herrmann et al., 2001). Similarly, a 2002 study from Taiwan compared 45 vegetarians with 45 nonvegetarians and found higher homocysteine levels in the vegetarians (Hung et al., 2002). In contrast to the population studies, an interventional study published in 2000 placed participants on a vegan diet, with moderate exercise, stress management, and exclusion of tobacco, alcohol, and caffeine. They found that after one week, participants' homocysteine levels had decreased by 13% (DeRose et al., 2000). The significance of any difference in homocysteine levels in vegetarians is unknown.

Body Weight

Studies have shown that vegetarians have lower body weights than nonvegetarians. Because obesity is a risk factor for the development of CAD, this leanness factor may contribute to a lower risk of CAD among vegetarians.

Vegetarian Diets and Treatment of Coronary Artery Disease

In addition to serving a preventive function, vegetarian diets have also been shown to be effective in reversing established CAD. In contrast to the results seen with vegetarian diets, studies have found that in the majority of patients on more traditional low-fat, "heart-friendly" diets, which allow meat and up to 30% fat, coronary artery lesions continue to progress (Esselstyn, 1999; Ornish, 1990).

Ornish compared the effect of diet, exercise, and stress management on a group of 46 patients with CAD who were studied for 24 days. One-half of the patients underwent stress management training, participated in a physical exercise program, and consumed an essentially vegan diet (minimal amounts of nonfat yogurt were allowed) with an average daily cholesterol content of 5 mg. The control group was not asked to make any lifestyle changes. Compared with the control group, the lifestyle-change group demonstrated a 44% mean increase in duration of exercise, improved heart muscle function, and a 91.0% mean reduction in frequency of anginal episodes. At the completion of the study, the average cholesterol level of the experimental group had gone from 229 mg/dl to 182 mg/dl and that of the control group had gone from 221 mg/dl to 215 mg/dl (Ornish et al., 1983).

In a later study, patients with coronary artery disease were studied by injecting dye into their blood vessels and then taking X-rays to visualize the coronary arteries (angiography). The 28 patients assigned to the experimental group consumed a low-fat vegetarian diet (no animal products except egg whites and minimal amounts of nonfat milk or yogurt) that contained 10% calories as fat (polyunsaturated: saturated ratio greater than 1) and restricted cholesterol to less than 5 mg/day. They also stopped smoking and participated in stress management training and exercise programs. Control-group patients were not asked to make any lifestyle changes, although they were free to do so. On average, the diet of the control-group patients contained about 30% of calories as fat and 190 mg of cholesterol daily. Overall, after one year, 82% of the experimental group had regression of their coronary artery stenosis (decreases in the blockage in the arteries around the heart); 17% had slight progression; and 1 patient, who had poor adherence to the program, had progression. Average percent diameter stenosis of the coronary arteries regressed from 40.0% to 37.8%. In the control group, 53% showed progression, 42% showed regression, and 5% showed no change. Also, in the control group, average percent diameter stenosis progressed from 42.7% to 46.1%. Patients in the experimental group reported a 91% reduction in the frequency of angina, a 42% reduction in the duration of angina, and a 28% reduction in the severity of angina. In contrast, control-group patients reported a 165% increase in frequency, a 95% increase in duration, and a 39% increase in the severity of their angina. In the experimental group, LDL cholesterol decreased by 40%, versus 1.2% in the control group. After 12 months, the average blood cholesterol level of the experimental group fell from 227mg/dl to 172 mg/dl and that of the control group fell from 245 mg/dl to only 231 mg/dl (Ornish et al., 1990).

This group of patients was studied again at five years. Again, the experimental group participated in the same lifestyle changes detailed for the first study. Control-group patients were asked to follow the advice of their personal physicians, with the result that their average diet had about 25% of calories from fat. In the experimental group, the average percent diameter stenosis had decreased by 3.1%, whereas in the control group it had increased by 11.8%. At five years, there was no statistical difference in the LDL cholesterol levels between the two groups (about 20% below baseline in both groups); however, 9 (60%) of the control-group participants had begun taking cholesterol-lowering drugs. Patients in the control group who did not take lipid-lowering drugs showed more than three times as much progression in stenosis. No experimental-group patient took lipid-lowering drugs, yet they showed better response in cholesterol levels than the control-group patients who did. Notably, HDL cholesterol levels decreased in the experimental group, although the ratio of LDL cholesterol to HDL cholesterol was improved and CAD decreased (Ornish et al., 1998).

Gould et al. reported on a group of 35 patients with known CAD, of whom 20 were placed on the same near-vegan diet as described above, as well as being placed on programs for exercise and stress management. Control-group patients remained under the care of their regular physicians for treatment and lifestyle recommendations. Both at the start of the study and after five years, the blood flow to the heart was studied. The researchers found that the blood flow to the heart had improved in the experimental group, but had worsened in the control group. The average serum cholesterol of the experimental group had decreased from 225 mg/dl to 175 mg/dl; that of the control group decreased from 250 mg/dl to 230mg/dl (Gould et al., 1995).

Ellis reported on four individuals with severe angina who were treated with a vegan diet. All experienced complete relief of their symptoms by the fifth or sixth month of the study. A follow-up after five years showed no return of their symptoms (Ellis & Sanders, 1977). Similarly, Ryde (1996) reported on two patients treated with a vegetarian diet who had significant relief of their angina.

In the Leiden Intervention Trial, 39 patients with known CAD were placed on a vegetarian diet that had a cholesterol content of less than 100 mg per day, a polyunsaturated:saturated fat ratio of at least 2, and 6.6% of calories from saturated fat. (Adherence to the diet could not be documented for several patients.) There were no other lifestyle changes. After 24 months, the patients' coronary arteries were reassessed by angiography. Eighteen (46%) of the patients showed no lesion progression and 21 (54%) of the patients had progression of the lesions. The researchers noted that in comparison to those who had lesion progression, the 18 patients with no progression had significantly lower values than the controls for total blood cholesterol and total/HDL cholesterol both at the beginning of the study (total cholesterol of 248 mg/dl vs. 287 mg/dl and total/HDL cholesterol of 5.8 vs. 8.1) and during the two years of intervention (total cholesterol of 224 mg/dl vs. 252 mg/dl and total/HDL cholesterol of 5.7 vs. 7.1). In addition, no progression was observed in those who had lower values for total/HDL cholesterol (<6.9) throughout the trial or who had high values (>6.9) that were significantly lowered by dietary intervention (Arntzenius et al., 1985).

Another study reported on 11 patients with known cardiac disease who were treated with a cholesterol-lowering drug and a vegetarian diet that derived less than 10% of calories from fat and eliminated all animal products except skim milk and nonfat yogurt. Patients did not participate in regular stress management or exercise programs. After an average follow-up of 5.5 years, the mean serum cholesterol had dropped from 246 mg/dl to 132 mg/dl. When the total of 25 coronary lesions were analyzed by percent stenosis, 11 had regressed and 14 had remained stable. Angina, initially reported by nine patients, was eliminated in two and reduced in seven. In contrast, of 5 patients who

were released from the project after 12 and 15 months because they did not adhere to the diet, all had further heart-related acute events. Of the patients who did adhere to the diet, all but one had no acute heart-related events (Esselstyn et al., 1995; Esselstyn & Favaloro, 1998).

This same author reported a further follow-up seven years after the conclusion of the five-year study. All but one patient had continued to adhere to the diet and medication. The group's mean serum cholesterol remained low, at 145 mg/dl. Adherent patients had experienced no extension of clinical disease, no coronary events, and no procedural interventions such as angioplasty (procedure to unblock the blood vessels that supply the heart). This is especially compelling given that the entire group of patients had experienced multiple coronary events in the eight years before the study began (Esselstyn, 1999).

The Indian Health Study followed two groups of patients, all with a definite or possible heart attack or angina. Both groups were advised to follow a fat-reduced diet. In addition, one group was given a semi-vegetarian diet and advised to eat more fruits, vegetables, nuts, and grain products. The semi-vegetarian diet reduced coronary death by 41% and nonfatal myocardial infarction (MI) by 38% after one year (Singh et al., 1992).

In general, these studies show that vegetarian diets that are very low in saturated fat and cholesterol and that eliminate most animal products can be part of an effective program to treat CAD. The best results were obtained when serum cholesterol levels approached 150 mg/dl (Gould, 1994). In many of these studies, the improvement in CAD was obtained using a low-fat vegetarian diet in combination with stress management and/or exercise programs. It would be interesting to study the effectiveness of vegetarian and vegan diets that are not necessarily low in total fat, but that are low in cholesterol and saturated fat.

Practical Aspects

A well-balanced vegetarian diet low in saturated fats, trans fats, and cholesterol is protective against CAD. Saturated fats, trans fats, and cholesterol are not essential nutrients and need not be included in any diet. Eliminating meat from the diet significantly reduces the intake of saturated fat and cholesterol, thereby reducing the risk for CAD. Saturated fats and cholesterol can also be found in nonmeat products, such as dairy products, oils, fats, and eggs. For best reduction of CAD risk, these foods, if eaten at all, should be used in limited amounts. The tropical oils (coconut oil, palm oil, and palm kernel oil) also contain saturated fat and should be used sparingly. Vegetable oils contain some, but much less, saturated fat. Trans fats, which act like saturated fat in that they increase the body's cholesterol level, should be avoided.

The optimal percentage of total fat in the diet is currently a matter of debate within the scientific community. The World Health Organization recommends a lower limit of 15% and an upper limit of 30% on total dietary fat for the general population (James et al., 1991). Some healthy populations do regularly consume diets very low in fat. Dietary fat consumption in rural counties of China varies from 6% to 24%, with an average of 14.5% (Campbell & Junshi, 1994). In rural China, animal product consumption is low, heart disease is uncommon, and the average serum cholesterol is 127 (Campbell, Parpia, & Chen, 1998). Native Japanese derived 15% of calories from fat, and in Taiwan in 1950 fat consumption was 16% (Lichtenstein & Van Horn, 1998). Also, as noted in the previous section, Ornish used a diet of approximately 10% fat in his studies that have shown reversal of CAD. However, the American Heart Association has voiced concerns about recommending a diet containing less than 15% fat for the general population, because of concerns that definitive data are lacking on the nutritional adequacy of very-low-fat diets (less than 15% fat) for young children, pregnant women, the elderly, and after long-term adherence (Lichtenstein & Van Horn, 1998).

There is also compelling evidence to suggest that the type of fat in the diet may be more important than the amount of fat consumed. Monounsaturated and polyunsaturated fats have many effects that protect against CAD, whereas saturated and trans fats have effects that contribute to CAD. The World Health Organization puts a lower limit of 3% and an upper limit of 7% on the amount of polyunsaturated fat that should be in the diet. The World Health Organization does not place either an upper or a lower limit on monounsaturated fat, but states that the amount of monounsaturated fat should make up the difference between the recommended total fat in the diet and the rest of the fats in the diet (James et al., 1991).

Recent epidemiologic studies suggest that the long-chain n-3 fatty acids (EPA and DHA), and possibly their parent compound, alpha-linolenic acid, decrease the risk of CAD. Because the primary sources of EPA and DHA are fish and seafood, vegetarians should make conscious efforts to get good sources of alpha-linolenic acid. For lacto-ovo vegetarians, eggs can provide a limited amount of DHA. Also, a small amount of DHA can be converted to EPA. Because there is no EPA or DHA in plant-based foods, except for sea plants such as microalgae and seaweed, vegans must rely on the synthesis of these n-3 long-chain fatty acids from alpha-linolenic acid. Some reports recommend that vegetarians consume at least double the standard recommended intake for alpha-linolenic acid. Good plant sources of alpha-linolenic acid are flaxseed, soybeans, and walnuts, as well as flaxseed oil, soybean oil, walnut oil, and canola oil (Davis & Kris-Etherton, 2003; Kris-Etherton et al., 2000).

In addition to limiting saturated fat and cholesterol, a healthy vegetarian diet should be well balanced and contain plenty of fruits and vegetables, fiber, folate, and antioxidant-rich foods for optimal heart health. Total calorie intake should be that which maintains optimal body weight. Plant foods rich in phytosterols, such as vegetable oils, may offer further benefit. Foods rich in phytoestrogens (such as soy) and other phytochemicals may also offer further benefit. Vitamin B12 intake should be adequate.

Conclusion

Vegetarian diets offer protection against the development of CAD. They have also been successful in reversing established CAD. Many factors may contribute to these benefits. The lower saturated fat and cholesterol content of a vegetarian diet, as opposed to a nonvegetarian diet, as well as its higher content of unsaturated fat and dietary fiber, probably play important roles. In addition, their lower rates of hypertension and decreased incidence of obesity may serve to protect vegetarians. The presence of fruits, vegetables, and soy products in the vegetarian diet may be other contributing factors.

Science is also studying additional potentially protective factors, such as antioxidants and phytochemicals. Preliminary evidence suggests that blood-clotting parameters in vegetarians may offer some protection. Although vegetarians do tend to have lower iron stores than omnivores, the benefit of this is unclear because any relationship between iron and increased CAD remains unproven.

References

Ågren JJ, Törmälä ML, Nenonen MT, Hänninen OO. Fatty acid composition of erythrocyte, platelet, and serum lipids in strict vegans. *Lipids*. 1995; 30(4):365–369.

Anderson JW, Johnstone BM, Cook-Newell ME. Meta-analysis of the effects of soy protein intake on serum lipids. *N Engl J Med*. 1995;333(5):276–282.

Andreotti F, Burzotta F, Manzoli A, Robinson K. Homocysteine and risk of cardiovascular disease. *J Thromb Thrombolysis*. 2000;9(1):13–21.

Anthony MS. Phytoestrogens and cardiovascular disease: Where's the meat? *Arterioscler Thromb Vasc Biol*. 2002;22(8):1245–1247.

Arntzenius AC, Kromhout D, Barth JD, et al. Diet, lipoproteins, and the progression of coronary atherosclerosis: The Leiden Intervention Trial. *N Engl J Med*. 1985;312(13):805–811.

Ascherio A, Willett WC, Rimm EB, et al. Dietary iron intake and risk of coronary disease among men. *Circulation*. 1994;89(3):969–974.

Asplund K. Antioxidant vitamins in the prevention of cardiovascular disease: A systematic review. *J Intern Med*. 2002;251(5):372–392.

Barnard ND, Scherwitz LW, Ornish D. Adherence and acceptability of a low-fat, vegetarian diet among patients with cardiac disease. *J Cardiopulmonary Rehabil*. 1992;12:423–431.

Baylin A, Kabagambe E, Ascherio A, et al. Adipose tissue a-linolenic acid and nonfatal acute myocardial infarction in Costa Rica. *Circulation*. 2003;107: 1586.

Bazzano LA, He J, Ogden LG, et al. Fruit and vegetable intake and risk of cardiovascular disease in U.S. adults: The first National Health and Nutrition Examination Survey Epidemiologic Follow-up Study. *Am J Clin Nutr*. 2002; 76(1):93–99.

Beilin LJ. Vegetarian diets, alcohol consumption, and hypertension. *Ann NY Acad Sci*. 1993;676: 83–91.

Berenson GS, Wattigney WA, Tracy RE, et al. Atherosclerosis of the aorta and coronary arteries and cardiovascular risk factors in persons aged 6 to 30 years and studied at necropsy (The Bogalusa Heart Study). *Am J Cardiol*. 1992;70(9): 851–858.

Berkel J, de Waard F. Mortality pattern and life expectancy of Seventh-Day Adventists in the Netherlands. *Intl J Epidemiol*. 1983;12(4):455–459.

Burr ML, Butland, BK. Heart disease in British vegetarians. *Am J Clin Nutr.* 1988;48(3, Suppl): 830-832.

Burr ML, Sweetnam PM. Vegetarianism, dietary fiber, and mortality. *Am J Clin Nutr.* Nov 1982;36(5): 873-877.

Campbell TC, Junshi C. Diet and chronic degenerative diseases: Perspectives from China. *Am J Clin Nutr.* 1994;59(5, Suppl):1153S-1161S.

Campbell TC, Parpia B, Chen J. Diet, lifestyle, and the etiology of coronary artery disease: The Cornell China study. *Am J Cardiol.* 1998;82(10B): 18T-21T.

Cassidy A. Potential risks and benefits of phytoestrogen-rich diets. *Intl J Vit Nutr Res.* 2003; 73(2):120-126.

Castelli WP. The new pathophysiology of coronary artery disease. *Am J Cardiol.* 1998;82(10B): 60T-65T.

Castelli WP. Epidemiology of coronary heart disease: The Framingham Study. *Am J Med.* 1984; 76(2A):4-12.

Chang-Claude J, Frentzel-Beyme R, Eilber U. Mortality pattern of German vegetarians after 11 years of follow up. *Epidemiology.* 1992;3(5):395-401.

Clarkson TB. Soy, soy phytoestrogens and cardiovascular disease. *J Nutr.* 2002;132(3):566S-569S.

Coulston AM. The role of dietary fats in plant-based diets. *Am J Clin Nutr.* 1999;70(3, Suppl):512S-515S.

Czernichow S, Hercberg S. Interventional studies concerning the role of antioxidant vitamins in cardiovascular diseases: A review. *J Nutr Health Aging.* 2001;5(3):188-195.

Davis B, Kris-Etherton PM. Achieving optimal essential fatty acid status in vegetarians: Current knowledge and practical implications. *Am J Clin Nutr.* 2003;78(3, Suppl):640S-646S.

DeRose DJ, Charles-Marcel ZL, Jamison JM, et al. Vegan diet-based lifestyle program rapidly lowers homocysteine levels. *Prev Med.* 2000;30(3): 225-233.

deValk B, Marx JJ. Iron, atherosclerosis, and ischemic heart disease. *Arch Intern Med.* 1999;159(14): 1542-1548.

Draper A, Lewis J, Malhotra N, Wheeler E. The energy and nutrient intakes of different types of

vegetarian: A case for supplements? *Br J Nutr.* 1993;69(1):3-19 [published erratum appears in *Br J Nutr.* 1993;70(3):812].

Dutta-Roy AK. Dietary components and human platelet activity. *Platelets.* 2002;13(2):67-75.

Dwyer J. Overview: Dietary approaches for reducing cardiovascular disease risks. *J Nutr.* 1995; 125(3, Suppl):656S-665S.

Ellis FR, Sanders TA. Angina and vegan diet. *Am Heart J.* 1977;93(6):803-805.

Enos WF, Holmes RH, Beyer J. Coronary disease among United States soldiers killed in action in Korea. *JAMA.* 1986;256(20):2859-2862.

Erikkila A, Lehto S, Pyorala K, Uusitupa M. n-3 fatty acids and 5-y risks of death and cardiovascular disease events in patients with coronary artery disease. *Am J Clin Nutr.* 2003;78(1):65-71.

Ernst E, Pietsch L, Matrai A, Eisenberg J. Blood rheology in vegetarians. *Br J Nutr.* 1986;56(3): 555-560.

Esselstyn CB Jr. Updating a 12-year experience with arrest and reversal therapy for coronary heart disease (an overdue requiem for palliative cardiology). *Am J Cardiol.* 1999;84(3):339-341.

Esselstyn CB, Ellis SG, Medendorp SV, Crowe TD. A strategy to arrest and reverse coronary artery disease: A 5-year longitudinal study of a single physician's practice. *J Fam Prac.* 1995;41(6): 560-568.

Esselstyn CB, Favaloro R. Introduction: More than coronary artery disease. *Am J Cardiol.* 1998; 82(10B):5T-9T.

Falk E, Zhou J, Moller J. Homocysteine and atherothrombosis. *Lipids.* 2001;36(Suppl):S3-S11.

Fernandez ML. Soluble fiber and nondigestible carbohydrate effects on plasma lipids and cardiovascular risk. *Curr Opin Lipidol.* 2001;12(1):35-40.

Fisher M, Levine PH, Weiner B, et al. The effect of vegetarian diets on plasma lipid and platelet levels. *Arch Intern Med.* 1986;146(6):1193-1197.

Food and Nutrition Board, Institute of Medicine. *Dietary Reference Intakes for Energy, Carbohydrate, Fiber, Fat, Fatty Acids, Cholesterol, Protein, and Amino Acids (Macronutrients).* Washington, DC: National Academy Press, 2002.

Ford ES, Mokdad AH, Giles WH, Mensah GA. Serum total cholesterol concentrations and awareness, treatment, and control of hypercholesterolemia among US adults. *Circulation.* 2003;107(17): 2185–2189.

Fraser GE. Diet and coronary heart disease: Beyond dietary fats and low-density-lipoprotein cholesterol. *Am J Clin Nutr.* 1994;59(5, Suppl):1117S–1123S.

Fraser GE, Shavlik DJ. Risk factors for all-cause and coronary heart disease mortality in the oldest-old. *Arch Intern Med.* 1997;157(19):2249–2258.

Garg A. High-monounsaturated-fat diets for patients with diabetes mellitus: A meta-analysis. *Am J Clin Nutr.* 1998;67(3, Suppl):577S–582S.

Glore SR, Van Treeck D, Knehans AW, Guild M. Soluble fiber and serum lipids: Literature review. *J Am Dietetic Assoc.* 1994;94(4):425–436.

Glueck CJ. Dietary fat and atherosclerosis. *Am J Clin Nutr.* 1979;32(12, Suppl):2703–2711.

Gould KL. Reversal of coronary atherosclerosis: Clinical promise as the basis for noninvasive management of coronary artery disease. *Circulation.* 1994;90(3):1558–1571.

Gould KL, Ornish D, Scherwitz L, et al. Changes in myocardial perfusion abnormalities by positron emission tomography after long-term, intense risk factor modification. *JAMA.* 1995;274(11): 894–901.

Grundy SM, Balady GJ, Criqui MH, et al. Primary prevention of coronary heart disease: Guidance from Framingham: A statement for healthcare professionals from the AHA Task Force on Risk Reduction. American Heart Association. *Circulation.* 1998;97(18):1876–1887.

Guthikonda S, Haynes WG. Homocysteine as a novel risk factor for atherosclerosis. *Curr Opin Cardiol.* 1999;14(4):283–291.

Haidari M, Javadi E, Sanati A, et al. Association of increased ferritin with premature coronary stenosis in men. *Clin Chem.* 2001;47(9):1666–1672.

Haines AP, Chakrabarti R, Fisher D, et al. Haemostatic variables in vegetarians and nonvegetarians. *Thromb Res.* 1980;19(1–2):139–148.

Heath AM, Fairweather-Tait SJ. Health implications of iron overload: The role of diet and genotype. *Nutr Rev.* 2003;61(2):45–62.

Hermanscn K, Dinesen B, Hoie IH, et al. Effects of soy and other natural products on LDL:HDL ratio and other lipid parameters: A literature review. *Adv Ther.* 2003;20(1):50–78.

Herrmann W, Schorr H, Purschwitz K, et al. Total homocysteine, vitamin B(12), and total antioxidant status in vegetarians. *Clin Chem.* 2001;47(6): 1094–1101.

Hirayama, T. Mortality in Japanese with life-styles similar to Seventh-Day Adventists: Strategy for risk reduction by life-style modification. *Natl Cancer Inst Monographs.* 1985;69:143–153.

Hostmark A, Lystad E, Vellar OD, et al. Reduced plasma fibrinogen, serum peroxides, lipids, and apolipoproteins after a 3-week vegetarian diet. *Plant Foods Hum Nutr.* 1993;43(1):55–61.

Hu FB. Plant-based foods and prevention of cardiovascular disease: An overview. *Am J Clin Nutr.* 2003;78(3, Suppl):544S–551S.

Hu FB, Willett WC. Optimal diets for prevention of coronary heart disease. *JAMA.* 2002;288(20): 2569–2578.

Hung CJ, Huang PC, Lu SC, et al. Plasma homocysteine levels in Taiwanese vegetarians are higher than those of omnivores. *J Nutr.* 2002;132(2): 152–158.

James WP (Chair), Beaton G, Chung-Ming C, et al. for the World Health Organization (excerpted by editors of *Nutrition Review*). Diet, nutrition, and the prevention of chronic diseases: A report of the WHO Study Group on Diet, Nutrition and Prevention of Noncommunicable Diseases. *Nutr Rev.* Oct 1991;49(10):291–301.

Jones P, Kubow S. Lipids, sterols, and their metabolites. In: Shils M, Olson J, Shihe M, Ross A, eds. *Modern Nutrition in Health and Disease.* Baltimore, MD: Lippincott Williams and Wilkins; 1999.

Jones PJ, MacDougall D, Ntanios F, Vanstone C. Dietary phytosterols as cholesterol-lowering agents in humans. *Can J Physiol Pharmacol.* 1997;75(3):217–227.

Joshipura KJ, Hu FB, Manson JE, et al. The effect of fruit and vegetable intake on risk for coronary heart disease. *Ann Intern Med.* 2001;134(12): 1106–1114.

Kannel W, D'Agostino RB, Belanger AJ. Fibrinogen, cigarette smoking, and risk of cardiovascular disease: Insights from the Framingham study. *Am Heart J.* 1987;113(4):1006–1010.

Kark JD, Kaufmann NA, Binka F, et al. Adipose tissue n-6 fatty acids and acute myocardial infarction in a population consuming a diet high in polyunsaturated fatty acids. *Am J Clin Nutr.* 2003; 77(4):796-802.

Katan MB, Grundy SM, Jones P, et al. Efficacy and safety of plant stanols and sterols in the management of blood cholesterol levels. *Mayo Clin Proc.* 2003;78(8):965-978.

Kenney JJ, Barnard RJ, Inkeles S. Very-low-fat diets do not necessarily promote small, dense LDL particles. *Am J Clin Nutr.* 1999;70(3):423-424.

Key TJ, Appleby PN, Davey GK, et al. Mortality in British vegetarians: Review and preliminary results from EPIC-Oxford. *Am J Clin Nutr.* 2003; 78(3, Suppl):533S-538S.

Key TJ, Fraser GE, Thorogood M, et al. Mortality in vegetarians and non-vegetarians: A collaborative analysis of 8300 deaths among 76,000 men and women in five prospective studies. *Public Health Nutr.* 1998;1(1):33-41.

Kinlen LJ, Hermon C, Smith PG. A proportionate study of cancer mortality among members of a vegetarian society. *Br J Cancer.* 1983;48(3): 355-361.

Kris-Etherton PM, Krummel D, Russell ME, et al. The effect of diet on plasma lipids, lipoproteins, and coronary heart disease. *J Am Diet Assoc.* 1988; 88(11):1373-1400.

Kris-Etherton PM, Taylor DS, Yu-Poth S, et al. Polyunsaturated fatty acids in the food chain in the United States. *Am J Clin Nutr.* 2000;71(1, Suppl): 179S-188S.

Kuratsune M, Ikeda M, Hayashi T. Epidemiologic studies on possible health effects of intake of pyrolyzates of foods, with reference to mortality among Japanese Seventh-Day Adventists. *Envir Health Persp.* 1986;67:143-146.

Kushi LH, Lew RA, Stare FJ, et al. Diet and 20-year mortality from coronary heart disease: The Ireland-Boston Diet-Heart Study. *N Engl J Med.* 1985;312(13):811-818.

Kwok TK, Woo J, Ho S, Sham A. Vegetarianism and ischemic heart disease in older Chinese women. *J Am Coll Nutr.* 2000;19(5):622-627.

Lada AT, Rudel LL. Dietary monounsaturated versus polyunsaturated fatty acids: Which is really better for protection from coronary heart disease? *Curr Opin Lipidol.* 2003;14(1):41-46.

Leaf, A. Management of hypercholesterolemia: Are preventive interventions advisable? *N Engl J Med.* 1989;321(10):680-684.

Lichtenstein AH. Atherosclerosis. In: Ziegler EE, Filer LJ, eds. *Present Knowledge in Nutrition.* Washington, DC: ILSI Press; 1996.

Lichtenstein AH, Van Horn L. Very low fat diets. *Circulation.* 1998;98(17):1828.

Lin CL, Fang TL, Gueng MK. Vascular dilatory functions of ovo-lacto vegetarians compared with omnivores. *Atherosclerosis.* 2001;158(1):247-251.

Liu S, Lee IM, Ajani U, et al. Intake of vegetables rich in carotenoids and risk of coronary heart disease in men: The Physicians' Health Study. *Intl J Epidemiol.* 2001;30(1):130-105.

Liu S, Manson JE, Lee IM, et al. Fruit and vegetable intake and risk of cardiovascular disease: The Women's Health Study. *Am J Clin Nutr.* 2000; 72(4):922-928.

Lopez PM, Ortega RM. Omega-3 fatty acids in the prevention and control of cardiovascular disease. *Eur J Clin Nutr.* 2003;57(Suppl 1):S22-S25.

Mann JL, Appleby PN, Key TJ, Thorogood M. Dietary determinants of ischaemic heart disease in health conscious individuals. *Heart.* 1997;789(15): 450-455.

Mann NJ, Sinclair AJ, Dudman NP, et al. The effect of diet on plasma homocysteine concentrations in healthy male subjects. *Eur J Clin Nutr.* 1999; 53(11):895-899.

Marchioli R, Schweiger C, Levantesi G, et al. Antioxidant vitamins and prevention of cardiovascular disease: Epidemiological and clinical trial data. *Lipids.* 2001;36 (Suppl):S53-S63.

Marckmann P, Sandstrom B, Jespersen J. Favorable long-term effect of a low-fat/high-fiber diet on human blood coagulation and fibrinolysis. *Arterioscler Thromb.* 1993;13(4):505-511.

Masarei JR, Rouse IL, Lynch WJ, et al. Vegetarian diets, lipids and cardiovascular risk. *Australia/ New Zealand J Med.* 1984;14(4):400-404.

McGill HC, McMahan CA. Pathobiological Determinants of Atherosclerosis in Youth (PDAY) Research Group. *Am J Cardiol.* 1998;82(10B): 30T-36T.

McNamara JJ, Molot MA, Stremple JF, Cutting RT. Coronary artery disease in combat casualties in Vietnam. *JAMA*. 1971;216(7):1185-1187.

Meade TW. Factor VII and ischaemic heart disease: Epidemiological evidence. *Haemostasis*. 1983; 13(3):178-185.

Meade TW, North WR, Chakrabarti R, et al. Haemostatic function and cardiovascular death: Early results of a prospective study. *Lancet*. 1980; 1(8177):1050-1054.

Merz-Demlow BE, Duncan AM, Wangren KE, et al. Soy isoflavones improve plasma lipids in normocholesterolemic, premenopausal women. *Am J Clin Nutr*. 2000;71(6):1462-1469.

Messina M, Messina V. *The Dietitian's Guide to Vegetarian Diets: Issues and Applications*. Gaithersburg, MD: Aspen Publishers; 1996.

Mezzano D, Munoz X, Matincez C, et al. Vegetarians and cardiovascular risk factors: Hemostasis, inflammatory markers and plasma homocysteine. *Thromb Haemostasis*. 1999;81(16):913-917.

Mojzisova G, Kuchta M. Dietary flavonoids and risk of coronary heart disease. *Physiol Res*. 2001; 50(6):529-535.

Murphy KJ, Chronopoulos AK, Singh I, et al. Dietary flavanols and procyanidin oligomers from cocoa (*Theobroma cacao*) inhibit platelet function. *Am J Clin Nutr*. 2003;77(6):1466-1473.

Ness AR, Powles JW. Fruit and vegetables, and cardiovascular disease: A review. *Intl J Epidemiol*. 1997;26(1):1-13.

Nestel P. Role of soy protein in cholesterol-lowering: How good is it? *Arterioscler Thromb Vasc Biol*. 2002;22(11):1743-1744.

Ornish D. *Dr. Dean Ornish's Program for Reversing Heart Disease*. New York: Random House; 1990: 25, 262.

Ornish D, Brown SE, Scherwitz LW, et al. Can lifestyle changes reverse coronary heart disease? The Lifestyle Heart Trial. *Lancet*. 1990;336(8708): 129-133.

Ornish D, Scherwitz LW, Billings JH, et al. Intensive lifestyle changes for reversal of coronary heart disease. *JAMA*. 1998;280(23):2001-2007.

Ornish D, Scherwitz LW, Doody RS, et al. Effects of stress management training and dietary changes in treating ischemic heart disease. *JAMA*. 1983; 249(1):54-59.

Pais P, Pogue J, Gerstein H, et al. Risk factors for acute myocardial infarction in Indians: A case-control study. *Lancet*. 1996;348(9024):358-363.

Pan WH, Chin CJ, Sheu CT, Lee MH. Hemostatic factors and blood lipids in young Buddhist vegetarians and omnivores. *Am J Clin Nutr*. 1993; 58(3):354-359.

Pandya DP. Oxidant injury and antioxidant prevention: Role of dietary antioxidants, minerals, and drugs in the management of coronary heart disease (Part II). *Compr Ther*. 2002;28(1):62-73.

Pasceri V, Willerson JT. Homocysteine and coronary heart disease: A review of the current evidence. *Semin Interv Cardiol*. 1999;4(3):121-128.

Pereira MA, O'Reilly E, Augustsson K, et. al. Dietary fiber and risk of coronary heart disease: A pooled analysis of cohort studies. *Arch Intern Med*. 2004; 164(4):370-376.

Pereira MA, Pins JJ. Dietary fiber and cardiovascular disease: Experimental and epidemiologic advances. *Curr Atheroscler Reps*. 2000;2(6):494-502.

Perez-Jimenez F, Lopez-Miranda J, Mata P. Protective effect of dietary monounsaturated fat on arteriosclerosis: Beyond cholesterol. *Atherosclerosis*. 2002;163(2):385-398.

Phillips RL, Lemon FR, Beeson WL, Kuzma JW. Coronary heart disease mortality among Seventh-Day Adventists with differing dietary habits: A preliminary report. *Am J Clin Nutr*. 1978;31(10, Suppl):S191-S198.

Pietinen P, Ascherio A, Korhonen P, et al. Intake of fatty acids and risk of coronary heart disease in a cohort of Finnish men: The Alpha-Tocopherol, Beta-Carotene Cancer Prevention Study. *Am J Epidemiol*. 1997;145(10):876-887.

Prior R. Fruits and vegetables in the prevention of cellular oxidative damage. *Am J Clin Nutr*. 2003; 78(3, Suppl):570S-578S.

Rajaram S. The effect of vegetarian diet, plant foods, and phytochemicals on hemostasis and thrombosis. *Am J Clin Nutr*. 2003;78(3, Suppl):552S-558S.

Rastogi T, Reddy KS, Vaz M, et al. Diet and risk of ischemic heart disease in India. *Am J Clin Nutr*. 2004;79(4):582-592.

Renaud S, Godsey F, Dumont E, et al. Influence of long-term diet modification on platelet function and composition in Moselle farmers. *Am J Clin Nutr.* 1986;43(1):136–150.

Renaud S, Lanzmann-Petithory D. Dietary fats and coronary heart disease pathogenesis. *Curr Atheroscler Reps.* 2002;4(6):419–424.

Renaud S, Lanzmann-Petithory D. Coronary heart disease: Dietary links and pathogenesis. *Public Health Nutr.* 2001;4(2B):459–474.

Resnicow K, Barone J, Engle A, et al. Diet and serum lipids in vegan vegetarians: A model for risk reduction. *J Am Diet Assoc.* 1991;91(4):447–453. Erratum in *J Am Diet Assoc.* 1991; 91(6):655.

Roberts WC. Preventing and arresting coronary atherosclerosis. *Am Heart J.* 1995;130(3, Pt. 1):580–600.

Ryde D. The challenge of angina. *Br J Gen Pract.* Dec 1996;46(413):759.

Sacks FM, Ornish D, Rosner B, et al. Plasma lipoprotein levels in vegetarians: The effect of ingestion of fats from dairy products. *JAMA.* 1985;254(10):1337–1341.

Sanders TA, Roshanai F. Platelet phospholipid fatty acid composition and function in vegans compared with age- and sex-matched omnivore controls. *Eur J Clin Nutr.* 1992;46(11):823–831.

Schaefer EJ. Lipoproteins, nutrition and heart disease. *Am J Clin Nutr.* 2002;75(2):191–212.

Setchell KD. Soy isoflavones—Benefits and risks from nature's selective estrogen receptor modulators (SERMs). *J Am Coll Nutr.* 2001;20(5, Suppl):354S–362S.

Shrapnel WS, Calvert GD, Nestel PJ, Truswell AS. Diet and coronary heart disease: The National Heart Foundation of Australia. *Med J Australia.* 1992; 156 (Suppl):S9–S16.

Singh RB, Rastogi SS, Laxmi VR, et al. Randomised controlled trial of cardioprotective diet in patients with recent acute myocardial infarction: Results of one year follow up. *Br Med J.* 1992; 304(6833):1015–1019.

Snowdon DA, Phillips RL, Fraser GE. Meat consumption and fatal ischemic heart disease. *Preven Med.* 1984;13(5):490–500.

St. Onge MP, Jones PJ. Phytosterols and human lipid metabolism: Efficacy, safety, and novel foods. *Lipids.* 2003;38(4):367–375.

Steffen LM, Jacobs DR, Stevens J, et al. Associations of whole-grain, refined-grain, and fruit and vegetable consumption with risks of all-cause mortality and incident coronary artery disease and ischemic stroke: The Atherosclerosis Risk in Communities (ARIC) study. *Am J Clin Nutr.* 2003; 78(3):383–390.

Steinberg FM, Guthrie NL, Villablanca AC, et al. Soy protein with isoflavones has favorable effects on endothelial function that are independent of lipid and antioxidant effects in healthy postmenopausal women. *Am J Clin Nutr.* 2003;78(1):123–130.

Stone NJ (Chair), Nicolosi RJ, Kris-Etherton P, Ernst ND, Krauss, RM, Winston M., for the American Heart Association. *Summary of the Scientific Conference on the Efficacy of Hypocholesterolemic Dietary Interventions.* Dallas, TX: American Heart Association; 1996.

Stone NJ, Van Horn L. Therapeutic lifestyle change and Adult Treatment Panel III: Evidence then and now. *Curr Atheroscler Reps.* 2002;4(6):433–443.

Taylor BV, Oudit GY, Evans M. Homocysteine, vitamins, and coronary artery disease: Comprehensive review of the literature. *Can Fam Physician.* 2000;46:2236–2245.

Tribble DL. AHA Science Advisory. Antioxidant consumption and risk of coronary heart disease: Emphasis on vitamin C, vitamin E, and beta-carotene. A statement for health care professionals from the American Heart Association. *Circulation.* 1999; 99(4):591–595.

Truswell AS. Cereal grains and coronary heart disease. *Eur J Clin Nutr.* 2002;56(1):1–14.

Van Horn L. Fiber, lipids, and coronary heart disease. A statement for healthcare professionals from the Nutrition Committee, American Heart Association. *Circulation.* 1997;95(12):2701–2704.

Visioli F, Borsani L, Galli C. Diet and prevention of coronary heart disease: The potential role of phytochemicals. *Cardiovasc Res.* 2000;47:419–425.

von Schacky C. The role of omega-3 fatty acids in cardiovascular disease. *Curr Atheroscler Reps.* 2003;5(2):139–145.

Vos E, Cunnane SC. Alpha-linolenic acid, linoleic acid, coronary artery disease, and overall mortality. *Am J Clin Nutr.* 2003;77(2):521-522.

Waaler HT, Hjort PF. Longevity among Norwegian Adventists 1960-77: A message on lifestyle and health. *Tidsskr Nor Laegeforen.* 1981;101(11): 623-627.

Wangen KE, Duncan AM, Xu X, Kurzer MS. Soy isoflavones improve plasma lipids in normocholesterolemic and mildly hypercholesterolemic postmenopausal women. *Am J Clin Nutr.* 2001; 73(2):225-231.

Willett, W, Sacks FM. Chewing the fat—how much and what kind? *N Engl J Med.* 1991;324(2):121-123.

Wilmink HW, Stroes ES, Erkelens WD, et al. Influence of folic acid on postprandial endothelial dysfunction. *Arterioscler Thromb Vasc Biol.* 2000; 20(1):185-188.

Wiseman H, O'Reilley J, Adlercreutz H, Mallet A, et al. Isoflavone phytoestrogens consumed in soy decreased F^2-isoprostane concentrations and increased resistance of low-density lipoprotein to oxidation in humans. *Am J Clin Nutr.* 2000; 72(2):395-400.

Wolfram G. Dietary fatty acids and coronary heart disease. *Eur J Med Res.* 2003;8(8):321-324.

11

Cancer

Peggy Carlson, MD

Introduction

Cancer is the second leading cause of death in the United States. Diet is one factor that can affect one's risk of cancer. This chapter looks at the relationships between dietary factors, vegetarian diets, and cancer risk.

Summary of the Scientific Literature: Cancer Rates among Vegetarians

There is evidence from several, but not all, studies that a vegetarian diet decreases the risk of cancer in general and the risk of a number of specific-site cancers (World Cancer Research Fund [WCRF]/American Institute for Cancer Research [AICR], 1997). Some of these studies have looked at groups of vegetarians. Others have been studies of Seventh-Day Adventists (SDAs). Because about half of SDAs are vegetarian, they provide a unique opportunity to investigate the effects of a vegetarian diet on cancer risk among people with similar lifestyles.

This chapter presents different types of epidemiologic studies. Ecological (observational,

correlation) studies compare large populations, such as in different countries or locales. Case-control studies focus on a group of individuals with a particular disease and then look back at the histories of those individuals to see if there is a common causal factor. In cohort (prospective) studies, researchers follow a large group of people over time to see who develops what diseases and whether the individuals who do develop a particular disease had something in common. Although prospective studies are generally considered the most rigorous and dependable, all three study types have limitations that can affect the results.

Studies of Vegetarian Groups and the Risk of Cancer

- Among 6,115 British vegetarians followed for 12 years, there was an approximately 40% reduction in mortality from cancer among the vegetarians as compared to meat eaters. This reduction persisted even after adjustment for smoking, body mass index, and social class (Thorogood et al., 1994).

- A 17-year study looked at the causes of death from cancer in a group of 10,771 British men and women recruited through health food shops, vegetarian societies, and health food magazines. Forty-three percent of the study participants were vegetarian. The authors found that in the men, the all-cancer standard mortality ratio (SMR)—that is, the observed number of deaths/ expected number of deaths—was 50% that of the general population. In women, the all-cancer SMR was 76%. For men, the SMRs were statistically lower than in the general population for all cancers combined (50%), and for cancers of the stomach (37%), colorectum (64%), and lung (27%). In women, the mortality rate was lower for cancer of the lung (37%). The lower risk of lung cancer in this cohort was attributed mainly to a lower proportion of smokers (19%). In the study, however, persons who described themselves as vegetarian were not found to be at lower risk of cancer. In fact, in women, being vegetarian was associated with increased risk of dying of breast cancer (relative risk of 1.7). The authors hypothesized that this increase in breast cancer risk may have been due to chance or to differences in parity between vegetarians and nonvegetarians (Key, Thorogood, Appleby, & Burr, 1996).

- A group of 1,904 German vegetarians was followed for 11 years. Researchers found lower all-cancer SMRs among the vegetarians when compared with the general German population. Rates were 48% (significant) of expected for men and 74% (nonsignificant) for women. The rate for lung cancer in men was only 8% of the expected rate. Total intestinal system cancers were 56% (nonsignificant) of expected for men and 49% (significant) for women.

There were no statistical differences in the SMRs for stomach and colon cancer individually. Breast and prostate cancer were not investigated. Being on a vegetarian diet for more than 20 years was associated with approximately half the risk of all-cancer mortality, as compared with being vegetarian for less than 20 years. The vegetarians making up this cohort were almost all nonsmokers, which would explain the extremely low rate of lung cancer (Frentzel-Beyme & Chang-Claude, 1994).

- A study investigated causes of death of 759 members of a British vegetarian society and compared them with expected death rates for England and Wales. They found no evidence of a reduction in mortality from cancer among the vegetarians (Kinlen, Hermon, & Smith, 1983).

- Researchers in a Swedish study compared the number of new cases of cancer among 9,000 health-food journal subscribers to the national average. The authors estimated that about 54% of the study group was vegetarian. There was a significant (82% of expected) reduction in the number of cancers among the study participants. The low risk was mainly due to a decreased risk of cancer of the digestive system (60% of expected). The only single-site cancer that came out significantly different was pancreatic (14% of expected); however, there were nonsignificant but noticeably lower risks of cancer of the biliary passages and liver (28% of expected) and of the colon (60% respectively) (Halling & Carstensen, 1984).

- A pooled analysis of five prospective studies of vegetarians presented mortality data for the five most common cancers: lung, colorectal, breast, prostate, and stomach. Mortality among the vegetarians did not differ significantly from that of the non-vegetarians for any of these cancer sites, although there was a slight, nonsignificant decrease for lung, breast, and prostate cancer. Mortality from colorectal cancer did not vary according to the length of time for which vegetarians had followed their current diets. In these studies, the mortality rates for both the vegetarians and the nonvegetarians used for comparison were substantially below national rates (Key et al., 1998).

- Ina case-control study of 689 women with breast cancer, compared with 711 controls, there was no statistical difference between the breast cancer rates in the vegetarians versus the nonvegetarians (Rao, Ganesh, & Desai, 1994).

- The EPIC-Oxford study followed 65,429 men and women, of whom 32% were vegetarian. Participants were sent a follow-up questionnaire five years after entry into the study. No significant difference between the vegetarians and nonvegetarians was found as to mortality from all malignant neoplasms combined (Key, Appleby, et al., 2003).

Studies of Seventh-Day Adventists and the Risk of Cancer

California Seventh-Day Adventist Study

Beginning in the late 1950s, the California Adventist Study has looked at cancer (and other health problems) among a group of about 25,000–35,000 Seventh-Day Adventists (SDAs) living in that state. From this study, several investigative projects have emerged.

About half of SDAs are vegetarian, and a few are vegan. Other SDA lifestyle factors that can affect cancer risk are fairly uniform among SDAs: namely, almost all are nonsmoking and most avoid alcohol, coffee, tea, and spices. Therefore, studies of SDAs can offer insight into the cancer risk of vegetarians versus nonvegetarians in a population where other lifestyle factors are somewhat constant.

- The 1958–1965 cancer mortality data for California SDAs showed that the SMR for all cancers combined was 53% of general population rates for males, and 67% for females. Rates were less than 50% of general population for cancers related to smoking and alcohol (mouth, pharynx, esophagus, bladder). For cancers classified by the authors as unrelated to smoking or alcohol (stomach, pancreas, colon, breast, and ovary), rates generally ranged from 50%–70% of expected. The rates of kidney and central nervous system (CNS) cancers and lymphomas were the same as seen in the general population (Phillips, 1975).

- The question of whether length of membership in the SDA church affects cancer risk was investigated in the same study. Although not significant, the trend was toward a decreased risk of stomach cancer and possibly all cancers combined in those who had joined the church when less than 18 years of age, as compared with those who had joined at a later age. For the other individual cancers studied (colorectal and breast), there was no difference. It was also found that, when considered in terms of length of church membership, again there was a decrease in stomach cancer among those who had been members for the longest time; for the other cancers and for all cancers combined, there was no difference (Phillips, 1975).

- When cancer SMRs were compared between 22,940 California SDAs followed for

17 years and 112,725 non-SDAs followed for 13 years, the SDAs were found to have lower rates of cancer in general (61%), stomach cancer in females (67%), colorectal cancer (53%), lung cancer (15%), and other smoking-related cancers (defined as cancer of the mouth, pharynx, esophagus, larynx, bladder and other urinary organs, and pancreas) (45%). There was a slight but nonsignificant decrease in breast and prostate cancers. When cancer mortality rates were compared between members of the California Seventh-Day Adventists study group and a group of non-SDA Californians of similar educational attainment, among the SDAs the risk for all cancers combined was still lower (66%–76%), as were the risks of death from lung cancer (14%–24%), other smoking-related cancers (60%–68%), and colorectal cancer (54%–55%). The difference in mortality between SDAs and all U.S. whites for other cancer sites was substantially reduced when SDAs were compared with a population of non-SDAs who were socioeconomically similar to SDAs, suggesting that high socioeconomic status or other factors that characterize persons who choose to join the SDA Church primarily account for the apparent low risk among SDA for those cancers. The fact that there was no attenuation in the colorectal cancer risk suggests that this difference can be attributed to some preventive factor in the typical SDA diet or lifestyle (Phillips, Garfinkel, et al., 1980; Phillips, Kuzma, et al., 1980).

- The SMRs for cancers among 22,940 SDAs followed from 1960 to 1976 were compared with the mortality rates of American Cancer Society Study non-SDAs and all U.S. whites. Results showed that mortality due to lung cancer among all nonsmoking SDAs was about half that of comparable non-smoking non-SDAs. Among the other cancers included in this report (colorectal, breast, prostate, stomach, lymphoma, and leukemia), fatal colorectal cancer was the only one that had a substantially lower risk among nonsmoking SDAs compared to nonsmoking non-SDAs of both sexes (females, 56%, and males, 67%). For breast cancer, the risk became lower for the SDAs among postmenopausal, as opposed to premenopausal, women (Phillips et al., 1980).

- The risk of colon cancer was found to be substantially reduced among the SDAs when compared to the risk for comparable non-SDAs and for all U.S whites (33% vs. 51% and 57.5%, respectively) in a study of 21,295 SDAs. SDAs also showed a minimum reduction in mortality from breast and prostate cancer. The deaths from colon cancer were unrelated to meat consumption (Phillips & Snowdon, 1983).

- Investigators compared breast cancer survival rates among 282 SDAs and 1,675 other white females. The SDA women had a more favorable five-year survival than the other women (69.7% vs. 62.9%), as well as a higher probability of not dying of breast cancer. However, the differences were not statistically significant when stage at diagnosis was taken into account. It appears likely that the lower breast cancer death rates for the SDA women resulted, at least in part, from earlier diagnosis and treatment. Among the small number of women who provided dietary data, survival rates did not differ significantly between SDA vegetarians and SDA nonvegetarians (Zollinger, Phillips, & Kuzma, 1984).

- A 7-year study of pancreatic cancer among 34,000 SDAs found that, compared to all U.S. whites, SDAs experienced decreased risk of pancreatic cancer death (SMR was

0.72 for men and 0.90 for women), although the difference was not statistically significant (Mills et al., 1988).

- A suggestive relationship between increasing animal product consumption and increased risk of prostate cancer was found in a group of approximately 14,000 SDA men followed from 1976 to 1982. The increased risk did not persist after accounting for the influence of fruit and vegetable consumption, nor was exposure to vegetarian diets during childhood associated with a change in risk (Mills et al., 1989a).
- Breast cancer incidence among 20,341 SDA women was monitored in a 6-year follow-up study. In this study, *lacto-ovo vegetarians* were defined as those who consumed meat, poultry, or fish less than once per week and consumed whole milk, eggs, or cheese in any amount. *Pure vegetarians* were defined as those consuming meat, poultry, fish, whole milk, eggs, or cheese less than one time per week. In comparison to omnivores (relative risk or RR of 1.0), the risk for breast cancer among lacto-ovo vegetarians (RR 0.86) and the risk for pure vegetarians (RR 0.34) were less; however, the results were not statistically significant. This study found no decrease in breast cancer risk among those who had begun their practice of vegetarianism during childhood and early adulthood as compared to those who had begun later (Mills et al., 1989b).
- In an evaluation of 34,000 California SDAs (1976–1982), the cancer SMR for all sites combined showed rates that were 73% of the general population (significant) for men and 92% (nonsignificant) for women. For men, rates were significantly lower for cancers of the mouth (24%), stomach (50%), esophagus (no cases), colon (64%), rectum (51%), bronchus and lung (25%),

bladder (59%), kidney (37%), and biliary and liver (24%); rates for prostate cancer were higher (126%). For women, rates were lower for cancers of the stomach (16%), colon (76%), and bronchus and lung (36%). For women, the decrease in risk of several cancers came close to statistical significance, including for cancers of the mouth (41%), rectum (71%), breast (91%), bladder (59%), and kidney (38%). The rate for endometrial cancer was higher (191%). The substantially lower rates of smoking-related cancers (lung, pancreas, bladder, and mouth) were expected (Mills et al., 1994).

Studies of Seventh-Day Adventists Other than the California Seventh-Day Adventist Study

- Inpatients with cancer at eight U.S. SDA hospitals were separated on the basis of SDA membership or non-SDA membership in a large investigatory study. The cancers studied included smoking-related cancers, leukemia, lymphoma, and cancers of the colon, breast, prostate, uterus, cervix, pancreas, stomach, and central nervous system. The observed rates for all cancer sites in male SDAs and for 9 of 12 sites in female SDAs (not adenocarcinoma of the lung, uterine cancer, and "miscellaneous" cancers) tended to be below the expected rate. However, the difference was statistically significant only for smoking-related cancers in men, miscellaneous cancers in men, and cervical cancer in women (Wynder, Lemon, & Bross, 1959).
- Among approximately 3,200 SDAs in the Netherlands, followed for 10 years, SMRs for all cancers combined were 50% of the general population. Risk of death from all individual cancers (except pancreas) were

also significantly lower among the SDAs, including breast cancer (50%), lung cancer (45%), colorectal cancer (43%), and stomach cancer (59%—borderline significant). Smoking was virtually nonexistent among the SDAs, which would explain the lower lung cancer rates (Berkel & de Waard, 1983).

- Ina Danish study, 781 Danish male SDAs were compared with 808 members of other temperance societies (lifelong nondrinkers or reformed alcoholics). For cancers of all sites, a significantly reduced risk was observed among SDAs (69%). For colon, lung, and bladder cancer, the risk among the SDAs was only 10% that of the members of other temperance societies. For other cancers, including stomach, rectum, pancreas, and kidney, there were no differences. For all but colon cancer, the difference was felt to be due to the avoidance of smoking among the SDAs (Jensen, 1983).

- Ina study of 7,693 Japanese SDAs followed from 1975 to 1981, deaths due to all cancers combined were 30% of expected (significant) for men and 78% (nonsignificant) for women when compared with the general Japanese population. For both men and women, the death rate due to stomach cancer was significantly lower than the general population rates (32% for men and 26% for women). Deaths due to respiratory cancers were also significantly lower for males (no observed cases among the SDAs). For other cancers (including esophagus, intestine, rectum, liver, pancreas, and breast), there were no statistical decreases among the SDAs (Kuratsune, Ikeda, & Hayashi, 1986).

- Whenlooking at cancer mortality data for 7,253 Norwegian SDAs in a 1961–1986 study, the investigators found that all-

cancer mortality for male and female SDAs was not significantly different from that of the general population. Site-specific incidences showed few differences between SDAs and non-SDAs. Among those less than 75 years old, respiratory cancer was lower among the SDAs (Fonnebo & Helseth, 1991). Cancer of the uterus in those less than 75 years old was more common in SDAs.

Study of Individuals with Lifestyles Similar to Seventh-Day Adventists

- A 16-year follow-up study tabulated the SMRs for cancer among 122,261 Japanese men with lifestyles similar to those of Seventh-Day Adventists (i.e., no smoking, no drinking, no daily meat consumption, and daily consumption of green and yellow vegetables). Their cancer risk was compared to that of Japanese men of opposite lifestyles. The Japanese with SDA-like lifestyles had one-fifth or less the risk for cancer of the mouth, pharynx, esophagus, and lung. Risks were less than half for cancer of all sites, stomach, and liver (Hirayama, 1985).

Conclusions

Several general impressions about cancer risk among vegetarians can be garnered from these studies. Almost all studies show a decreased risk of cancer among vegetarians as compared with the general public. Much of this decrease can be attributed to a decrease in lung cancer and other smoking-related cancers. The majority of studies showed decreases among vegetarians for gastrointestinal cancers, especially colon cancer and possibly stomach cancer. A few, but not all, studies showed some reduction in breast cancer among vegetarians. The data regarding prostate cancer are equivocal. Leukemia, lymphoma, and central nervous system cancers do not seem to be decreased among vegetarians.

The Relationship Between Diet and Cancer

Introduction

The fact that environmental factors strongly contribute to one's risk of developing cancer is suggested by studies showing that cancer incidences vary from one country to another; that the cancer risk in persons who migrate to another country soon approaches that of the new country; that variations over time in the incidence of cancer exist within particular communities; and actual identification of many specific causes of cancer or preventive factors (Doll & Peto, 1981). Numerous studies point to diet being a significant determinant of cancer risk (Milner, 2002). Mortality from many cancers, including colon, breast, and prostate cancers, rise among populations as diets "Westernize"—that is, become higher in fat, meat, dairy, and processed foods and lower in plant-based foods (WCRF/AICR, 1997). Doll and Peto, in their classic study, estimated that 35% of cancer deaths may be attributable to diet, with a wide range of acceptable estimates from 10%–70% (Doll & Peto, 1981). Wynder and Gori (1977) estimated that approximately 50% of cancers may be attributable to diet. The National Institutes of Health (NIH), United Kingdom Department of Health, National Cancer Institute, and American Cancer Society (2000) have also suggested that diet may be related to one-third of all cancer deaths.

What Causes Cancer

Cancer is believed to begin when a cell's DNA is exposed to an agent (a *carcinogen*) that changes that DNA, resulting in a abnormal (cancerous) cell that can multiply and spread. More than 500 dietary compounds have been identified as potential modifiers of cancer (Milner, 2002). Dietary factors may affect the development and spread of cancer by several mechanisms (Milner, 2002; Go, Wong, & Butrum, 2001). Some dietary components can block the formation or activation of a carcinogen or change its concentration within the body. Other dietary factors can affect the processes whereby a cell becomes carcinogenic and then spreads. Dietary factors may also influence cancer by shifting hormonal balances or affecting the immune system. In addition, some substances in foods are themselves suspected carcinogens.

Dietary Factors That May Affect Cancer Risk

The relationship between specific dietary factors and cancer is an area of increasing interest for science. Although much is known, there is also much that remains unknown. Current information is based on population studies, human clinical studies, and experimental and physiological studies, as well as theories based on biologic plausibility.

This section reviews what we know today about how cancer risk is affected by the dietary factors that appear to have the greatest potential influence on cancer risk. Specifically, it investigates fruits and vegetables, vitamins, antioxidants, phytochemicals, fiber, fats, meat, cooking methods, and soy products.

Much of the knowledge about the relationship between diet and cancer is summarized in Figure 11.1. This chart is taken from *Food, Nutrition and the Prevention of Cancer: A Global Perspective*, published by the World Cancer Research Fund in association with the American Institute for Cancer Research (2007). Much of the information in that book was taken from case-control studies and a few prospective studies. Several prospective studies done since the publication of that book have weakened a few of the associations noted on the table. These are noted in the discussions that follow.

Fruits and Vegetables

Many factors and components in fruits and vegetables may potentially decrease cancer risk. These include vitamins, antioxidants, phytochemicals, and fiber. These substances have the potential to interfere with the carcinogenic process at almost all stages in the development of a cancer, from the formation of and contact with a carcinogen, to the cancerous conversion of a cell, to the development and spread of a tumor (La Vecchia, Altieri, & Tavani, 2001). In addition, part of the protective effect of fruits and vegetables may be attributable to their low fat content, because fat itself may be a risk factor for cancer. Also, diets high in fruits and vegetables may prevent weight gain, thereby protecting against cancers for which obesity is a risk factor.

There is consistent evidence from case-control studies that fruits and vegetables serve an important function in decreasing one's risk of developing cancer (WCRF/AICR, 1997; Potter & Steinmetz, 1996). According to the 1997 World Cancer Research Fund report, at least 247 (14 ecological, 196 case-control, and 37 cohort) studies have investigated the relationship between fruit and vegetable consumption and cancer risk. When studies for all cancer sites were combined, it was found that 78% have shown a significant decrease in risk with higher intake of at least one vegetable and/or fruit category (WCRF/AICR, 1997). Steinmetz and Potter reviewed nearly 200 (174 case-control and 21 cohort) studies and concluded that increased fruit and vegetable consumption is consistently associated with a reduced risk of cancer at nearly all sites. They noted that prostate cancer is the only cancer for which the majority of studies have not reported at least one statistically significant inverse association for some fruit or vegetable category (Potter & Steinmetz, 1996; Steinmetz & Potter, 1991). Block reviewed 156 case-control and prospective studies and found a statistically significant protective effect of fruit and vegetable consumption demonstrated in 128 (82%) (Block, Patterson, & Subar, 1992).

Until recently, much of the evidence showing a protective role for fruits and vegetables had been drawn from case-control studies (Key et al., 2004). Since the mid-1990s, the evidence from several large prospective studies, however, has not been as supportive of an across-the-board protective effect of fruits and vegetables against all cancers (WCRF/AICR, 2007; La Vecchia, Altieri, & Tavani, 2001; Terry, Terry, & Wolk, 2001). In 2003, Riboli and Norat analyzed case-control and prospective studies on fruit and vegetable intake and risk of cancer. They concluded that case-control studies overall support a significant reduction in the risks of cancer of the esophagus, lung, stomach, and colorectum associated with both fruits and vegetables; a decrease in breast cancer risk with vegetable consumption; and an inverse association of bladder cancer with fruit consumption. They found that prospective studies suggest a protective effect of both fruits and vegetables for most of the cancer sites considered, but found that the risk reduction

Figure 11.1   Food Nutrition and the Prevention of Cancer: An Overview

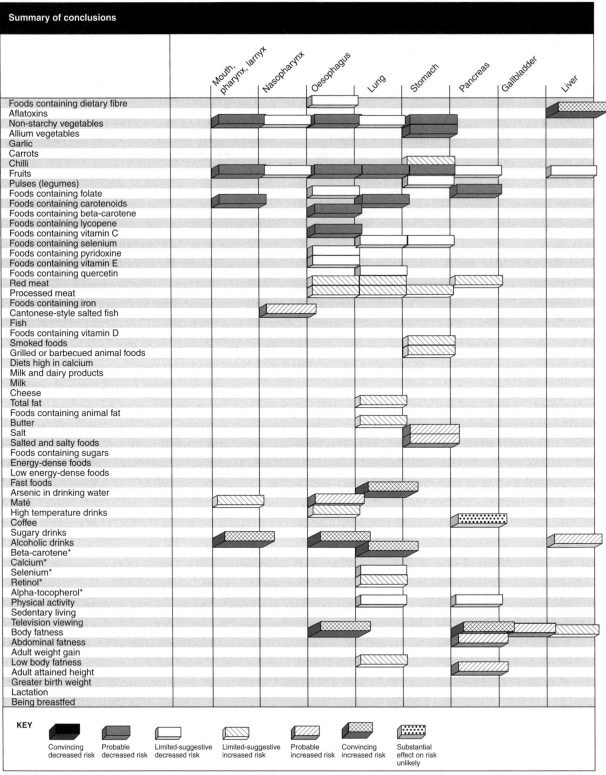

Source: World Cancer Research Fund/American Institute for Cancer Research. *Food, Nutrition and the Prevention of Cancer: A Global Perspective.* Washington, DC: American Institute for Cancer Research, 2007. Reprinted with permission from the American Institute for Cancer Research.

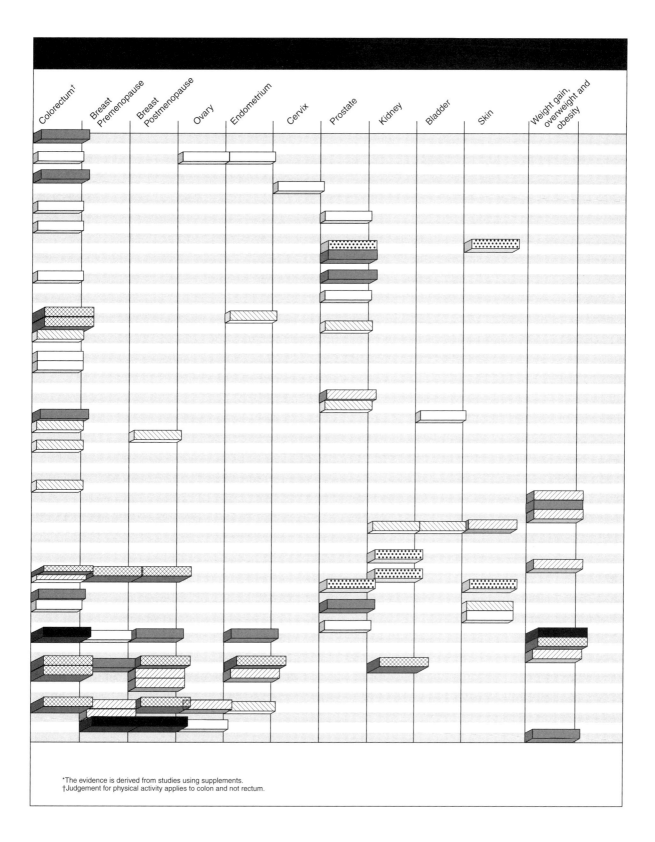

Table 11.1 Protective Effects of Fruit and Vegetable Consumption on Specific Cancers: Risk Reduction

Strength of the Evidence	Exposure	Cancer Site
Convincing		
Probable	Non-starchy vegetables	Mouth, pharynx, larynx, esophagus, stomach
	Allium vegetables	Stomach
	Garlic	Colorectum
	Fruits	Mouth, pharynx, larynx, esophagus, lung, stomach
	Foods containing folate	Pancreas
	Foods containing carotenoids	Mouth, pharynx, larynx, lung
	Foods containing beta-carotene	Esophagus
	Foods containing lycopene	Prostate
	Foods containing vitamin C	Esophagus
	Foods containing selenium	Prostate
Limited—suggestive	Non-starchy vegetables	Nasopharynx, lung, colorectum, ovary, endometrium
	Carrots	Cervix
	Fruits	Nasopharynx, pancreas, liver, colorectum
	Pulses (legumes)	Stomach, prostate
	Foods containing folate	Esophagus, colorectum
	Foods containing pyridoxine	Esophagus
	Foods containing vitamin E	Esophagus, prostate
	Foods containing selenium	Lung, stomach, colorectum
	Foods containing quercetin	Lung
Substantial effect on risk unlikely	Foods containing beta carotene	Prostate, skin (nonmelanoma)

is significant only for cancers of the lung and bladder and only for fruit (Riboli & Norat, 2003).

Although recent prospective studes have weakened the evidence for a general protective role of fruits and vegetables against cancer, the 2007 World Cancer Research Fund report concluded that specific fruits and vegetables, as well as some vitamins, micronutrients, and other compounds found in fruits and vegetables, may protect against individual cancers. These effects are summarized in Table 11.1.

Despite the fact that the results of more recent prospective studies have weakened the findings of previous studies, fruits and vegetables may still likely play a role in protecting the body against most cancers (Key et al., 2004). Also, there is no cancer site for which evidence supports an increase in cancer with an increase in fruit and vegetable consumption (WCRF/AICR, 1997).

Antioxidants

Antioxidants are currently enjoying much interest from researchers. Plant foods contain hundreds of different antioxidants, including nutrient (substances essential to the body) antioxidants, such as vitamin C, vitamin E, and beta-carotene; and nonnutrient (nonessential) phytochemicals that have antioxidant properties, such as flavonoids, carotenoids, hydroxycinnamic acid, and phenolic acids (Halliwell, 1999; Dreosti, 1998; Johnson, 1998). It is hypothesized that the ability of antioxidants to inhibit free-radical damage to DNA, or to scavenge free radicals, may give antioxidants their cancer-

Table 11.2   Some Common Phytochemicals with Anti-Cancer Effects

Examples of Phytochemicals with Potential Anti-Cancer Effects	Main Food Sources
Fiber	Whole grains, fruits, and vegetables
Flavonoids	Vegetables, citrus fruits, wine, tea
Isoflavonoids	Soybeans and soy products
Saponins	Legumes
Lignans	Flaxseed
Isothicyanates	Cruciferous vegetables (broccoli, cabbage, brussel sprouts)
Carotenoids	Deep orange fruits and vegetables, dark green vegetables
Terpenoids	Citrus fruits, cherries
Allium compounds	Garlic, onions, leeks
Phytosterols	Vegetable oils
Hydroxycinnamic acids	Apples, pears, mustard, curry
Ellagic acid	Grapes, strawberries, raspberries, nuts
Glucarates	Citrus, grains, solanaceous vegetables (tomatoes, eggplant, bell peppers)

prevention properties (Tamimi et al., 2002; Dreosti, 1998; Johnson, 1998; Halliwell, 2002). Although there is compelling evidence that oxidative damage may lead to cancer, studies to prove this contention have not been done (Halliwell, 2002). In addition to their antioxidant potential, many of these compounds may inhibit cancer formation by other mechanisms as well.

Phytochemicals

Phytochemicals are nonnutritive (nonessential) substances in plants that possess health-protective effects. Thousands of different phytochemicals are present in plant foods (Liu, 2003). Many phytochemicals have shown anticancer effects in laboratory experiments, and it is felt that these effects may play a role in preventing human cancers. Some of the different classes of phytochemicals with potential anticancer effects are listed in Table 11.2 (Craig, 1997; Rowland, 1999).

Phytochemicals may act as anticancer agents via several different mechanisms occurring anywhere in the multistep sequence of events leading to carcinogenesis (LeMarchand, 2002; Lopez-Lazaro, 2002; Kris-Etherton et al., 2002; Birt, Hendrich, & Wang, 2001), including:

- Inhibiting the formation of carcinogens
- Reducing the activation of carcinogens
- Increasing the detoxification of carcinogens
- Blocking the access of carcinogenic compounds to target tissues
- Interacting with various hormonal actions that are associated with the development of cancer
- Preventing the cancerous conversion of cells by:
  ○ antioxidant effects
  ○ effects on DNA
  ○ effect on enzymatic pathways
  ○ effects on cellular mechanisms, structure, and growth
- Decreasing the spread of cancer by decreasing blood vessel growth
- Increasing anti-inflammatory effects
- Exerting antiviral effects
- Increasing immune surveillance

There are only limited data on whether these potential anticancer mechanisms translate into decreased cancer risk in humans. The isoflavonoids found in soy have received perhaps the greatest attention in studies investigating the effects of phytochemicals on cancer risk. Isoflavonoids are phytoestrogens. The possibility that isoflavonoids may decrease the risk of breast and prostate cancer has been intriguing, but the evidence remains conflicting. Isoflavonoids have also demonstrated anticancer effects not related to their estrogenic effects (Birt, Hendrich, & Wang, 2001; Ren et al., 2001; Sarkar & Yiwei, 2003). Hundreds of *in vitro* studies have demonstrated that genistein (an isoflavone) can inhibit a wide range of both hormone-dependent and hormone-independent cancer cells, including breast and prostate cells (Ren et al., 2001; Messina et al., 1994).

There are only very limited epidemiological data on the effect of other flavonoids on cancer risk. Although a few relationships have emerged, there are no conclusive data (Tamimi et al., 2002; LeMarchand, 2002; Kampman, Arts, & Hollman, 2003).

Phytoestrogens

Phytoestrogens are phytochemicals that are structurally similar to human estrogens, and thus can bind to estrogen receptors. By binding to the receptors, they cause a modest estrogen-like response, but at the same time they block the binding of more potent estrogens. Therefore, phytoestrogens have some estrogenic and some anti-estrogenic properties (Birt, Hendrich, & Wang, 2001; Ren et al., 2001; Peeters et al., 2003). The specific effect that any particular phytoestrogen might have may depend on the phytoestrogen concentration or the tissue of action (Ren et al., 2001).

Phytoestrogens can be found in a number of legumes, fruits, and vegetables. The two main classes of phytoestrogens are the isoflavones and the lignans. Isoflavones are found in greatest concentration in soybeans and soy products. Lignans are found primarily in flaxseed.

Because higher estrogen levels are associated with increased breast cancer risk, it has been hypothesized that an anti-estrogenic effect of phytoestrogens may protect against breast cancer. Most of the epidemiology and dietary intervention studies concerning phytoestrogens have been conducted with soy or flaxseed rather than phytoestrogens per se. The results of these studies have been conflicting, with no clear effect of phytoestrogens on breast cancer risk being proven (Peeters et al., 2003; Magee & Rowland, 2004; Adlercreutz, 2002).

It has also been theorized that phytoestrogens may afford some protection against prostate cancer (Magee & Rowland, 2004; Messina, 2003) and colon cancer (McIntosh et al., 2003). As yet, human studies to support this hypothesis have been too few in number and inconclusive. Phytoestrogens also have other anticancer effects not related to their anti-estrogenic properties, including antioxidant effects, inhibition of blood vessel formation, effects on DNA, and effects on enzymatic and cellular mechanisms (Birt, Hendrich, & Wang, 2001; Magee & Rowland, 2004).

Fiber

Fiber may affect the risk of several cancers. Several different mechanisms of action have been proposed. Many, but not all, case-control and observational studies suggest that diets high in fiber can protect against colorectal cancer (Martinez, Marshall, & Alberts, 1999). Several meta-analyses have been done. These studies are listed in Table 11.3.

Many prospective studies have also been supportive of a protective effect of fiber on colorectal cancer (Heilbrun et al., 1989; Stein-

Table 11.3 Meta-Analyses of Case Control and Observational Studies Investigating Fiber and Risk of Colon Cancer

- In a combined analysis of 13 case-control studies, Howe et al. (1992) found that the risk of colon cancer decreased as fiber intake increased, with a relative risk of 0.53 at the highest quintile of intake.
- Shankar and Lanza (1991) reviewed 32 observational and case-control studies and found that 25 supported an inverse association between fiber intake and colon cancer.
- Another review of 37 observational studies and 23 case-control studies found that 57% showed a protective effect of fiber with regard to colon cancer (Trock, Lanza, & Greenwald, 1992).
- Another meta-analysis of 13 case-control studies showed that high-fiber foods reduce the risk of colon cancer by one-half (Friedenreich, Brant, & Riboli, 1994).
- Kim (2000) concluded that most of the published case-control studies showed a significant inverse relationship between dietary fiber and colorectal cancer.
- Sengupta, Tjandra, and Gibson (2001) reviewed the 1986–2000 literature and found that 13 of 24 case-control studies demonstrated a protective effect of dietary fiber against colorectal cancer.

metz et al., 1994, WCRF/AICR, 2007), although some studies have disagreed (Heilbrun et al., 1989; Steinmetz et al., 1994; Fuchs et al., 1999; Giovannucci et al., 1994). The 2007 World Cancer Research Fund report concluded that prospective studies have generally been consistent in finding a protective effect of fiber against colon cancer, although confounding factors could not be excluded. Kim summarized the results from six large prospective studies and concluded that the relationship between fiber and colon cancer was equivocal, but also reported that a large prospective study (Cancer Prevention Study II), involving more than 1 million subjects, showed a 30% reduction in colorectal cancer among those consuming the highest amount of fiber (Kim, 2000). In Sengupta's review, only 3 of 13 prospective studies found a protective effect of fiber (Sengupta, Tjandra, & Gibson, 2001). It is possible that in some of these prospective studies, the range of dietary fiber might have been too narrow to detect an effect (Kim, 2000). A few more recent interventional studies have looked at whether dietary fiber can affect the occurrence or size of colonic adenomas, precursors to colonic cancer. The results of these studies, by and large, have not supported any effect of dietary fiber

(Sengupta, Tjandra, & Gibson, 2001; Ferguson, Chavan, & Harris, 2001).

Fiber may protect against breast cancer. Many case-control studies have supported such a relationship; however, some have not. In 1997, a review of nine case-control studies and three cohort studies found a slightly decreased risk of breast cancer with greater amounts of dietary fiber in the case-control studies, but not in the prospective studies, although the reviewers did find a fair amount of discrepancy among the studies (Clavel-Chapelon, Niravong, & Joseph, 1997). In 1998, Gerber reviewed 10 case-control studies and found that 8 showed an inverse relationship of fiber intake with breast cancer risk; however, the differences were significant in only 5. Of four prospective studies reviewed, Gerber found no change in two and found a nonsignificant decrease in breast cancer risk with increasing fiber intake in two. She also noted that when there was a reduction, it appeared to be dose-dependent, giving some credence to the significance of the risk reduction (Gerber, 1998). A 2002 Canadian study, which followed 49,536 women for about 16 years, found no association between breast cancer risk and the amount or type of dietary fiber, including soluble or insoluble, cereal fiber, or fiber from fruit and vegetables (Terry et al., 2002).

There are limited data regarding the effect of fiber on other cancers (WCRF/AICR, 1997; Baghurst & Rohan, 1994; Clavel-Chapelon, Niravong, & Joseph, 1997; Aronson, Yip, & Dekernion, 1999). Jacob reviewed more than 50 case-control studies on various gastrointestinal and hormone-related tumors, and found that 43 supported an inverse association with high intake of whole grains (Jacob et al., 1998). In a review of 12 studies of fiber and risk of esophageal cancer, there was some suggestion that dietary fiber may offer protection (WCRF/AICR, 2007). There has been very limited research into the effect of fiber on prostate cancer. A couple of studies on the effect of dietary fiber on prostate specific antigen (PSA) levels in men without cancer yielded conflicting results (Moyad & Carroll, 2004a, 2004b).

There are several hypotheses on how fiber might reduce colon cancer risk (Kim, 2000; Sengupta, Tjandra, & Gibson, 2001) (see Figure 11.2). In the colon, fiber may bind or dilute carcinogens; it may also decrease colonic transit time, thereby reducing the time during which carcinogens are in contact with the colon. The short-chain fatty acids (SCFAs) produced by the fermentation of fiber may themselves be anticarcinogenic. In addition, SCFAs decrease colonic pH, which, in turn, decreases the production and availability of toxic bile acids. Fiber may also change the existence or activity of bacteria that can affect the presence of carcinogens in the colon. Fiber also contains phytochemicals, some of which have phytoestrogenic effects, which may decrease the risk of colon cancer (McIntosh et al., 2003).

Fiber could, theoretically, decrease breast cancer risk, both because it reduces serum estrogen (which is known to increase the risk of breast cancer) and because it contains phytoestrogens (which can inhibit the effect and

amount of estrogen in the body) (Baghurst & Rohan, 1994; Goldin et al., 1994; Griffiths et al., 1996). Similarly, fiber can decrease testosterone levels, which have been hypothesized to increase prostate cancer risk (Aronson, Yip, & Dekernion, 1999; Griffiths et al., 1996).

Fiber may also reduce the incidence of cancer due to the anticarcinogenic properties of other phytochemicals present in fiber-rich foods.

Fats

Although hundreds of studies have been conducted to investigate the role of fat in cancer risk, any possible connections remain unproven. Studies point to a possible link between diets high in total fat and saturated fat and cancers of the lung, colon, breast, and prostate (WCRF/AICR, 2007; Key et al., 2004; Zock, 2001; Kushi & Giovannucci, 2002).

Although the exact biologic mechanisms behind any possible associations between fat intake and cancer remain unknown, several mechanisms have been put forth as possible explanations. Increased fat intake can lead to obesity, which may be a risk factor for endometrial, breast, colon, kidney, esophageal, pancreatic, and liver cancer (WCRF/AICR, 2007; Levi, 1999; Johnson, 2004; Gatof & Ahnen, 2002; Giovannucci, 2002; McTiernan, 2003; Key, Allen, et al., 2003; Key, Allen, et al., 2002). Obesity, and possibly dietary fat, can alter hormone levels, which may increase the risk of breast cancer (McTiernan, 2003; Key, Allen, et al., 2002; Goldin & Gorbach, 1994). Dietary fat may also increase testosterone, which has been hypothesized to increase prostate cancer risk (WCRF/AICR, 1997). Additionally, dietary fat can increase the colonic concentration of the secondary bile acids that act as colon carcinogens. Dietary fat also increases the amount of intestinal free fatty acids, which have been shown to damage

Figure 11.2   Mechanisms by Which Fiber May Protect against Cancer

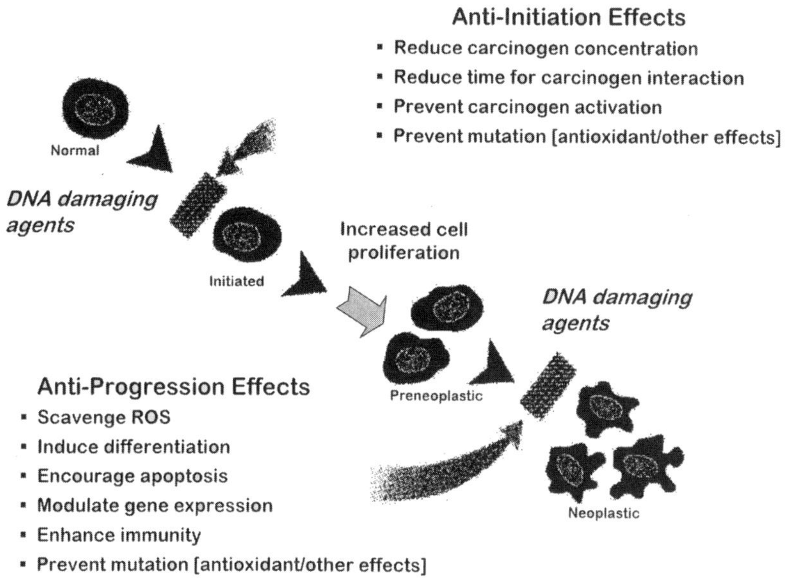

Source: Ferguson LR, Chavan RR, Harris PJ. Changing concepts of dietary fiber: Implications for carcinogenesis. *Nutr Cancer.* 2001;39(2):155–169.
ROS, reactive oxygen species.

bowel mucosa (Key et al., 2004). Fat intake may also alter immune function, cell membranes, cellular mechanisms, oxidative stress, genetic pathways, prostaglandin production, and angiogenesis, all of which may affect cancer risk (Clavel-Chapelon, Niravong, & Joseph, 1997; Lipkin et al., 1999; Kolonel, Nomura, & Cooney, 1999).

Meat

There is evidence that consumption of red meat is linked to an increased risk of colon cancer. The 2007 World Cancer Research Fund report reviewed 16 cohort and 71 case-control studies and found substantial evidence for an increased risk of colorectal cancer with increased red meat consumption (WCRF/AICR, 2007). A meta-analysis of 48 studies found that total meat consumption was weakly, but not significantly, associated with colorectal cancer, but that con-

sumption of red meat and processed meat were both significantly associated with colorectal cancer risk (Norat et al., 2002). A conflicting study by Truswell, however, found that 20 of 30 case-control studies and 12 of 15 prospective studies showed no association between meat consumption and colon cancer (Truswell, 2002).

Meat intake, especially of processed meats (WCRF/AICR, 2007), may also increase the risk of prostate cancer, although not all studies have agreed (Kushi & Giovannucci, 2002; Nelson, De Marzo, & Isaacs, 2003; Dagnelie et al., 2004; Clinton & Giovannucci, 1998). There may also be a connection between meat consumption and increases in esophageal, lung, pancreatic, endometrial, and breast cancer (WCRF/AICR, 2007; Kushi & Giovannucci, 2002; Bingham, 1999; Thomson et al., 2003).

There are a number of reasons to explain how meat might increase the risk of cancer.

The high fat content of meat may increase risk. The process of cooking or curing meat may lead to the production of potentially carcinogenic compounds such as N-nitroso compounds, polycyclic aromatic hydrocarbons, and heterocyclic amines (Key et al., 2004). These compounds may increase the risk for several types of cancer (WCRF/AICR, 2007; Cummings & Bingham, 1998; LeMarchand et al., 2002). It has also been theorized that the iron in meat may increase the formation of cancer-causing free radicals (Kushi & Giovannucci, 2002; Norat et al., 2002; Lund et al., 1999). In addition, if meat is consumed at the expense of other potentially protective foods, such as fruits, vegetables, and grains, this could increase cancer risk.

Cooking and Food Preservation Methods

Grilling, barbecuing, and frying of meats and fish produce chemicals (polycyclic aromatic hydrocarbons and heterocyclic amines) that may have carcinogenic properties in humans. These chemicals have been implicated in increased risks of stomach and colorectal cancers (LeMarchand et al., 2002) and may increase the risk of other cancers as well (WCRF/AICR, 2007; Cummings & Bingham, 1998).

Curing is a method for preserving meat and fish. Cured meats are a source of N-nitroso compounds, which may be carcinogenic, particularly in the stomach and possibly in the colon (WCRF/AICR, 2007; Key, Schatzkin, et al., 2004).

Data are convincing that diets high in Chinese-style salted fish increase the risk of nasopharyngeal cancer. Regular consumption of highly salted or pickled meats, fish, vegetables, and other foods may increase the risk of stomach cancer (WCRF/AICR, 2007; Yamaguchi & Abe, 1999).

Soy Products

Several mechanisms have been hypothesized by which soy products could exert a protective effect against cancer. Soy has one of the highest concentrations of isoflavonoids. Isoflavonoids have been shown *in vitro* to demonstrate several anticancer effects through many mechanisms, including effects on enzymes and cellular factors that control the growth and differentiation of cells, as well as antioxidant effects and effects on blood vessels (Birt, Hendrich, & Wang, 2001; Willis & Wians, 2003). Isoflavonoids are also phytoestrogens and, as such, may have anticancer properties. Isoflavonoids have been shown to inhibit the growth of a wide range of hormone-dependent and hormone-independent cancer cells in culture (Ren et al., 2001; Messina et al., 1994). Soybeans also contain other compounds with anticarcinogenic effects, such as protease inhibitors, phytosterols, saponins, fiber, and other phytochemicals (Birt, Hendrich, & Wang, 2001).

Despite these numerous theoretical protective effects, to date there is no conclusive evidence showing that soy actually does decrease cancer risk. Numerous epidemiologic studies have given conflicting results on the potential protective effects of soy products on breast and prostate cancer (LeMarchand, 2002; Peeters et al., 2003; Magee & Rowland, 2004; Adlercreutz, 2002; Messina, 2003; Sirtori, 2001). Although it has been theorized that the increased soy consumption in Asian countries may explain the substantially lower rates of breast and prostate cancer in those countries, this remains an unproven hypothesis (Magee & Rowland, 2004; Sirtori, 2001). One article that evaluated 13 epidemiological studies found that the data relating soy products to risk of colorectal cancer were inconclusive, but did point to a possible inverse relationship (Spector et al., 2003). Messina reviewed the studies that examined associations between soy products and cancer risk and concluded that although the literature suggests a protective effect of nonfermented soy products, inconsistencies prohibit a stronger conclusion (Messina et al., 1994).

Obesity

Obesity is probably a significant risk factor for cancers of the colon (Gatof & Ahnen, 2002; Giovannucci, 2002), breast (Key, Allen, et al., 2003; Key, Allen, et al., 2002), endometrium, kidney (WCRF/AICR, 2007; Key, Allen, et al., 2002), esophagus, pancreaa, and liver (WCRF/AICR, 2007). It may be a risk factor for prostate cancer as well (Moyad & Carroll, 2004a, 2004b). The underlying reason(s) for the apparent association between obesity and cancer are unclear, but may include excess energy consumption, lack of exercise, specific dietary factors, and metabolic or hormonal changes.

Common Cancers and Related Dietary Factors

The most common cancers in the United States are lung (28%), colon (12%), breast (9%), and prostate (6%). With the exception of lung cancer, 85% of which is directly attributable to cigarette smoking, no one particular environmental factor is known to cause these cancers. However, it appears certain that dietary factors can influence risk. This section summarizes the dietary factors that are thought at this time to possibly contribute to the risk of these four common cancers.

Lung Cancer

- Cigarette smoking causes the vast majority of lung cancers.

- There is convincing evidence that fruits and vegetables can decrease the risk of lung cancer, although the results of prospective studies have not been as consistent in showing the protection from fruits and vegetables shown by case-control studies (WCRF/AICR, 2007; Key, Schatzkin, et al., 2004; Terry, Terry, & Wolk, 2001; Riboli & Norat, 2003; Smith-Warner & Giovannucci, 1999).
- Epidemiologicaldata suggest that increased dietary intake of carotenoids can decrease the risk of lung cancer (WCRF/AICR, 2007; Omenn, 1996; Alavanja et al., 1993).
- Studiesalso point to a possible increase in risk from total fat, and a possible decrease in risk from selenium (WCRF/AICR, 2007; Alavanja et al., 1993).

Colon Cancer

Of all the major cancers, a role for dietary factors affecting risk is strongest for colon cancer.

- There is strong evidence from case-control studies that vegetables, and possibly fruits, can protect against the development of colon cancer. More recent large prospective studies, however, have found less evidence of a protective effect of fruits and vegetables (WCRF/AICR, 2007; Terry, Terry, & Wolk, 2001; Kampman, Arts, & Hollman, 2003; Sengupta, Tjandra, & Gibson, 2001; Key et al., 2004; Giovannucci, 2003). When the study types were pooled, a moderate but significantly decreased risk of colorectal cancer with high intake of vegetables and fruits was found (Riboli & Norat, 2003).
- There is evidence from case-control and some prospective studies that fiber can decrease the risk of colorectal cancer (WCRF/AICR, 2007; Howe et al., 1992; Shankar &

Lanza, 1991; Trock, Lanza, & Greenwald, 1992; Sengupta, Tjandra, & Gibson, 2001; Ferguson, Chavan, & Harris, 2001; Giovannucci, 2003;Turini & DuBois, 2002; Hawk, Limburg, & Viner, 2002).

- Intervention studies have not supported a protective effect of fruits, vegetables, and fiber on the formation of colonic adenomas thought to be sites of early cancer development (Turini & DuBois, 2002; Hawk, Limburg, & Viner, 2002).

- There is no consistent evidence that diets high in total fat increase the risk of colon cancer (Zock, 2001; Kushi & Giovannucci, 2002; Hawk, Limburg, & Viner, 2002). Saturated fat may increase the risk of colon cancer (WCRF/AICR, 2007). Whether any other particular subtype of fat, such as the n-6 or n-3 polyunsaturated fats, can influence colon cancer risk is unknown (Johnson, 2004; McEntree & Whelan, 2002).

- There is fairly convincing evidence that obesity and physical inactivity are risk factors for colon cancer (WCRF/AICR, 2007; Gatof & Ahnen, 2002; Giovannucci, 2002; Giovannucci, 2003; Hawk, Limburg, & Viner, 2002).

- Red meat consumption may be carcinogenic in the colon (WCRF/AICR, 1997; Key, Schatzkin, et al., 2004; Kushi & Giovannucci, 2002; Truswell, 2002; Chao et al., 2005). One review shed doubt on any such relationship with its finding that only 10 of 30 adequate case-control studies and only 3 of 15 prospective studies had found an association between meat consumption and colon cancer (Truswell, 2002). Another review found that consumption of red meat and processed meat, but not total meat consumption, were significantly associated with increased risk of colorectal cancer (Norat et al., 2002). Heterocyclic aromatic amines and polycyclic aromatic amines formed during cooking of meats are carcinogenic and may increase the rate of colorectal cancer (LeMarchand et al., 2002). In addition, nitrosamines, which are found in cured meats, are also carcinogenic and may increase colorectal cancer risk (Key et al., 2004).

- Although the data regarding any relationship between soy products and colorectal cancer is inconclusive, a possible decreased risk with increased consumption of soy has been suggested (Spector et al., 2003).

- There is some support for the hypotheses that dietary iron and/or iron stores may increase the risk of colorectal cancer (Nelson, 2001).

Breast Cancer

- It has been hypothesized that dietary fiber, by reducing estrogen levels, might reduce the risk of breast cancer. Several case-control studies have shown that fiber can reduce the risk of breast cancer; however, prospective studies have not generally supported this theory (Baghurst & Rohan, 1994; Key, Allen, et al., 2003; Duncan, 2004).

- Although phytoestrogens may protect against breast cancer, the data have been somewhat inconsistent (Peeters et al., 2003; Magee & Rowland, 2004; Key, Allen, et al., 2003).

- Meat may be a risk factor for breast cancer, although the results of studies vary (Kushi & Giovannucci, 2002; Gerber et al., 2003). Any effect of meat may possibly be due to the fat content and/or the presence of heterocyclic amines and N-nitroso compounds (Cummings & Bingham, 1998).

- Total fat intake may increase the risk of breast cancer (WCRF/AICR, 2007).

Prostate Cancer

- In contrast to all other cancers, the evidence for a protective effect of fruits and vegetables is very weak with regard to prostate cancer, although there may be some protection, especially with fruits and vegetables containing lycopene (WCRF/AICR, 2007; Terry, Terry, & Wolk, 2001; Dagnelie et al., 2004; Clinton & Giovannucci, 1998; Smith-Warner & Giovannucci, 1999).
- Although numerous case-control studies have found an increase in prostate cancer risk with increasing fat consumption, more recent prospective studies have not agreed with this (WCRF/AICR, 2007; Kushi & Giovannucci, 2002; Dagnelie et al., 2004; Moyad, 2002; Thomas, 1999).
- There is some evidence that meat, especially processed meat, may increase the risk of prostate cancer, but the results of studies are not consistent (WCRF/AICR, 2007; Kushi & Giovannucci, 2002; Dagnelie et al., 2004; Gronberg, 2003).
- It has been hypothesized that increased hormone levels may be a risk factor for prostate cancer. Both high dietary fiber and possibly low dietary fat can decrease serum hormone levels; therefore, it is thought that both may decrease prostate cancer occurrence (Yip, Heber, & Aronson, 1999; Ross, Pusateri, & Shultz, 1990; Fair, Fleshner, & Heston, 1997; Pusateri et al., 1990). An additional theory suggests that phytoestrogens may protect against prostate cancer by acting as antiandrogens (Magee & Rowland, 2004; Messina, 2003).
- Studies investigating the effect of soy on prostate cancer risk have been inconsistent but intriguing (Messina, 2003; Willis & Wians, 2003).

- Several lines of evidence suggest that antioxidants may have a protective effect against prostate cancer (Willis & Wians, 2003; Sikka, 2003).
- Several studies have suggested a protective role for tomatoes and/or tomato sauce, but many studies have not found this relationship (Moyad & Carroll, 2004a, 2004b; Dagnelie et al., 2004).

The Relationship Between Vegetarian Diets and Dietary Factors That May Affect Cancer Risk

As discussed throughout this chapter, many dietary factors have potential links to cancer risk. Each of these factors also provides plausible links between vegetarian diets and cancer risk.

Fruits and Vegetables

Evidence suggests that fruit and vegetable consumption may decrease the risk of many, if not most, cancers. It seems reasonable to assume that vegetarians consume large amounts of fruits and vegetables and that this might serve to decrease the risk of cancer among vegetarians. Vegetarians appear to have both higher carotenoid intakes and higher serum carotenoid levels than nonvegetarians. They also commonly consume more vitamin C than nonvegetarians. Folate intakes appear to be similar or better in vegetarians than in nonvegetarians.

Antioxidants

Antioxidants serve many potentially anticarcinogenic functions. Antioxidants are abundant in fruits, vegetables, and grains, thereby affording potential protection against cancer for vegetarians.

Phytochemicals

Phytochemicals have shown many potential anticarcinogenic mechanisms in the laboratory. Vegetarians, because they tend to consume more plant foods, will typically have higher intakes of phytochemicals than nonvegetarians, thereby potentially lowering their cancer risk. Those vegetarians who consume foods high in phytoestrogens, especially soy and flaxseed, may enjoy yet another potential protective factor. Compared to omnivores, vegetarians have higher levels of isoflavonoids and phytoestrogens in plasma and urine (Adlercreutz, 2002).

Fiber

Fiber probably plays a protective role against colorectal cancer and may protect against other cancers as well. Because vegetarians consume more fiber than nonvegetarians, it is plausible that this may be one mechanism whereby a vegetarian diet could lower cancer risk.

Fats

Although much controversy exists surrounding the potential role of dietary fat in cancer risk, there is evidence to suggest a possible connection. Vegetarian diets are slightly lower in total fat and considerably lower in saturated fat than omnivorous diets, thus providing yet another potential protective mechanism.

Meat

It is possible that meat consumption is linked to an increased risk of colon cancer. Meat may also increase the risk of other cancers. Vegetarians, by definition, consume no meat, and this may give them an advantage against cancer.

Cooking and Food Preservation Methods

Vegetarians would not be exposed to the potentially carcinogenic compounds produced when meat is grilled, barbecued, or fried or when meat is cured. Vegetarians who regularly consume highly salted or pickled vegetables may increase their risk of stomach cancer.

Soy Products

Although, to date, there is no conclusive evidence that soy reduces cancer risk, there are many theoretical mechanisms that make it a possibility. Vegetarians who consume soy may be getting some protection against cancer from it.

Common Cancers and Vegetarian Diets

Lung Cancer

It is probably true that vegetarians tend to be more health conscious and, therefore, less likely to smoke, thereby eliminating the predominant risk factor for lung cancer. A vegetarian diet may afford protection from lung cancer by virtue of its increased quantity of fruits, vegetables, and carotenoids, and lower amounts of fat.

Colon Cancer

Of all cancers, it appears that a vegetarian diet has the greatest chance of decreasing the risk of colon cancer. Fiber may decrease the risk of colon cancer. Because vegetarians consume no meat and less fat than nonvegetarians, their risk for colon cancer may be lowered even further. Their lower incidence of obesity may also protect vegetarians from colon cancer. Furthermore, several studies have shown that the colonic environment in vegetarians differs from that of omnivores in ways that may be protective against colon cancer (Messina & Messina, 1996).

- Vegetarians have lower colonic concentrations of the potentially carcinogenic secondary bile acids (WCRF/AICR, 1997; Reddy, 1999; Turjman et al., 1984; Korpela, Adlercreutz, & Turunen, 1988).
- The bacteria in the colon of vegetarians may differ in ways that decrease the production of secondary bile acids (Korpela, Adlercreutz, & Turunen, 1988; Willett et al., 1990).
- The colonic pH of vegetarians appears to be lower, which in turn would decrease the production of potentially carcinogenic secondary bile acids (van Dokkum et al., 1983).
- Vegetarians tend to have larger, softer stools and decreased transit time in the colon, thereby lessening the time that potentially carcinogenic compounds spend in the body.
- Several studies have shown that vegetarians have lower levels of fecal mutagens (Kuhnlein, Bergstrom, & Kuhnlein, 1981; Nader, Potter, & Weller, 1981).
- Vegetarians have decreased colonic cell proliferation; more rapid proliferation is common among those at high risk of colon cancer (WCRF/AICR, 1997).

Breast Cancer

Several attributes of a vegetarian diet may decrease the risk of breast cancer, including higher intake of fruits and vegetables, fiber, and phytoestrogens, and decreased intake of fat and meat. Vegetarians tend to be leaner than nonvegetarians, and this may afford some protection against breast cancer.

Increased exposure to estrogen appears to increase the risk of breast cancer. Similarly, early age of menarche is an established risk for breast cancer, possibly because it increases a woman's lifetime exposure to estrogen. Several studies have reported that vegetarians have lower blood estrogen levels (Goldin et al., 1994; Goldin & Gorbach, 1994; Rose et al., 1991; Howie & Shultz, 1985; Barbosa et al., 1990; Adlercreutz et al., 1986), perhaps because of their lower fat and greater fiber consumption. Vegetarians also have later age of menarche (Griffiths et al., 1996; Sanchez, Kissinger, & Phillips, 1981), which would decrease lifetime exposure to estrogen. In addition, vegetarians have higher levels of phytoestrogens (Griffiths et al., 1996; Adlercreutz et al., 1995), which may act as anti-estrogens.

Prostate Cancer

The lower fat content and lack of meat, especially processed meats, in a vegetarian diet may decrease the risk of prostate cancer. Higher intakes of fiber, phytoestrogens, and foods containing lycopene might also offer some protection.

Hormones such as testosterone are thought to be important determinants of the risk of prostate cancer. Some, but not all, studies have found that vegetarian men have lower levels of free testosterone in the blood (Pusateri et al., 1990; Belanger et al., 1989), possibly due to differences in dietary fat and/or fiber.

Practical Aspects

Many aspects of a vegetarian diet may offer protection from cancer. To maximize protection, a vegetarian diet should include an abundance of and a variety of fruits and vegetables.

Current recommendations are for five or more servings per day of fruits and vegetables. One should consume other plant-based foods, such as grains, pasta, cereals, rice, or beans, several times each day. Vitamin intake should be adequate. One should assure that there is adequate fiber in the diet. The National Cancer Institute recommends that individuals consume 20 to 35 grams of fiber per day to decrease cancer risk. One should limit total fats to between 15% and 30% of total calories, with particular attention to limiting fats of animal origin (WCRF/AICR, 2007; Adlercreutz et al., 1995). Consumption of soy products may offer further protection from cancer.

Conclusion

The World Cancer Research Fund and the American Institute for Cancer Research (2007) recommend, for maximal cancer protection, a predominately plant-based diet rich in a variety of vegetables, fruits, and legumes, which limits intake of red meat and avoids processed meats, and which contains a minimal amount of processed starchy foods. The American Cancer Society (2000) recommends reducing cancer risk by choosing foods primarily from plant sources and limiting the intake of high-fat foods, particularly those from animal sources.

A well-balanced vegetarian diet is in line with these recommendations. Thus, many aspects of a vegetarian diet may decrease cancer risk. In fact, when it comes to cancer protection, a vegetarian diet offers many potential advantages over an omnivorous diet, including greater consumption of fruits and vegetables, fiber, vitamins, antioxidants, phytochemicals, and soy products, as well as decreased consumption of fat and absence of meat.

Evidence suggests that vegetarians do have a decreased risk of cancer. Even after eliminating smoking-related cancers, it appears that vegetarians have a decreased cancer risk. Evidence is strongest for a decreased risk of gastrointestinal (especially colon) cancer among vegetarians. Vegetarians may also be protected to some degree by diet from other cancers, such as breast cancer and possibly prostate cancer.

When it comes to cancer, the first and best tool is prevention. Consuming a vegetarian diet is an excellent way of providing the body with the many dietary factors that may offer protection from cancer.

References

Adlercreutz CH, Goldin B, Gorbach SL, et al. Soybean phytoestrogen intake and cancer risk. *J Nutr.* 1995;125(3, Suppl):757S–770S.

Adlercreutz H. Phytoestrogens and breast cancer. *J Steroid Biochem Mol Biol.* 2002;83(1–5): 113–118.

Adlercreutz H, Fotsis T, Bannwart C, et al. Urinary estrogen profile determination in young Finnish vegetarian and omnivorous women. *J Steroid Biochem.* 1986;24(1):289–296.

Alavanja MC, Brown CL, Swanson C, Brownson RC. Saturated fat intake and lung cancer risk among nonsmoking women in Missouri. *J Natl Cancer Inst.* 1993;85(23):1906–1916.

American Cancer Society. *Nutrition and Prevention Topics: The Importance of Nutrition in Cancer Prevention.* Retrieved March 25, 2000, from http://www2.cancer.org/prevention/index.cfm?prevention=1.

Aronson W, Yip I, Dekernion J. Prostate cancer. In: Herber D, Blackburn G, Go V, eds. *Nutritional Oncology.* San Diego: Academic Press; 1999: 453–461.

Baghurst PA, Rohan TA. High-fiber diets and reduced risk of breast cancer. *Intl J Cancer.* 1994;56(2): 173–176.

Barbosa J, Shultz TD, Filley SJ, Nieman DC. The relationship among adiposity, diet, and hormone concentrations in vegetarian and nonvegetarian postmenopausal women. *Am J Clin Nutr.* 1990; 51(5):798–803.

Belanger A, Locong A, Noel C, et al. Influence of diet on plasma steroid and sex plasma binding globulin levels in adult men. *J Steroid Biochem.* 1989;32(6):829–833.

Berkel J, de Waard F. Mortality pattern and life expectancy of Seventh-Day Adventists in the Netherlands. *Intl J Epidemiol.* 1983;12(4):455–459.

Bingham SA. High-meat diets and cancer risk. *Proc Nutr Soc.* 1999;58(2):243–248.

Birt DF, Hendrich S, Wang W. Dietary agents in cancer prevention: Flavonoids and isoflavonoids. *Pharmacol Ther.* 2001;90(2–3):157–177.

Block G, Patterson B, Subar A. Fruit, vegetables, and cancer prevention: A review of the epidemiological evidence. *Nutr Cancer.* 1992;18(1):1–29.

Chao A, Thun MJ, Connell CJ, et al. Meat consumption and risk of colorectal cancer. *JAMA.* 2005; 293(2):172–182.

Clavel-Chapelon F, Niravong M, Joseph RR. Diet and breast cancer: Review of the epidemiologic literature. *Cancer Detect Preven.* 1997;21(5): 426–440.

Clinton SK, Giovannucci E. Diet, nutrition, and prostate cancer. *Ann Rev Nutr.* 1998;18:413–440.

Craig WJ. Phytochemicals: Guardians of our health. *J Am Diet Assoc.* 1997;97(10, Suppl 2):S199–S204.

Cummings JH, Bingham SH. Diet and the prevention of cancer. *Br Med J.* 1998;317(7173): 1636–1640.

Dagnelie PC, Schuurman AG, Goldbohm RA, Van den Brandt PA. Diet, anthropometric measures and prostate cancer risk: A review of prospective cohort and intervention studies. *BJU Int.* 2004;93(8):1139–1150.

Doll R, Peto R. The causes of cancer: Quantitative estimates of avoidable risks of cancer in the United States today. *J Natl Cancer Inst.* 1981; 66(6):1191–1308.

Dreosti IE. Nutrition, cancer, and aging. *Ann NY Acad Sci.* Nov 20, 1998;854:371–377.

Duncan AM. The role of nutrition in the prevention of breast cancer. *AACN Clin Issues.* 2004;15(1): 119–135.

Fair WR, Fleshner NE, Heston W. Cancer of the prostate: A nutritional disease? *Urology.* 1997;50(6): 840–848.

Ferguson LR, Chavan RR, Harris PJ. Changing concepts of dietary fiber: Implication for carcinogenesis. *Nutr Cancer.* 2001;39(2):155–169.

Fonnebo V, Helseth A. Cancer incidence in Norwegian Seventh-Day Adventists 1961 to 1986. Is the cancer-life-style association overestimated? *Cancer.* 1991;68(3):666–671.

Frentzel-Beyme R, Chang-Claude J. Vegetarian diets and colon cancer: The German experience. *Am J Clin Nutr.* 1994;59(Suppl):1143S–1152S.

Friedenreich CM, Brant RF, Riboli E. Influence of methodologic factors in a pooled analysis of 13 case-control studies of colorectal cancer and dietary fiber. *Epidemiology.* 1994;5(1):66–79.

Fuchs CS, Giovannucci EL, Colditz G, et al. Dietary fiber and the risk of colorectal cancer and adenoma in women. *N Eng J Med.* 1999;340(3): 169–176.

Gatof D, Ahnen D. Primary prevention of colorectal cancer. *Gastroenterol Clin N Am.* 2002;31(2): 587–623.

Gerber B, Muller H, Reimer T, et al. Nutrition and life-style factors on the risk of developing breast cancer. *Breast Cancer Res Treat.* 2003;79(2):265–276.

Gerber M. Fibre and breast cancer. *Eur J Cancer Preven.* 1998;7(Suppl 2):S63–S67.

Giovannucci E. Diet, body weight, and colorectal cancer: A summary of the epidemiologic evidence. *J Women's Health.* 2003;12(2):173–182.

Giovannucci E. Modifiable risk factors for colon cancer. *Gastroenterol Clin N Am.* 2002;31(4): 925–943.

Giovannucci E, Rimm EB, Stampfer MJ, et al. Intake of fat, meat, and fiber in relation to risk of colon cancer in men. *Cancer Res.* 1994;54(9):2390–2397.

Go VL, Wong DA, Butrum R. Diet, nutrition and cancer prevention: Where are we going from here? *J Nutr.* 2001;131(11, Suppl):3121S–3126S.

Goldin B, Gorbach S. Hormone studies and the diet and breast cancer connection. In: American Institute for Cancer Research, ed. *Diet and Breast Cancer.* New York: Plenum Press; 1994.

Goldin BR, Woods MN, Spiegelman DL, et al. The effect of dietary fat and fiber on serum estrogen concentrations in premenopausal women under controlled dietary conditions. *Cancer.* 1994;74 (3, Suppl):1125-1131.

Griffiths K, Adlercreutz H, Boyle P, Denis L, Nicholson R, Morton M. *Nutrition and Cancer.* Oxford, UK: Isis Medical Media Ltd; 1996.

Gronberg H. Prostate cancer epidemiology. *Lancet.* 2003;361(9360):859-864.

Halling H, Carstensen J. Cancer incidence among a group of Swedish vegetarians. *Cancer Detect Preven.* 1984;7:425.

Halliwell B. Effect of diet on cancer development: Is oxidative DNA damage a biomarker? *Free Radical Biol Med.* 2002;32(10):968-974.

Halliwell B. Establishing the significance and optimal intake of dietary antioxidants: The biomarker concept. *Nutr Rev.* 1999;57(4):104-113.

Hawk ET, Limburg PJ, Viner, JL. Epidemiology and prevention of colorectal cancer. *Surg Clin N Am.* 2002;82(5):905-941.

Heilbrun LK, Nomura A, Hankin JH, Stemmermann GN. Diet and colorectal cancer with special reference to fiber intake. *Intl J Cancer.* 1989;44(1): 1-6.

Hirayama T. Mortality in Japanese with life-styles similar to Seventh-Day Adventists: Strategy for risk reduction by life-style modification. *Natl Cancer Inst Monographs.* 1985;69:143-153.

Howe GR, Benito E, Castelleto R, et al. Dietary intake of fiber and decreased risk of cancers of the colon and rectum: Evidence from the combined analysis of 13 case-control studies. *J Natl Cancer Inst.* 1992;84(24):1887-1896.

Howie B, Shultz TD. Dietary and hormonal interrelationships among vegetarian Seventh Day Adventists and nonvegetarian men. *Am J Clin Nutr.* 1985;42(1):127-134.

Jacob DR, Marquart L, Slavin J, Kushi LH. Whole-grain intake and cancer: An expanded review and meta-analysis. *Nutr Cancer.* 1998;30:85-96.

Jensen OM. Cancer risk among Danish male Seventh-Day Adventists and other temperance society members. *J Natl Cancer Inst.* 1983;70(6):1011-1014.

Johnson IT. New approaches to the role of diet in the prevention of cancers of the alimentary tract. *Mutat Res.* 2004;551(1-2):9-28.

Johnson IT. Antioxidants and anticarcinogens. *Eur J Cancer Preven.* 1998;7(Suppl 2):S55-S62.

Kampman E, Arts IC, Hollman PC. Plant foods versus compounds in carcinogenesis: Observational versus experimental human studies. *Intl J Vit Nutr Res.* 2003;73(2):70-78.

Key TJ, Allen NE, Spencer EA, Travis RC. Nutrition and breast cancer. *Breast.* 2003;12(6):412-416.

Key TJ, Allen NE, Spencer EA, Travis RC. The effect of diet on risk of cancer. *Lancet.* 2002;360(9336): 861-868.

Key TJ, Appleby PN, Davey GK, et al. Mortality in British vegetarians: Review and preliminary results from EPIC-Oxford. *Am J Clin Nutr.* 2003; 78(3, Suppl):533S-538S.

Key TJ, Fraser GE, Thorogood M, et al. Mortality in vegetarians and non-vegetarians: A collaborative analysis of 8300 deaths among 76,000 men and women in five prospective studies. *Public Health Nutr.* 1998;1(1):33-41.

Key TJ, Schatzkin A, Willett WC, et al. Diet, nutrition and the prevention of cancer. *Public Health Nutr.* 2004;7(1A):187-200.

Key TJ, Thorogood M, Appleby PN, Burr ML. Dietary habits and mortality in 11,000 vegetarians and health conscious people: Results of a 17 year follow up. *Br Med J.* 1996;313(7060):775-779.

Kim YI. AGA technical review: Impact of dietary fiber on colon cancer occurrence. *Gastroenterology.* 2000;118(6):1235-1257.

Kinlen LJ, Hermon C, Smith PG. A proportionate study of cancer mortality among members of a vegetarian society. *Br J Cancer.* 1983;48(3):355-361.

Kolonel LN, Nomura AM, Cooney RV. Dietary fat and prostate cancer. *J Natl Cancer Inst.* 1999;91(5): 414-428.

Korpela J, Adlercreutz H, Turunen MJ. Fecal free and conjugated bile acids and neutral sterols in vegetarians, omnivores, and patients with colorectal cancer. *Scand J Gastroenterol.* 1988;23(3): 277-283.

Kris-Etherton PM, Hecker KD, Bonanome A, et al. Bioactive compounds in foods: Their role in the prevention of cardiovascular disease and cancer. *Am J Med.* 2002;113(Suppl 9B):71S–88S.

Kuhnlein U, Bergstrom D, Kuhnlein H. Mutagens in feces from vegetarians and non-vegetarians. *Mutat Res.* 1981;85(1):1–12.

Kuratsune M, Ikeda M, Hayashi T. Epidemiologic studies of possible health effects of intake of pyrolyzates of foods, with reference to mortality among Japanese Seventh-Day Adventists. *Envir Health Persp.* 1986;67:143–146.

Kushi L, Giovannucci E. Dietary fat and cancer. *Am J Med.* 2002;113(Suppl 9B):63S–70S.

La Vecchia C, Altieri A, Tavani A. Vegetables, fruit, antioxidants and cancer: A review of Italian studies. *Eur J Nutr.* 2001;40:261–267.

LeMarchand L. Cancer preventive effects of flavonoids—A review. *Biomed Pharmacother.* 2002;56(6):296–301.

LeMarchand L, Hankin JH, Pierce LM, et al. Well-done red meat, metabolic phenotypes and colorectal cancer in Hawaii. *Mutat Res.* 2002;506–507:205–214.

Levi F. Cancer prevention: Epidemiology and perspectives. *Eur J Cancer.* 1999;35(7):1046–1058.

Lipkin M, Reddy B, Newmark H, Lamprecht S. Dietary factors in human colorectal cancer. *Ann Rev Nutr.* 1999;19:545–586.

Liu RH. Health benefits of fruit and vegetables are from additive and synergistic combinations of phytochemicals. *Am J Clin Nutr.* 2003;78(3, Suppl):517S–520S.

Lopez-Lazaro M. Flavonoids as anticancer agents: Structure-activity relationship study. *Curr Med Chem Anti-Cancer Agents.* 2002;2(6):691–714.

Lund EK, Wharf SG, Fairweather-Tate SJ, Johnson IT. Oral ferrous sulfate supplements increase the free radical-generating capacity of feces from healthy volunteers. *Am J Clin Nutr.* 1999;69(2):250–255.

Magee PJ, Rowland IR. Phyto-oestrogens, their mechanism of action: Current evidence for a role in breast and prostate cancer. *Br J Nutr.* 2004;91(4):513–531.

Martinez M, Marshall J, Alberts D. Dietary fiber, carbohydrates, and cancer. In: Heber D, Blackburn G, Go V, eds. *Nutritional Oncology*. San Diego: Academic Press; 1999:185–194.

McEntree MF, Whelan J. Dietary polyunsaturated fatty acids and colorectal neoplasia. *Biomed Pharmacother.* 2002;56(8):380–387.

McIntosh GH, Noakes M, Royle PJ, Foster PR. Whole-grain rye and wheat foods and markers of bowel health in overweight middle-aged men. *Am J Clin Nutr.* 2003;77(4):967–974.

McTiernan A. Behavioral risk factors in breast cancer: Can risk be modified? *Oncologist.* 2003;8(4):326–334.

Messina M, Messina V. *The Dietitian's Guide to Vegetarian Diets: Issues and Applications.* Gaithersburg, MD: Aspen Publishers; 1996.

Messina MJ. Emerging evidence on the role of soy in reducing prostate cancer risk. *Nutr Rev.* 2003;61(4):117–131.

Messina MJ, Persky V, Setchell KD, Barnes S. Soy intake and cancer risk: A review of the in vitro and in vivo data. *Nutr Cancer.* 1994;21(2):113–131.

Mills PK, Beeson WL, Abbey DE, et al. Dietary habits and past medical history as related to fatal pancreas cancer among Adventists. *Cancer.* 1988;61(12):2578–2585.

Mills PK, Beeson WL, Phillips RL, Fraser GE. Cancer incidence among California Seventh-Day Adventists, 1976–1982. *Am J Clin Nutr.* 1994;59(5, Suppl):1136S–1142S.

Mills PK, Beeson WL, Phillips RL, Fraser GE. Cohort study of diet, lifestyle, and prostate cancer in Adventist men. *Cancer.* 1989a;64(13):598–604.

Mills PK, Beeson WL, Phillips RL, Fraser GE. Dietary habits and breast cancer incidence among Seventh-Day Adventists. *Cancer.* 1989b;64(3):582–590.

Milner JA. Strategies for cancer prevention: The role of diet. *Br J Nutr.* 2002;87(Suppl 2):S265–S272.

Moyad MA. Dietary fat reduction to reduce prostate cancer risk: Controlled enthusiasm, learning a lesson from breast or other cancers, and the big picture. *Urology.* 2002;59(4, Suppl):51–62.

Moyad MA, Carroll PR. Lifestyle recommendations to prevent prostate cancer, part I: Time to redirect our attention? *Urol Clin N Am.* 2004a;31(2):289–300.

Moyad MA, Carroll PR. Lifestyle recommendations to prevent prostate cancer, part II: Time to redirect our attention? *Urol Clin N Am.* 2004b;31(2): 301–311.

Nader C, Potter J, Weller R. Diet and DNA-modifying activity in human fecal extracts. *Nutr Reps Intl.* 1981;23(1):113–117.

Nelson RL. Iron and colorectal cancer risk: Human studies. *Nutr Rev.* 2001;59(5):140–148.

Nelson W, De Marzo A, Isaacs W. Mechanisms of disease: Prostate cancer. *N Engl J Med.* 2003;349(4): 366–381.

Norat T, Lukanova A, Ferrari P, Riboli E. Meat consumption and colorectal cancer risk: Dose-response meta-analysis of epidemiological studies. *Intl J Cancer.* 2002;98(2):241–256.

Omenn G. Micronutrients (vitamins and minerals) as cancer-preventive agents. In: Stewart B, McGregor D, Kleihues P, eds. *Principles of Chemoprevention.* Lyon, France: International Agency for Research on Cancer; 1996:33–45.

Peeters PH, Keinan-Boker L, van der Schouw YY, Grobbee DE. Phytoestrogens and breast cancer risk. *Breast Cancer Res Treat.* 2003;77(2):171–183.

Phillips RL. Role of life-style and dietary habits in risk of cancer among Seventh-Day Adventists. *Cancer Res.* 1975;35(11, Pt.2):3513–3522.

Phillips RL, Garfinkel L, Kuzma JW, et al. Mortality among California Seventh-Day Adventists for selected cancer sites. *J Natl Cancer Inst.* 1980; 65(5):1097–1107.

Phillips RL, Kuzma JW, Beeson WL, Lotz T. Influence of selection versus lifestyle on risk of fatal cancer and cardiovascular disease among Seventh-Day Adventists. *Am J Epidemiol.* 1980;112(2): 296–314.

Phillips RL, Snowdon DA. Association of meat and coffee use with cancers of the large bowel, breast, and prostate among Seventh-Day Adventists: Preliminary results. *Cancer Res.* 1983;43(5, Suppl): 2403S–2408S.

Potter J, Steinmetz K. Vegetables, fruit and phytoestrogens as preventive agents. In: Stewart B, McGregor D, Kleihues P, eds. *Principles of Chemoprevention.* Lyon, France: International Agency for Research on Cancer; 1996:61–90.

Pusateri D, Roth WT, Ross JK, Shultz TD. Dietary and hormonal evaluation of men at different risks

for prostate cancer: Plasma and fecal hormone-nutrient interrelationships. *Am J Clin Nutr.* 1990; 51(3):371–377.

Rao DN, Ganesh B, Desai PB. Role of reproductive factors in breast cancer in a low-risk area: A case-control study. *Br J Cancer.* 1994;70(1):129–132.

Reddy BS. Role of dietary fiber in colon cancer: An overview. *Am J Med.* 1999;106(1A):16S–19S.

Ren MO, Kuhn G, Wegner J, Chen J. Isoflavones, substances with multi-biological and clinical properties. *Eur J Nutr.* 2001;40(4):135–146.

Riboli E, Norat T. Epidemiologic evidence of the protective effect of fruit and vegetables on cancer risk. *Am J Clin Nutr.* 2003;78(3, Suppl):559S–569S.

Rose DP, Goldman M, Connolly JM, Strong LE. High-fiber diet reduces serum estrogen concentrations in premenopausal women. *Am J Clin Nutr.* 1991; 54(3):520–525.

Ross JK, Pusateri DJ, Shultz TD. Dietary and hormonal evaluation of men at different risks for prostate cancer: Fiber intake, excretion, and composition, with in vitro evidence for an association between steroid hormones and specific fiber components. *Am J Clin Nutr.* 1990;51: 365–370.

Rowland I. Optimal nutrition: Fibre and phytochemicals. *Proc Nutr Soc.* 1999;58(2):415–419.

Sanchez A, Kissinger D, Phillips R. A hypothesis on the etiological role of diet and age of menarche. *Med Hypotheses.* 1981;7:1339–1345.

Sarkar F, Yiwei L. Soy isoflavones and cancer prevention. *Cancer Investig.* 2003;21(5):744–757.

Sengupta S, Tjandra JJ, Gibson PR. Dietary fiber and colorectal neoplasia. *Dis Colon Rectum.* 2001; 44(7):1016–1033.

Shankar S, Lanza E. Dietary fiber and cancer prevention. *Hematol Oncol Clin N Am.* 1991;5(1):25–41.

Sikka SC. Role of oxidative stress response elements and antioxidants in prostate cancer pathobiology and chemoprevention—A mechanistic approach. *Curr Med Chem.* 2003;10(24):2679–2692.

Sirtori CR. Risks and benefits of soy phytoestrogens in cardiovascular diseases, cancer, climacteric symptoms and osteoporosis. *Drug Safety.* 2001; 24(9):665–682.

Smith-Warner S, Giovannucci E. Fruit and vegetable intake and cancer. In: Herber D, Blackburn G, Go V, eds. *Nutritional Oncology*. San Diego: Academic Press; 1999:153-183.

Spector D, Anthony M, Alexander D, Arab L. Soy consumption and colorectal cancer. *Nutr Cancer*. 2003;47(1):1-12.

Steinmetz KA, Kushi LH, Bostick RM, et al. Vegetables, fruit, and colon cancer in the Iowa Women's Health Study. *Am J Epidemiol*. 1994;139(1):1-15.

Steinmetz KA, Potter J. Vegetables, fruit, and cancer. I. Epidemiology. *Cancer Causes Control*. 1991;2(5):325-357.

Tamimi RM, Lagiou P, Adami H, Trichopoulos D. Prospects for chemoprevention of cancer. *J Intern Med*. 2002;251(4):286-300.

Terry P, Jain M, Miller AB, et al. No association among total dietary fiber, fiber fractions, and risk of breast cancer. *Cancer Epidemiol Biomarkers Preven*. 2002;11(11):1507-1508.

Terry P, Terry JB, Wolk A. Fruit and vegetable consumption in the prevention of cancer: An update. *J Intern Med*. 2001;250(4):280-290.

Thomas J. Diet, micronutrients, and the prostate gland. *Nutr Rev*. 1999;57(4):95-103.

Thomson CA, LeWinn K, Newton TR, et al. Nutrition and diet in the development of gastrointestinal cancer. *Curr Oncol Reps*. 2003;5(3):192-202.

Thorogood M, Mann J, Appleby PN, McPherson K. Risk of death from cancer and ischaemic heart disease in meat and non-meat eaters. *Br Med J*. 1994;308(6945):1667-1671.

Trock B, Lanza E, Greenwald P. Dietary fiber, vegetables, and colon cancer: Critical review and meta-analysis of 13 case-control studies. *J Natl Cancer Inst*. 1992;84:1887-1896.

Truswell AS. Meat consumption and cancer of the large bowel. *Eur J Clin Nutr*. 2002;56(Suppl 1): S19-S24.

Turini ME, DuBois RN. Primary prevention: Phytoprevention and chemoprevention of colorectal cancer. *Hematol Oncol Clin N Am*. 2002;16(4): 811-840.

Turjman N, Goodman GT, Jaeger B, Nair P. Diet, nutrition intake, and metabolism in populations at high and low risk for colon cancer. *Am J Clin Nutr*. 1984;40(4, Suppl):937-941.

van Dokkum W, de Boer BC, van Faassen A, et al. Diet, faecal pH and colorectal cancer. *Br J Cancer*. 1983;48(1):109-110.

Willett W, Stampfer MJ, Colditz GA, et al. Relation of meat, fat, and fiber intake to the risk of colon cancer in a prospective study among women. *N Engl J Med*. 1990;323(24):1664-1672.

Willis MS, Wians FA. The role of nutrition in preventing prostate cancer: A review of the proposed mechanism of action of various dietary substances. *Clin Chim Acta*. 2003;330(1-2): 57-83.

World Cancer Research Fund (WCRF)/American Institute for Cancer Research (AICR). *Food, Nutrition and the Prevention of Cancer: A Global Perspective*. Washington, DC: American Institute for Cancer Research; 2007.

World Cancer Research Fund (WCRF)/American Institute for Cancer Research (AICR). *Food, Nutrition and the Prevention of Cancer: A Global Perspective*. Washington, DC: American Institute for Cancer Research; 1997.

Wynder EL, Gori GB. Contribution of the environment to cancer incidence: An epidemiologic exercise. *J Natl Cancer Inst*. 1977;58(4):825-832.

Wynder EL, Lemon FR, Bross IJ. Cancer and coronary artery disease among Seventh-Day Adventists. *Cancer*. 1959;12(5):1016-1028.

Yamaguchi N, Abe K. Gastric cancer. In: Herber D, Blackburn G, Go V, eds. *Nutritional Oncology*. San Diego: Academic Press; 1999:477-487.

Yip I, Heber D, Aronson W. Nutrition and prostate cancer. *Urol Clin N Am*. 1999;26(2):403-411.

Zock PV. Dietary fats and cancer. *Curr Opin Lipidol*. 2001;12(1):5-10.

Zollinger TW, Phillips RL, Kuzma JW. Breast cancer survival rates among Seventh-Day Adventists and non-Seventh-Day Adventists. *Am J Epidemiol*. 1984;119(4):503-509.

12

Hypertension

James Craner, MD, MPH*

Introduction

Hypertension (high blood pressure) is a major public health problem and one of the most prevalent chronic diseases in the United States and other Westernized nations. Long-standing hypertension contributes to the development of a variety of atherosclerotic and other vascular diseases, including coronary artery disease (CAD) and cerebrovascular disease (stroke). Hypertension affects adults of all ages and both sexes, and to some extent disproportionately affects certain minority populations and individuals above the age of 60. The clinical manifestations of hypertension typically develop after many years of relatively silent disease—hence its reputation as the "silent killer."

At least 60 million Americans currently have a diagnosis of hypertension, and many more have the disease but have not been diagnosed. More than 30 million Americans, nearly 60%–75% of individuals with hypertension, receive drug therapy for hypertension (Oparil, 1993),

with total annual costs for medication, complications, and treatment of complications exceeding $15 billion as of 1996 (Barrie, 1996). In addition, diseases with risk factors that include hypertension, especially coronary artery disease and stroke, collectively constitute many of the major chronic diseases and causes of early loss of life, and contribute significantly to health care costs in the United States and other Westernized nations. A multitude of epidemiological and clinical studies have been conducted in the past 40 years to elucidate the contributory factors and outcomes of hypertension and the impact of treatment. Despite the high prevalence and economic costs of hypertension, however, in nearly all (95%) cases the specific etiology of "essential hypertension" remains unknown.

Although the specific cause and mechanism of hypertension as a disease still remain incompletely understood, epidemiological and clinical research has consistently established that diet and lifestyle are significant contributory or causal factors to the risk for development and progression of hypertension, as well as important but often underemphasized methods

---

* The author wishes to thank Peggy Carlson, MD, for her review of and suggestions for this chapter.

of primary treatment of the disease. Understanding the specific relationships between certain dietary factors and hypertension is an area of active medical research, in terms of both epidemiological investigation and treatment interventions. This chapter summarizes the scientific knowledge and current medical practice regarding the prevention and treatment of hypertension. It then presents the current scientific evidence for the role of diet, particularly vegetarian diets, in the prevention and treatment of hypertension.

Summary of the Scientific Literature

Etiology and Epidemiology of Hypertension

Etiology of Hypertension

Why certain people—and why so many people—develop hypertension remains unanswered. The interplay between genetic influences and environmental factors is not well understood, not unlike the situation with many other chronic diseases. In populations in which the incidence of hypertension is low, migration to Westernized nations is associated with increasing incidence of hypertension (Messina & Messina, 1996; Sacks & Kass, 1988). This observation suggests that environmental factors, specifically changes in lifestyle, have a significant effect on the risk of essential hypertension. Little research information is available about the potential for reversing (as opposed to controlling or "managing") hypertension.

Diseases Associated with Hypertension

The relationship between hypertension and vascular diseases has been extensively investigated in large epidemiological investigations.

Well-designed, prospective epidemiological studies that measure the health outcomes of a large group (*cohort*) of participants (*subjects*) over many years offer some of the most reliable information about cause-and-effect relationships between "exposures," such as diet and lifestyle factors, and the frequency (*incidence*) of new cases of disease and the death (*mortality*) rate attributable to the disease. Such studies require significant resources and time, and thus are much less common than observational (*cross-sectional*) epidemiological studies that measure associations between disease and various factors at a single point in time.

Coronary Artery Disease (CAD)

The Multiple Risk Factor Intervention Trial (MRFIT) was one of the largest studies ever undertaken to examine the role of various lifestyle factors in the incidence and progression of hypertension, CAD, and other prevalent chronic diseases in the United States (Stamler, Neaton, & Wentworth, 1989). Nearly 350,000 men between the ages of 35 and 57 in the United States were enrolled in the study, and their health status was followed for an average of 12½ years. Records of death from CAD and all causes were compiled. The risk of CAD—myocardial infarction (heart attack) and angina, and complications thereof—was found to be directly proportional to elevations in both systolic (top number) and diastolic (bottom number) blood pressure. Compared with men who had optimal blood pressure at the outset of the study, individuals with progressively higher blood pressure readings had a commensurately increased risk of death from CAD; men with borderline blood pressure elevation had more than double the risk, while those with the highest (above 180 mm Hg) systolic blood pressures (SBP) had 6 times the risk of death as those with normal blood pressure. Notably, 67% of all

CAD deaths in the study population occurred in men whose blood pressure was considered average (i.e., 120–140/70–90 mm Hg), leading the authors of the study to conclude that "the observed population average SBP and diastolic blood pressure (DBP) levels cannot be regarded as 'normal' or desirable" (Stamler, Stamler, & Neaton, 1993). The individuals with elevated blood pressure who also had at least one other significant risk factor for CAD, such as elevated serum cholesterol and/or cigarette smoking, accounted for 75% of the total men in the study and had even greater risk of death from CAD (34–64 times as likely to die from CAD) than those with no risk factors. The authors found that in the very small number of subjects (3.3%) who had no risk factors, the risk of death from CAD was virtually nil.

Other large, prospective studies have confirmed the MRFIT data in adult men; studies of women, the elderly, African Americans, and younger individuals have corroborated similar trends in terms of CAD risk and hypertension in these individuals. In a compilation of the data from nine major prospective studies, it was found that DBPs that were lower than average by 5, 7.5, and 10 mm Hg were associated with reductions in CAD morbidity of at least 21%, 29%, and 37%, respectively (McMahon et al., 1990). Furthermore, throughout the range of DBP studied (70–100 mm Hg), as the DBP declined, so too did the risk of developing symptomatic coronary heart disease.

Stroke (Cerebrovascular Accident, CVA)

Large cohort studies, notably the MRFIT (Stamler, Neaton, & Wentworth, 1989) and the Framingham (Kannel, Wolf, & Garrison, 1987) studies, have demonstrated a strong, direct relationship between the extent of hypertension and risk of stroke. In the MRFIT study, those individuals with SBP in the "high-normal" range (130–139 mm Hg) had 3 times the risk of stroke as those with SBP in the "desirable" range (less than 110 mm Hg). This risk increased steadily to 20 times for men with SBP of 180 mm Hg, even after age, race, income, serum cholesterol levels, smoking, and diabetes were statistically adjusted as confounding variables. The MRFIT study probably underestimated the true risk relationship, because it was based on a limited number of blood pressure readings at the outset of the study and did not account for the fact that some individuals were already receiving drug treatment for hypertension.

In the aforementioned analysis of data from 9 major studies (McMahon et al., 1990), the same relative decrements in DBP of 5, 7.5, and 10 mm Hg were associated with 34%, 46%, and 56% lower risks of stroke, respectively. As with CAD, throughout the range of DBP studied (70–100 mm Hg), the lower the DBP, the lower the risk of stroke.

Congestive Heart Failure (CHF)

Chronic elevations in SBP and DBP are directly related to increased risk of CHF due to hypertensive heart disease (Stamler, Stamler, & Neaton, 1993).

Chronic Renal Failure (CRF)

One-quarter (25%) of all cases (men and women) of dialysis-dependent, end-stage CRF are directly caused by long-standing hypertension (Whelton & Klag, 1989).

Peripheral Vascular Disease (PVD)

Hypertension, particularly elevated SBP, is a major risk factor for PVD, including atherosclerosis of the arteries of the legs, which can lead to symptoms of leg pain known as *intermittent claudication* (Stamler, Stamler, & Neaton,

1993). Other peripheral vascular diseases associated with long-standing hypertension include aortic aneurysm, carotid stenosis, and ischemic bowel disease. All these diseases lead to significant morbidity (illness rate) and mortality, and often require intensive surgical procedures to forestall fatal or disabling complications. The leading causes of impotence (erectile dysfunction) in middle-aged men are peripheral vascular disease and hypertension (including side effects from blood pressure medications).

All-Cause Mortality

Cardiovascular-related deaths represent roughly 50% of all deaths in adult Americans. Data from the large MRFIT study demonstrated that for every 10 mm Hg increase in SBP, all-cause mortality (primarily due to CAD and stroke) increased progressively, even when statistically adjusted for other risk factors, with men in the "high-normal" range having a 34% greater chance of early death, and those in the highest range an 85% increased risk in comparison with normotensive individuals (Stamler, Stamler, & Neaton, 1993). Similarly, in another study, a difference of only 4 mm Hg in lower blood pressure was found to be associated with a marked reduction in mortality from all causes (Hypertension Detection and Follow-up Program Cooperative Group, 1979). Most excess deaths attributable to hypertension were in those who had "high-normal" or slightly elevated blood pressure, even among those who received medical treatment.

Comorbid Conditions and Contributory Factors

Though the specific etiology and mechanism of essential hypertension remain unknown, several lifestyle-related factors, including diet, have been consistently identified as strongly associated with, and contributory to, the risk of developing hypertension.

Overweight/Obesity. Numerous studies have established that being overweight, and specifically being obese (i.e., more than 20% above ideal body weight) is a significant risk factor for hypertension (Huang et al., 1998; McCarron & Reusser, 1999; Appel, 1999; Hermansen, 2000). It is estimated that 33%–60% of hypertensive individuals in the United States are overweight (Pietinen & Aro, 1990). Being overweight is associated with a twofold to sixfold increase in the risk of developing hypertension (Dickey & Janick, 2001). In overweight and obese hypertensive subjects, weight loss by any means—including diet pills and short-term "starvation" diets, as well as more balanced diets—usually produces blood pressure reduction (Hermansen, 2000; Stevens, Corrigan, & Obarzanek, 1993; Whelton et al., 1998). Because most weight-loss efforts are usually unsustainable, the long-term impact of short-term weight loss in obese/overweight hypertensive populations has not been systematically studied.

Alcohol Consumption. Excessive alcohol consumption (typically three or more drinks per day) increases blood pressure in certain individuals (McCarron & Reusser, 1999; Appel, 1999; Alderman, 1994; Nurminen, Korpela, & Vapaatalo, 1998). Alcohol consumption can elevate blood pressure even in normotensive individuals, though the effects may be transient and reversible. It is not known whether regular, excessive alcohol consumption results in chronic hypertension. Among those who drink, alcohol reduction or abstinence can produce normalized blood pressure (Puddey, Beilin, & Vandongen, 1987).

Psychological Stress. The role of stress in relation to blood pressure and the management of hypertension remains unclear. In studies investigating the cause of hypertension, stress may be a confounding variable for other unhealthy lifestyle behaviors. Most intervention trials indicate that relaxation methods alone yield little, if any, benefit in producing sustained lowering of elevated blood pressures (Dickey & Janick, 2001; Beilin, 1999).

Exercise. Research has consistently shown that physical exercise is associated with lower blood pressures (McCarron & Reusser, 1999; Appel, 1999; Dickey & Janick, 2001). However, physical fitness is also associated with being slim, which itself is associated with lower blood pressure. Not all studies of exercise have demonstrated an independent effect on blood pressure (Beilin, 1999; Blumenthal & Siegel, 1991). Exercise is known to have a therapeutic role in control of hypertension among those who are overweight (Whelton et al., 2002). In the presence of overweight or obesity, the weight loss due to exercise appears to be the principal mechanism of this effect. It is unclear whether exercise without weight loss lowers blood pressure, or if exercise in non-overweight hypertensive individuals is independently an effective primary treatment for any degree of hypertension (Whelton et al., 1998).

Cigarette Smoking. There is no evidence that cigarette smoking directly increases blood pressure (Dickey & Janick, 2001). In the presence of elevated blood pressure, however, smoking contributes strongly to increased risks of CAD, PVD, and other vascular diseases.

Caffeine. There is no clear, substantiated relationship between caffeine consumption and blood pressure (Nurminen, Korpela, & Vapaatalo, 1998).

Current Treatment Approaches

Current national recommendations for the treatment of hypertension call for nonpharmacological intervention—namely lifestyle modifications—as first-line treatment of mild to moderate hypertension (e.g., blood pressure in the range of 140–159/90–100 mm Hg) (Joint National Committee, 2000). The typical diet "prescribed" by physicians is the DASH diet (see later discussion) promoted by the National Cholesterol Education Program (NCEP) and the American Heart Association (AHA) as the "Eating Plan for Healthy Americans" (National Institutes of Health, 2001; Krauss et al., 2000). Most individuals with high-normal blood pressure or hypertension are advised to follow this type of diet, including those who need to lose weight. DASH diets encourage or permit consumption of chicken, fish, pork, and "lean" red meats, as well as allowing dairy products and eggs, with specific recommendations to limit calories from fat to 27%–30% of total calories; to limit dietary cholesterol to 150–300 mg per day; and to minimize intake of saturated fats and salt. Alcohol "moderation" and regular exercise are also part of these recommendations. Notably, none of these guidelines contains any mention of the term "vegetarian diet" in its preamble or as an alternative. The efficacy of these dietary guidelines in actually reducing CAD and other vascular disease endpoints (i.e., morbidity and mortality) has never been directly studied or validated (Hermansen, 2000), whereas many research studies (discussed later in this chapter) have demonstrated that other, more aggressive dietary regimens offer greater therapeutic benefits. Advocates of stronger dietary recommendations, including vegetarian diets, have criticized the relative ineffectiveness of the AHA/NCEP dietary approach.

It is well recognized that a substantial majority of individuals "fail" these nonpharmacological dietary measures as a first step in management of hypertension. These individuals are almost always then treated with one or more antihypertensive medications. Diuretics, beta blockers, calcium channel blockers, ACE inhibitors, and other classes of antihypertensive drugs, used alone or in combination, work by various mechanisms to lower blood pressure. Although these medications can lower blood pressure and have been shown to reduce CAD, stroke risk, and mortality, no scientific evidence exists that any drug actually reverses (i.e., cures) the disease. It is unlikely that any of these drugs actually treats the underlying cause of the hypertension. Once blood pressure is controlled with medication, dietary measures are then often ignored or minimized by the physician and/or the patient. Thus, most individuals who receive blood pressure medication will continue to take it for life. As of 1995, 12.6% of U.S. adults—more than 23 million people—were taking one or more prescribed antihypertensive medications (Burt et al., 1995). Nonetheless, only an estimated 27% of such individuals actually had acceptable blood pressure control (i.e., blood pressure readings consistently below 140/90 mm Hg). The incidence of adverse side effects due to antihypertensive medications is substantial, as are the resultant numbers of doctor visits, diagnostic tests, and hospitalizations (Dimsdale, 1992; Pickering, 1992). The costs of treatment of side effects in some cases exceed the costs of the drugs themselves (Weber & Laragh, 1993). As discussed later, the literature on reversal of hypertension, however, demonstrates that with effective dietary interventions, many individuals can safely reduce or eliminate altogether the need for medication to bring their blood pressure to desirable levels.

Hypertension and Vegetarian Diets

Prevalence of Hypertension among Vegetarians

Seventh-Day Adventist Vegetarians. From a health perspective, the best-studied population of vegetarians is the Seventh-Day Adventists (SDAs). As one of its principal religious tenets, the SDA religion advocates that its members eat a lacto-ovo vegetarian (LOV) diet (i.e., a diet that prohibits animal flesh but permits dairy and egg products). The SDA religion also proscribes smoking and consumption of alcohol and caffeinated beverages. Approximately 50% of American SDAs (as of the early 1990s) adhere to a LOV diet. The SDA LOV population is therefore most suitable for studying the long-term health status of vegetarians in comparison to both nonvegetarian SDAs (who commonly follow the other, nondietary tenets), and to omnivores in the United States and other Western countries.

Several studies have consistently found lower blood pressures and lower incidence of high blood pressure among SDA vegetarians when compared with SDA nonvegetarians and non-SDA nonvegetarians.

- The relationship between blood pressure and diet and lifestyle among 98 SDA LOVs, 82 SDA omnivores, and 113 Mormon omnivores aged 25 to 44 years was examined in one study (Rouse, Armstrong, & Beilin, 1983). The latter group practices similar (if not stricter) nondietary lifestyle behaviors than SDAs, and therefore serves as an excellent control group to isolate the effects of diet. Average blood pressures among SDA vegetarians were significantly lower than either SDA omnivores or Mormon omnivores, even after statistically controlling for other dietary and lifestyle factors. After statistical adjustment for the greater prevalence of obesity observed among the Mormons, average differences of 5–7 mm Hg in SBP were measured in SDA LOVs when compared to Mormon omnivores (Beilin, 1986). Only 1%–2% of SDA vegetarians had hypertension (blood pressure greater than 140/90 mm Hg), in comparison to 8.5% of SDA omnivores and 10% of Mormon omnivores. Those SDA LOVs who self-reported as being "less strict" about their diets tended to have blood pressures that were intermediate between the adherent vegetarians and the meat-eating Mormons. This study, albeit cross-sectional in nature, demonstrated a lower prevalence of hypertension among vegetarians, even when other lifestyle behaviors were optimized.

- In a large study of 34,192 California SDAs, the prevalence of hypertension was approximately twofold greater in the nonvegetarians than in the vegetarians (Fraser, 1999).

- A smaller cross-sectional study compared 779 SDAs with 18,188 controls from the general population (Webster & Rawson, 1979). Among the SDAs in the study, 39% never ate meat, 51% ate it only seldom, and only 4% ate meat regularly. Systolic blood pressure in the SDAs was lower in early adult life and rose less with aging than in the controls.

- In a study of 167 African American Seventh-Day Adventist vegetarians, semi-vegetarians, and nonvegetarians, 16% of the vegetarians were hypertensive compared with 35.7% of the semi-vegetarians and 31.1% of the nonvegetarians (Melby, Toohey, & Cebrick, 1994). In a previous study comparing African American and Caucasian vegetarians and nonvegetarians,

44% of the African American nonvegetarians were on antihypertensive medications, compared to only 18% of the African American vegetarians, 7% of SDA white vegetarians, and 22% of white SDA non-vegetarians (Melby et al., 1989).

- A study of (white) Seventh-Day Adventists over the age of 60 found that systolic, but not diastolic, blood pressure was lower among the vegetarians than the nonvegetarians. The lower systolic blood pressure was best explained by the lower body weight of the vegetarians (Melby, Lyle, & Poehlman, 1988).

- In contrast, blood pressures among SDA adolescents have not been shown to differ from those of non-SDA peers, which suggests that the beneficial effects of a vegetarian diet may not manifest until adulthood (Kuczmarski, Anderson, & Koch, 1994).

- A study of blood pressures in Australian SDA vegetarians also demonstrated that vegetarians had significantly lower blood pressures (averages of 128/76 mm Hg vs. 139/84 mm Hg) when compared with nonvegetarians from the same locale (Armstrong, van Merwyk, & Coates, 1977). The differences in blood pressure were not explained by alcohol, tobacco, caffeine consumption, physical activity, or socioeconomic status.

Non-Seventh-Day Adventist Vegetarians. Numerous cross-sectional studies of other (non-SDA) vegetarian and vegan populations have also shown significantly lower blood pressure measurements and less incidence of hypertension than among nonvegetarians.

- In a study that compared 226 "strict" vegetarians (i.e., those who ate few or no animal products) with 63 LOVs and 521 omnivorous (nonvegetarian) controls, average systolic and diastolic blood pressures in both vegetarian groups generally were 10–15 mm Hg lower than in the nonvegetarian controls, and blood pressures in the strict vegetarians were slightly lower than in the LOV group (Sacks & Kass, 1988).

- A comparison of 98 vegetarians with an age- and gender-matched group of nonvegetarians found that the average blood pressure was 126/77 mm Hg for the vegetarians versus 147/88 mm Hg for the controls (Ophir et al., 1983). Of the nonvegetarians studied, 41% had hypertension, compared with only 13% of the vegetarians. Also, the prevalence of blood pressure higher than 160/95 mm Hg was 13 times greater (26% vs. 2%) among the nonvegetarians than among the vegetarians. These differences were maintained when the findings were statistically adjusted for body weight.
- A retrospective study of 439 vegetarians culled from 37 Buddhist temples, compared with the same number of nonvegetarians chosen from 12 surrounding communities, showed that the vegetarians had significantly lower blood pressures (approximately 5–6 mm Hg in SBP) than the nonvegetarian controls (Ko, 1983). In addition, the Buddhist vegetarians did not experience the degree of increase in blood pressure with age that was seen among the omnivore controls. The author found that among Buddhist vegetarians, the longer the person had been vegetarian, the lower the systolic blood pressure tended to be.
- In a cross-sectional study of vegetarians and omnivores in England, self-reported diagnosis of hypertension and measured blood pressure were both significantly lower among vegetarians than nonvegetarians, in the following ascending rank order: vegans < vegetarians (LOV) < fish eaters < meat eaters (Appleby, Davey, & Key, 2002).
- Finally, in a prospective study of risk factors for ischemic heart disease, lower blood pressure levels were measured in vegetarians compared with meat eaters (Haines et al., 1980).

Only a few small studies have not shown any advantage of a vegetarian diet in terms of blood pressure. One of these was a study of Tanzanian villagers that compared "mainly vegetarians" with fish-eating individuals (Pauletto et al., 1996). The authors' focus and intent were to demonstrate the putative beneficial effects of fish oils. They concluded that a diet based on freshwater fish was superior to the "near-vegetarian" diet in terms of blood pressure levels. The results are of questionable validity, as the "vegetarians" did not follow a true vegetarian diet, and observer bias may have contributed significant error. A study of 181 Trappist monks who lived on a frugal vegetarian diet, compared to 168 Benedictine monks who lived on a mixed "Western" diet, found no significant difference in average diastolic pressure; however, average systolic pressure was slightly higher among the Trappist monks, and this difference was hypothesized to be due to difference in ages between the two groups (Groen et al., 1962). A study of 22 vegans found that, when compared with matched controls, the blood pressures of the vegans, although normal, tended to be higher than that of the controls (Sanders & Key, 1987). The authors of this study hypothesized that some of the differences between the two groups may have been obliterated by the fact that the controls ate a diet that was higher in protein and vitamin C, but lower in total fat than the national average. Finally, a study of 300 subjects with a special interest in "health foods" found no consistent differences between the blood pressures of the 85 vegetarians and the 214 nonvegetarians. Presumably, the nonvegetarians in this study were healthier than typical omnivores (Burr et al., 1981).

In summary, the vast majority of epidemiological studies consistently demonstrates that vegetarians have statistically significantly lower blood pressures and a lower prevalence of diagnosed hypertension than nonvegetarians. Messina and Messina (1996) summarized the myriad of cross-sectional studies that have compared the blood pressures of vegetarians with those of omnivores, and concluded that the blood pressures of vegetarians were lower than those of omnivores by approximately 5–10 mm Hg. Differences of this magnitude translate epidemiologically into a substantially positive impact in terms of reducing the risk of hypertension-related chronic diseases. They also found that significant differences between vegetarians and nonvegetarians remained after controlling for body weight.

Vegetarian Diets for Treatment of Hypertension

The foregoing wealth of observational data that have demonstrated significantly lower blood pressure and lower prevalence of hypertension among vegetarians has prompted various investigations of the effect of a vegetarian diet on people with elevated blood pressure.

- In a study of nonhypertensive omnivores aged 25–63, subjects were randomly allocated to receive a LOV diet either before or after eating an omnivorous (meat- and dairy-based) diet (Rouse et al., 1983). Both experimental groups experienced significant reductions (approximately 6 mm Hg) in blood pressure while on the LOV diet for 6 weeks, with blood pressure elevating back to baseline upon reversion to the omnivorous diet. Control subjects who ate omnivorously throughout the study had no change in their blood pressure. Dietary changes in sodium and potassium intake were not statistically related to the changes.

- Twenty-one normotensive, nonvegetarian males were placed on a LOV diet for six weeks (Sciarrone et al., 1993). Their blood pressures were significantly lower while on the LOV diet.

- A similar intervention trial involved 24 omnivore volunteers who consumed a vegetarian diet for 6 weeks (Burstyn, 1982). Their SBP fell 1% (a statistically nonsignificant finding), while diastolic pressures fell 4.5% (a significant finding). Both values returned to baseline after the vegetarian diet was discontinued.

- The effect of 6 weeks of a LOV diet on 58 untreated individuals with mild hypertension was compared with controls who ate their usual meat- and dairy-based diet (Margetts et al., 1985). Subjects on the LOV diet experienced significant reductions in their SBP (but not DBP); the reduction was not related to weight loss or reduction of sodium intake.

- A residential study employing yoga, meditation, and a low-fat, lacto vegetarian diet resulted in substantial weight loss, improved cholesterol levels, and lower blood pressures, particularly in those individuals whose blood pressure was elevated at the outset of the study (Schmidt et al., 1997). The effects of meditation and yoga were not differentiated from the dietary changes.

Fewer studies have focused on implementation of a completely animal-product-free (i.e., vegan) diet.

• Perhaps the most aggressive and successful vegetarian program that has been implemented and studied is that of McDougall et al. in northern California (1995). Five hundred hypercholesterolemic subjects with a variety of health problems attended a 12-day residential lifestyle modification program, during which they were maintained on a very-low-fat (5% of calories from fat), completely vegan diet. No limits were placed on the amount of food the subjects ate. They also exercised and practiced stress management techniques. In most cases, all blood pressure medications were stopped shortly after lifestyle treatment began. Within 11 days, subjects experienced an average decline of –9/–4 mm Hg in blood pressure; those with higher blood pressures on admission had the greatest reductions (–17/–13 mm Hg). Lipid profiles and weight similarly improved. Most individuals left the program free of medication for hypertension. More than any other study performed to date, this investigation demonstrated that rapid, significant reductions in blood pressure are achieved with an optimized vegan diet that restricts only the type but not the amount of food consumed, and that blood pressure medication can be safely discontinued in favor of a substantive dietary intervention as the primary form of treatment.

• Aone-year regimen of a very-low-fat, lacto vegetarian (near-vegan) diet, combined with regular exercise and meditation, in 28 individuals with advanced CAD and risk factors, including hypertension, reduced the extent of CAD as measured by angio-grams (radiographic studies of the blood vessels supplying the heart) (Ornish et al., 1990). However, average blood pressure values (which were relatively low at baseline in both groups) decreased equivalently in controls and experimental subjects. This lack of an effect may have been due to the ongoing use of medication in both groups, as CAD itself, and not risk factors, was the targeted endpoint for measurement.

• Ina study of 29 individuals who had been on drug treatment for hypertension for at least 8 years, all were "treated" with a vegan diet for one year (Lindahl et al., 1984). In nearly all cases, blood pressure medication was withdrawn or drastically reduced after a year on the vegan diet, with significant reductions in both SBP and DBP. The subjects also had significant improvements in their overall well-being (perhaps reflecting loss of medication side effects).

Comparison of Vegetarian Diets and Nonvegetarian Diets for Treatment of Hypertension

No head-to-head study comparing conventional (nonvegetarian) diets with a vegetarian diet for treatment of hypertension has ever been conducted. There have been numerous interventional studies using conventional dietary recommendations (i.e., the AHA and NCEP recommendations, which promote the DASH diet) in populations of individuals with borderline or mild hypertension, or with multiple CAD risk factors. The methodologies and results from these nonvegetarian dietary studies are nonetheless informative in assessing the relative (potential) impact of certain dietary modifications on the risk for development or progression of hypertension and related diseases.

One of the longest, randomized, controlled trials of primary prevention of hypertension enrolled 200 men and women aged 30–44 with "high-normal" blood pressure (Stamler et al., 1989). Half the subjects were randomized to modify their diet, reduce alcohol and salt intake, and increase physical activity to reduce blood pressure (without the use of medication) through an "intensive individualized approach" involving physicians and nutrition counselors; the other half received "usual care" (i.e., no dietary or lifestyle instruction or intervention). At the start of the study, all subjects were an average of 20% above ideal body weight. Those randomized to modify their diets were placed on an AHA "Step I" diet, eating "lean meat," chicken, fish, and pork, as well as vegetables and fruits, with a goal of consuming no more than 30% of calories from fat, and up to 300 milligrams of cholesterol per day (comparable to the same AHA recommendations currently promoted). After 5 years, the incidence of hypertension, defined as persistent diastolic blood pressure above 90 mm Hg, was 19.2% in the control group versus 8.8% in the intervention group; when only nonsmokers were considered, however, the results were 11.5% versus 7.8%—a statistically nonsignificant difference. Intervention subjects lost an average of only 4.4 pounds after 5 years. Although the results were interpreted by the authors as "modest benefits" of the dietary intervention, the more evident conclusion is that the AHA Step I dietary recommendations are ineffective for treatment of hypertension or clinically meaningful weight loss.

The Dietary Approaches to Stop Hypertension (DASH) study compared 3 different diets with respect to their effect on the blood pressures of 459 adults with systolic blood pressures less than 160 mm Hg and diastolic blood pressures of 80–95 mm Hg (i.e., high-normal and borderline values). Subjects were randomized into one of the three dietary intervention groups (Vogt et al., 1999). All foods were provided to the participants at caloric requirements calculated for each individual (a "feeding study" design). The control diet was close to a typical American diet. The second (fruit-and-vegetable diet) was rich in fruits and vegetables (18.5 servings per day), and dietary sources of potassium, magnesium, and fiber. The third (combination diet) was rich in fruits and vegetables, potassium, magnesium, and calcium; had 2.7 servings of low-fat dairy per day; and was lower in saturated fat and total fat than the fruit-and-vegetable diet. The combination diet was more than 10% lower in total fat (26% vs. 35.1% and 35.5%), had half the dietary cholesterol (150 vs. 300 and 300 mg per day), and a higher percentage of carbohydrate (55% vs. 48% and 48%) than the fruit-and-vegetable and control diets, respectively.

In the DASH study, after 8 weeks, the combination diet reduced SBP and DBP by a mean (average) of 5.5 and 3.0 mm Hg, respectively, more than the control diet. The fruit-and-vegetable diet reduced SBP by 2.8 mm Hg and diastolic blood pressure by 1.1 mm Hg more than the control diet (Appel et al., 1997). Among those participants with hypertension (blood pressure higher than 140/90 mm Hg), the combination diet reduced SBP and DBP by 11.4 mm Hg and 5.5 mm Hg, respectively, more than the control diet. Among those without hypertension, the corresponding reductions were 3.5 mm Hg and 2.1 mm Hg.

Among hypertensive subjects entering the study with SBP of more than 140 mm Hg or DBP of more than 90 mm Hg, the combination diet controlled blood pressure in 70% of participants, versus 25% of those on the control diet (Appel et al., 1997). In subjects with a diagnosis of hypertension at the start of the study, the reduction in blood pressure with the combination diet was similar in magnitude to that observed in trials of drug monotherapy for mild hypertension (Conlin, 2001). Subgroup analysis indicated that hypertensive African Americans appeared to derive the most benefit from the combination diet (Svetky et al., 1999). A subsequent study combining the DASH diet with reduced dietary sodium demonstrated even further blood pressure reductions (Sacks et al., 2001). In another study of overweight adults taking a single blood pressure medication, the impact of a lowered-calorie, low-sodium, DASH-style diet, along with supervised exercise and weight loss, produced significant blood pressure reductions as well as lowered serum cholesterol (Miller et al., 2002).

It is noteworthy that the blood pressure-lowering effect of vegetarian diets provided some original inspiration for the DASH study. Also of note is the fact that, in designing these tiered interventions, the authors of the DASH study acknowledged that "the only consistently positive findings [of dietary blood pressure reduction] have come from the few trials that have tested the effects of vegetarian dietary patterns, which have shown consistent systolic blood pressure reduction of 5-6 mm Hg" (Vogt et al., 1999). However, the planning group for the study "strongly intended that the results of the trial would be acceptable to the U.S. population, and opted against testing a vegetarian diet" (Sacks et al., 1999).

When comparable, DASH-style diets were investigated in "free-living" subjects (as opposed to those who received all their foods completely prepared); in these circumstances, the short-term results on blood pressure reduction were far less impressive (Nowson et al., 2004). Addition of dietary calcium through low-fat dairy foods actually resulted in *increases* in blood pressure in comparison with controls, whereas the low-sodium, high-potassium (i.e., more fruits and vegetables) diet resulted in decreased (–3.5/–1.9 mm Hg) blood pressures.

Mechanism of Protective/Therapeutic Effect of Vegetarian Diet

Many researchers have attempted to isolate and define the specific dietary factors that contribute to blood pressure control and reduction. Several factors of a vegetarian diet have been suggested as possibly contributing to the blood pressure-lowering effect of a vegetarian diet (Sacks & Kass, 1988).

Weight Loss

Numerous studies have established that obesity and excess body weight increase the risk of hypertension (McCarron & Reusser, 1999; Appel, 1999; Hermansen, 2000). As discussed earlier in this chapter, in overweight/obese, hypertensive subjects, weight loss by any means—including diet pills and short-term "starvation" diets, as well as more balanced diets—usually produces blood pressure reduction. Reduction in insulin resistance is thought to be a major mechanism for this change due to weight loss (Denker & Pollock, 1992). However, the blood pressure-lowering effect of vegetarian diets cannot be totally accounted for by the lower body weights of vegetarians, as blood pressures in nonvegetarians have been found to be higher than those in vegetarians with similar body weights (Ophir et al., 1983). In fact, in most studies that found blood pressures to be lower in vegetarians, weight loss was statistically controlled for, and in the two studies where it was not, weight differences were thought to have little, if any, impact (Messina & Messina, 1996).

Minerals: Sodium (Salt), Potassium, Calcium

Sodium. The notion that reduction of dietary sodium (salt) intake can reduce blood pressure in hypertensive individuals has been promoted for decades by physicians and public health advocates. This conventional wisdom remains a mainstay of first-line, nonpharmacological treatment recommendations (often in conjunction with medications) by doctors and dietitians for hypertension. The evidence of the relationship between salt content and hypertension, however, is controversial (Zozaya, 2000; McCarron, 1998). Numerous trials of salt reduction as part of nonpharmacological intervention have demonstrated no significant benefit of salt reduction, whether used alone or in combination with other dietary measures or medications (Trials of Hypertension Prevention [TOHP] Collaborative Research Group, 1997). A meta-analysis of 56 intervention trial studies on dietary sodium intake reduction concluded that the decreases in blood pressure attributable to dietary salt reduction were relatively minor except in the elderly (Midgley et al., 1996). However, other meta-analyses have concluded that a reduced-sodium diet does result in a fall in blood pressure (Nurminen, Korpela, & Vapaatalo, 1998; Appel, 2000; Kotchen & McCarron, 1998). In addition, the DASH-sodium trial compared the effect on blood pressures at different levels of sodium intake alone and in combination with the DASH diet. Both the DASH diet alone and reduced sodium intake alone were associated with significant reductions in blood pressure, and the combination produced the greatest reduction (Conlin, 2001).

These data collectively indicate that there may be groups of individuals who are particularly sensitive to the effects of salt on blood pressure, particularly the elderly and the obese, type 2 diabetics, those with kidney disease, and African Americans (Appel, 1999; Hermansen, 2000; Zozaya, 2000). Although attempts to generalize these findings into recommendations that every member of the general public reduce sodium intake continue to generate debate, it is generally accepted that more specific recommendations, stating that hypertensive individuals who are salt-sensitive should restrict their sodium intake, are reasonable.

The question as to the significance of salt reduction has been addressed within the context of vegetarian diets. One observational study comparing vegetarians with nonvegetarians and two interventional studies comparing ovo-lacto vegetarian diets with omnivorous diets found that low dietary sodium was not related to the protective, blood pressure-lowering effect of a vegetarian diet (Rouse et al., 1983; Armstrong et al., 1979; Beilin, 1994). Also, the sodium intake of vegetarians in industrialized countries is similar to that of omnivores (Messina & Messina, 1996). Therefore, sodium intake does not appear to account for the lower blood pressures of vegetarians compared with nonvegetarians.

Potassium. Another current area of interest among researchers seeking to find the "magic bullet" of nutritional blood pressure control is dietary potassium. Population studies have found an inverse association between dietary potassium and blood pressure (McCarron & Reusser, 1999; Hermansen, 2000; TOHP Collaborative Research Group, 1997; Kotchen & McCarron, 1998; Whelton et al., 1997). Although the results of clinical intervention studies have been somewhat less consistent and persuasive (TOHP Collaborative Research Group, 1997), the majority of well-designed clinical trials and a meta-analysis have shown that an increase in dietary potassium is associated with a decrease in blood pressure (McCarron & Reusser, 1999; Whelton et al., 1997). Further evidence for a blood pressure-lowering effect of dietary potassium comes from the results of meta-analyses of clinical trials, which concluded that oral potassium supplementation lowers both systolic and diastolic blood pressure (Cappuccio & McGregor, 1991). In hypertensive individuals on medication, an increase in potassium intake from natural foods has also been shown to decrease the amount of antihypertensive medication needed (Whelton et al., 1998).

In vegetarian diets, where potassium intake is inherently higher than in animal-based diets, the effects of potassium appear much less significant in terms of explaining the lower blood pressures observed in vegetarians. The potential role of potassium in lowering blood pressure was examined in a population of older (mean age 60) Israeli LOVs who had followed this diet for an average of 19 years, as compared to meat-eating controls (Ophir, Peer, & Gilad, 1983). As discussed earlier, this study found that vegetarians had significantly lower mean blood pressure (126/77 mm Hg vs. 147/88 mm Hg) when compared with omnivores at every age group, with only 2% of vegetarians receiving a diagnosis of hypertension (greater than 160/95) and 26% of controls being so diagnosed. The differences remained after statistical adjustment for body weight, caffeine intake, and smoking. The finding that vegetarians excreted significantly more potassium led the authors to conclude that the high intake of potassium is a protective factor. However, the authors did not discuss the possibility that high potassium intake may simply be a marker for a vegetarian diet, as plant-based foods contain relatively large amounts of potassium, and thus potassium may be a confounding variable in the vegetarian diet–blood pressure relationship.

Calcium.   The most recent area of interest in the dietary nutrient–blood pressure-lowering quest is calcium. Low dietary calcium intake has been fairly consistently associated with an increase in the prevalence of hypertension in cross-sectional epidemiological studies (Hermansen, 2000). However, the results from clinical studies have been less consistent and less

impressive (McCarron & Reusser, 1999; Hermansen, 2000; Nurminen, Korpela, & Vapaatalo, 1998). Two meta-analyses of the results of calcium supplementation on blood pressure in nonvegetarians calculated very small but nonetheless statistically significant (0.53–1.68 mm Hg) reductions in systolic blood pressure, but no changes in diastolic blood pressure (Hermansen, 2000; Kotchen & McCarron, 1998). Presently there is no convincing research evidence that dietary calcium is a major factor in blood pressure control, particularly in light of the fact that long-time vegan vegetarians, whose calcium intake is relatively lower than that of omnivores, enjoy significantly lower blood pressures than nonvegetarians.

Vitamins and Antioxidants

Although vegetarian diets contain large quantities of many vitamins, including the antioxidant vitamins C and E, these factors do not appear to principally account for the blood pressure-lowering effect of a vegetarian diet (Rouse et al., 1986).

Fiber

Although dietary fiber is abundant in vegetarian diets, it is unclear whether high fiber intake alone produces an antihypertensive effect (Swain et al., 1990). Indirect epidemiological evidence of a positive association is the fact that there has been a population-wide trend toward a decrease in dietary fiber intake over the past 50 years, while the incidence of hypertension has increased. In most cross-sectional general population studies, fiber intake has been associated with decreased risk of hypertension (Beilin & Burke, 1995; He & Whelton, 1999). In the Heath Professional's Follow-up Study of 30,681 men followed for 4 years, fiber consumption was associated with a lower risk of hypertension (Ascherio et al., 1992). The Nurses' Health Study of 41,541 women found that among those who developed hypertension during the 4 years of the study, fiber intake was not associated with hypertension; however, among women who did not report hypertension during the study, fiber intake was associated with lower blood pressures (Ascherio et al., 1996). In contrast, controlled interventional trials of increased fiber intake have yielded inconsistent results regarding any effect of dietary fiber intake on blood pressure (Nurminen, Korpela, & Vapaatalo, 1998; Beilin & Burke, 1995; He & Whelton, 1999).

Fruits and Vegetables

Several studies have shown a decrease in blood pressure with diets in which fruit and vegetable consumption is high. The DASH trial compared the effects of 3 diets on blood pressure in 459 adults with high-normal blood pressure or mild hypertension. Both SBP and DBP were significantly reduced by the two diets with fruits and vegetables when compared with a control diet (Appel et al., 1997). A 6-month study of 690 individuals found that when participants were encouraged to increase their consumption of fruits and vegetables, blood pressure was decreased (John et al., 2002). Prospective epidemiological studies in the United States have also been supportive of a protective effect of fruits and vegetables. In the Health Professionals Follow-up study, consumption of fruit fiber, but not vegetable fiber, was inversely associated with blood pressure (Ascherio et al., 1992). The Nurses' Health study found that diets rich in fruits and vegetables were associated with lower blood pressures (Ascherio et al., 1996). Collectively, these and other studies suggest that the higher amounts of fruits and vegetables in a vegetarian diet may be at least partly re-

sponsible for the blood pressure-lowering effect of vegetarian diets.

Flavonoids

Flavonoids are phytochemicals found in a variety of plant foods, including fruits and vegetables, legumes, and soy. It has been hypothesized that flavonoids may reduce the risk of hypertension, perhaps through antioxidant effects that block the formation of atherosclerotic plaques in blood vessels (Moline et al., 2000). Currently, no direct research studies have been published to support or refute this hypothesis.

Dietary Protein, Cholesterol, and Fat

Many cross-sectional epidemiological studies, including the INTERSALT study of 10,020 men and women from 32 countries and the MRFIT study of 11,342 men, have found that higher dietary protein intake is associated with small decreases in blood pressure (He & Whelton, 1999; Elliott, 2003). These results seem paradoxical given that vegetarian diets, which are typically lower in protein than nonvegetarian diets, are highly associated with lower blood pressures (Hermansen, 2000). Most published interventional trials have not shown a decrease in blood pressure with increased dietary protein intake, and prospective studies of dietary protein and blood pressure have not shown consistent results either (Nurminen, Korpela, & Vapaatalo, 1998; He & Whelton, 1999; Elliott, 2003).

A handful of cross-sectional studies that have investigated the effects on blood pressure of animal proteins and vegetable proteins separately have yielded inconsistent results (Elliott, 2003). However, an eight-year, longitudinal study in nonvegetarians found an inverse association between vegetable protein and change in both systolic and diastolic blood pressure, and a direct association between animal protein and change in systolic blood pressure (Stamler et al., 2002).

Two interventional studies have investigated the effect of replacing meat protein with plant protein. No effect on blood pressure was found for meat versus plant protein. The studies concluded that avoidance of meat itself is not responsible for the blood pressure-lowering effect of a vegetarian diet (Prescott et al., 1988; Kestin et al., 1989).

Several interventional investigations into the potential antihypertensive effects of certain dietary proteins have been conducted (Sacks & Kass, 1988). In one study, egg protein was added to the diet of vegetarians in a three-week study, with no resultant effect on blood pressure. Another study compared the addition of milk protein or soy protein to the diets of strict vegetarians (those who ate few, if any, animal products) and found no difference in blood pressure with either addition. A study of the effect of protein supplementation in 18 vegetarians who consumed a high-protein supplement of soy and wheat protein for 6 weeks and then an isocaloric, low-protein diet supplement of rice for another 6 weeks, also showed no significant change in blood pressure due to changes in protein content. In contrast, several recent trials have demonstrated a blood pressure-lowering effect of soy supplementation (Elliott, 2003). It is unknown which component(s) of soy might be responsible for this effect. In summary, in vegetarian diets, dietary protein intake does not appear to be a significant, independent factor in producing the documented blood pressure-lowering effect.

Studies of cholesterol, total dietary fat, and dietary fat types (saturated, polyunsaturated, unsaturated) also have not demonstrated any consistent relationship with blood pressure

(McCarron & Reusser, 1999; Hermansen, 2000; Nurminen, Korpela, & Vapaatalo, 1998; Beilin & Burke, 1995; Sacks & Kass, 1988; Iacono et al., 1983). Indirect epidemiological evidence suggests a direct association between diets high in saturated fats and elevated blood pressure, as many populations that have low blood pressure levels do consume diets low in total fat and saturated fatty acids. However, clinical trials have failed to show a significant effect on blood pressure from total fat or saturated or polyunsaturated fat intake (Hermansen, 2000; Appel, 2000; Margetts et al., 1985; Margetts et al., 1988). The Health Professionals Follow-up study also found no significant associations of hypertension with total fat, or saturated, trans-saturated, and polyunsaturated fats (Ascherio et al., 1992). Conversely, the MRFIT study (of 11,342 men followed for 6 years) found that consumption of saturated fats was positively related to blood pressure, and that the ratio of dietary polyunsaturated to saturated fats was inversely related to blood pressure (Stamler et al., 1996). Two interventional studies observed that, compared with a higher-fat diet with a lower polyunsaturated fat/saturated fat ratio, a diet low in fat (24%) and with a relatively high polyunsaturated fat/saturated fat ratio (ratio 0.9–1.2) lowered blood pressure (Iacono et al., 1983; Puska et al., 1985). A third interventional study found that a diet with a high (1:1) polyunsaturated fat/saturated fat ratio lowered blood pressure regardless of total fat intake (Iacono et al., 1981). Some studies have shown that a diet rich in monounsaturated fats lowers blood pressure, but other studies have not found any such effect (Hermansen, 2000; Nurminen, Korpela, & Vapaatalo, 1998; Ferrara et al., 2000; Beilin et al., 1987).

Vegetarian diets are lower in saturated fat and higher in unsaturated fats than nonvegetarian diets. Whether these differences contribute to the blood pressure-lowering effect of a vege-tarian diet remains unknown.

Conclusions

Appel et al. (1997) reviewed several possible explanations for the discrepancy between the positive associations with hypertension and some dietary factors observed in population studies and in vegetarian diets, and the incon-sistent results from studies that modified sin-gle nutrients and looked for an effect on blood pressure. They concluded that the effect of any individual nutrient in lowering blood pressure may be too small to detect in trials of limited size. However, if several dietary constituents with blood pressure-lowering effects are com-bined, the cumulative effect may be greater and, therefore, noticeable. Another explanation could be that nutrients other than those tested in trials or in observational studies may be re-sponsible for lowering blood pressure. A final explanation these researchers proposed was that nutrients in dietary supplements may not reduce blood pressure to the same extent as nutrients in foods, because of interaction with other dietary components or because of altered bioavailability.

Among the many studies of vegetarians and vegetarian diets, no single nutrient source has yet been identified as a principal blood pressure-lowering factor (Beilin & Burke, 1995). There is most likely a combination of related factors in a vegetarian diet that collectively results in lower blood pressure (Messina & Messina, 1996). It may also be simply that vegetarian diets are effective in reducing or eliminating the blood pressure-raising/hypertensive effects of the animal-product-based, typical Western diet.

Practical Aspects

Because no single dietary factor has been found to account for the blood pressure-lowering effect of a vegetarian diet, it is prudent to eat a general, well-balanced vegetarian diet. Such a diet should contain the number of calories needed to achieve or maintain an ideal body weight. It should include generous amounts of fruits and vegetables, fiber, vitamins and antioxidants, and potassium and calcium. Soy products may have additional beneficial effects on blood pressure. Those who have hyperten-sion that is responsive to salt restriction should limit their intake of salty foods and table salt.

Individuals who are currently under treat-ment with antihypertensive medications will most likely benefit from a change to a vegetar-ian (and preferably vegan or near-vegan) diet and, under proper medical supervision, may be able to reduce or eliminate their need for medications. Other comorbid conditions and risk factors, such as hyperlipidemia, coronary artery disease, stroke, peripheral vascular dis-ease, and hypertensive-induced renal insuffi-ciency, are similarly likely to benefit as a result. A caveat is that the diseases in some individu-als, with long-standing hypertension or active vascular disease complications, may be too advanced to benefit from solely nonpharma-cological interventions; therefore, these indi-viduals will probably continue to require some medication.

Individuals who attempt to make only small changes toward a vegetarian diet, rather than moving directly to a vegetarian (and preferably vegan or near-vegan) diet, should understand that the benefits of these minor changes (albeit well intended) may be commensurately small or negligible in terms of blood pressure reduc-tion, as demonstrated by the scientific studies cited herein that were designed around this incremental approach. In addition, the medical literature currently available shows no benefit from attempts to supplement a primarily animal-based diet with potassium, fiber, or antioxidant vitamins rather than switching to a true vegetarian diet.

Conclusion

The general consensus in the medical literature and profession is that "[n]onpharmacologic approaches have enormous potential as a means to reduce blood pressure and control hypertension, thereby preventing the occurrence of atherosclerotic coronary and other vascular disease" (Appel, 1999). Although medication-based treatment continues to dominate the management of hypertension, the scientific evidence collected over the past 30 years regarding the effect of a vegetarian diet on prevention and treatment of hypertension has shown consistently strong, positive benefits. A vegetarian diet, and preferably a vegan diet, represents the most effective form of primary, nonpharmacological treatment to prevent the development, progression, or complications of hypertension, and potentially to reverse the disease and thereby prevent complications. Adopting and maintaining a vegetarian diet significantly increases the opportunity for individuals with advanced stages of hypertension, or who have been taking antihypertensive medication, to reduce or eliminate the need for such medication.

Twenty years ago, Beilin et al. concluded that:

[T]here is now convincing evidence from epidemiological studies and randomized controlled trials that adoption of an ovo-lacto vegetarian diet leads to blood pressure reduction in both normotensive and hypertensive subjects. This effect appears to be indepen-

dent of both dietary sodium and weight loss but additive to effects of weight reduction. Long-term adherence to a vegetarian diet is associated with less of a rise of blood pressure with age and a decreased prevalence of hypertension. The nutrients responsible for these effects have not been clearly identified and the mechanisms involved are unknown (Beilin et al., 1987).

Since that time, the scientific evidence in favor of the blood pressure-lowering benefits of a vegetarian diet as a primary form of treatment and prevention has continued to mount. Recent dietary research indicates that switching to and adhering to a vegetarian diet is not only feasible, but actually easier than adopting a conventional, DASH-style diet (Barnard et al., 2004). Although the reason(s) for the blood pressure-lowering effect of a vegetarian diet remain elusive, it is clear that such a diet is highly effective and safe.

References

Alderman M. Non-pharmacological treatment of hypertension. *Lancet.* 1994;344:307–311.

Appel L. The role of diet in the prevention and treatment of hypertension. *Curr Atheroscler Reps.* 2000;2:521–528.

Appel L. Nonpharmacologic therapies that reduce blood pressure: A fresh perspective. *Clin Cardiol.* 1999;22(Suppl 3):III-1 to III-5.

Appel LJ, Moore TJ, Obarzanek E, et al. A clinical trial of the effects of dietary patterns on blood pressure. DASH Collaborative Research Group. *N Engl J Med.* 1997;336:1117–1124.

Appleby PN, Davey GK, Key TJ. Hypertension and blood pressure among meat eaters, fish eaters, vegetarians and vegans in EPIC-Oxford. *Public Health Nutr.* 2002;5:645–654.

Armstrong B, Clarke H, Martin C, et al. Urinary sodium and blood pressure in vegetarians. *Am J Clin Nutr.* 1979;32:2472–2476.

Armstrong B, van Merwyk A, Coates H. Blood pressure in Seventh-day Adventist vegetarians. *Am J Epidemiol.* 1977;105:444-449.

Ascherio A, Hennekens C, Willett W, et al. A prospective study of nutritional factors, blood pressure, and hypertension among U.S. women. *Hypertension.* 1996;27:1065-1072.

Ascherio A, Rimm E, Giovannucci E, et al. A prospective study of nutritional factors, blood pressure, and hypertension among U.S. men. *Circulation.* 1992;86:1475-1484.

Barnard ND, Scialli AR, Turner-McGrievy G, Lanou AJ. Acceptability of a low-fat vegan diet compares favorably to a step II diet in a randomized controlled trial. *J Cardiopulm Rehab.* 2004;24:229-235.

Barrie W. Cost-effective therapy for hypertension. *W J Med.* 1996;164:303-309.

Beilin L. Lifestyle and hypertension—An overview. *Clin Exper Hypertension.* 1999;21:749-762.

Beilin L. Vegetarian and other complex diets, fats, fiber and hypertension. *Am J Clin Nutr.* 1994;59(Suppl):1130S-1135S.

Beilin L. Vegetarian approach to hypertension. *Can J Physiol Pharmacol.* 1986;64(6):852-855.

Beilin L, Burke V. Vegetarian diet components, protein and blood pressure: Which nutrients are important? *Clin Exper Pharm Physiol.* 1995;22:195-198.

Beilin LJ, Armstrong BK, Margetts BM, et al. Vegetarian diet and blood pressure. *Nephron.* 1987;47(Suppl 1):37-41.

Blumenthal S, Siegel N. Failure of exercise to reduce blood pressure in patients with mild hypertension: Results of a randomized controlled trial. *JAMA.* 1991;266:2098-2104.

Burr M, Bates C, Fehily A, St. Leger AS. Plasma cholesterol and blood pressure in vegetarians. *J Hum Nutr.* 1981;35:437-441.

Burstyn P. Effect of meat on blood pressure. *JAMA.* 1982;248:29-30.

Burt VL, Cutler JA, Higgins M, et al. Trends in the prevalence, awareness, treatment, and control of hypertension in the adult U.S. population. *Hypertension.* 1995;26:60-69.

Cappuccio F, McGregor G. Does potassium supplementation lower blood pressure: A meta-analysis of published trials. *J Hypertension.* 1991;9:465-473.

Conlin P. Dietary modification and changes in blood pressure. *Curr Opin Nephrol Hypertension.* 2001;10:359-363.

Denker PS, Pollock VE. Fasting serum insulin levels in essential hypertension. A meta-analysis. *Arch Intern Med.* 1992;152:1649-1651.

Dickey R, Janick J. Lifestyle modifications in the prevention and treatment of hypertension. *Endocr Pract.* 2001;7:392-399.

Dimsdale J. Reflections on the impact of antihypertensive medications on mood, sedation, and neuropsychological functioning. *Arch Intern Med.* 1992;152:35-39.

Elliott P. Protein intake and blood pressure in cardiovascular disease. *Proc Nutr Soc.* 2003;62:495-504.

Ferrara L, Raimondi S, d'Episcopa L, et al. Olive oil and reduced need for antihypertensive medications. *Arch Intern Med.* 2000;160:837-842.

Fraser GE. Associations between diet and cancer, ischemic heart disease, and all-cause mortality in non-Hispanic white California Seventh-day Adventists. *Am J Clin Nutr.* 1999;70(Suppl):532S-538S.

Groen J, Tijong K, Koster M, et al. The influence of nutrition and ways of life on blood cholesterol and the prevalence of hypertension and coronary heart disease among Trappist and Benedictine monks. *Am J Clin Nutr.* 1962;10:456-470.

Haines AP, Chakrabarti R, Fisher D, et al. Hemostatic variables in vegetarians and nonvegetarians. *Thromb Res.* 1980;19(1-2):139-148.

He J, Whelton P. Effect of dietary fiber and protein intake on blood pressure: A review of epidemiologic evidence. *Clin Exper Hypertension.* 1999;21:785-796.

Hermansen K. Diet, blood pressure and hypertension. *Br J Nutr.* 2000;83(Suppl 1):S113-S119.

Huang Z, Willett W, Manson J, et al. Body weight, weight change, and risk for hypertension in women. *Ann Intern Med.* 1998;128:81-88.

Hypertension Detection and Follow-up Program Co-operative Group. Five-year findings of the hypertension detection and follow-up program. *JAMA.* 1979;242:2562–2571.

Iacono J, Judd J, Marshall M, et al. The role of dietary essential fatty acids and prostaglandins in reducing blood pressure. *Prog Lipid Res.* 1981;20:349–364.

Iacono J, Puska P, Dougherty R, et al. Effect of dietary fat on blood pressure in a rural Finnish population. *Am J Clin Nutr.* 1983;38:860–869.

John J, Ziebland S, Yudkin P, et al. Effects of fruit and vegetable consumption on plasma antioxidant concentrations and blood pressure: A randomized controlled trial. *Lancet.* 2002;359:1969–1974.

Joint National Committee on Prevention, Detection, Evaluation, and Treatment of High Blood Pressure (JNC VII). *The Seventh Report of the Joint National Committee on Prevention, Detection, Evaluation, and Treatment of High Blood Pressure.* NIH Publication 03-5233. Washington, DC: U.S. Department of Health and Human Services; Dec 2000.

Kannel W, Wolf P, Garrison R, eds. *Section 34: Some Risk Factors Related to the Annual Incidence of Cardiovascular Disease and Death Using Pooled Repeated Biennial Measurements. Framingham Heart Study, 30-Year Follow-Up.* NIH Publication 87-2703. Bethesda, MD: National Institutes of Health; 1987.

Kestin M, Rouse I, Correll R, Nestel P. Cardiovascular disease risk factors in free-living men: Comparison of two prudent diets, one based on lacto-ovo-vegetarianism and the other allowing lean meat. *Am J Clin Nutr.* 1989;50:280–287.

Ko Y. Blood pressure in Buddhist vegetarians. *Nutr Reps Intl.* 1983;28:1375–1383.

Kotchen T, McCarron D. Dietary electrolytes and blood pressure. A statement for healthcare professionals from the American Heart Association Nutrition Committee. *Circulation.* 1998;98:613–617.

Krauss RM, Eckel RH, Howard B, et al. AHA Dietary Guidelines, Revision 2000: A statement for healthcare professionals from the nutrition committee of the American Heart Association. *Circulation.* 2000;102:2296–2311.

Kuczmarski R, Anderson J, Koch G. Correlates of blood pressure in Seventh-Day Adventists (SDA) and non-SDA adolescents. *J Am Coll Nutr.* 1994;13:165–173.

Lindahl O, Lindwal L, Spanber A, et al. A vegan regimen with reduced medication in the treatment of hypertension. *Br J Nutr.* 1984;52:11–20.

Margetts B, Beilin L, Armstrong B, et al. Blood pressure and dietary polyunsaturated and saturated fats: A controlled trial. *Clin Sci.* 1985(Suppl 3);69:165–175.

Margetts B, Beilin L, Armstrong B, Vandongen R. Vegetarian diet in mild hypertension: Effects of fat and fiber. *Am J Clin Nutr.* 1988;48:801–805.

Margetts B, Beilin L, Armstrong B, Vandongen R. Vegetarian diet in the treatment of mild hypertension: A randomized controlled trial. *J Hypertension.* 1985;3(Suppl 3):S429–S431.

McCarron D, Reusser M. Nonpharmacologic therapy in hypertension: From single components to overall dietary management. *Prog Cardiol Dis.* 1999;41:451–460.

McCarron DA. Diet and blood pressure—The paradigm shift. *Science.* 1998;281:933–934.

McDougall J, Litzau K, Haver E, Saunders V, Spiller GA. Rapid reduction of serum cholesterol and blood pressure by a twelve-day, very low fat, strictly vegetarian diet. *J Am Coll Nutr.* 1995;14(5):491–496.

McMahon S, Peto R, Cutler J, et al. Blood pressure, stroke, and coronary heart disease. Part I, prolonged differences in blood pressure: Prospective studies corrected for the regression dilution bias. *Lancet.* 1990;325:765–774.

Melby C, Goldflies D, Hyner G, Lyle R. Relation between vegetarian/nonvegetarian diets and blood pressure in black and white adults. *Am J Public Nutr.* 1989;79:1283–1288.

Melby C, Lyle R, Poehlman E. Blood pressure and body mass index in elderly long-term vegetarians and nonvegetarians. *Nutr Reps Intl.* 1988;37:47–55.

Melby C, Toohey M, Cebrick J. Blood pressure and blood lipids among vegetarian, semivegetarian, and nonvegetarian African Americans. *Am J Clin Nutr.* 1994;59:103–109.

Messina M, Messina V. *The Dietitian's Guide to Vegetarian Diets: Issues and Applications.* Gaithersburg, MD: Aspen Publishers; 1996.

Midgley J, Matthew A, Greenwood C, Logan A. Effect of reduced dietary sodium on blood pressure: A meta-analysis of randomized controlled trials. *JAMA.* 1996;275:1590–1597.

Miller ER, Erlinger TP, Young DR, et al. Results of the diet, exercise, and weight loss intervention trial (DEW-IT). *Hypertension.* 2002; 40:612–618.

Moline J, Bukharovich F, Wolff M, Phillips R. Dietary flavonoids and hypertension: Is there a link? *Med Hypotheses.* 2000;55:306–309.

National Institutes of Health. *Third Report of the National Cholesterol Education Panel (NCEP) Expert Panel on Detection, Evaluation, and Treatment of High Blood Cholesterol in Adults* [executive summary]. NIH Publication 01-3670. Washington, DC: National Cholesterol Education Program, National Heart. Lung, and Blood Institute; May 2001.

Nowson C, Worsley A, Margerison C, et al. Blood pressure response to dietary modifications in free-living individuals. *J Nutr.* 2004;134:2322–2329.

Nurminen M, Korpela R, Vapaatalo H. Dietary factors in the pathogenesis and treatment of hypertension. *Ann Med.* 1998;30:143–150.

Oparil S. Antihypertensive therapy—Efficacy and quality of life [editorial]. *N Engl J Med.* 1993;328: 959–961.

Ophir O, Peer (Peresecenschi) G, Gilad J, et al. Low blood pressure in vegetarians: The possible role of potassium. *Am J Clin Nutr.* 1983;37:755–762.

Ornish D, Brown SE, Scherwitz LW, et al. Can lifestyle changes reverse coronary heart disease? The Lifestyle Heart Trial. *Lancet.* 1990;336(8708): 129–133.

Pauletto P, Puato M, Angeli M, et al. Blood pressure, serum lipids, and fatty acids in populations on a lake-fish diet or on a vegetarian diet in Tanzania. *Lipids.* 1996;31(Suppl):S309–S312.

Pickering TG. Predicting the response to nonpharmacologic treatment in mild hypertension [editorial]. *JAMA.* 1992;267:1256–1257.

Pietinen P, Aro A. The role of nutrition in the prevention and treatment of hypertension. In: Draper H, ed. *Advances in Nutrition Research.* New York: Plenum Press; 1990:35–78.

Prescott S, Jenner D, Beilin L, et al. A randomized controlled trial of the effect on blood pressure of dietary non-meat protein vs. meat protein in normotensive omnivores. *Clin Sci.* (London) 1988; 74:665–672.

Puddey IB, Beilin LJ, Vandongen R. Regular alcohol use raises blood pressure in treated hypertensive subjects. *Lancet.* 1987;1:647–651.

Puska P, Iacono J, Nissinen A, et al. Dietary fat and blood pressure: An intervention study on the effects of a low-fat diet with two levels of polyunsaturated fat. *Preven Med.* 1985;14:573–584.

Rouse I, Armstrong B, Beilin L. The relationship of blood pressure to diet and lifestyle in two religious populations. *J Hypertension.* 1983;1:65–71.

Rouse I, Beilin L, Armstrong B, Vandongen R. Blood-pressure-lowering effect of a vegetarian diet: Controlled trial in normotensive subjects. *Lancet.* 1983;1:5–10.

Rouse I, Beilin L, Mahoney D, et al. Nutrient intake, blood pressure, serum and urinary prostaglandins and serum thromboxane B2 in a controlled trial with a lacto-ovo-vegetarian diet. *J Hypertension.* 1986;4:241–250.

Sacks F, Appel L, Moore T, et al. A dietary approach to prevent hypertension: A review of the Dietary Approaches to Stop Hypertension (DASH) study. *Clin Cardiol.* 1999;22(Suppl 3):III6–III10.

Sacks F, Kass E. Low blood pressure in vegetarians: Effects of specific foods and nutrients. *Am J Clin Nutr.* 1988;48(Suppl):795–800.

Sacks FM, Svetky LP, Vollmer WM, et al. Effects on blood pressure of reduced dietary sodium and the Dietary Approaches to Stop Hypertension (DASH) diet. DASH-Sodium Collaborative Research Group. *N Engl J Med.* 2001;344:3–10.

Sanders T, Key T. Blood pressure, plasma rennin activity and aldosterone concentrations in vegans and omnivore controls. *Hum Nutr Appl Nutr.* 1987;41A:204–211.

Schmidt T, Wilga A, Von Zur Huhlen A, et al. Changes in cardiovascular risk factor and hormones during a comprehensive residential three month kriya yoga training and vegetarian nutrition. *Acta Physiol Scand.* 1997;640(Suppl):158–162.

Sciarrone S, Strahan M, Beilin L, et al. Ambulatory blood pressure and heart rate responses to vegetarian meals. *J Hypertension.* 1993;11:277–285.

Stamler J, Caggiula A, Grandits G, et al. Relationship to blood pressure of combinations of dietary macronutrients. *Circulation.* 1996;94:2417–2423.

Stamler J, Liu K, Ruth K, et al. Eight-year blood pressure change in middle-aged men. *Hypertension.* 2002;39:1000–1006.

Stamler J, Neaton J, Wentworth D. Blood pressure (systolic and diastolic) and risk of fatal coronary heart disease. *Hypertension.* 1989;13:2–12.

Stamler J, Stamler R, Neaton J. Blood pressure, systolic and diastolic, and cardiovascular risks: U.S. population data. *Arch Intern Med.* 1993;153:598–615.

Stamler R, Stamler J, Gosch R, et al. Primary prevention of hypertension by nutritional-hygienic means. Final report of a randomized, controlled trial. *JAMA.* 1989;262:181–187.

Stevens V, Corrigan S, Obarzanek E. Weight loss intervention in phase 1 of the trials of hypertension prevention. *Arch Intern Med.* 1993;153:849–858.

Svetky LP, Simons-Morton D, Vollmer WM, et al. Effects of dietary patterns on blood pressure: Subgroup analysis of the Dietary Approaches to Stop Hypertension (DASH) randomized clinical trial. *Arch Intern Med.* 1999;159:285–293.

Swain J, Rouse I, Curley C, Sacks F. Comparison of the effects of oat bran and low-fiber wheat on serum lipoprotein levels and blood pressure. *N Engl J Med.* 1990;322:147–152.

Trials of Hypertension Prevention (TOHP) Collaborative Research Group. *Arch Intern Med.* 1997;157:657.

Vogt TM, Appel LJ, Obarzanek E, et al. Dietary approaches to stop hypertension: Rationale, design, and methods. *J Am Diet Assoc.* 1999;99(Suppl):S12–S18.

Weber M, Laragh J. Hypertension: Steps forward and steps backward. The Joint National Committee Fifth Report [editorial]. *Arch Intern Med.* 1993;1:65–71.

Webster I, Rawson G. Health status of Seventh-Day-Adventists. *Med J Aust.* 1979;1:417–420.

Whelton P, Appel L, Espeland M, et al. Sodium reduction and weight loss in the treatment of hypertension in older persons: A randomized control trial of nonpharmacologic interventions in the elderly (TONE). *JAMA.* 1998;279:839–846.

Whelton P, He J, Cutler J, et al. Effects of oral potassium on blood pressure. *JAMA.* 1997;227:1624–1632.

Whelton P, Klag M. Hypertension as a risk factor for renal diseases: A review of clinical and epidemiological evidence. *Hypertension.* 1989;13(Suppl 5):I19–I27.

Whelton SP, Chin A, Xin X, He J. Effect of aerobic exercise on blood pressure: A meta-analysis of randomized, controlled trials. *Ann Intern Med.* 2002;136:493–503.

Zozaya I. Nutritional factors in high blood pressure. *J Hum Hypertension.* 2000;14(Suppl 1):S100–S104.

13

Stroke

Peggy Carlson, MD

Introduction

Each year in the United States, approximately 750,000 people suffer a stroke. It is the third leading cause of death in this country. Unlike heart disease, where a connection to diet has been well documented for many years, the relationship between stroke and diet is still not clear. However, research in this area is beginning to show many potential connections.

This chapter starts with some background information about stroke that will help in understanding the current research regarding the relationship between stroke and diet. We then review studies that have investigated the risk of stroke among groups of people consuming different types of diets. Lastly, we examine many individual dietary factors that may affect the risk of stroke and how these relate to a vegetarian diet.

Summary of the Scientific Literature

Background Information

Types of Strokes

A *stroke* is an injury to the brain that occurs either because of a sudden lack of blood flow to the brain (*thromboembolic stroke*) or because of sudden, spontaneous bleeding into or around the brain (*hemorrhagic stroke*). The resulting brain injury can cause many symptoms, including paralysis on one side of the body, difficulty in speaking or understanding speech, weakness of an arm or leg, difficulty in walking, and even death.

Thromboembolic strokes (also known as *ischemic* strokes), account for about 70%–80% of the strokes in the United States. Thromboembolic strokes can be classified into two categories: thrombotic strokes and embolic strokes. *Thrombotic strokes* are caused by the narrowing and eventual blockage of a vessel that supplies blood to a part of the brain. The blood vessels involved can be either the larger blood vessels leading to the brain or the smaller blood vessels within the brain. An *embolic stroke* results when a blood clot or piece of debris breaks free and lodges in a vessel, thereby blocking blood flow to the brain. These traveling clots or debris are called *emboli* and typically originate either from a diseased heart or from atherosclerotic blood vessels leading to the brain (such as the carotid arteries).

Hemorrhagic strokes account for about 20%–30% of the strokes in the United States. These strokes result from blood vessels that leak or rupture. Hemorrhagic strokes are classified into those that result in spontaneous bleeding around the brain (*subarachnoid hemorrhage*) or bleeding inside the brain (*intracerebral hemorrhage*).

Some research studies use the term *cerebrovascular disease*. This term includes all diseases of the blood vessels supplying the brain. Stroke is a major type of cerebrovascular disease.

Risk Factors for Stroke

Much research is currently being conducted to determine what factors increase the chance that an individual will suffer a stroke and the relative importance of each of these factors. In addition to nonmodifiable traits such as age, sex, heredity, and race, the following factors are currently felt to be the primary risk factors for stroke:

- Hypertension (high blood pressure)
- Heart disease
- High blood lipids
- Atherosclerosis of the carotid arteries
- Smoking
- Diabetes
- Excessive alcohol consumption
- Obesity

Studies of Different Diets and Stroke

Limitations of Studies of Diet and Stroke

There have not been a great number of studies on the relationship between different diets and stroke. The studies that have been done face the problem of separating the effects of diet from the effects of other factors such as smoking or alcohol use. Also, because strokes are caused by several different mechanisms, diet may have an effect on one type of stroke but not on another. The studies that have been done often lump different types of strokes together. This may limit the researchers' ability to detect an effect that a particular diet may have on one type of stroke, but not another.

Additionally, even though differentiating between types of strokes may be important in diet studies, it has not always been done. Until the mid-1970s, when the CAT scan machine became fairly widely available, and the 1980s, when the MRI machine came into use, it was difficult to diagnose a stroke and accurately differentiate among different types of strokes. Even today, studies do not always differentiate among the different types of strokes. Furthermore, in those studies where an attempt is made to differentiate among stroke types, accuracy may be elusive. For example, even with the help of CAT scans and MRIs, it can often be difficult to state with certainty whether a stroke is due to an atherosclerotic narrowing of a vessel or to an embolism. Confounding the situation further is the fact that many thromboembolic strokes occur without producing symptoms.

Throughout this chapter, when the general term *stroke* is used, it refers to all types of stroke combined.

Studies of Vegetarian Diets and Stroke

- A study of death certificates dated from 1936–1970 for members of a vegetarian society in England found no difference in the risk of death due to cerebrovascular disease among vegetarian society members as compared with the general population of England and Wales (Kinlen, Hermon, & Smith, 1983).
- A study by Key, conducted over a 10- to 12-year period ending in 1985, followed 4,627 vegetarians and 6,144 nonvegetarian customers of health food shops in Great Britain. Both groups had a lower-than-expected number of deaths due to cerebrovascular disease, though there was little or no difference between the vegetarians and the nonvegetarians (Burr & Butland, 1988). A follow-up in 1995 continued to find no difference in mortality from cerebrovascular diseases among the vegetarians compared with the nonvegetarians; however, the researchers did find that consumption of fresh fruit daily was associated with a significant reduction (32%) in deaths due to cerebrovascular disease (Key et al., 1996).
- The risk of death from cerebrovascular disease was studied in a group of 1,904 German "strict" and "moderate" vegetarians. The strict vegetarians ate no fish or meat. The moderate vegetarians were customers of health food stores who ate fish or meat occasionally. Compared with the general German population, the risk of death from cerebrovascular disease was reduced by 29% for strict vegetarians. For the near-vegetarians, risk was reduced by 35%. Nei-

ther reduction was statistically significant. Differences in socioeconomic status, smoking, and body weight were not factored into the data (Chang-Claude, Frentzel-Beyme, & Eilber, 1992).

Studies of Seventh-Day Adventists and Stroke

Seventh-Day Adventists (SDAs) are prohibited by their religion from smoking and consuming alcohol, and are discouraged from consuming meat, fish, and eggs. Because about 50% or more of SDAs do not eat meat, but otherwise have similar lifestyles, they offer a unique opportunity to study the effects of vegetarian diets.

- Phillips compared 22,940 SDAs with 112,726 non-SDAs in California. There was a significant reduction in cerebrovascular disease among the SDAs. This reduction persisted even when SDA non-smokers were compared with non-SDA nonsmokers (Phillips et al., 1980).
- During a 10-year period, Berkel studied the causes of death of 482 SDAs in the Netherlands and found a significant (nearly 50%) decrease in the death rate from cerebrovascular disease among the SDAs as compared with the general Dutch population. These results were not, however, adjusted for differences in alcohol consumption and smoking (Berkel & de Waard, 1983).
- Hirayama conducted a 16-year follow-up study of 122,261 men in Japan, comparing those with a lifestyle similar to SDAs (no smoking, no drinking, no daily meat consumption, daily consumption of green and yellow vegetables) to a group with opposite lifestyles. Those with a lifestyle similar to SDAs had a decreased risk of sub-

arachnoid hemorrhage and thrombotic strokes. Among those who smoked and drank alcohol, adding meat and removing daily vegetables significantly increased the risk of subarachnoid hemorrhage and slightly increased the risk of thrombotic stroke (Hirayama, 1985).

• Snowdon (1988) reported on a study conducted in California, which compared 18,858 SDAs who had never smoked with 50,217 California non-SDAs who had never smoked. The SDAs had lower mortality rates from stroke. Among the SDAs, meat consumption itself did not seem to increase the risk of death due to stroke.

Studies of Individual Dietary Factors and Stroke

Cholesterol and Dietary Fats

Although the connection between elevated serum cholesterol and increased risk of coronary artery (heart) disease has been well documented for many years, the connection between cholesterol and risk of stroke remains debatable. In recent years, however, evidence has been mounting that serum cholesterol does affect the risk of some types of stroke.

Problems with Studies of Cholesterol and Stroke. The studies that have been done on the relationship between cholesterol and stroke have been plagued by many of the same problems associated with studies of diet and stroke, such as small numbers of participants and lack of differentiation between types of strokes. In addition, there are other problems. There is evidence that atherosclerosis may be a factor in the etiology of strokes that result from disease in larger blood vessels (such as the carotid arteries), but may not be a factor in strokes due

to disease in the smaller vessels within the brain; in the latter, the primary association may be with hypertension (Benfante et al., 1994). Because it is often difficult to differentiate between large- and small-vessel strokes, they are frequently grouped together as thromboembolic strokes. Because strokes involving larger vessels may be responsible for only 9%–12% of strokes in this country, it may be difficult to document a causal role for cholesterol in large-vessel thromboembolic strokes through studies that include many types of stroke (Gillman et al., 1995; Crouse et al., 1997).

Adding to the confusion is the effect of cultural differences on strokes. For example, in Japanese and Chinese populations, the risk of hemorrhagic stroke is much higher proportionately than in the United States and other Western cultures. Also, strokes due to large- and medium-vessel disease may be much more common in Western cultures than in Japanese cultures, where small-vessel disease appears to be a more significant cause of stroke. Because of this difference, studies of risk factors for stroke in Japanese and Chinese cultures may be less relevant to Western cultures.

Keeping all of these concerns in mind, it is useful to look at the studies that have been done regarding cholesterol and stroke risk.

Low Serum Cholesterol and Possible Increased Risk of Hemorrhagic Stroke. Several studies have found that low serum cholesterol may be associated with an increased risk of hemorrhagic stroke (Yano, Reed, & MacLean, 1989; Neaton et al., 1992; Lindgren et al., 1992; Gatchev et al., 1993; Ueshima et al., 1980; Tanaka et al., 1982; Okada et al., 1976; Shimamoto et al., 1996). Some of these studies were conducted in Japanese populations, where the risk of hemorrhagic stroke is much higher than in Western populations (Ueshima et al., 1980; Tanaka et al., 1982; Okada et al., 1976; Shimamoto et al., 1996).

A few studies have been conducted in Western cultures. One of these, the Honolulu study, conducted among 7,850 Japanese-Americans in Hawaii, found significantly increased risk of intracerebral hemorrhage, but not of subarachnoid hemorrhage, among those with a serum cholesterol less than 189 mg/dl (Chapman et al., 1966). The Multiple Risk Factor Intervention Trial (MRFIT) study of approximately 350,000 U.S. men reported an increase in intracerebral hemorrhage, but not of subarachnoid hemorrhage, those with serum cholesterol levels less than 160 mg/dl (Neaton et al., 1992). In his Swedish population, Lindgren found an increased risk of hemorrhagic stroke in those with low serum cholesterol (Lindgren et al., 1992). In a Swedish population studied by Gatchev, low serum cholesterol was associated with an increased risk of subarachnoid hemorrhage in men, but not with intracerebral hemorrhage; no significant increase in either subarachnoid hemorrhage or intracerebral hemorrhage was found in women (Gatchev et al., 1993). The Eastern Stroke and Coronary Heart Disease Collaborative Research Group (1998) study of 124,774 participants from China and Japan also found a weak, nonsignificant increase in the risk of hemorrhagic stroke with decreased cholesterol levels.

Two prospective studies found that low intake of saturated fat and low intake of animal protein were associated with an increased risk of intracerebral brain hemorrhage. One study was the U.S. Nurses' Health Study, which followed 85,764 women for 14 years (Iso et al., 2001); the other was a 14-year study of 4,755 Japanese (Iso et al., 2003). In the Japanese study, the association with animal protein was nonsignificant.

It has been hypothesized that even if there is a true relationship between low cholesterol and risk of hemorrhagic stroke, it may not be a causal relationship. It may be that low cholesterol is merely a marker for individuals who are at risk of hemorrhagic stroke for other reasons, such as heavy alcohol use, systemic illness, poor nutrition, or a higher intake of polyunsaturated fats (which are known to reduce platelet clumping) (Iso et al., 1989). Additionally, a diet low in saturated fat may reduce platelet clumping (Iso et al., 2003). Alternatively, it has been proposed that low cholesterol may make blood vessels more vulnerable to rupture (Iso et al., 2003).

Still, some studies have cast doubt on the existence of any relationship between low cholesterol and hemorrhagic stroke. In 1989, Chen reported that prospective follow-up data on 9,021 Chinese subjects, from an area where more than half of fatal strokes are hemorrhagic, showed no excess of stroke risk in the lowest quintile of serum cholesterol, which had a mean cholesterol level of 160 mg/dl (Chen, Collins, & Peto, 1989). In a 1995 prospective study of 450,000 individuals with 5 to 30 years of follow-up, no increased stroke risk at low cholesterol levels was found even among Asian populations with generally low total cholesterol and high proportions of hemorrhagic stroke (Prospective Studies Collaboration, 1995). A 2001 6-year prospective study of 114,793 Korean men did not find cholesterol levels to be related to risk of hemorrhagic stroke (Suh et al., 2001).

Elevated Cholesterol and Possible Increased Risk of Ischemic Stroke. Dozens of studies have investigated the possibility of a relationship between elevated serum cholesterol and stroke. In addition to all of the problems inherent in studies of the relationship between cholesterol and stroke (as mentioned earlier), there is the additional problem of the possible relationship between low cholesterol and increased risk of hemorrhagic stroke. If real, this association could mask any relationship that

Table 13.1   Meta-Analyses of Studies, Primarily Published before 1990, Investigating a Relationship between Stroke and Cholesterol

- A 1995 meta-analysis of 45 prospective studies found no association between blood cholesterol and stroke in those older than 45; however, most studies did not distinguish between ischemic and hemorrhagic stroke. In those under 45 years of age, there was a significant increase in occurrence of stroke in those with increased serum cholesterol (Qizilbash et al., 1995).
- Qizilbash et al.(1992) reviewed the combined data of 10 epidemiologic studies, dating from 1966 to 1989, that had approximately equal cutoff points for total cholesterol. They found a significant association between risk of stroke and total cholesterol of more than 220 mg/dl. The researchers estimated that approximately 20% of the risk of stroke in Caucasians with cholesterol higher than 187–227 mg/dl could be attributed to elevated cholesterol.
- A 2002 analysis of 8 prospective studies, most of which had been published in the 1980s and that looked at a combined 24,343 women, found that for all women under 55 years of age, there was a significant independent, positive correlation between cholesterol and nonhemorrhagic stroke mortality. For those over 55 years of age, there was no relationship between stroke mortality and cholesterol level (Horenstein, Smith, & Mosca, 2002).

may exist between high serum cholesterol and elevated risk of ischemic stroke in studies that considered all types of stroke together. This would be especially true in studies of Japanese populations, where the risk of hemorrhagic stroke is proportionately much higher than in Western cultures.

Some studies published more than 15 years ago showed no connection between elevated serum cholesterol and stroke, although in a few of these there was a nonsignificant trend toward increased risk with increased cholesterol (Salonen & Puska, 1983; Salonen et al., 1982; Khaw et al., 1984; Welin et al., 1987; Chapman et al., 1966). However, a few studies did document a direct relationship between stroke and serum cholesterol (Westlund & Nicolaysen, 1972; Boysen et al., 1988; Johnson, Yano, & Kato, 1967). Many studies focused specifically on ischemic stroke and found no relationship with elevated cholesterol (Ueshima et al., 1980; Tanaka et al., 1982; Rossner et al., 1978; Szatrowski et al., 1984; Gertler et al., 1968; Sridharan, 1992; Noma et al., 1979); however, many of these studies involved only Japanese populations (Ueshima et al., 1980; Tanaka et al.,

1982; Szatrowski et al., 1984; Noma et al., 1979) in which, as mentioned previously, a greater proportion of ischemic strokes occurs secondary to disease in small vessels rather than to disease in larger vessels, where cholesterol may be more of a determining factor. Several studies conducted in non-Japanese populations did find a statistically nonsignificant trend relating elevated cholesterol and ischemic stroke (Tilvis et al., 1987; Aronow et al., 1988; Robinson, Higano, & Cohen, 1963; Fogelholm & Aho, 1973). Heyman, in his 1961 case-control study of 68 patients with cerebral infarctions, did document a direct relationship between ischemic stroke and serum cholesterol (Heyman, Nefzger, & Estes, 1961). Several meta-analyses of studies, most conducted before 1990, found a relationship between stroke and serum cholesterol level, particularly in certain subsets of the population (Table 13.1).

Several studies published within the past 15 years have looked specifically at the relationship between serum cholesterol and ischemic strokes. Many have found that elevated serum cholesterol does increase the risk of ischemic strokes (Table 13.2). A few studies, however,

Table 13.2   Studies Published Since 1990 Showing a Relationship between Serum Cholesterol and Ischemic Stroke

- The 1992 MRFIT study, which followed 350,977 men for 12 years, found no association between serum cholesterol level and total stroke. However, when the stroke types were examined separately, the researchers found that the higher the cholesterol level, the greater the risk of nonhemorrhagic stroke (Neaton et al., 1992).
- The 1994 study by Lindenstrom, which followed 19,698 men and women, found that total cholesterol was associated with increased risk of nonhemorrhagic stroke, but only at serum cholesterol levels greater than 309 mg/dl (Lindenstrom, Boysen, & Nyboe, 1994).
- The 1994 Honolulu Heart Program study of 6,352 Japanese-American men found that the risk of thromboembolic stroke was 1.7 times greater in those in the highest, compared to the lowest, quartile of serum cholesterol (Benfante et al., 1994).
- Hachinski's study of 90 patients with stroke or transient ischemic attack (TIA; stroke symptoms that resolve completely within a few hours) found significantly higher cholesterol levels among those with stroke or TIA as compared to controls (Hachinski et al., 1996).
- A study of 8,586 men followed for 21 years found a nonsignificant increase in ischemic stroke with increased total serum cholesterol (Tanne, Yaari, & Goldbourt, 1997).
- A 1998 study, which followed 2,805 men and women over 60 years of age for about 8 years, revealed an inverse relationship between HDL cholesterol and ischemic stroke, but no relationship between total cholesterol and ischemic stroke (Simons et al., 1998).
- In a 6-year follow-up study of 28,519 male smokers, an increased risk of cerebral infarction was found in those with the highest cholesterol levels (Leppala et al., 1999).
- A study of 11,177 patients followed for 6 to 8 years found a direct correlation between ischemic stroke and blood levels of total and LDL cholesterol (Koren-Morag et al., 2002).

have not found such a relationship (Lindgren et al., 1992; Simons et al., 1998; Harmsen et al., 1990).

Giving further credence to the hypothesis that elevated serum cholesterol is directly associated with some types of stroke is the fact that carotid artery atherosclerotic disease, a known risk factor for stroke, has been clearly related to elevated serum total cholesterol and low-density lipoprotein (LDL) cholesterol (Gorelick et al., 1997). Additionally, several studies have demonstrated that lowering serum cholesterol retards the rate of progression of carotid atherosclerosis (Gorelick et al., 1997; Crouse et al., 1995). Autopsy studies have also shown elevated cholesterol levels to be related to atherosclerosis of blood vessels to the brain (Tell, Crouse, & Furberg, 1988).

Additional support for the theory that elevated serum cholesterol increases the risk of some strokes comes from studies of stroke among those taking cholesterol-lowering medications (Hankey, 2002). Although two earlier meta-analyses by Atkins et al. (1993) and Herbert (Herbert, Gaziano, & Hennekens, 1995) showed that lowering serum cholesterol (primarily by using drugs) did not reduce the risk of stroke, more recent studies, using the more effective cholesterol-lowering statin drugs, have found an effect on stroke-risk reduction. Several meta-analyses of these studies investigating the effect of statin drugs on stroke risk have been done (Table 13.3). These analyses show a significant reduction in the risk of stroke among those on statin drugs. Also, the Heart Protection Study Collaborative Group (2002)

Table 13.3   Meta-Analyses of Studies Investigating the Effect of Statin Drugs on the Risk of Stroke

- Crouse reviewed 12 studies on the effect of statin drugs and found a highly significant 27% reduction in stroke in individuals taking the statin drugs. These studies also showed a 30%–40% reduction in cholesterol levels, as opposed to the 10%–12% reduction seen in the earlier studies reviewed by Adkins and Herbert, which did not show any stroke-risk reduction from cholesterol-lowering drugs (Crouse et al., 1997).
- Blauw conducted an analysis of 13 trials with statin drugs and found a 31% reduction in stroke risk in the participants who took the statin drugs (Blauw et al., 1997).
- DiMascio reviewed 41 clinical trials of cholesterol-lowering medications, including many studies that looked at the statin drugs, and found an approximately 16% reduction in risk of stroke over approximately 4 years for the cholesterol-lowering drugs (DiMascio, Marchioli, & Tognoni, 2000).
- A meta-analysis of 38 trials found that lipid-lowering drugs resulted in a significant (17%) reduction in the incidence of stroke; the best results came from use of the statin drugs, which lowered the risk of stroke by 26% (Corvol et al., 2003).

reported a lower incidence of stroke in those treated with statin drugs. One reason for this reduced stroke risk with the statin drugs is that, by lowering serum cholesterol, they may decrease or stop the progression of atherosclerosis in the large vessels leading to the brain. Other proposed mechanisms involve stabilization of the atherosclerotic plaque in blood vessels; protective effects on blood vessels themselves; or anti-inflammatory, antithrombotic (reducing blood clotting), or neuroprotective effects (Corvol et al., 2003; Rosenson & Tangney, 1998; Vaughan & Delanty, 1999).

Studies that have looked at the relationship between dietary monounsaturated and polyunsaturated fat and the risk of stroke have been few in number and have shown inconsistent results (He et al., 2003).

Sodium and Potassium

High sodium intake has been associated with hypertension, which, in turn, increases the risk of stroke. Several studies have found that increased potassium intake decreases the risk of both fatal and nonfatal strokes (Green et al., 2002) (see Table 13.4). This effect of potassium

may be due to its effect on lowering blood pressure; however, some studies have suggested that the effect of potassium on stroke is independent of blood pressure (Green et al., 2002). Other theories have been proposed, including effects of potassium on oxidative stress as well as blood-vessel and atherosclerotic changes (Green et al., 2002).

Homocysteine and Folate

Homocysteine is an amino acid produced by the body from the essential dietary amino acid methionine. Some studies suggested that elevated homocysteine levels may be associated with the development of atherosclerotic coronary heart disease, although more recent prospective studies cast some doubt on this (Falk, Zhou, & Moller, 2001).

Several studies suggest that elevated homocysteine may be associated with increased risk of stroke. Again, however, more recent prospective studies have been less supportive (Perry, 1999; Yoo, Chung, & Kang, 1998; Giles et al., 1998; Hankey & Eikelboom, 2001). Boushey et al. (1995) reviewed 11 studies addressing the association between homocysteine and risk of

Table 13.4   Studies of the Effect of Potassium Intake on the Risk of Stroke

- Khaw followed 859 adults for 12 years and concluded that a 10 mmoL increase in daily potassium intake was associated with a 40% decrease in stroke-associated death (Khaw & Barrett-Conner, 1987).
- A study of 9,866 individuals, followed for 16.7 years in the first National Health and Nutrition Examination Survey (NHANES I), found that increased dietary potassium was related to lower risk of death from stroke only among black men and hypertensive men, and not among white or nonhypertensive men, or among women (Fang, Madhavan, & Alderman, 2000).
- In another study out of NHANES I, in which 9,805 men and women were followed over an average of 19 years, researchers found that dietary potassium was inversely related to the risk of stroke (Bazzano et al., 2001).
- The Cardiovascular Health Study, which followed 5,600 men and women for 4 to 7 years, found that a lower serum potassium level in users of diuretic medications and low potassium intake in those not taking diuretics were associated with increased stroke incidence (Green et al., 2002).
- The Honolulu Heart Program, which followed 7,591 Japanese-American men, found an inverse relationship of potassium intake with fatal thromboembolic stroke, but not with nonfatal thromboembolic stroke or hemorrhagic stroke (Lee et al., 1988).
- The Health Professionals Follow-up Study, of 43,738 men followed for 8 years, found lower risk of stroke among those with greater potassium intake (Ascherio et al., 1998).

cerebrovascular disease, and found that 9 case-control studies supported the hypothesis that elevated homocysteine increases the risk of cerebrovascular disease; however, the two prospective studies lacked evidence of an association.

Elevated homocysteine levels have been associated with low levels of the vitamins folate, B6, and B12. Folate appears to be the main dietary determinant of homocysteine levels (Perry, 1999). Increasing folate consumption, and to a lesser degree intakes of B6 and B12, reduces homocysteine levels (Boushey et al., 1995). Increased serum folate levels have been shown to be associated with a decrease in carotid artery disease (Selhub et al., 1995). In addition to its effect of decreasing homocysteine, folate may have protective effects on blood vessels themselves (Wilmink et al., 2000).

A few studies have investigated the relationship between folate and risk of stroke. The first National Health and Nutrition Examination Survey Study (NHANES I), which followed 9,764 men and women over an average of 19 years,

found that dietary folate was inversely related to the risk of stroke (Bazzano et al., 2002a). The Health Professionals Follow-up Study looked at 43,732 men during a 14-year follow-up and found that increased folate and B12 intakes were associated with a decreased risk of ischemic stroke (He et al., 2004).

The mechanism by which homocysteine may increase the risk of stroke remains unclear (Bazzano et al., 2002a). Homocysteine may promote atherosclerosis and blood clotting and may affect blood vessels themselves (Hankey & Eikelboom, 2001; Kittner et al., 1999). There is also some evidence to suggest that elevated homocysteine levels may be the result of, rather than the cause of, vascular events such as strokes (Hankey & Eikelboom, 2001). It remains to be seen whether any association between homocysteine and stroke is causal by investigating whether lowering plasma homocysteine levels reduces the risk of stroke (Hankey & Eikelboom, 2001).

As noted in Chapter 10, on heart disease, a handful of studies have looked at homocysteine levels among vegetarians versus nonvegetarians. To date, most of the studies have found higher homocysteine levels in vegetarians. It is not known what difference, if any, this may have on the risk of stroke for vegetarians.

Antioxidants

Antioxidants protect the body from damaging free radicals. Examples of antioxidants include vitamins C and E, carotenoids (such as beta-carotene, which can be converted into vitamin A), and many phytochemicals, including the flavonoids. A few studies have investigated the relationship between antioxidants and the risk of stroke. These studies looked at antioxidants in food as well as those from supplements. Some of the studies found a protective effect (in some cases for one antioxidant and not another), and others did not (Yochum, Folsom, & Kushi, 2000; Keli et al., 1996; Eidelman et al., 2004; Voko et al., 2003; Barer et al., 1989; Lapidus et al., 1986).

It may be that a single antioxidant alone does not have an effect on the risk of stroke, whereas a mixture of antioxidants may be protective (Sauvaget et al., 2003). This could account for the fact that intake of fruits and vegetables, which contain a mixture of different antioxidants, appears to protect against stroke, but that, so far, no effect on stroke has been demonstrated for individual antioxidant supplements.

Fiber

Only a very few studies have focused on the association of fiber with risk of stroke. Ascherio looked at the effect of fiber on stroke risk among 43,738 men in the Health Professionals Follow-up Study and found that fiber intake protected against stroke (Ascherio et al., 1998). The Nurses' Health Study, which followed 75,521

women for 12 years, found that higher intake of whole-grain foods was associated with a lower risk of ischemic stroke, independent of known cardiovascular risk factors (Liu et al., 2000). The Atherosclerosis Risk in Communities (ARIC) Study, which followed 11,940 participants over an average of 11 years, found that whole-grain consumption was inversely related to the risk of ischemic stroke; however, the effect was attenuated after adjustment for several confounding factors (Steffen et al., 2003).

The effect of whole grains could be due to one or more of their many components, including not only fiber, but also antioxidants, minerals (such as potassium), phytochemicals, and vitamins (such as folate). Any effect of fiber may also be due to its effects on lipids, body weight, diabetes, heart disease, and/or blood pressure. Fiber was also shown in one study to decrease the level of factor VII in the blood-clotting scheme, which could theoretically decrease the risk of ischemic stroke (Rajaram, 2003).

Fruit and Vegetable Consumption

Many studies have looked at the relationship between intake of fruits and vegetables and the risk of stroke (see Table 13.5). Nearly universally, a protective effect has been found.

The reasons for a protective effect of fruits and vegetables are not known, though many possible mechanisms have been proposed. A diet rich in fruits and vegetables may be correspondingly lower in saturated fat. Fruits and vegetables are also rich in fiber, folate, antioxidants, and potassium. Phytochemicals are abundant in fruits and vegetabales, and many have demonstrated antiplatelet-clumping effects, as well as protective effects on the blood vessels themselves (Rajaram, 2003; Anthony, 2002; Dutta-Roy, 2002; Mojzisova & Kuchta, 2001). Consumption of fruits and vegetables has also

Table 13.5   Studies Investigating the Effect of Fruit and Vegetable Consumption on Risk of Stroke

- Vollset,in a study of 16,713 Norwegians, found decreased cerebrovascular disease mortality in those with greater consumption of fruits and vegetables (Vollset & Bjelke, 1983).
- Acheson andWilliams found that eating fresh fruits and green vegetables was associated with reduced risk of death from cerebrovascular disease in England.They studied the consumption of these foods in different geographical areas and compared this to the general cerebrovascular death rate in those areas (Acheson & Williams, 1983).
- A 20-year follow-up of 832 men in the Framingham study found that increased consumption of fruits and vegetables was associated with a decreased risk of all strokes combined, as well as ischemic and hemorrhagic strokes separately. For each increment of three daily servings of fruits and vegetables, there was a 22% decrease in the risk of all stroke (Gillman et al., 1995).
- Key studied 4,627 vegetarians and 6,144 nonvegetarians over a 10- to 12-year period and found that, although there was no difference in mortality from cerebrovascular disease among vegetarians when compared with nonvegetarians, daily fresh fruit consumption did confer a protective effect against stroke (Key et al., 1996).
- In 1997,Ness and Powles reviewed studies of diets that reported on the intake of either fresh fruits and vegetables or a nutrient that could serve as a marker for fruit and vegetable consumption (vitamin C, beta-carotene, folate, flavonoids, potassium, and dietary fiber from vegetables). For stroke, 9 of the 14 studies found a significant protective association with the consumption of fruits and vegetables (Ness & Powles, 1997).
- Artalejo concluded that increased fruit consumption and decreased wine consumption from 1964 to 1980 may have contributed to the decline in cerebrovascular mortality in Spain from 1975 to 1993 (Artalejo et al., 1998).
- A 1999 study looked at 75,596 women from the Nurses'Health Study, followed for 14 years, and 38,683 men from the Health Professionals Follow-up Study, followed for 8 years.The analysis found that fruit and vegetable consumption protected against ischemic stroke. Each increment of 1 serving per day of fruits and vegetables was associated with a 6% lower risk of ischemic stroke. Intake beyond 6 servings per day provided little further benefit (Joshipura et al., 1999).
- In a study of 26,593 male smokers followed for 6 years (theAlpha-Tocopherol, Beta-Carotene Cancer Prevention Study in Finland), consumption of vegetables was found to be inversely associated with the risk of cerebral infarction.The consumption of fruits was inversely associated with the risk of intracerebral hemorrhage (Hirvonen et al., 2000).
- The NHANES I trial,which studied 9,608 adults for an average of 19 years, found that consuming fruits and vegetables 3 times per day or more, compared with less than once per day, was associated with a 27% lower risk of stroke and a 42% lower stroke mortality (Bazzano et al., 2002b).
- A 2003 study followed 40,349 Japanese men and women for an average of 16 yearsThe researchers found that daily consumption of green-yellow vegetables and fruits was associated with a lower risk of death from stroke, intracerebral hemorrhage, and cerebral infarction (Sauvaget et al., 2003).
- The 2003 Danish Diet,Cancer and Health Study, of 54,506 men and women followed for a mean of 3 years, found a decreased risk of ischemic stroke from increased fruit consumption.This effect was most pronounced for citrus fruits.They found no clear association between the intake of vegetables and the risk of ischemic stroke (Johnsen et al., 2003).
- TheARIC study of 11,940 participants found no relationship between fruit and vegetable intake and the risk of ischemic stroke. In comparing the results of this study with the 24%–31% lower risk of stroke observed among those with higher fruit and vegetable consumption in the Nurses' Health Study, the Health Professionals Study, the Framingham Study, and the NHANES study, the authors noted that average fruit and vegetable consumption was higher in these other studies than in the ARIC study (Steffen et al., 2003).

been shown to lower blood pressure, which could decrease stroke risk.

Studies of Meat Consumption and Stroke

As noted earlier, Snowdon (1988) did not find that meat consumption among Seventh-Day Adventists increased the risk of death due to stroke. However, Hirayama (1985) found that adding meat and removing daily vegetables from the diet increased the risk of subarachnoid and thrombotic strokes. Jamrozik et al. (1994) studied 536 stroke victims in Australia and compared them with control subjects. These researchers found that consumption of meat more than four times weekly was associated with an increased risk of stroke. In the Health Professionals Follow-up Study, of 43,732 men followed for 14 years, there was no association of red meat intake with either ischemic or hemorrhagic stroke (He et al., 2003).

Putting It All Together with Vegetarian Diets

Because there have been an insignificant number of studies specifically concerning vegetarian diets and risk of stroke, one must, for now, look at the issue indirectly. To do this, one can look at stroke risk among Seventh-Day Adventists, and how known risk factors for stroke are affected by different components of vegetarian diets.

The consensus, supported by multiple studies, is that fruit and vegetable consumption decreases the risk of stroke. Also, evidence shows that Seventh-Day Adventists, who follow vegetarian diets, have a decreased incidence of stroke. These data suggest that vegetarian diets may protect against stroke.

Several medical conditions that are known risk factors for stroke are also affected by veg-

etarian diets. Hypertension (high blood pressure) is the strongest and most prevalent risk factor for stroke, and studies show that vegetarians have lower blood pressures and a decreased incidence of hypertension. Heart disease is also a major risk factor for stroke, and studies show a lower incidence of heart disease among vegetarians. There is some evidence that diabetes, another risk factor for stroke, may be less prevalent and/or more easily controlled in vegetarians. Lastly, obesity, which is considered to increase the risk of stroke, is less common among vegetarians.

Vegetarian diets may affect the risk of stroke because of specific dietary factors. Cholesterol is one of these factors. Vegetarians have lower serum cholesterols. There is significant evidence that elevated cholesterol does raise the risk of thromboembolic strokes, the most common type of stroke in Western cultures. Also, controlling cholesterol levels is important for reducing heart disease, which itself is a risk factor for stroke. Some studies have correlated low cholesterol levels (less than 160–180 mg/dl) with an increased risk of hemorrhagic stroke. Even if true, however, it is unclear whether the low cholesterol causes the increase in stroke risk or whether the increase in stroke incidence is due to some other factor that happens to be associated with lower cholesterol.

In addition to cholesterol, other dietary factors that may be associated with stroke can be affected by vegetarian diets. Some studies suggest that potassium intake may decrease the risk of stroke. Vegetarians tend to consume more potassium than nonvegetarians (Messina & Messina, 1996). A few studies suggest than antioxidants and folate may protect against stroke. Vegetarians tend to have higher consumption of antioxidants and folate than nonvegetarians. Another potential protective factor, which is consumed in greater quantity by vegetarians than by nonvegetarians, is fiber. Potential effects of vegetarian diets on decreasing blood clotting were summarized in Chapter 10 on cardiovascular issues; any correlation of these effects with the risk of stroke is purely speculative at this time.

The National Stroke Association concludes that, to reduce the risk of stroke, it remains prudent to limit excess saturated fat and sodium intake; maintain adequate intakes of vitamin B12, vitamin B6, and folate; and eat a diet rich in fruits and vegetable (Gorelick et al., 1999). A well-balanced vegetarian diet will help to accomplish these goals.

Practical Aspects

Several dietary factors may help in the prevention of stroke. Studies suggest that a diet rich in fruits and vegetables and potassium and low in saturated fats and cholesterol reduces the risk of stroke. Good sources of fiber and folate may be beneficial. Body weight should be kept normal. Sodium consumption should be limited in those with sodium-sensitive high blood pressure. Excessive alcohol consumption should be avoided. Dietary factors that help prevent or control other diseases associated with a higher risk of stroke, such as hypertension, heart disease, and diabetes, should be emphasized.

Conclusion

There have been far too few studies of the risk of stroke among vegetarians to be conclusive. Speculation remains as to whether low serum cholesterol may increase the risk of hemorrhagic stroke. This risk factor would, theoretically, be of greater importance to vegetarians, who tend to have lower serum cholesterol levels.

A large number of studies suggest that particular aspects of a vegetarian diet may decrease the risk of stroke. Many studies suggest that increased consumption of fruits and vegetables may decrease the risk of stroke. Many studies also suggest that lower serum cholesterol may offer some protection against ischemic stroke, the most common type of stroke in Western cultures. Other factors associated with vegetarian diets that may help protect against the risk of stroke include increased intake of fruits and vegetables, potassium, folate, antioxidants, and fiber. Also, lower incidences of hypertension, heart disease, diabetes, and obesity among vegetarians may help protect them from stroke.

References

Acheson RM, Williams DR. Does consumption of fruit and vegetables protect against stroke? *Lancet.* 1983;1(8335):1191–1193.

Anthony MS. Phytoestrogens and cardiovascular disease: Where's the meat? *Arterioscler Thromb Vasc Biol.* 2002;22(8):1245–1247.

Aronow W, Gutstein H, Lee N, Edwards M. Three-year follow-up of risk factors correlated with new atherothrombotic brain infarction in 708 elderly patients. *Angiology.* 1988;39(7, Pt 1): 563–566.

Artalejo F, Guallar-Castillón P, Banegas J, et al. Consumption of fruit and wine and the decline in cerebrovascular diseases mortality in Spain (1975–1993). *Stroke.* 1998;29:1556–1561.

Ascherio A, Rimm EB, Hernan MA, et al. Intake of potassium, magnesium, calcium, and fiber and risk of stroke among U.S. men. *Circulation.* 1998;98(12):1198–1204.

Atkins D, Psaty BM, Koepsell TD, et al. Cholesterol reduction and the risk for stroke in men: A meta-analysis of randomized, controlled trials. *Ann Intern Med.* 1993;119:136–145.

Barer D, Leibowitz R, Ebrahim S, et al. Vitamin C status and other nutritional indices in patients with stroke and other acute illnesses: A case-control study. *J Clin Epidemiol.* 1989;42(7):625–631.

Bazzano LA, He J, Ogden LG, et al. Dietary intake of folate and risk of stroke in U.S. men and women: NHANES I Epidemiologic Follow-Up Study. National Health and Nutrition Examination Survey. *Stroke*. 2002a;33(5):1183-1188.

Bazzano LA, He J, Ogden LG, et al. Fruit and vegetable intake and risk of cardiovascular disease in U.S. adults: The first National Health and Nutrition Examination Survey Epidemiologic follow-up study. *Am J Clin Nutr.* 2002b;76(1):93-99.

Bazzano LA, He J, Ogden LG, et al. Dietary potassium intake and risk of stroke in U.S. men and women. National Health and Nutrition Examination Survey I Epidemiologic Follow-Up Study. *Stroke.* 2001;32(7):1473-1480.

Benfante R, Yano K, Hwang L, et al. Elevated serum cholesterol is a risk factor for both coronary heart disease and thromboembolic stroke in Hawaiian Japanese men: Implications of shared risk. *Stroke.* 1994;25(4):814-820.

Berkel J, de Waard F. Mortality pattern and life expectancy of Seventh-Day Adventists in the Netherlands. *Intl J Epidemiol.* 1983;12(4):455-459.

Blauw GJ, Lagaay AM, Smelt AH, Westendorp RG. Stroke, statins, and cholesterol. A meta-analysis of randomized, placebo-controlled, double-blind trials with HMG-CoA reductase inhibitors. *Stroke.* 1997;28(5):946-950.

Boushey C, Beresford S, Omenn G, Motulsky A. A quantitative assessment of plasma homocysteine as a risk factor for vascular disease. Probable benefits of increasing folic acid intakes. *JAMA.* 1995;274(13):1049-1057.

Boysen G, Nyboe J, Appleyard M, et al. Stroke incidence and risk factors for stroke in Copenhagen, Denmark. *Stroke.* 1988;19(11):1345-1353.

Burr ML, Butland BK. Heart disease in British vegetarians. *Am J Clin Nutr.* 1988;48(3, Suppl):830-832.

Chang-Claude J, Frentzel-Beyme R, Eilber U. Mortality pattern of German vegetarians after 11 years of follow-up. *Epidemiology.* 1992;3(5):395-401.

Chapman J, Reeder L, Borun E, et al. Epidemiology of vascular lesions affecting the central nervous system: The occurrence of strokes in a sample population under observation for cardiovascular disease. *Am J Public Health.* 1966;56(2):191-201.

Chen Z, Collins R, Peto R. Serum cholesterol levels and stroke mortality. *N Engl J Med.* 1989;321(19):1339-1340.

Corvol JL, Bouzamondo A, Sirol M, et al. Differential effects of lipid-lowering therapies on stroke prevention: A meta-analysis of randomized trials. *Arch Intern Med.* 2003;163(6):669-676.

Crouse JR, Byington RP, Bond MG, et al. Pravastatin, lipids, and atherosclerosis in the carotid arteries (PLAC-II). *Am J Cardiol.* 1995;75(7):455-459.

Crouse JR, Byington RP, Hoen HM, Furberg CD. Reductase inhibitor monotherapy and stroke prevention. *Arch Intern Med.* 1997;157(12):1305-1310.

DiMascio R, Marchioli R, Tognoni G. Cholesterol reduction and stroke occurrence: An overview of randomized clinical trials. *Cerebrovascular Dis.* 2000;10(2):85-92.

Dutta-Roy AK. Dietary components and human platelet activity. *Platelets.* 2002;13(2):67-75.

Eastern Stroke and Coronary Heart Disease Collaborative Research Group. Blood pressure, cholesterol, and stroke in eastern Asia. *Lancet.* 1998;352(Dec 5):1801-1807.

Eidelman RS, Hollar D, Herbert P, et al. Randomized trials of vitamin E in the treatment and prevention of cardiovascular disease. *Arch Intern Med.* 2004;164(14):1552-1556.

Falk E, Zhou J, Moller J. Homocysteine and atherothrombosis. *Lipids.* 2001;36(Suppl):S3-S11.

Fang J, Madhavan S, Alderman MH. Dietary potassium intake and stroke mortality. *Stroke.* 2000;31(7):1532-1537.

Fogelholm R, Aho K. Ischaemic cerebrovascular disease in young adults. 2. Serum cholesterol and triglyceride values. *Acta Neurol Scand.* 1973;49(4):428-433.

Gatchev O, Rastam L, Lindberg G, et al. Subarachnoid hemorrhage, cerebral hemorrhage, and serum cholesterol concentration in men and women. *Ann Epidemiol.* 1993;3(4):403-409.

Gertler MM, Rusk HA, Whiter HH, et al. Ischemic cerebrovascular disease. The assessment of risk factors. *Geriatrics.* 1968;23(3):135-141.

Giles WH, Croft JB, Greenlund KJ, et al. Total homocyst(e)ine concentration and the likelihood of nonfatal stroke: Results from the Third National Health and Nutrition Examination Survey, 1988–1994. *Stroke.* 1998;29(12):2473–2477.

Gillman MW, Cupples LA, Gagnon D, et al. Protective effect of fruits and vegetables on development of stroke in men. *JAMA.* 1995;273(14):1113–1117.

Gorelick PB, Sacco RL, Smith DB, et al. Prevention of a first stroke: A review of guidelines and a multidisciplinary consensus statement from the National Stroke Association. *JAMA.* 1999;281(12):1112–1120.

Gorelick PB, Schneck M, Berglund LF, et al. Status of lipids as a risk factor for stroke. *Neuroepidemiology.* 1997;16(3):107–115.

Green DM, Ropper AH, Kronmal RA, et al. Serum potassium level and dietary potassium intake as risk factors for stroke. *Neurology.* 2002;59(3):314–320.

Hachinski V, Graffagnino C, Beaudry M, et al. Lipids and stroke: A paradox. *Arch Neurol.* 1996;53(4):303–308.

Hankey GJ. Role of lipid-modifying therapy in the prevention of initial and recurrent stroke. *Curr Opin Lipidol.* 2002;13(16):645–651.

Hankey GJ, Eikelboom JW. Homocysteine and stroke. *Curr Opin Neurol.* 2001;14(1):95–102.

Harmsen P, Rosengren A, Tsipogianni A, Wilhelmsen L. Risk factors for stroke in middle-aged men in Goteborg, Sweden. *Stroke.* 1990;21(2):223–229.

He K, Merchant A, Rimm EB, et al. Folate, vitamin B6, and B12 intakes in relation to risk of stroke among men. *Stroke.* 2004;35(1):169–174.

He K, Merchant A, Rimm EB, et al. Dietary fat intake and risk of stroke in male U.S. healthcare professionals: 14 year prospective cohort study. *Br Med J.* 2003;327(7418):777–782.

Heart Protection Study Collaborative Group. MRG/BHF Heart Protection Study of cholesterol lowering with simvastatin in 20,536 high-risk individuals: A randomized placebo-controlled trial. *Lancet.* 2002;360(9326):7–22.

Herbert PR, Gaziano JM, Hennekens CH. An overview of trials of cholesterol lowering and risk of stroke. *Arch Intern Med.* 1995;155(1):50–55.

Heyman A, Nefzger M, Estes EH. Serum cholesterol level in cerebral infarction. *Arch Neurol.* 1961 (Sept 5):264–268.

Hirayama T. Mortality in Japanese with life-styles similar to Seventh-Day Adventists: Strategy for risk reduction by life-style modification. *Natl Cancer Inst Monographs.* 1985;69:143–153.

Hirvonen T, Virtamo J, Korhonen P, et al. Intake of flavonoids, carotenoids, vitamins C and E, and risk of stroke in male smokers. *Stroke.* 2000;31(10):2301–2306.

Horenstein R, Smith D, Mosca L. Cholesterol predicts stroke mortality in the Women's Pooling Project. *Stroke.* 2002;33(7):1863–1868.

Iso H, Jacobs DR, Wentworth D, et al. Serum cholesterol levels and six-year mortality from stroke in 350,977 men screened for the Multiple Risk Factor Intervention trial. *N Engl J Med.* 1989;320(14):904–910.

Iso H, Sato S, Kitamura A, et al. Fat and protein intakes and risk of introparenchymal hemorrhage among middle-aged Japanese. *Am J Epidemiol.* 2003;157(1):32–39.

Iso H, Stampfer MJ, Manson J, et al. Prospective study of fat and protein intake and risk of introparenchymal hemorrhage in women. *Circulation.* 2001;103(6):856–863.

Jamrozik K, Broadhurst RJ, Anderson C, Stewart-Wynne EG. The role of lifestyle factors in the etiology of stroke: A population-based case-control study in Perth, Western Australia. *Stroke.* 1994;25(1):51–59.

Johnsen SP, Overvad K, Stripp C, et al. Intake of fruit and vegetables and the risk of ischemic stroke in a cohort of Danish men and women. *Am J Clin Nutr.* 2003;78(1):57–64.

Johnson KG, Yano K, Kato H. Cerebral vascular disease in Hiroshima, Japan. *J Chronic Dis.* 1967;20(7):545–559.

Joshipura KJ, Ascherio A, Manson JE, et al. Fruit and vegetable intake in relation to risk of ischemic stroke. *JAMA.* 1999;282(13):1233–1239.

Keli SO, Hertog MG, Feskens EJ, Kromhout D. Dietary flavonoids, antioxidant vitamins, and incidence of stroke. The Zutphen study. *Arch Intern Med.* 1996;156(6):637–642.

Key TJ, Thorogood M, Appleby PN, Burr ML. Dietary habits and mortality in 11,000 vegetarians and health conscious people: Results of a 17 year follow up. *Br Med J.* 1996;313(7060):775–779.

Khaw K, Barrett-Conner E. Dietary potassium and stroke-associated mortality. A 12-year prospective population study. *N Engl J Med.* 1987;316(5):235–240.

Khaw K, Barrett-Connor E, Suarez L, Criqui MH. Predictors of stroke-associated mortality in the elderly. *Stroke.* 1984;15(2):244–248.

Kinlen LJ, Hermon C, Smith PG. A proportionate study of cancer mortality among members of a vegetarian society. *Br J Cancer.* 1983;48(3):355–361.

Kittner SJ, Giles WH, Macko RF, et al. Homocyst(e)ine and risk of cerebral infarction in a biracial population: The stroke prevention in young women study. *Stroke.* 1999;30(8):1554–1560.

Koren-Morag N, Tanne D, Graff E, Goldbourt U. Low- and high-density lipoprotein cholesterol and ischemic cerebrovascular disease: The bezafibrate infarction prevention registry. *Arch Intern Med.* 2002;162(9):993–999.

Lapidus L, Andersson H, Bengtsson C, Bosaeus I. Dietary habits in relation to incidence of cardiovascular disease and death in women: A 12-year follow-up of participants in the population study of women in Gothenburg, Sweden. *Am J Clin Nutr.* 1986;44(4):444–448.

Lee CN, Reed DM, MacLean CJ, et al. Dietary potassium and stroke. *N Engl J Med.* 1988;318(15):995–996.

Leppala JM, Virtamo J, Fogelholm R, et al. Different risk factors for different stroke subtypes: Association of blood pressure, cholesterol and antioxidants. *Stroke.* 1999;30(12):2535–2540.

Lindenstrom E, Boysen G, Nyboe J. Influence of total cholesterol, high density lipoprotein cholesterol, and triglycerides on risk of cerebrovascular disease: The Copenhagen city heart study. *Br Med J.* 1994;309:11–15.

Lindgren A, Nilsson-Ehle P, Norrving B, Johansson BB. Plasma lipids and lipoproteins in subtypes of stroke. *Acta Neurol Scand.* 1992;86(6):572–578.

Liu S, Manson JE, Stampfer MJ, et al. Whole grain consumption and risk of ischemic stroke in women: A prospective study. *JAMA.* 2000;284(12):1534–1540.

Messina M, Messina V. *The Dietitian's Guide to Vegetarian Diets: Issues and Applications.* Gaithersburg, MD: Aspen Publishers; 1996.

Mojzisova G, Kuchta M. Dietary flavonoids and risk of coronary heart disease. *Physiol Res.* 2001;50(6):529–535.

Neaton JD, Blackburn H, Jacobs D, et al. Serum cholesterol level and mortality findings for men screened in the Multiple Risk Factor Intervention trial. *Arch Intern Med.* 1992;152(7):1490–1500.

Ness AR, Powles JW. Fruit and vegetables, and cardiovascular diseases: A review. *Intl J Epidemiol.* 1997;26(1):1–13.

Noma A, Matsushita S, Komori T, et al. High and low density lipoprotein cholesterol in myocardial and cerebral infarction. *Atherosclerosis.* 1979;32(3):327–331.

Okada H, Horibe H, Ohno Y, et al. A prospective study of cerebrovascular disease in Japanese rural communities, Akabane and Asahi. Part 1: Evaluation of risk factors in the occurrence of cerebral hemorrhage and thrombosis. *Stroke.* 1976;7(6):599–607.

Perry IJ. Homocysteine, hypertension and stroke. *J Hum Hypertension.* 1999;13(15):289–293.

Phillips RL, Kuzma JW, Beeson WL, Lotz T. Influence of selection versus lifestyle on risk of fatal cancer and cardiovascular disease among Seventh-Day Adventists. *Am J Epidemiol.* 1980;112(2):296–314.

Prospective Studies Collaboration. Cholesterol, diastolic blood pressure, and stroke: 13,000 strokes in 450,000 people in 45 prospective cohorts. *Lancet.* 1995;346(Dec. 23/30):1647–1653.

Qizilbash N, Duffy S, Warlow C, Mann J. Lipids are risk factors for ischaemic stroke: Overview and review. *Cerebrovascular Dis.* 1992;2:127–136.

Qizilbash N, Lewington S, Duffy S, et al. Cholesterol, diastolic blood pressure, and stroke: 13,000 strokes in 450,000 people in 45 prospective cohorts. *Lancet.* 1995;346:1647–1653.

Rajaram S. The effect of vegetarian diet, plant foods, and phytochemicals on hemostasis and thrombosis. *Am J Clin Nutr.* 2003;78(3, Suppl):552S–558S.

Robinson RW, Higano N, Cohen W. Comparison of serum lipid levels in patients with cerebral thrombosis and in normal subjects. *Ann Intern Med.* 1963;59(2):180–185.

Rosenson RS, Tangney CL. Antiatherothrombotic properties of statins: Implications for cardiovascular event reduction. *JAMA.* 1998;279(20):1643–1650.

Rossner S, Kjellin KG, Mettinger KC, et al. Normal serum-cholesterol but low H.D.L.-cholesterol concentration in young patients with ischaemic cerebrovascular disease. *Lancet.* 1978;1(8064):577–579.

Salonen JT, Puska P. Relation of serum cholesterol and triglycerides to the risk of acute myocardial infarction, cerebral stroke and death in Eastern Finnish male population. *Intl J Epidemiol.* 1983;12(1):26–31.

Salonen JT, Puska P, Tuomilehto J, Homan K. Relation of blood pressure, serum lipids, and smoking to the risk of cerebral stroke. A longitudinal study in Eastern Finland. *Stroke.* 1982;13(3):327–333.

Sauvaget C, Nagano J, Allen N, Kodama K. Vegetable and fruit intake and stroke mortality in the Hiroshima/Nagasaki Life Span study. *Stroke.* 2003;34(10):2355–2360.

Selhub J, Jacques PF, Bostom AG, et al. Association between plasma homocysteine concentrations and extracranial carotid-artery stenosis. *N Engl J Med.* 1995;332(5):286–291.

Shimamoto T, Iso H, Iida M, Komachi Y. Epidemiology of cerebrovascular disease: Stroke epidemic in Japan. *J Epidemiol.* 1996;6(3, Suppl):S43–S47.

Simons LA, McCallum J, Friedlander Y, Simons J. Risk factors for ischemic stroke: Dubbo Study of the elderly. *Stroke.* 1998;29(7):1341–1346.

Snowdon DA. Animal product consumption and mortality because of all causes combined, coronary heart disease, stroke, diabetes, and cancer in Seventh-Day Adventists. *Am J Clin Nutr.* 1988;48(3, Suppl):739–748.

Sridharan R. Risk factors for ischemic stroke: A case control analysis. *Neuroepidemiology.* 1992;11(1):24–30.

Steffen LM, Jacobs DR,. Stevens J, et al. Associations of whole-grain, refined-grain, and fruit and vegetable consumption with risks of all-cause mortality and incident coronary artery disease and ischemic stroke: The Atherosclerosis Risk in Communities (ARIC) study. *Am J Clin Nutr.* 2003;78(3):383–390.

Suh I, Jee SH, Kim HC, et al. Low serum cholesterol and haemorrhagic stroke in men: Korea Medical Insurance Corporation Study. *Lancet.* 2001;357(9260):922–925.

Szatrowski TP, Peterson AV, Shimizu Y, et al. Serum cholesterol, other risk factors, and cardiovascular disease in a Japanese cohort. *J Chronic Dis.* 1984;37(7):569–584.

Tanaka H, Ueda Y, Hayashi M, et al. Risk factors for cerebral hemorrhage and cerebral infarction in a Japanese rural community. *Stroke.* 1982;13(1):62–73.

Tanne D, Yaari S, Goldbourt U. High-density lipoprotein cholesterol and risk of ischemic stroke mortality. *Stroke.* 1997;28(1):83–87.

Tell GS, Crouse JR, Furberg CD. Relation between blood lipids, lipoproteins, and cerebrovascular atherosclerosis: A review. *Stroke.* 1988;19(4):423–430.

Tilvis RS, Erkinjuntti T, Sulkava R, et al. Serum lipids and fatty acids in ischemic strokes. *Am Heart J.* 1987;113(2, Pt 2):615–619.

Ueshima H, Iida M, Shimamoto T, et al. Multivariate analysis of risk factors for stroke. *Preven Med.* 1980;9(6):722–740.

Vaughan CJ, Delanty N. Neuroprotective properties of statins in cerebral ischemia and stroke. *Stroke.* 1999;30(9):1969–1973.

Voko Z, Hollander M, Hofman A, et al. Dietary antioxidants and the risk of ischemic stroke: The

Rotterdam study. *Neurology.* 2003;61(9):1273–1275.

Vollset SE, Bjelke E. Does consumption of fruit and vegetables protect against stroke? *Lancet.* 1983; 2(8352):742.

Welin L, Svardsudd K, Wilhelmsen L, et al. Analysis of risk factors for stroke in a cohort of men born in 1913. *N Engl J Med.* 1987;317(9):521–526.

Westlund K, Nicolaysen R. Ten-year mortality and morbidity related to serum cholesterol. A follow-up of 3,741 men aged 40–49. *Scand J Clin Lab Investig.* 1972;30(127, Suppl):1–24.

Wilmink HW, Stroes ES, Erkelens WD, et al. Influence of folic acid on postprandial endothelial dysfunction. *Arterioscler Thromb Vasc Biol.* 2000; 20(1):185–188.

Yano K, Reed DM, and MacLean CJ. Serum cholesterol and hemorrhagic stroke in the Honolulu Heart Program. *Stroke.* 1989;20(11):1460–1465.

Yochum LA, Folsom AR, Kushi LH. Intake of anti-oxidant vitamins and risk of death from stroke in postmenopausal women. *Am J Clin Nutr.* 2000; 72(2):476–483.

Yoo JH, Chung CS, Kang SS. Relation of plasma homocyst(e)ine to cerebral infarction and cerebral atherosclerosis. *Stroke.* 1998;29(12):2478–2483.

14

Obesity and a Vegetarian Diet

Sudha Raj, PhD, RD

Introduction

Vegetarians, in general, weigh less than their omnivore counterparts. This chapter reviews dietary and lifestyle factors that may contribute to the leanness of vegetarians. These dietary factors include total calories, carbohydrate, fat, protein, and fiber; lifestyle factors include physical activity. We also look at the potential of vegetarian diets to serve as weight-loss tools.

Summary of the Scientific Evidence

General Introduction on Obesity

The incidence and prevalence of obesity have been on the rise over the past three decades, and presently are at epidemic proportions. A common measure of the degree of obesity is body mass index (BMI), a number obtained by dividing weight in kilograms by the square of the height in meters. Preobesity (BMI of greater than 25-29.9) and obesity (BMI greater than 30) are prevalent. Worldwide statistics estimate that 400 million people suffer from obesity

and its consequences (World Health Organization, 2006). Results from the 1999–2002 National Health and Nutrition Examination Survey (NHANES) estimated that 65% of the adults in the United States are overweight or obese. An estimated 16% of children and adolescents are overweight (Centers for Disease Control and Prevention, 2007). Children in the 95th percentile for weight are likely to become overweight adults (Guo & Chumlea, 1999).

Regardless of age, excess body weight increases morbidity and mortality from chronic degenerative conditions such as diabetes, stroke, coronary heart disease, arthritis, gallbladder disease, respiratory problems, and cancer. Obese individuals are also vulnerable to a myriad of social, mental, and psychological problems, such as discrimination and low self-esteem.

Obesity is characterized as a multifactorial degenerative disease. Excess weight gain results from an interaction of genetic, metabolic, lifestyle/environmental, cultural, and psychological influences (Beamer, 2000; Kral et al., 2001; Speakman, 2004). The discovery of more than 70 gene loci that regulate body weight at the levels of metabolism and appetite signals suggests that the cause of obesity has a genetic component (Beamer, 2000). Unraveling the genetic basis of obesity could also help us understand ethnic differences in obesity.

Research suggests that the circulating hormone leptin may regulate body weight by monitoring energy reserves available to the body and reducing energy intake when body fat increases. Plasma concentrations of leptin parallel the amount of adipose tissue (fat cells) in the body and provide an inhibitory feedback circuit to the hypothalamus, a region of the brain that is important in appetite regulation. This suggests that leptin may play a role in regulating body weight by decreasing appetite (Margetic et al., 2002). Because obese individuals have higher circulating levels of leptin, it is speculated that one cause of obesity may be a functional resistance or decreased sensitivity to leptin (Cummings, Parham, & Strain, 2002).

A changing lifestyle has contributed to the obesity epidemic. Lives have become more sedentary for many reasons, including computer technology, television viewing, and labor-saving tools and devices. Diets have also changed, in part due to the immediate availability of low-cost, highly palatable convenience foods of high caloric density and increased portion sizes (Hill & Peters, 1998; Jennifer & Rosetta, 2004). Advertising and marketing strategies have successfully promoted sales of these products. Longer working hours with less time for meal planning and preparation have fostered increased reliance on these products.

Altered mood states such as depression, as well as many of the antidepressive medications themselves, can contribute to the obesity problem (Stunkard et al., 1990; Carpenter et al., 2000). Studies show that patients with depression may overeat or crave foods rich in carbohydrates in an effort to reduce depressive symptoms. Foods rich in carbohydrates but low in proteins can increase plasma levels of

tryptophan, an amino acid that is converted to serotonin, a chemical messenger that is involved in regulating mood and providing a calming effect (Cummings, Parham, & Strain, 2002). In addition, those trying to give up unhealthy behaviors, such as smoking, may overeat to compensate or as a substitute for the habit they are trying to quit.

Notwithstanding its multifaceted etiology, the expert consensus is that obesity results when caloric consumption exceeds caloric expenditure; in short, when people eat too much and exercise too little. These circumstances promote energy storage as lipid in the adipose tissue. Treatment of obesity has focused on addressing both behavioral and environmental factors, such as decreasing caloric intake, increasing physical activity, and making permanent healthy lifestyle changes. Successful treatment of obesity involves weight loss and long-term weight maintenance as well as treatment of associated diseases such as diabetes, hypertension, and cardiovascular disease.

Americans presently spend billions of dollars annually on products and services that promise fast and easy weight loss (Kruger et al., 2004). Overweight individuals, who often lose weight but then gain it back again, may find themselves caught in a vicious cycle of using these products and services. Commercial weight-loss programs can also be expensive, a fact that limits their usefulness and support of long-term weight maintenance (Cummings, Parham, & Strain, 2002).

Success stories from those who have maintained their weight loss note that persistent attempts are necessary for long-term success (Fletcher, 2003). Failure to maintain long-term weight loss is often due to such things as lack of motivation and consistency in following the weight-loss plan, and an inability to view diet as part of a comprehensive plan that includes physical activity and stress management. Programs

with a three-pronged approach, aimed at addressing diet, behavior, and physical activity simultaneously, are credited with providing better
benefits and results than programs that deal
with any one of these facets in isolation. Helping individuals achieve a healthier weight is
best done by encouraging and assisting them
to adopt healthier lifestyles, including making
healthier food choices, adjusting caloric intake,
and getting exercise.

Vegetarians and Obesity

Vegetarian diets have been suggested as a possible dietary strategy to treat or prevent obesity.
Vegetarians are leaner than their omnivore
counterparts. Studies comparing Seventh-
Day Adventist vegetarians and nonvegetarians,
both in the United States and abroad, note
the prevalence of lower body mass indexes
among vegetarians regardless of age or gender
(Fraser, 1999; Appleby et al., 1999; Brathwaite
et al., 2003). Studies comparing omnivores
and vegetarians indicate that lacto-ovo vegetarians and vegans who had followed such
diets for more than five years had lower body
weights than omnivores (Brathwaite et al.,
2003). Several Slovakian investigations found
an absence of obesity in vegetarian study subjects (Krajcovivova-Kudlackova et al., 1994;
Krajcovivova-Kudlackova, Simoncic, Cerna
et al., 1993; Krajcovivova-Kudlackova, Simoncic, Babinska, & Bederova, 1993). Another evaluation of vegetarians indicated that body mass
index was 36% lower in men and 31% lower in
women than in their meat-eating counterparts
(Appleby et al., 1998).

There is some evidence that the higher consumption of plant foods, such as vegetables,
may prevent the development of abdominal
obesity. A 10-year longitudinal study of 79,000
individuals showed that those who consumed

19 or more servings of vegetables per week
had less central girth than omnivores who ate
meat more than 7 times per week (Kahn et al.,
1997).

The lower BMI of vegetarians cannot, however, be attributed solely to their diets. Vegetarians may be more health-conscious in general,
and are also known to adopt other healthy lifestyle habits, such as regular exercise, that potentially affect their tendency toward leanness.
Research has not been able to separate out the
effects of these various lifestyle practices.

Reports indicate that the BMI of vegetarian
children is within normal standards for height
and weight (Hebbelinck & Clarys, 2001). This
is an advantage in view of the current childhood obesity epidemic. Vegetarian children also
have higher intakes of fruits, vegetables, and
fiber (Perry et al., 2002). With guidance in meal
planning, healthy vegetarian diets for children
and adolescents can form the basis for lifelong
healthy eating patterns.

Several diet-related factors can help explain
the lower body mass index of vegetarians compared to omnivores. These include an overall
reduction in energy consumption; higher intake of fiber and complex carbohydrates; differences in amino acid patterns of plant proteins;
and differences in the type and quantity of dietary fat.

Calorie Intake

A vegetarian diet may prevent obesity by virtue of its lower caloric density. Nonnutritive
fiber in plant foods such as fruits and vegetables contributes bulk, thereby reducing the
number of calories per unit volume of food.
Therefore, a vegetarian diet may be greater in
volume, but still lower in calories. A study of
vegetarian and nonvegetarian diets among free-
living individuals found that vegetarians had a
significantly lower caloric intake, a lower total

dietary fat and saturated fat intake, and a higher carbohydrate intake compared to their omnivore counterparts (Kennedy et al., 2001). The lower caloric density of a vegetarian diet can also be beneficial with regard to chronic disease risk and longevity (Blackburn, 2003). One should, however, always take care that children and adolescents get the calories they need for growth (Donovan & Gibson, 1996).

Higher Fiber Intake

The higher fiber content of a vegetarian diet may be beneficial in achieving and/or maintaining weight loss. The fiber intake of the average nonvegetarian is about 15 grams per day, for ovo-lacto vegetarians is about 20–35 grams per day, and for vegans is between 25–50 grams per day (Fiber and Health, 2000).

High-fiber diets can facilitate calorie control by reducing hunger at subsequent meals (Levine et al., 1989). Inclusion of small quantities of fruits or soluble fiber, such as pectin, along with other foods has been shown to be an effective appetite suppressant (Tiwary, Ward, & Jackson, 1997). Fiber, being resistant to digestion, adds bulk and provides a feeling of fullness and satiety.

Nuts are advantageous, not only because they are good sources of dietary fiber, but also because they are excellent sources of desirable fats and protein. Dietary intervention studies using different types of nuts in moderate to large amounts report positive effects of nut consumption on body weight (Sabaté, 2003). Although nuts are energy-dense, the caloric contribution from nuts is limited by the presence of lipase inhibitors that interfere with fat absorption. This effect is small, but it can make a difference over time. Nuts also provide sensory and satiety appeal, thereby facilitating compliance with dietary schemes, particularly in weight-loss regimens.

Higher Carbohydrate Intake

Vegetarian (particularly vegan) diets contain significant quantities of complex carbohydrates, such as whole grains, nuts, legumes, fruits, and vegetables. Such diets are advantageous to those trying to lose weight and keep it off. Foods rich in complex carbohydrates contribute to satiety. There is some evidence that fiber in whole foods slows the digestion and absorption of carbohydrates, which is beneficial in reducing blood glucose spikes and the resultant increases in insulin secretion. The latter can help with weight control because insulin is lipogenic, meaning that it promotes fat storage (McCarty, 1986). Carbohydrate ingestion can also enhance the synthesis and release of serotonin, which can act as an appetite suppressant (Leibowitz & Alexander, 1998). The inefficiency of metabolic conversion of carbohydrates to fat, as well as the ability of carbohydrates to boost metabolism by activating thyroid hormone, are additional benefits (Messina & Messina, 1996, pp. 238-241). In a study by Toth and Poehlman (1994), young male vegetarians had an 11% higher resting metabolic rate than nonvegetarians, in spite of similar energy intake. The major dietary differences between the two groups were higher ingestion of carbohydrates and less fat intake by the vegetarians. When the researchers used statistical methods to control for these differences, the metabolic advantage disappeared, indicating that the composition of the diet was responsible for the observed increase in resting metabolic rate.

Lower Protein Intakes and Specific Amino Acid Profiles

Vegetarian diets that contain a variety of plant foods meet all protein requirements. Also, vegetarian diets may, because of their specific amino acid patterns, offer an advantage in weight management over diets containing meat products. Amino acids, the building blocks of dietary protein, can influence the secretion of insulin (a lipogenic hormone) and glucagon (an anti-lipogenic hormone). Plant proteins, including soy proteins, contain a higher fraction of non-essential amino acids that can down-regulate insulin and up-regulate glucagon responses, both after meals and in fasting states (McCarty, 2000).

Another mechanism by which plant proteins may affect weight control is through fatty acid oxidation. It is known that hepatic fatty acid oxidation promotes appetite control. Plant proteins may promote fatty acid oxidation and in this way control appetite. The higher glucagon response in vegan diets may also down-regulate insulin-like growth factor (IGF-1), thereby inhibiting fat storage and therefore protecting against obesity (McCarty, 2001).

Type of Fat

In general, a high-fat diet appears to promote obesity (Alfieri, Pomerleau, & Grace, 1997). There also appears to be a tendency for obese adults and children to ingest more fat, often as a result of their inability to initiate satiety signals (Prentice, 1998). Because fats contain twice as many calories as carbohydrates and proteins, a common strategy for weight loss is to lower fat intake so as to reduce calorie intake. This translates into limiting fats and fatty foods. However, diets that severely limit all fats are not beneficial and may even be harmful. Severe fat restriction can result in elimination of healthful fats such as polyunsaturated and monounsaturated fats, which have been shown to have cardioprotective effects (Coulston, 1999). The low satiety of low-fat diets may also decrease long-term compliance. Nuts, seeds, and plant oils are good sources of monounsaturated

and polyunsaturated fats such as oleic and linolenic acids. Unsaturated fats are prone to oxidation and therefore, by being metabolized, are less likely than saturated fats to contribute to the obesity picture (Delaney et al., 2000). Unsaturated fats also often coexist in plant foods with other beneficial substances, such as phytochemicals and antioxidants. Including higher-fat plant foods that are palatable, such as nuts, nut butters, and olive oil, while keeping calorie intake moderate, may be part of an effective strategy for long-term weight control (Sabaté, 2003).

Vegetarian diets, because they are usually lower in fat than omnivorous diets, are sometimes chosen by those attempting to lose weight. However, a vegetarian diet does not always equate with a low-fat diet. Certain vegetarian regimens, such as lacto- and ovo-lacto-vegetarian patterns, do include animal products (such as whole milk, eggs, and butter) that are major sources of saturated fat in the American diet. Also, immigrant populations, who are exposed to a new food supply and often confronted with the unavailability of traditional foods and ingredients, may make inappropriate dietary changes and consume high-fat vegetarian foods in place of traditional food items (Satia-Abouta et al., 2002).

Other Issues

The reasons for the imbalance of calories consumed versus calories expended that causes obesity are complicated. Experts have argued that long-term food choices are influenced by the easy accessibility of highly palatable, low-cost, energy-dense foods. However, the relationship between diet quality and cost warrants further study. Research is also needed to identify specific genes and variants in the DNA sequences related to obesity, the relationship between genetic and environmental factors in obesity, and the habit-forming characteristics of foods and ingredients in the development of food preferences (Jennifer & Rosetta, 2004).

There are also unresolved issues regarding the efficiency and effectiveness of manipulating the content of carbohydrate, fat, and protein in the diet to achieve weight loss. Although there is some evidence that certain dietary combinations, such as a high-protein, low-carbohydrate diet, can produce greater short-term weight losses than a low-fat diet (Buchholz & Schoeller, 2004), this conclusion requires further elucidation. Also, as mentioned earlier, plant protein, as opposed to animal protein, may confer benefits regarding body weight (McCarty, 2000). Further study in this area is needed.

In general, the reasons for the lower body weights experienced by vegetarians remain unclear. Possible explanations include the higher intakes of fiber and complex carbohydrates, the lower intakes of total calories and saturated fat, and the beneficial role of plant proteins. Also, the possibility of a generally healthier lifestyle among vegetarians may be significant. For example, many vegetarians engage in regular physical activity that can greatly affect weight loss and weight maintenance (Brathwaite et al., 2003). It is likely that many of these factors have an additive effect in contributing to the leanness of vegetarians.

Dieting with a Vegetarian Diet

A well-planned vegetarian diet, rich in a variety of whole grains, fruits, vegetables, and legumes, is undoubtedly a good starting point in planning a healthy weight-loss or weight-maintenance diet. Several studies point to the effectiveness of a vegetarian diet in maintaining leanness (Fletcher, 2003; Fraser, 1999; Ap-

pleby et al., 1999; Brathwaite et al., 2003); others have observed changes in body composition, such as reduction in skin-fold thickness, upon changing from a nonvegetarian to a vegetarian diet. A fairly recent noncontrolled study evaluating the efficiency of a nonprescribed, self-selected vegetarian diet that included fish showed significant reductions in the weight-to-height ratio and skin-fold thickness, although no significant changes were observed in body weights (Phillips et al., 2004). Also, one study comparing young adults' experiences with vegetarian and weight-loss diets reported a higher degree of compliance with the vegetarian diets than with weight-loss diets, although the reasons for this were unclear (Smith, Burke, & Wing, 2000).

Weight-loss regimens do not, however, consistently give an edge to a vegetarian approach. Although one investigation showed that patients placed on a vegetarian diet lost an average of 7 pounds, while their omnivore controls lost only 3.5 pounds (Brestrich, Vlaus, & Blumchen, 1996), another study found that the 12-month weight loss among women randomly assigned to either a lacto-vegetarian or a regular mixed 1,300-calorie weight-loss diet was slightly more for the regular diet group than for the lacto vegetarian group (23 pounds vs. 20 pounds) (Hakala & Karvetti, 1989).

Even in vegetarian diets, inappropriate food selection (e.g., high-calorie snacks, vegetables in butter-drenched sauces, etc.) and method of food preparation (frying rather than steaming) can add extra calories and, therefore, extra pounds. Regardless of macronutrient manipulations, any diet will be of limited success if it does not lower the calorie intake. Any weight-loss diet, even a vegetarian diet, can be unhealthy if there are poor food choices. Those consuming very restrictive vegetarian diets should be especially careful to include good sources of vitamin B12, zinc, and calcium (Mangels, Messina, & Melina, 2003).

Practical Aspects

Dietary Changes

Here are some practical suggestions for planning a vegetarian diet as a healthy basis for weight loss efforts.

1. Emphasize consumption of vegetables, fruits, and whole grains such as barley, rye, and oats. In addition to providing higher fiber intakes and a favorable blood glucose response, these foods supply bulk that can improve overall satiety. Be wary of processed grain products that are made with lots of saturated or trans fats (e.g., muffins, biscuits, etc.).
2. Adopt a plant-based diet with a full complement of whole grains, nuts, legumes, fruits, and vegetables (including vegetable oils), to ensure that the diet contains phytochemicals, antioxidants, vitamins, minerals, and fiber, all of which help fight disease and contribute to good health.
3. Find plant-based protein foods, such as beans, legumes, and nuts, that offer alternatives to animal-based protein sources high in saturated fats. Plant proteins may be more effective than animal proteins in keeping hunger at bay. However, certain plant foods that are rich in saturated fat, such as coconut oil and palm kernel oil, should be used in moderation. Even commercial vegetarian foods can contain high amounts of fat, so try to find and select low-fat alternatives.
4. Aim for optimal fat intake by making healthy choices such as non-fat or reduced-fat dairy products or nondairy alternatives. Avoid trans fatty acids. Include mono-unsaturated and polyunsaturated fats, found in olives, nuts, and seeds, and essential fatty acid sources such as walnuts and flax-seeds. Use healthful cooking oils for sautéing vegetables or other foods for flavor and taste. Experiment with the use of vegetable juices as a sautéing medium and fresh herbs to improve flavor and sensory appeal; both strategies can add variety to meals.
5. Frequent small meals rather than three large meals a day can minimize hunger pangs. Practice portion control and be conscious of becoming super-sized!

Lifestyle Changes

A lifestyle change that complements the benefits accrued with dietary changes is regular physical activity. Physical activity can promote weight loss and pave the way for successful, long-term weight management. Physical activity can also have other benefits, such as improved lipid profiles, improved blood glucose control in diabetics, endorphin-mediated positive mood responses, lowered levels of anxiety and stress, stronger bones, improved cognition and mental function, a reduced risk of chronic degenerative diseases, and an increased immune capacity (Brooks et al., 2004). There is growing evidence that sedentary, inactive lifestyles lead to atrophy and dysfunction of cells and metabolic systems (Landers & Petruzzello, 1994).

The minimal amount of accumulated physical activity generally recommended to prevent chronic diseases is 30 minutes per day; current recommendations indicate an equivalent of 60 minutes of physical activity per day to prevent undesirable fat accretion and maintain a BMI in the normal range (from 18.5 to less than 25) (Saris et al., 2003). In the long run, increasing exercise can be a more healthful way of losing weight than consuming an excessively restrictive weight-loss diet that may not be nutritionally sound.

Conclusion

Vegetarians are less likely to suffer from obesity and tend to be slimmer than nonvegetarians. Well-planned vegetarian diets can be used as nutrient-dense weight-loss diets. The overweight individual will likely need to make several lifestyle changes to complement dietary changes.

Research has shown that well-planned vegetarian diets can provide significant health benefits, such as a favorable body weight and lower chronic disease risk. These benefits may accrue because the plant-food choices that form the basis of the vegetarian diet are generally low in saturated fat and cholesterol and rich in complex carbohydrates, dietary fiber, healthful fats, antioxidants, and phytochemicals.

The efficacy of a vegetarian diet as a weight-loss tool remains to be determined. Preliminary results are promising; however, long-term weight loss requires lifestyle changes such as balancing caloric intake and expenditure, evaluating emotional reasons for overeating, and getting enough physical exercise. A vegetarian diet well balanced in calories is an excellent place to start.

References

Alfieri M, Pomerleau J, Grace DM. A comparison of fat intake of normal weight, moderately obese and severely obese subjects. *Obes Surg.* Feb 1997;7(1):9-15.

Appleby PN, Thorogood M, Mann JI, Key TJ. The Oxford Vegetarian Study. An overview. *Am J Clin Nutr.* 1999;70:525S-531S.

Appleby PN, Thorogood M, Mann JL, Key TJ. Low body mass index in non meat eaters: The possible roles of animal fat, dietary fiber and alcohol. *Intl J Obes Related Metab Disord.* May 1998; 22(5):454-460.

Beamer BA. Genetic influences on obesity. In: Anderson RE, ed. *Obesity: Etiology, Assessment, Treatment and Prevention.* Champaign, IL: Human Kinetics; 2000:43-46.

Blackburn JL. "Vegging out" for better health? Vegetarians may have healthier, longer lives than their carnivorous counterparts. *Health News.* Nov 2003;9(11):8-9.

Brathwaite N, Fraser HS, Modeste N, Broome H, King R. Are vegetarians at less risk for obesity, diabetes, and hypertension? Obesity, diabetes, hypertension, and vegetarian status among Seventh-Day Adventists in Barbados: Preliminary results. *Ethnic Dis.* Winter 2003;13(1):148.

Brestrich M, Vlaus J, Blumchen G. Lactovegetarian diet: Effect on changes in body weight, lipid status, fibrinogen and lipoprotein (a) in cardiovascular patients during inpatient rehabilitation treatment. *Z Kardiol.* Jun 1996;85(6):418-427.

Brooks GA, Butte N, Rand W, et al. Chronicle of the Institute of Medicine physical activity recommendation: How a physical activity recommendation came to be among dietary recommendations. *Am J Clin Nutr.* 2004;70(Suppl):921S-930S.

Buchholz A, Schoeller DA. Is a calorie a calorie? *Am J Clin Nutr.* 2004;79(Suppl):899S-906S.

Carpenter KM, Hasin DS, Allison BB, Faith MS. Relationships between obesity and DSM-IV major depressive disorder, suicide ideation, and suicide attempts: Results from a general population study. *Am J Public Health.* 2000;90:251-257.

Centers for Disease Control and Prevention (CDC). Overweight and obesity. May 2007. Available at http://www.cdc.gov/nccdphp/dnpa/obesity/index.htm. Accessed July 5, 2007.

Coulston AM. The role of dietary fats in plant-based diets. *Am J Clin Nutr.* 1999;70(3, Suppl):512S-515S.

Cummings S, Parham E, Strain G. Position of the American Dietetic Association: Weight management. *J Am Diet Assoc.* 2002;102(8):1145-1155.

Delaney JP, Windhauser MM, Champagne CM, Bray GA. Differential oxidation of individual dietary fatty acids in humans. *Am J Clin Nutr.* Oct 2000;72(4):905-911.

Donovan UM, Gibson R. Dietary intakes of adolescent females consuming vegetarian, semi-vegetarian and omnivorous diets. *J Adolesc Health.* 1996;18: 292-300.

Fiber and Health. *Veg Nutr Health Lett.* Oct 2000; 1(9):1-8.

Fletcher A. Learning from losers: Lessons from people who have maintained weight loss. *Weight Mgmt Newsl.* 2003;1(2):1-3.

Fraser GE. Associations between diet and cancer, ischemic heart disease, and all-cause mortality in non-Hispanic white California Seventh-day Adventists. *Am J Clin Nutr.* 1999;70(Suppl):532S-538S.

Guo SS, Chumlea WC. Tracking the body mass index in children in relation to overweight in adulthood. *Am J Clin Nutr.* 1999;70:145S-148S.

Hakala P, Karvetti RL. Weight reduction on lacto-vegetarian and mixed diets: Changes in weight, nutrient intake, skinfold thickness and blood pressure. *Eur J Clin Nutr.* Jun 1989;43(6):421-430.

Hebbelinck M, Clarys P. Physical growth and development of vegetarian children and adolescents. In Sabaté J, ed. *Vegetarian Nutrition.* Boca Raton, FL: CRC Press; 2001:173-193.

Hill JO, Peters JC. Environmental contributions to the obesity epidemic. *Science.* 1998;280:1371-1374.

Jennifer M, Rosetta N. Solving the obesity conundrum. *Food Technol.* 2004;58(6):32-37.

Kahn HS, Tatham LM, Rodriguez C, et al. Stable behaviors associated with adults' ten year change in body mass index and likelihood of gain at the waist. *Am J Public Health.* May 1997;87(5): 747-754.

Kennedy ET, Bowman SA, Spence JT, et al. Popular diets: Correlation to health, nutrition and obesity. *J Am Diet Assoc.* 2001;101(4):411-420.

Krajcovivova-Kudlackova M, Simoncic R, Babinska K, Bederova A. Lipid parameters in blood of vegetarians. *Cor Vasa.* 1993;35(6):224-229.

Krajcovivova-Kudlackova M, Simoncic R, Bederova A, et al. Selected parameters of lipid metabolism in young vegetarians. *Ann Nutr Metab.* 1994; 38(6):331-335.

Krajcovivova-Kudlackova M, Simoncic R, Cerna O, et al. Biochemical and hematologic indicators in the blood of young vegetarians. *Bratisl Lek Listy.* Dec 1993;94(12):621-625.

Kral JG, Buckley MC, Kissileff HR, Schaffner F. Metabolic correlates of eating behavior in severe obesity. *Intl J Obes Related Metab Disord.* Feb 2001;25(2):258-264.

Kruger J, Galuska DA, Serdula MK, Jones DA. Attempting to lose weight: Specific practices among U.S. adults. *Am J Preven Med.* Jun 2004;26(5): 402-406.

Landers DM, Petruzzello SJ. Physical activity, fitness and anxiety. In: Bouchard C, Shephard RJ, Stevens T, eds. *Physical Activity, Fitness and Health.* Champaign, IL: Human Kinetics; 1994:868-882.

Leibowitz SF, Alexander JT. Hypothalmic serotonin in control of eating behavior, meal size, and body weight. *Biol Psychiatr.* Nov 1998;44(9):851-864.

Levine AS, Tallman JR, Grace MK, et al. Effect of breakfast cereals on short-term food intake. *Am J Clin Nutr.* Dec 1989;50(6):1303-1307.

Mangels AR, Messina V, Melina V. Position of the American Dietetic Association and Dietitians of Canada: Vegetarian diets. *J Am Diet Assoc.* 2003; 103(6):748-765.

Margetic S, Gazzola G, Pegg GG, Hill RA. Leptin: A review of its peripheral actions and interactions. *Intl J Obes Res.* 2002;26:1407-1433.

McCarty MF. Modulation of adipocyte lipoprotein lipase expression as a strategy for preventing or treating visceral obesity. *Med Hypotheses.* Aug 2001;57:192-200.

McCarty MF. The origins of western obesity: A role for animal protein? *Med Hypotheses.* Mar 2000; 54(3):488-494.

McCarty MF. The unique merits of a low fat diet for weight control. *Med Hypotheses.* Jun 1986;20(2): 183-197.

Messina V, Messina M. *The Vegetarian Way.* New York: Three Rivers Press; 1996.

Perry CL, McGuire MT, Neumark-Sztainer D, Story M. Adolescent vegetarians. How well do their dietary patterns meet the Healthy People 2010 objectives? *Arch Pediatr Adolesc Med.* 2002;156:431-437.

Phillips F, Hackett AF, Stratton G, Billington D. Effect of changing to a self-selected vegetarian diet on anthropometric measurements in U.K. adults. *J Hum Nutr Diet.* 2004;17:249-255.

Prentice AM. Manipulation of dietary fat and energy density and subsequent effects on substrate flux and food intake. *Am J Clin Nutr.* Mar 1998;67(3, Suppl):535S–541S.

Sabaté J. Nut consumption and body weight. *Am J Clin Nutr.* 2003;78(Suppl):647S–650S.

Saris WH, Blair SN, vanBank MA, et al. Outcome of the IASO First Stock Conference and consensus statement. *Obes Rev.* 2003;4:101–114.

Satia-Abouta J, Patterson R, Neuhouser M, Elder J. Dietary acculturation: Applications to nutrition research and dietetics. *J Am Diet Assoc.* 2002; 102(8):1105–1118.

Smith CF, Burke LE, Wing RR. Vegetarian and weight-loss diets among young adults. *Obes Res.* Mar 2000;8(2):123–129.

Speakman JR. Obesity: The integrated roles of environment and genetics. *J Nutr.* Aug 2004;134(8, Suppl):2090S–2105S.

Stunkard AJ, Fernstrom MH, Frank E, Kupfer DJ. Direction of weight change in recurrent depression: Consistency across episodes. *Arch Gen Psychiatr.* 1990;47:857–860.

Tiwary CM, Ward JA, Jackson BA. Effect of pectin on satiety in healthy US Army adults. *J Am Coll Nutr.* Oct 1997;16(5):423–428.

Toth MJ, Poehlman ET. Sympathetic nervous system activity and resting metabolic rate in vegetarians. *Metabolism.* 1994;43(5):621–625.

World Health Organization. Obesity and overweight. Fact Sheet No. 311. September 2006. Available at http://www.iotf.org/popout.asp?linkto=http://www.who.int/nut/obs.htm. Accessed July 5, 2007.

15

Diabetes and Vegetarian Diets

Peggy Carlson, MD

Introduction

Diabetes mellitus afflicts about 18 million people in the United States and is the sixth leading cause of death in this country (Centers for Disease Control and Prevention [CDC], 2003). Furthermore, the incidence of diabetes in the United States is increasing rapidly.

Diabetes results when there is not enough effective insulin in the body. Insulin, a hormone produced by the pancreas, is involved in the regulation of many metabolic processes. Without enough insulin, there are alterations in carbohydrate, lipid, and protein metabolism. One of the consequences of these changes is an elevated blood glucose (blood sugar) level.

There are two types of diabetes. Type 1 diabetes results when the pancreas does not produce enough insulin. Type 2 diabetes begins with a resistance to the action of insulin and later involves a decline in insulin production (Steyn et al., 2004). Type 1 diabetes typically has its onset in childhood or adolescence and requires daily insulin injections for treatment. Type 2 diabetes typically begins in adulthood and can often be controlled by diet and/or oral medication alone, although in some cases insulin injections may be required. Based on these differences, type 1 diabetes is referred to as *insulin-dependent diabetes mellitus* (IDDM) and type 2 diabetes is commonly called *non-insulin-dependent diabetes mellitus* (NIDDM). In the United States, about 90%–95% of diabetics have NIDDM (Edelman, 1998).

The cause of diabetes is unknown and is most likely multifactorial, with both genetic and environmental (including lifestyle and dietary) components. Obesity is the most common predisposing factor for the development of NIDDM.

Diabetics may develop any of a number of complications as a result of the disease. Cardiovascular diseases are the major causes of mortality in both IDDM and NIDDM (Edelman, 1998; Nutrition Subcommittee, 1992). When compared to the general population, both IDDM and NIDDM diabetics have an increased risk of heart disease. Diabetics show a two- to four-fold higher risk of coronary artery disease (CAD) than matched nondiabetic individuals (CDC, 2003).

Although rates of elevated total cholesterol in IDDM and NIDDM diabetics in the United

States are the same or only slightly higher than in those without diabetes, high or borderline high total cholesterol levels may be present in as many as 70% of adults with diabetes (Franz et al., 1994; Kern, 1987). Elevated LDL cholesterol levels also appear to occur with the same frequency in IDDM and NIDDM individuals as in nondiabetic individuals, meaning a frequency of about 40% (Franz et al., 1994; Kern, 1987). Both elevated total cholesterol and LDL cholesterol are risk factors for CAD.

IDDM individuals who are treated with insulin generally have plasma triglyceride levels similar to those found in the general public, and have normal or higher-than-normal HDL cholesterol levels (Franz et al., 1994; Kern, 1987). However, in NIDDM, hypertriglyceridemia and low HDL cholesterol values are seen more commonly than in nondiabetics. There is some debate as to whether hypertriglyceridemia puts one at increased risk of CAD; however, it appears that in the case of diabetics, a high blood triglyceride level may increase CAD risk (Franz et al., 1994; Snehalatha et al., 2000). The Framingham study concluded that individuals with high triglyceride levels should be considered at high risk for CAD, with the only exception being those with a very low total/HDL cholesterol ratio (Castelli, 1986).

In diabetics, the elevation in triglycerides and LDL cholesterol may be at least partially reversible with good blood sugar control (Franz et al., 1994; American Diabetes Association, 1999b). In general, glucose-lowering agents do not change or have only a modest effect on raising HDL cholesterol levels (American Diabetes Association, 1999b).

In addition to CAD, diabetics are also at increased risk of other health problems, such as high blood pressure. Approximately 73% of adults with diabetes have high blood pressure (CDC, 2003). This contributes to their increased risk for CAD. Diabetics also are at increased risk

of kidney disease, which afflicts 30%–50% of those with IDDM and more than 20% of those with NIDDM (Shils et al., 1999). Diabetics also suffer from a higher rate of peripheral vascular disease, which can lead to poor blood flow to the legs. These circulation problems can sometimes be severe enough to necessitate amputation. Vascular disease also contributes to the two to four times higher risk of stroke among diabetics (CDC, 2003). Eye problems in diabetics (*diabetic retinopathy*) are also a common complication and may lead to blindness. Diabetes may also cause nerve damage (*neuropathy*), which can lead to symptoms such as numbness in the legs.

Some diabetics may develop complications at an accelerated rate despite reasonable control of their blood sugar. However, in general, keeping blood sugar levels as close to normal as possible has been shown to reduce the risk of several of the complications of diabetes. The Diabetes Control and Complications Trial Study, a large, multicenter study conducted by the National Institutes of Health and carried out in 29 diabetes centers in the United States and Canada, showed that in IDDM, maintaining good control of blood sugar slows the onset and progression of retinopathy by 76%, of kidney disease by about 50%, and of neuropathy by 60% (Diabetes Control and Complications Trial Research Group, 1993). Likewise, there is also good evidence that improved blood sugar control in NIDDM diabetics also reduces their risk of development or progression of retinopathy, kidney disease, and neuropathy (Edelman, 1998; American Diabetes Association, 1999a).

This chapter discusses many facets of diet in relation to diabetes. It includes an investigation of dietary risk factors for diabetes; the occurrence of diabetes among vegetarians versus non-vegetarians; dietary fat, fiber, carbohydrates, and protein in diets for diabetics; current diet recommendations for diabetics; factors in a vegetarian diet that are beneficial to diabetics; and the effect of a vegetarian diet on diabetes control. In the "Practical Aspects" section, we discuss how to plan a vegetarian diet for diabetics.

Summary of the Scientific Literature

Dietary Risk Factors for Diabetes

Some information about the relative impact of lifestyle and diet on the causation of diabetes can be gleaned from population studies. There are striking variations in the prevalence of diabetes throughout the world. In some populations it is rare or almost nonexistent, whereas in others as much as 50% of the population is thought to be diabetic (Messina & Messina, 1996). Although in some cases genetic susceptibility appears to play a large role, lifestyle and diet are also contributing factors.

Evidence that environmental factors (including diet and lifestyle) play a role in the prevalence of diabetes has emerged from several studies. For example, evidence has shown that ethnically Japanese persons who live in Hawaii or Washington demonstrate a greater prevalence of diabetes than Japanese who continue to live in Japan (Kawate et al., 1979; Tsunehara, Leonetti, & Fujimoto, 1990). A similar increased risk of diabetes is seen among Yemenites who migrate to Israel (Messina & Messina, 1996). A large difference between the prevalence of glucose intolerance among Chinese in Da Qing (3%) and the Chinese in Mauritius (33%) has also been documented and is unlikely to be due principally to genetic factors (King & Rewers, 1991). A World Health Organization study concluded that the wide range in prevalence of diabetes arising in different parts of the world (0%–50%) is probably greater than that of any other chronic disease and is a strong in-

dication of the importance of environmental factors (King & Rewers, 1991). There have also been dramatic increases in the incidence of NIDDM within some populations over relatively short time periods, again suggesting that environmental factors contribute heavily to the etiology of diabetes.

Diet has been shown to be one of the environmental factors that varies in populations with changing diabetes rates (Kawate et al., 1979). As diets Westernize—that is, include greater amounts of fat and animal products and less fiber—the occurrence of diabetes increases (Lichtenstein & Schwab, 2000; Addanki, 1981). International comparisons generally show that the prevalence of diabetes increases with greater intake of total fat, saturated fat, animal fat, protein, and animal protein and decreases with greater intakes of fiber and vegetable fat (Messina & Messina, 1996; Tsunehara, Leonetti, & Fujimoto, 1990; Addanki, 1981; West & Kalbfleisch, 1971; Vessby, 1995). The prevalence of diabetes is increasing in emerging and developing countries and parallels the increase in obesity; the rates of both diabetes and obesity increase progressively as the percentage of energy from fat in the diet increases (Shils et al., 1999). A 40-country study that looked at the incidence of type 1 diabetes in children younger than 15 years old found that energy from animal sources (particularly meat and dairy products) was positively related to the risk of diabetes, and that energy from plant sources (particularly cereals) was inversely related (Muntoni et al., 2000).

A few studies have found an increased risk of diabetes among those who eat meat. In a study of 25,698 Seventh-Day Adventists followed for 21 years, meat consumption was positively associated with self-reported diabetes prevalence in both males and females. In that same study, meat consumption was positively associated with mention of diabetes on death certificates for males, but not for females (Snowdon & Phillips, 1985). Also, populations with higher cholesterol intake and higher serum cholesterol levels have shown higher incidences of diabetes (Tsunehara, Leonetti, & Fujimoto, 1990; West & Kalbfleisch, 1971). (Cholesterol is found only in animal products.) A more recent study found that heme iron intake from red meat was associated with an increased risk of type 2 diabetes, but the study was unable to determine whether the association was due to heme iron per se or to other components of red meat (Jiang et al., 2004).

A few studies have found that processed meats increase the risk of diabetes. In a study of 339 children with IDDM and 528 control children, Dahlquist found an increased risk of IDDM among those consuming greater amounts of nitrosamines (chemicals found in cured meats) (Dahlquist et al., 1990). The Health Professional's Follow-up Study, which followed 42,504 men for 12 years, found that frequent consumption of processed meat was associated with higher risk of type 2 diabetes (van Dam et al., 2002). Consumption of processed meat, but not other meats, was positively associated with risk of type 2 diabetes in the Nurses' Health Study of 84,360 women followed for 6 years (Colditz et al., 1992). In the Women's Health Study, where 37,309 women aged 45 years or older were followed for 8.8 years, meat consumption was found to increase the incidence of type 2 diabetes. In that study, the risk was greatest for those who frequently consumed processed meats. The researchers also found a direct relationship between diabetes and intakes of both heme iron and cholesterol (Song et al., 2004).

Prospective studies generally have not supported a positive association between total fat consumption and prevalence of diabetes, although different types of fats may be related to an increased risk of diabetes. A 14-year follow-up of the Nurse's Health Study found that total fat, saturated fat, and monounsaturated fat were not associated with risk, but that there was a decreased risk with increased intake of polyunsaturated fat (Salmeron et al., 2001). The Health Professionals Follow-up Study found that animal fat, total fat, saturated fat, monounsaturated fat, long-chain n-3 fats, and alpha-linolenic acid (a polyunsaturated fat) were not appreciably associated with risk of NIDDM. Linoleic acid was associated with a decreased risk in lean men and men under 65 years of age (van Dam et al., 2002). The Iowa Women's Health Study, which followed 35,988 women for 11 years, found that total fat, saturated fat, and monounsaturated fats were not related to NIDDM risk, but that there was an inverse relationship of NIDDM incidence with vegetable fat consumption and with polyunsaturated fat when substituted for saturated fat and cholesterol (Meyer et al., 2001). The Women's Health Study found no association between saturated, monounsaturated, polyunsaturated, or vegetable fat and risk of NIDDM (Song et al., 2004). Other smaller prospective studies have yielded conflicting results; however, several have found increased risk of NIDDM with saturated fat and decreased risk with unsaturated fat (Parillo & Riccardi, 2004).

In metabolic studies, a high saturated fat intake has been associated with higher risk of impaired glucose metabolism, higher fasting glucose, and higher insulin levels (Steyn et al., 2004; Hu, van Dam, & Liu, 2001; Feskens & van Dam, 1999). (High fasting insulin levels, a marker for insulin resistance, precede the appearance of glucose intolerance in NIDDM.) Conversely, higher vegetable fat (unsaturated fat) and polyunsaturated fat intake have, in turn, been associated with lower fasting glucose concentrations (Steyn et al., 2004; Feskens & van Dam, 1999). Additionally, higher proportions of saturated fatty acids in serum lipids and muscle phospholipids have been associated with impaired insulin sensitivity, whereas higher proportions of long-chain polyunsaturated fatty acids in skeletal muscle phospholipids have been associated with improved insulin sensitivity (Steyn et al., 2004). The data with regard to monounsaturated fatty acids are inconsistent (Steyn et al., 2004).

In general, available epidemiological data suggest a possible beneficial effect of vegetable (unsaturated) fat and a potentially adverse effect of animal (saturated) fat on the risk of diabetes (Parillo & Riccardi, 2004; Rivellese & Lilli, 2003). Total fat intake does not seem to be related to the risk of type 2 diabetes (Parillo & Riccardi, 2004; Hu, van Dam, & Liu, 2001). The differences in the effects of different types of fat are most likely linked to their effects on insulin sensitivity (Parillo & Riccardi, 2004).

A few studies have found that fruit and vegetable consumption may decrease the risk of diabetes (Parillo & Riccardi, 2004; Ford & Mokdad, 2001). The National Health and Nutrition Examination Survey I (NHANES I), which followed 9,665 participants for about 20 years, found a significant inverse relationship between fruit and vegetable intake and diabetes incidence among women, but not among men (Ford & Mokdad, 2001). The Nurse's Health Study found that intake of vegetables, but not fruit, was inversely related to the risk of diabetes (Colditz et al., 1992). In a 20-year follow-up study of 338 men, Feskens found that increases in vegetable and legume intake (but not baseline fruit and vegetable intake) were inversely associated with blood glucose abnormalities indicative of diabetes (Feskens et al., 1995).

Most prospective epidemiologic studies indicate that low fiber intake correlates with a higher prevalence of diabetes (Parillo & Riccardi, 2004). Diabetes was rare among the primitive people living in rural East Africa who had high fiber intakes, but became prevalent as their food became more highly processed (Trowell & Woodgreen, 1975). A 2004 ecological study using nutrient consumption data in the United States between 1909 and 1997 found that increasing intakes of refined carbohydrate with decreasing intakes of fiber paralleled the upward trend in the prevalence of type 2 diabetes (Gross et al., 2004). The Nurses' Health Study found that cereal fiber intake was associated with a decreased risk of NIDDM (Schulze et al., 2004). Similarly, the Health Professionals Follow-up Study found that intakes of whole grains, particularly cereal fiber, were inversely associated with risk of NIDDM (Fung et al., 2002). A prospective study of 35,988 women in the Iowa Women's Health Study showed a decreased risk of diabetes among those consuming greater amounts of total grains, whole grains, total fiber, and cereal fiber. In this study, women in the highest quintile of dietary fiber intake had a 22% lower risk of developing diabetes than did women in the lowest quintile (Meyer et al., 2000). A 10-year Finnish study of 4,316 men and women found that whole-grain consumption and cereal fiber intake were associated with a decreased risk of type 2 diabetes (Montonen et al., 2003). Total dietary fiber was not associated with a decreased risk of diabetes in a 9-year study of 12,251 adults; however, cereal fiber was inversely associated with risk of diabetes in Caucasians, but not African Americans (Stevens et al., 2002). In prospective studies that have examined associations between different types of dietary fiber and risk of type 2 diabetes, cereal, more than soluble, fiber appears to be most strongly associated with a decreased risk of diabetes (Steyn et al., 2004; Schulze et al., 2004). A few studies have not demonstrated an association of dietary fiber and diabetes (Parillo & Riccardi, 2004). In addition, the beneficial effect of whole grains may be due to other constituents instead of or in addition to fiber (Liu et al., 2000; Liese et al., 2003). For example, whole grains contain antioxidants that may improve insulin action. Magnesium in whole grains may also improve insulin sensitivity. Phytochemicals may also play a role.

The Occurrence of Diabetes among Vegetarians versus Nonvegetarians

Snowdon has investigated the risk of diabetes among Seventh-Day Adventists (SDAs). About half of SDAs are vegetarian; therefore, this population can offer insights into the effect of a vegetarian diet on, among other things, the risk of diabetes. Snowdon studied a population of 25,698 adult Caucasian SDAs who were followed for 21 years. During this time, the risk of diabetes as an underlying cause of death among the SDAs was only 45% of the risk for all U.S. Caucasians. Also, in this same study, within the male SDA population, vegetarians had a substantially lower risk than nonvegetarians of diabetes as an underlying or contributing cause of death. Within both the male and female SDA populations, the prevalence of self-reported diabetes was lower among vegetarians than nonvegetarians. In this study, meat consumption was positively associated with self-reported diabetes in both males and females. Meat consumption was also positively associated with mention of diabetes on the death certificate in males, but not females (Snowdon & Phillips, 1985).

In a study of 56 vegetarians and 264 nonvegetarians, Gear found lower blood glucose levels among the vegetarians (Gear et al., 1980). Another study of 30 lacto-ovo vegetarians and 30 meat eaters found that the vegetarians were more insulin-sensitive (Hua, Stoohs, & Facchini, 2001).

Dietary Fat, Fiber, Carbohydrate, and Protein in Diets for Diabetics

General Considerations

Dietary recommendations for diabetics have changed over time. Table 15.1 summarizes the changes in diabetic dietary recommendations in America since 1930 (Shils et al., 1999).

In the past, dietary recommendations for diabetics limited the intake of carbohydrates. However, this reduction in calories from carbohydrates was accompanied by an increase in the percent of calories from fat and protein. As evidence accumulated showing the detrimental health effects of saturated fat and excessive protein in the diet of diabetics, recommendations moved toward increasing the amount of carbohydrate in the diet and decreasing the amount of fat. Dietary recommendations are now more tailored for each individual and, in general, recommend increasing fiber intake, limiting excessive dietary protein, limiting saturated fat intake, and replacing saturated fat with carbohydrates or monounsaturated fats.

Dietary Fat

In 1928, Dr. Elliott Joslin stated that "with an excess of fat diabetes begins and from an excess of fat diabetics die" (Joslin, 1928). There is some wisdom in these words. Dietary saturated fat has a twofold detrimental effect. Both of these detrimental effects of saturated fat on general health and on blood glucose control are important considerations for diabetics.

Dietary fat, because it is higher in calories per gram than carbohydrates or protein, may contribute to obesity. Obesity is the primary risk factor for the development of NIDDM. In addition, obesity increases the risk for other health problems that have an increased incidence

Table 15.1 Nutritional Recommendations for Persons with Diabetes: 1930–1997*

Nutrient	1930	1955	1970	1990	1997
Carbohydrates, total g/day	70	176	225	290	280
% of energy	14	35	45	58	56
Simple, g/day	40	71	112	130	90
Complex, g/day	30	105	113	160	190
Fat, total, g/day	153	99	82	60	67
% of energy	69	45	37	27	30
Saturated, g/day	87	46	35	14	18
Monounsaturated, g/day	50	37	31	26	31
Polyunsaturated, g/day	9	11	13	17	18
Cholesterol, mg/day	1060	690	550	150	150
Protein, g/day	85	101	90	75	70
% of energy	17	20	18	15	14
Dietary fiber, g/day	8	15	20	40	35

*Values for a 2,000-kcal diet.
Source: Shils M, Olson J, Shike M, Ross A, eds. *Modern Nutrition in Health and Disease*. Philadephia, PA: Lippincott/Williams & Wilkins; 1999.

among diabetics, such as hypertension, heart disease, and stroke. Dietary saturated fat also contributes directly to an increased risk of CAD, vascular disease, hypertension, and stroke, all of which disproportionately affect diabetics.

Evidence also indicates that diets high in saturated fat decrease tissue sensitivity to insulin, thereby worsening blood glucose control (Lichtenstein & Schwab, 2000; Rivellese & Lilli, 2003). Accumulating evidence suggests that monounsaturated fats may enhance insulin sensitivity and blood sugar control in diabetics (Meyer et al., 2001; Luscombe, Noakes, & Clifton, 1999; Franz et al., 2002). Also, monounsaturated fats, when they replace saturated fats in the diet, lower total serum cholesterol and LDL cholesterol levels, resulting in decreased cardiovascular risk. Limited data suggest that monounsaturated fats may decrease blood pressure and may also protect against blood clotting (Perez-Jimenez, Lopez-Miranda, & Mata, 2002). Monounsaturated fats may also reduce the susceptibility of LDL cholesterol to oxidation, thereby decreasing the formation of atheroscle-

rotic plaque in blood vessels (Perez-Jimenez, Lopez-Miranda, & Mata, 2002). Collectively, these findings suggest that high-monounsaturated-fat diets may confer benefits for both diabetes control and cardiovascular risk.

Fiber

Dietary fiber has benefits for the general health of the diabetic as well as for improving blood glucose control. Based on solubility in water, dietary fiber can be divided into two types, soluble and insoluble.

Soluble fiber has been shown to be effective in reducing coronary artery disease, a major cause of death and disability among diabetics. One way in which dietary fiber reduces coronary artery disease risk is by reducing total serum cholesterol and LDL cholesterol levels (Van Horn, 1997). Fiber may also have an effect on lowering blood pressure (Van Horn, 1997), which in turn decreases the risk of CAD. Although not proven, dietary fiber may contribute to decreasing obesity, which is crucial not only in terms of decreasing the risk of development of NIDDM, but also in terms of decreasing the risk of CAD.

Evidence suggests that a high-fiber diet can improve blood sugar control in diabetics (Liu et al., 2000; Chandalia et al., 2000; Jenkins et al., 2003). Of 53 studies that have examined the effects of a high-fiber diet in diabetics, 62% showed evidence of improved glucose control, 15% reported no change, and 4% found a worsening of control (Anderson & Akanji, 1993). Also, in several studies, intake of whole grains and dietary fiber has been associated with increased insulin sensitivity (Liese et al., 2003; Pereira et al., 2002). Table 15.2 summarizes the advantages and disadvantages of a high-fiber diet for diabetics (Shils et al., 1999).

As shown in this table, many mechanisms have been proposed to account for the beneficial effect of fiber, especially soluble fiber, on blood glucose control (Pereira et al., 2002; Ha & Lean, 1998). Soluble fiber causes slower gastric emptying and decreased intestinal absorption, which can dampen the rise of blood glucose after a meal. Fiber may also have the effect of increasing insulin sensitivity and increasing insulin receptor binding. It has also been proposed that the effects of fiber on the secretion of several gastrointestinal hormones may play a role in improving blood glucose levels. Furthermore, it has been hypothesized that a lower rise in blood glucose after a high-fiber meal may be the result of the longer time it takes to eat a meal with greater amounts of fiber. Short-chain fatty acids, a byproduct of the intestinal fermentation of soluble fiber, have effects on liver and muscle metabolism that may affect blood glucose levels. The role of the short-chain fatty acids in glucose utilization and insulin secretion is currently under study. Dietary fiber may also contribute to decreased obesity, which can, in and of itself, improve blood sugar control.

Table 15.2 High Fiber Intakes: Advantages and Disadvantages

Advantages
- Slow nutrient digestion and absorption
- Decrease postprandial plasma glucose
- Increase tissue insulin sensitivity
- Increase insulin receptor number
- Stimulate glucose use
- Attenuate hepatic glucose output
- Decrease counterregulatory hormone release (e.g., glucagon)
- Lower serum cholesterol
- Lower fasting and postprandial serum triglycerides
- May attenuate hepatic cholesterol synthesis
- May increase satiety between meals

Disadvantages
- Increase intestinal gas
- May cause temporary abdominal discomfort or gastrointestinal distress
- May alter pharmacokinetics of certain drugs

Source: Shils M, Olson J, Shike M, Ross A, eds. *Modern Nutrition in Health and Disease.* Philadephia, PA: Lippincott/Williams & Wilkins; 1999.

Carbohydrates

Foods containing different carbohydrates cause different magnitudes of increase in blood glucose even when the amount of carbohydrate is held constant. The term *glycemic index* describes the magnitude of rise in blood glucose level that a food produces relative to a reference standard. Foods with a higher glycemic index cause a greater elevation in blood sugar and, in diabetics, may adversely affect blood glucose control. To date, nearly 1,300 foods have been assessed in terms of their glycemic index (Foster-Powell, Holt, & Brand-Miller, 2002).

Many different factors can affect the glycemic index of a food (Ha & Lean, 1998; Hollenbeck, Coulston, & Reaven, 1988). Variations in the rate of absorption of the carbohydrates in different foods is almost certainly the primary explanation for why foods have different glycemic indexes (Wolever, 1990). Factors such as the amount of fat, fiber, and protein in the food can also affect the glycemic index of a food. In addition, particle size, ingestion time, ripeness, and methods of processing and cooking also affect the glycemic index. Less refined foods tend to have lower glycemic indexes. Classification as a simple or complex carbohydrate is not relevant to a food's glycemic index; some complex carbohydrates have higher glycemic indexes than some simple carbohydrates, and vice versa (Steyn et al., 2004).

A number of studies have shown that, compared to high-glycemic-index diets, consumption of low-glycemic-index diets, similar in fiber and macronutrient composition (fat, protein, carbohydrate), improves glycemic control (Miller, 1994). Willett et al. found that in 8 of 9 studies conducted among persons with both type 1 and type 2 diabetes, glycemic control was significantly improved when subjects consumed low-glycemic-index diets (Willett, Manson, & Liu, 2002). Anderson et al. (2004) did a meta-analysis of 9 studies comparing the effects of low-glycemic-index diets and high-glycemic-index diets in diabetic patients. These researchers found that fasting plasma glucose values were significantly lower in persons on the low-glycemic-index diets. Hemoglobin A1c levels (a measure of blood glucose control) were improved also, but not significantly.

There have, however, been some criticisms of the use of the glycemic indexes in meal planning. For instance, the fact that so many factors can affect the glycemic index of a food can be confusing. Some people feel that the use of glycemic indexes makes meal planning too complex. Another criticism is the problem of the large variations in glucose response to foods in different individuals. Some debate continues regarding whether the rest of the foods consumed at a meal can affect the glyce-

mic index of individual foods, making the glycemic indexes less useful.

A 1997 review paper on the use of glycemic indexes in diabetes management outlined the practical applications of glycemic indexes, but stressed that macronutrient recommendations remain the primary consideration. Within those recommendations, however, the glycemic index is a useful tool (Perlstein et al., 1997). A 2003 review paper also concluded that although other nutritional intervention methods can lead to greater improvements in overall glycemic control, there may be a small beneficial effect on glucose control from using a low-glycemic-index diet rather than a high-glycemic-index diet. The authors suggested that low-glycemic-index diets may be used as dietary adjuncts to "fine-tune" glycemic control (Franz, 2003). Franz et al. concluded in 2002 that the use of low-glycemic foods may reduce glucose levels after meals; however, these researchers did not feel there was sufficient evidence of long-term benefit to recommend general use of low-glycemic diets for diabetics (Franz et al., 2002). Nevertheless, several major diabetes associations around the world do endorse the use of the glycemic index in meal planning for diabetics (Anderson et al., 2004).

Protein

Very little data are available as to whether variations in dietary protein intake affect blood glucose control or insulin and/or oral hypoglycemic medication requirements in diabetics (Henry, 1994). Hence, recommendations for the amount of protein in the diet are the same for diabetics and nondiabetics. However, because dietary protein can adversely affect kidney function, diabetics should probably aim for the lower end of the range of acceptable protein intake (Shils et al., 1999).

For diabetics with kidney disease, protein restriction is of value for two reasons. For one, it reduces some symptoms of kidney failure, such as nausea, vomiting, and itching, by reducing nitrogenous waste products of protein metabolism. Secondly, and more importantly, protein restriction can slow and/or limit the progression of kidney failure.

Numerous studies indicate that dietary protein restriction may limit the progression of kidney disease in both nondiabetic (Maschio et al., 1983; Ihle et al., 1989; Rosman et al., 1984; El Nahas et al., 1984; Levey et al., 1996; Alvestrand, Ahlberg, & Bergstrom, 1983) and diabetic (Wiseman, Bognetti et al., 1987; Percheron et al., 1995; Barsotti, Ciardella et al., 1988; Zeller et al., 1991; Walker et al., 1989; Evanoff et al., 1987; American Diabetes Association, 1999a; Brouhard & LaGrone, 1990; Cohen, Dodds, & Viberti, 1987) individuals (Franz et al., 2002; Henry, 1994). In these studies, the protein contents of the diets generally were in the range of 0.4–0.8 grams per kilogram of body weight per day (g/kg/day), with most in the area of 0.6 g/kg/day. Henry reviewed 32 original articles related to protein restriction for IDDM and NIDDM diabetics with renal disease. Virtually all studies reported that protein restriction helped slow the progression of renal disease in diabetic patients (Henry, 1994). Pedrini performed a meta-analysis of the effects of protein-restricted diets on the progression of renal disease in IDDM diabetics and nondiabetics. The study concluded that protein restriction slowed the progression of renal disease in both diabetics with IDDM and the nondiabetics (Pedrini et al., 1996).

The reason for the deleterious effect of protein on the progression of kidney failure has been postulated to be the high filtration rate (glomerular filtration rate or GFR) and high renal plasma flow that occur when the kidneys handle an increased protein load (Henry, 1994; Percheron et al., 1995). The result of this increased GFR and renal plasma flow is an increased pressure gradient within the kidney, which can damage the kidney.

Although studies suggest that protein-restricted diets may limit the progression of kidney disease, it is still unclear whether such diets can serve a protective effect in the absence of kidney disease (Henry, 1994). The earliest stage at which diabetic kidney disease will respond to protein restriction remains to be determined (Henry, 1994).

Several studies have suggested that plant protein may be less harmful to the kidneys than animal protein (Henry, 1994; Kontessis et al., 1990; Nakamura et al., 1989; D'Amico et al., 1992; Jibani et al., 1991; Barsotti, Navalesi et al., 1988; Wiseman, Hunt et al., 1987). In the EURODIAB IDDM Complications Study of 2,696 diabetics with IDDM, increased albumin excretion (a sign of kidney disease) was correlated with intakes of total protein and animal protein, but not vegetable protein (Toeller et al., 1997). A handful of studies have investigated the effects of soy protein (a plant protein) intake compared with animal protein intake on urinary protein loss (*proteinuria*) and on the progression of kidney disease. A vegetarian diet in which soy protein replaced all animal protein was shown to favorably affect kidney function, in terms of decreased proteinuria, in patients with nephrotic kidney disease. The vegetarian diet in this study did, however, contain less overall protein (D'Amico et al., 1992). Some research indicates that soy protein, when substituted for animal protein, tends to lower GFRs or renal blood flow (Kontessis et al., 1990; Nakamura et al., 1989; Kontessis et al., 1995). (As noted, increased GFR and renal blood flow are postulated to be the mechanism behind the deleterious effect of excess protein on kidney function.) Therefore, it is felt that substituting soy protein for animal protein may decrease the risk of developing kidney failure in diabetics, as well as slow the progression of that kidney failure (Kontessis et al., 1990; Nakamura et al., 1989; Jibani et al., 1991; Anderson et al., 1998). Further work is required to establish whether a higher protein intake is acceptable with regard to kidney function if that protein comes from vegetable sources (Shils et al., 1999).

It is unclear whether it is the quality of the vegetable protein itself or some other related factor, such as dietary fiber, the reduced intake of saturated fat, the cholesterol-lowering effect of vegetable protein, or the presence of phytochemicals, that may be responsible for the beneficial effects of soy protein on kidney function (Ha & Lean, 1998; D'Amico et al., 1992). For those with end-stage kidney disease, other issues that must be considered when soy protein is used in place of animal protein are the higher potassium, and to a lesser extent phosphorus, content of soy foods, which may be important because of high potassium and phosphorus blood levels that may already exist in those with severe kidney disease (Messina & Messina, 2000).

Several studies have investigated the effects of a vegetarian diet on diabetic renal function. In his study of eight IDDM diabetics, Barsotti reported that a vegetarian diet slowed the progression of renal disease (Barsotti, Navalesi et al., 1988). Jibani studied the effect of a predominantly vegetarian diet on eight patients with IDDM and found that those who consumed the near-vegetarian diet showed some improvements in terms of decreased albumin excretion. However, it could not be determined if this was due to a reduction in the amount of protein of animal origin or to the lower total protein content of the vegetarian diet (Jibani et al., 1991). In another study, when individuals with IDDM were placed on a near-vegetarian diet, kidney function was favorably affected (in terms of lower GFR and renal plasma flow) when com-

pared to those consuming a nonvegetarian diet containing a similar amount of protein (Garg, 1998). Lower levels of GFR and urinary albumin excretion have been described in vegans and lacto vegetarians compared with omnivores (Kontessis et al., 1990; Wiseman, Hunt et al., 1987; Bosch et al., 1983).

There are several possible reasons for the beneficial effect of a vegetarian diet on renal disease. Since it is thought that kidney failure results from a chronic increase in GFR and increased renal plasma flow, perhaps one explanation for the beneficial effect of a vegetarian diet is its resultant decrease in GFR and renal plasma flow. The lower GFR and renal plasma flow may be the result of one or more factors of a vegetarian diet, including lower overall dietary protein content, substitution of plant protein for animal protein, and lower saturated fat content (which can decrease vascular disease in the kidney).

Phytoestrogens

Only a very limited number of studies have been done on the effect of soy and flaxseed on diabetic glycemic parameters. Emerging evidence, though not always consistent, suggests that they may have beneficial effects on glucose control in diabetics (Jayagopal et al., 2002; Bhathena & Velasquez, 2002). It is not clear whether it is the phytoestrogens or some other component of soy and flaxseeds that cause the effect (Bhathena & Velasquez, 2002).

High-Carbohydrate, Low-Fat, High-Fiber Diets

The preceding information suggests that diets low in fat, high in fiber, and without excessive protein would be advantageous for diabetics. Calories in the diet are derived from fat (9 kcal/g), protein (4 kcal/g), and carbohydrate

(4 kcal/g). Since daily calorie intake stays fairly constant, diabetics who keep dietary fat and protein low will get a relatively greater amount of their calories from carbohydrates. Several studies have reported on the use of such high-carbohydrate, low-fat, high-fiber diets in diabetics.

There has been considerable success in the management of diabetic patients with high-carbohydrate, low-fat, high-fiber diets, including reductions in insulin usage, serum glucose levels, and blood lipids. In 2004, Anderson did a meta-analysis of 13 studies of high-carbohydrate, high-fiber diets (defined as carbohydrate greater than or equal to 60% of energy and fiber greater than or equal to 20 g/1,000 kcal) and found that, when compared to baseline measurements, the high-carbohydrate, high-fiber diets significantly decreased fasting plasma glucose levels (14%), plasma glucose levels after meals (14%), and average daily plasma glucose levels (13%). The decrease in HgbA1c was also significant. The diets also reduced all serum lipid measurements, including total cholesterol (19%), LDL cholesterol (16%), and fasting triglycerides (13%). HDL cholesterol was non-significantly decreased (6%), yet the LDL/HDL cholesterol was decreased about 10.9%. Additionally, the researchers found that moderate-carbohydrate, high-fiber diets significantly improved glycemic control compared to moderate-carbohydrate, low-fiber diets. (Moderate carbohydrate was defined as 30%–59.9% of energy. Low fiber was defined as less than 10 g/1,000 kcal.) Also, the high-carbohydrate, high-fiber diets provided greater benefits in terms of glucose and lipid values when compared to low- or moderate-carbohydrate, low- or moderate-fiber diets (Anderson et al., 2004). In 1987, Anderson had done a meta-analysis of 9 studies of high-carbohydrate, high-fiber diets and got results similar to his 2004 analysis. In addition, in the earlier analysis he reported that 5 of the 9 studies reported decreases in insulin dosage, with an average reduction of 40% (Anderson et al., 1987).

Studies have shown that diets that are high in carbohydrate but low in fiber do not yield the beneficial effects for glucose control and insulin requirements that are derived from diets high in carbohydrate and high in fiber (Riccardi et al., 1984; Rivellese et al., 1980). Therefore, it appears likely that high-carbohydrate diets are most effective for diabetes control if they are also high in fiber.

Some short-term controlled studies have shown that diets high in carbohydrate (60%) and low in fat (20%–25%) may result in increased levels of blood triglycerides and decreased HDL cholesterol levels. Some have suggested that these changes may be transitory (Lichtenstein & Schwab, 2000; Mann, 2000); however, other reports indicate that higher triglyceride levels tend to persist (Coulston et al., 1989; Reaven, 1980; Jones et al., 1987; Garg et al., 1994). Either way, several studies suggest that this increase in triglycerides and decrease in HDL that may accompany high-carbohydrate, low-fat diets may be prevented if the diet is also high in fiber (Stone & Van Horn, 2002). In the meta-analysis done by Anderson, the high-carbohydrate, high-fiber diets showed a nonsignificant decrease in HDL cholesterol and a decrease in triglycerides (Anderson et al., 2004).

Lower-Carbohydrate, Higher-Monounsaturated-Fat Diets

Because of the evidence suggesting that a high-carbohydrate, low-fat diet (especially one that is low in fiber) may increase serum triglyceride levels and decrease HDL cholesterol levels, some investigators have looked at diets for diabetics that replace some of the carbohydrate in the high-carbohydrate diets with monounsaturated fat, as a way of preventing these triglyceride and HDL cholesterol changes.

Increasing the amount of monounsaturated fat in the diet can also have other benefits. There is some evidence that dietary monounsaturated fats, as opposed to saturated fats, may improve blood glucose control. Additionally, monounsaturated fats, when replacing saturated fats in the diet, decrease total blood cholesterol and LDL cholesterol levels. There is also some evidence that monounsaturated fats reduce the susceptibility of LDL cholesterol to oxidation, and thereby reduce its atherogenic potential (Perez-Jimenez, Lopez-Miranda, & Mata, 2002). All these improvements in blood lipids translate into lower risk of CAD and other vascular diseases.

Several studies have reported on the use of these lower-carbohydrate, higher-monounsaturated fat diets in diabetics. Garg did a meta-analysis of nine studies that compared high-carbohydrate, low-saturated-fat diets with high-monounsaturated-fat diets in patients with NIDDM. In these studies, the high-carbohydrate diets contained about 50%–60% carbohydrate and 20%–30% fat, whereas the higher-monounsaturated-fat diet contained about 35%–40% carbohydrate and 40%–50% fat, of which about 25%–33% was monounsaturated fats. The amount of fiber in the diets was not listed. The authors found that, compared with high-carbohydrate, low-saturated-fat diets, high-monounsaturated-fat diets improved lipid profiles (decreased triglycerides and increased HDL cholesterol, without adversely affecting LDL cholesterol) and improved glucose control. However, the omission from the analysis of dietary fiber content may be significant (Garg, 1998).

The reason for the improvements in blood glucose control from the high-monounsaturated-fat diets could be twofold. First, monounsaturated fats may themselves improve insulin sensitivity. Second, improvements in glucose control may be due to the lower carbohydrate load in the monounsaturated-fat diets (Garg, 1998).

A few studies have compared high-carbohydrate, low-fat, high-fiber diets with lower-carbohydrate, higher-monounsaturated-fat diets (Table 15.3). In general, these studies have not shown a significant difference between the two diets in terms of blood glucose control.

Because monounsaturated fats contain more calories per gram than carbohydrates, increasing dietary monounsaturated fats at the expense of carbohydrates may increase the risk of obesity for some individuals. This could be disadvantageous because obesity itself worsens glycemic control and is a risk factor for several complications of diabetes, such as high blood pressure, coronary artery disease, peripheral vascular disease, and stroke. Some investigators, however, have not noted weight gain with diets high in monounsaturated fats when compared with high-carbohydrate, low-fat diets (Walker et al., 1995). Also, although low-fat, high-carbohydrate diets have been found to be advantageous in preventing and treating coronary artery disease, there is insufficient information regarding the effect of diets high in monounsaturated fats on prevention and treatment of coronary artery disease.

Current Diet Recommendations for Diabetics

As the preceding sections have shown, the content of fiber, fat, carbohydrate, and protein in the diet is of great importance for diabetics. Currently, no one specific diet is recommended for diabetics; instead, there are recommended guidelines. Following these guidelines can both improve blood sugar control and help prevent some of the health complications that can result from diabetes. The current guidelines from

Table 15.3 Studies Comparing High-Carbohydrate, High-Fiber Diets with Lower-Carbohydrate, Higher-Monounsaturated-Fat Diets

- Two studies compared low-fat,high-carbohydrate diets with high-monounsaturated-fat diets in diabetic patients. Both diets consisted of "natural food"; stressed moderation in consumption of red and processed meat, eggs, and whole-fat dairy products; and emphasized consumption of vegetables and fruits. Also, the fiber content was kept constant. The difference in total fat between the diets was less than in the studies in Garg's analysis (Ros, 2003). Both studies found similar glycemic (blood glucose) control and lipid profiles between the diets (Ros, 2003; Rodriguez-Villar et al., 2004; Rodriguez-Villar et al., 2000).
- In another study,70 subjects with NIDDM were randomly assigned to one of three diets: a weight maintenance diet (no advice on the specific distribution of nutrients); a high-carbohydrate, high-fiber diet (55% carbohydrate, 30% fat, 30 or more grams of fiber per day); or a modified-fat diet (45% carbohydrate and 36% fat, with equal amounts of saturated fat, monounsaturated fat, and polyunsaturated fat). Both the high-carbohydrate, high-fiber diet and the modified-fat diet resulted in similar improvements in LDL cholesterol and glycemic control (Milne et al., 1994).
- Another study compared a high-carbohydrate (60%),low-fat (20%) diet with a lower-carbohydrate (40%), fat-modified (40% fat) diet in both IDDM and NIDDM subjects. In these studies, the fat-modified diet was obtained by substituting monounsaturated fat for carbohydrates. In both the IDDM and the NIDDM subjects, glucose control was worse and triglyceride levels were higher in the high-carbohydrate diet. However, in these cases, the high-carbohydrate, low-fat diet was not a high-fiber diet.

  Therefore, the researchers then compared a fat-modified diet, in which monounsaturated fats were the major source of fat, with a high-carbohydrate, low-fat diet in which the carbohydrate sources were also high in fiber. In this trial, for both diabetics with NIDDM and those with IDDM, the high-carbohydrate, low-fat, high-fiber diet resulted in better glucose control than the fat-modified diet. There were no significant differences in triglyceride levels between the two groups. Compared with the fat-modified group, however, there were reductions in both HDL cholesterol and LDL cholesterol in the high-carbohydrate, low-fat, high-fiber diet (Riccardi & Rivellese, 1991).
- Walker compared a high-carbohydrate,low-fat diet (50% carbohydrate, 23% fat) with a monounsaturated-fat-enriched diet (40% carbohydrate, 36% fat, of which half was monounsaturated fat) in 24 NIDDM patients. Both diets were relatively rich (43 g vs. 25 g per day) in fiber. They found little difference in glycemic or lipid control between the diets (Walker et al., 1995).
- Campbell compared a high-carbohydrate,low-fat diet (52% carbohydrate, 24% fat) with a high-monounsaturated-fat diet (40% carbohydrate, 38% fat, 21% of which was monounsaturated fat). Both diets were moderately high in fiber (more than 30 g per day). The higher-monounsaturated-fat diet resulted in better glucose control and lower fasting triglycerides. LDL cholesterol, HDL cholesterol, and triglyceride levels did not vary (Campbell et al., 1994).
- Gerhard compared a low-fat,high-carbohydrate diet with a high-monounsaturated-fat diet for 6 weeks in 11 type 2 diabetics. The low-fat diet was higher in fiber. They found no difference in glycemic control or lipid response between the diets (Gerhard et al., 2004).

several major diabetes organizations around the world are listed in Table 15.4 (Anderson et al., 2004).

The total calories in the diet should be the amount that maintains optimum weight. Obesity is the most common factor predisposing individuals to NIDDM. Maintaining a proper weight through diet and exercise reduces the incidence of type 2 diabetes in high-risk persons by 40% to 60% over 3 to 4 years (Primary Working Group, 2004). For diabetics who are overweight, moderate weight loss has been

Table 15.4 International Recommendations for Medical Nutrition Therapy for Persons with Diabetes

Parameter	ADA [3]	BDA [4]	CDA [5]	EASD [6]
Weight Reduction	Modest weight loss (5-7%)	BMI to approach desirable weight	Maintain healthy weight (7-10%)	BMI 18.5-25 desirable weight
Carbohydrate	50-60%	50-55%	50-60%	45-60% (55-60% with low GI foods)
Polysaccharides	Whole grains, fruits, vegetables	Most of CHO, rich in fiber or resistant starch	Whole grain cereals & legumes	Low GI foods
Mono- & Disaccharides	No restriction	<25 g/d	≤10% added	<10% calories
Glycemic index	Does not recommend for general use	Discusses	Includes low GI foods	With meals, low GI foods recommended
Fiber, total	As for general population	>30 g/d	25-35 g/d	Increase with low GI foods
Protein	15-20%	10-15%	11%, 0.86 g/kg/d	10-20%
Total fat	25-35%	30-35%	≤30%	<35%
Saturated/Trans Fatty Acids	<10%	<10%	<10%	<10%
Monounsaturated Fatty Acids	10-20%	10-15%	10-15% favored	10-20% favored
Polyunsaturated FattyAcids	~10%	<10%	≤10%	≤10%
Cholesterol	<300 mg/d	<300 mg/d		≤300 mg

Abbreviations:
    ADA—American Diabetes Association
    AHA—American Heart Association
    BDA—British Diabetic Association
    CDA—Canadian Diabetes Association

Japan [8]	S Africa [9]	India [7]	AHA [10]	NCEP [11]
Attain & maintain desirable weight	Achieve & maintain reasonable weight	19–23 BMI desirable weight	Achieve & maintain desirable weight	Maintain desirable weight
60%	55–60%	>65%	45–55%	50–60%
Vegetables 300 g	Whole grain cereals & legumes	Vegetables, fruits, legumes —40 g/d; cereal— 40 g		Grains, whole grains, fruits, vegetables
1 serving fruit	<10% added sugar	From foods	No comment	No comment
Recommended	Quotes supportive references			No comment
1 fruit, 400 g vegetables	40 g/d	From fruits, vegetables, legumes	≥25 g/d	20–30 g/d
15–20%	12–20%		~15%	~15%
20–25%	<30%	<21%	<30%	25–35%
	<10%	<7%	<10%	<7%
	<13%	<7%	<11%	up to 20%
	6–8%	<7%	<10%	up to 10%
			<200 mg	<200 mg

EASD—European Association for the Study of Diabetes

NCEP—National Cholesterol Education Program

Source: Anderson JW, Randles KM, Kendall CW, Jenkins DJ. Carbohydrate and fiber recommendations for individuals with diabetes: A quantitative assessment and meta-analysis of the evidence. *J Am Coll Nutr.* 2004;23(1):5–17.

>ery polyunsaturated fat (James et al., 1991).
ery polyunsaturated fat (James et al., 1991).

shown to improve glucose control, lipid profiles, and blood pressure (American Diabetes Association, 1999c).

Dietary fiber is an important component of a healthful diabetic diet. Evidence suggests that dietary fiber improves blood sugar control. In addition, fiber has other beneficial health effects that are important to diabetics. Dietary fiber reduces total cholesterol and LDL cholesterol levels, reduces the risk of CAD, and may also have an effect on lowering blood pressure and preventing obesity. The American Diabetes Association recommends that diabetics consume 20–35 g of fiber daily and include sources of both soluble and insoluble fiber (American Diabetes Association, 1999c). Nearly all studies on the effect of high-fiber diets in diabetics have used fiber contents of at least 20 g per day. Many of these studies have used fiber contents of 50–90 g per day, and internationally, high fiber intakes are in this range. By comparison, the typical American diet contains only about 10–20 grams of fiber per day.

Diabetics do not need more protein than the general population. For those diabetics without evidence of kidney disease, there is no scientific evidence to support a diet different in protein content from that of the general public. This would mean a protein intake of 10%–20% of total daily calories (American Diabetes Association, 1999c). The Recommended Daily Allowance (RDA) for protein for the general population is 0.8 g/kg/day (about 10% of daily calories). Because of the theoretical role that protein may play in the development of kidney disease, it may be advisable for diabetics to stay closer to this RDA rather than the higher range of the average protein intake for the population. For diabetics who already have kidney disease, there is significant evidence that excessive protein intake can cause further deterioration in kidney function; therefore, it is

recommended that diabetics with kidney disease limit their protein intake to 0.8 g/kg/day (about 10% of total calories). Some studies suggest that further restriction to 0.6 g/kg/day may be beneficial (Ha & Lean, 1998; American Diabetes Association, 1999c). Also, these guidelines do not take into consideration the different effects of plant and animal proteins. As noted earlier, there is evidence to suggest that plant proteins may not be as detrimental to the kidneys as animal proteins and, therefore, may not have to be limited to the same degree.

This leaves 80%–90% of calories to be divided between dietary fats and carbohydrates. The ADA recommends that less than 10% of these calories be from saturated fat (less than 7% for those with elevated LDL cholesterol levels). Of course, because saturated fat is not a necessary dietary requirement, and because it increases the risk of CAD, the dietary content of saturated fat should probably be kept as close to zero as possible. The ADA and the European Association for the Study of Diabetes recommend that less than or equal to 10% of calories be from polyunsaturated fats (American Diabetes Association, 1999c; Diabetes and Nutrition Study Group [DNSG], 1995). The World Health Organization puts a lower limit of 3% and an upper limit of 7% on the amount of dietary polyunsaturated fat (James et al., 1991).

This would leave about 70%–80% of calories to be divided between monounsaturated fats and carbohydrates. Fruits, vegetables, legumes, and cereals are the preferred sources of carbohydrate, as they are rich in fiber, micronutrients, and vitamins (DNSG, 1995).

Both high-carbohydrate, low-fat, high-fiber diets and lower-carbohydrate, higher-monounsaturated-fat diets for diabetics have been discussed. The high-carbohydrate, low-fat, high-fiber diets that have been studied typically contained about 50%–75% carbohydrate, 15%–

30% fat, and 25–80 g of fiber per day. The high-monounsaturated-fat diets typically contained about 35%–40% carbohydrate and 40%–50% fat, of which about 24%–33% was monounsaturated fat. For comparison, in the United States the average total monounsaturated fat content is about 13%–14% (Kris-Etherton, 1999). In some Mediterranean countries, the percent of dietary fat can reach 40%, with most of the fat coming from plant sources (Grundy, 1999). Evidence shows that both high-carbohydrate, low-fat, high-fiber diets and lower-carbohydrate, high-monounsaturated-fat diets improve blood sugar control and decrease cholesterol levels. Both diets can be appropriate for diabetics. Because monounsaturated fats are higher in calories per gram than carbohydrates, diabetics who need to lose weight may want to tend more toward a high-carbohydrate, low-fat, high-fiber diet. Because of some concerns that high-carbohydrate diets (especially those that are low in fiber) may increase serum triglyceride levels, diabetics with elevated triglycerides may want to favor a lower-carbohydrate, higher-monounsaturated-fat diet. Consideration should also be given to the fact that although low-fat, high-carbohydrate, high-fiber diets have been shown to prevent and treat coronary artery disease, there is as yet no conclusive evidence that monounsaturated fats have the same effects.

When deciding what type of carbohydrates to consume, the evidence mentioned above shows that diets containing carbohydrates with lower glycemic indexes may improve glucose control, as compared to diets with higher glycemic indexes. Extensive tables are available that list the glycemic indexes of hundreds of foods (Foster-Powell, Holt, & Brand-Miller, 2002). Diabetics may want to increase their consumption of low-glycemic-index foods and decrease their consumption of higher-glycemic-index foods.

Factors in a Vegetarian Diet That Are Beneficial to Diabetics

Many aspects of a healthful vegetarian diet fit well with the current dietary recommendations for diabetics, as noted earlier. In addition, it is easy to design a healthful vegetarian diet for diabetes, whether it is a high-carbohydrate, low-fat, high-fiber diet or a lower-carbohydrate, higher-monounsaturated-fat diet.

The ADA recommends that diabetics consume 20–35 grams of fiber per day. The typical American omnivorous diet contains only about 10–20 g per day. Lacto-ovo vegetarians typically consume 20–35 g per day, whereas most vegans consume 25–50 g per day. Therefore, in terms of fiber content, a vegetarian diet meets and often exceeds the daily recommended amount of dietary fiber and is much closer to the recommended intake than is an omnivorous diet.

Additionally, carbohydrate intake is higher among vegetarians. Lacto-ovo vegetarians consume about 50%–55% of their calories as carbohydrates and vegans roughly 50%–65%, whereas omnivores generally consume less than 50% of their calories as carbohydrates (Messina & Messina, 1996).

Vegetarians tend to weigh less than their omnivorous counterparts, offering benefits for the prevention and control of diabetes as well as for the prevention of some health complications of diabetes.

The lower protein content of a vegetarian diet may also be advantageous for diabetics. The RDA for protein is 0.8 g/kg/day (about 10% of calories). It is recommended that all diabetics, especially those with kidney disease, stay at about this level. Although the typical U.S. diet contains between 14% and 18% of calories as protein, lacto-ovo vegetarian diets contain about 12%–14% of calories as protein and vegan diets

Table 15.5 Comparison of Vegetarian and Nonvegetarian Intakes of Protein, Fat, Carbohydrate, Cholesterol, and Fiber

Nutrient	Nonvegetarian	Vegetarian	Vegan
Fat (% total calories)	34–38	30–36	28–33
Cholesterol (total grams)	300–500	150–300	0
Carbohydrate (% total calories)	<50	50–55	50–65
Dietary fiber (total grams/day)	10–12	20–35	25–50
Protein (% total calories)	14–18	12–14	10–12
Animal protein (% total protein)	60–70	40–60	0

Source: Messina M, Messina V. *The Dietitian's Guide to Vegetarian Diets: Issues and Applications.* Gaithersburg, MD: Aspen Publishers; 1996.

about 10%–12% (Messina & Messina, 1996). This puts vegetarian, and especially vegan, diets more in line with the dietary protein recommendations for diabetics. Additionally, there is some evidence to suggest that plant protein may not have the detrimental effects on kidney function seen with animal protein. Vegetarians, of course, consume more plant protein and less animal protein than omnivores, in whose diets 65% of protein is of animal origin (Messina & Messina, 1996) (Table 15.5).

The lower total fat and saturated fat content of a vegetarian diet also may improve the blood sugar control, blood lipid profiles, and risk of CAD of diabetics. In addition, the higher unsaturated fat content of vegetarian diets, as well as soy and flaxseed, could also offer benefits for both diabetes control and decreased CAD risk.

All of this means that vegetarians consume a relatively high-carbohydrate, low-fat, high-fiber diet, a diet that evidence indicates improves the glucose control and lipoprotein profile among diabetics. The higher content of unsaturated (vegetable) fats in vegetarian diets may also prove useful for blood sugar control and the lipoprotein profile of diabetics.

Finally, diabetics have an increased risk of CAD and stroke over nondiabetics. For this rea-

son, dietary factors that affect the risk of these diseases are very important to diabetics. Many factors in a vegetarian diet can reduce the risk of CAD: lower cholesterol and saturated fat content, and higher contents of unsaturated fat, fiber, antioxidants, soy protein, and phytochemicals. Many factors in a vegetarian diet may also contribute to a lower risk of some types of stroke, including a greater content of fruits and vegetables, fiber, antioxidants, and a lower content of cholesterol and saturated fat.

The Effect of a Vegetarian Diet on Diabetes Control

Only a few studies have investigated the effect of a vegetarian diet on diabetics. Nicholson et al. compared seven individuals with NIDDM who were placed on a low-fat vegan diet with four subjects placed on a conventional low-fat diet. The vegan diet provided 14% of calories from protein, 75% from carbohydrate, and 11% from fat, and contained 26 g of fiber. The conventional low-fat diet provided 18% of calories from protein, 51% from carbohydrate, and 31% from fat, and contained 20 g of fiber per day. Those on the vegan diet had a 28% reduction in fasting serum glucose, which was significantly different from the 12% reduction seen in the control group. Among the six individuals in the vegan diet group on oral hypoglycemics, medication was discontinued in one and reduced in three. Insulin doses decreased in both individuals on insulin in the vegan diet group. Of the four individuals on the conventional low-fat diet, all of whom had required oral hypoglycemic medications, none reduced medication use (Nicholson et al., 1999).

In another study, 21 individuals with diabetic neuropathy were placed on a low-fat vegetarian diet and an exercise program. Seventeen had a remission of pain due to the neuropathy in less than 2.5 weeks. In addition, there was a decrease in average fasting blood sugar levels, and six individuals were able to discontinue either their insulin or hypoglycemic medication (Crane & Sample, 1994).

In 1982 and 1983, Barnard reported on two studies involving individuals with NIDDM who were placed on the Pritikin near-vegetarian diet and an exercise program. The diet contained 13% of calories from protein, less than 10% from fat, and the remainder from carbohydrate. The diet also included 10–20 g of fiber per day. The protein was derived entirely from plant sources, with the exception of nonfat milk and small amounts of fish or fowl that were served weekly. In the first part of the study, 60 individuals with NIDDM were followed for 26 days. At the end of this period, of the 23 who were taking oral hypoglycemic agents, all but 2 were off medication by the end of the period. Of the 17 who were on insulin, all but 4 were off medication at the end of the study. Average fasting blood glucose, as well as serum cholesterol and triglyceride levels, were reduced. In the second phase of the study, 69 individuals with NIDDM were placed on a diet and exercise program similar to that of the first study, except that the diet now contained 35–40 g of

fiber per day. During the first 26 days of the study, average fasting glucose was reduced, oral hypoglycemic medications were discontinued in 24 of 31 individuals, and insulin was discontinued in 13 of 18 individuals. One person was placed on insulin. Two to three years later, the individuals were contacted by phone and blood tests were checked. Fasting glucose levels were not significantly different from the values at the end of the 26-day period. However, compared with the end of the 26-day period, 7 more individuals were taking oral agents and 4 more were on insulin. The authors found that the main difference between those individuals who had to go back on medication and those remaining off medication was adherence to the diet and percent of calories derived from fat (17% vs. 10%) (Barnard et al., 1982; Barnard et al., 1983).

In 1994, Barnard reported on 652 diabetics followed for 3 weeks on a very-low-fat vegetarian diet plus exercise. Of those using insulin, 39% were able to stop insulin use, and 71% of those on oral hypoglycemic drugs were able to discontinue the medication. Serum cholesterol fell by a little more than 20% and triglycerides decreased by 33%. HDL cholesterol fell by 11%–14% (Barnard, Jung, & Inkeles, 1994).

All of these studies may have been confounded by weight loss among those on the experimental diets. Because weight loss itself improves glycemic control, further study is needed to see how much, if any, of the improvement in metabolic values in these studies was due to weight loss alone and how much was due to the effects of specific individual dietary factors independent of weight loss.

As noted previously in the section on protein, several studies have looked at the effects of a vegetarian diet on diabetic renal function. These studies have found beneficial effects.

Practical Aspects: How to Plan a Vegetarian Diet for Diabetics

The studies presented in this chapter indicate that diabetics who switch to a vegetarian diet may experience decreases in blood glucose and diabetic medication requirements. Because of this, changes in the diet of diabetics should be done under the supervision of a physician. Blood sugar measurements should be done regularly when dietary changes are made. In addition, changing to a vegetarian diet may result in decreases in blood pressure and serum lipids, necessitating changes in dosages of blood pressure and lipid-lowering medications also.

There is no one ideal vegetarian diet for diabetics. General dietary guidelines for diabetics were discussed earlier. These guidelines can easily be used to guide diabetics in planning vegetarian diets.

In general, total calories should be the amount that maintains ideal body weight. Daily fiber intake should ideally be at least 20–35 g. Many studies of diets for diabetics have used 50–70 g of fiber per day.

Total protein intake should probably be the RDA for the general population, which is 0.8 g/kg/day (about 10% of total calories). Some studies suggest that diabetics with kidney disease may benefit from further protein restrictions to 0.6 g/kg/day. That said, there is some evidence that plant protein may not have the detrimental effects on the kidneys seen with animal protein. Although further studies are needed, the intake of plant protein may not have to be limited to the same degree as animal protein.

The ADA recommends that less than 10% of calories be from saturated fat (less than 7% for those with elevated LDL cholesterol levels). Ideally, saturated fat intake should be as close to zero as possible, because saturated fat intake translates into higher cholesterol levels and increased risk of CAD and other vascular diseases. The amount of polyunsaturated fat in the diet should range from 3% at the lower end to 7%–10% at the upper limit.

This leaves roughly 80%–90% of calories to be divided between carbohydrate and monounsaturated fat. The healthiest sources of dietary carbohydrates are fruits, vegetables, legumes, and cereals. Typically the high-carbohydrate, low-fat, high-fiber diets for diabetics have consisted of about 50%–75% carbohydrate, 15%–30% fat, and 26–80 g of fiber per day. Diets with higher monounsaturated fat intake have used about 35%–40% carbohydrate and 40%–50% fat, of which about 25%–33% was monounsaturated fat. Both dietary plans have shown success in improving blood glucose control and blood lipid profiles. Individual diabetics can also combine the two plans. Diabetics with weight problems may want to use less monounsaturated fats because of their higher caloric content. Because of some concerns that high-carbohydrate diets that are low in fiber may increase triglyceride levels, diabetics with elevated triglycerides may want to choose a higher monounsaturated-fat intake. Consideration should also be given to the fact that low-fat, high-carbohydrate, high-fiber diets have been shown beneficial in preventing and treating coronary heart disease; there is as yet no definitive proof of such effects with high-monounsaturated-fat diets. Lastly, some evidence suggests that carbohydrates with lower glycemic indexes may improve blood sugar control, when compared with carbohydrates with higher glycemic indexes.

Because diabetics are at greater risk of CAD and stroke than the general population, diets for diabetics should limit or eliminate dietary cholesterol and saturated fats. Healthy diets for diabetics should supply generous amounts of the dietary factors that may reduce the risk of these diseases: fruits and vegetables, antioxidants, phytochemicals, soy protein, and folate.

Conclusion

Diabetes and diet are intrinsically linked, in terms of both prevention and treatment. The cause of diabetes is likely multifactorial, but evidence suggests that diet may play a role. As diets in populations "westernize," the incidence of diabetes increases. Studies suggest that diets high in saturated fat may increase the risk of developing diabetes. Some preliminary studies also indicate that diets high in fiber, high in fruits and vegetables, low in animal products, and higher in unsaturated fats may decrease the risk of diabetes. Although few in number, studies have indicated that vegetarians may have a lower incidence of diabetes than nonvegetarians.

There is no one recommended "diabetic diet." Instead, there are dietary guidelines that diabetics can use to improve blood sugar control and improve blood lipoprotein profiles. Total calories should be at a level that maintains ideal body weight. Diets should contain generous amounts of fiber, fruits, and vegetables and limited or no saturated fat and cholesterol. It is recommended that protein intake for diabetics be the daily RDA. Slightly greater protein restriction may be of value for diabetics with kidney disease. Within these guidelines, both high-carbohydrate, low-fat, high-fiber diets and lower-carbohydrate, higher-monounsaturated-fat diets have been used successfully by diabetics.

Vegetarian diets come closer to these recommended guidelines than does the typical U.S. omnivorous diet. Therefore, vegetarian diets can easily serve as a baseline from which to devise a healthful diabetic diet. Although limited in number, some studies have indicated that vegetarian diets can improve blood glucose control and kidney function. In addition, other beneficial effects of a vegetarian diet, including decreased risk of CAD, lower risk of hypertension, decreased incidence of obesity, and possibly a decreased incidence of stroke, are important

to diabetics because of the greater incidence of these diseases in diabetics as compared with nondiabetics.

Any dietary changes undertaken by a diabetic should be done under the strict supervision of a physician. Improvements in diet may decrease blood sugar levels, change blood lipid profiles, and lower blood pressure, necessitating changes in medications. Good diabetes control requires an appropriate balance between good nutrition, adequate physical exercise, and careful medication use. Consuming a vegetarian diet can result in improved diabetic control and health protection.

References

Addanki S. Roles of nutrition, obesity, and estrogens in diabetes mellitus: Human leads to an experimental approach to prevention. *Preven Med.* 1981;10(5):577–589.

Alvestrand A, Ahlberg M, Bergstrom J. Retardation of the progression of renal insufficiency in patients treated with low-protein diets. *Kidney Intl Suppl.* 1983;24(Suppl 16):S268–S272.

American Diabetes Association. Diabetic nephropathy. *Diabetes Care.* 1999a;22(Suppl 1):S66–S69.

American Diabetes Association. Management of dyslipidemia in adults with diabetes. *Diabetes Care.* 1999b;22(Suppl 1):S56–S59.

American Diabetes Association. Nutrition recommendations and principles for people with diabetes mellitus. *Diabetes Care.* 1999c;22(Suppl 1):S42–S45.

Anderson J, Akanji A. Treatment of diabetes with high fiber diets. In: Spiller GA, ed. *Handbook of Dietary Fiber in Human Nutrition.* Boca Raton, FL: CRC Press; 1993.

Anderson JW, Blake JE, Turner J, Smith B. Effects of soy protein on renal function and proteinuria in patients with type 2 diabetes. *Am J Clin Nutr.* 1998;68(6, Suppl):1347S–1353S.

Anderson JW, Gustafson NJ, Bryant CA, Tietyen-Clark J. Dietary fiber and diabetes: A comprehensive review and practical application. *J Am Diet Assoc.* 1987;87(9):1189–1197.

Anderson JW, Randles KM, Kendall CW, Jenkins DJ. Carbohydrate and fiber recommendations for individuals with diabetes: A quantitative assessment and meta-analysis of the evidence. *J Am Coll Nutr.* 2004;23(1):5–17.

Barnard RJ, Jung T, Inkeles SB. Diet and exercise in the treatment of NIDDM. *Diabetes Care.* 1994; 17(12):1469–1472.

Barnard RJ, Lattimore L, Holly RG, et al. Response of non-insulin-dependent diabetic patients to an intensive program of diet and exercise. *Diabetes Care.* 1982;5(4):370–374.

Barnard RJ, Massey MR, Cherny S, et al. Long-term use of a high-complex-carbohydrate, high-fiber, low-fat diet and exercise in the treatment of NIDDM patients. *Diabetes Care.* 1983;6(3): 268–273.

Barsotti G, Ciardella F, Morelli A, et al. Nutritional treatment of renal failure in type 1 diabetic nephropathy. *Clin Nephrol.* 1988;29(6):280–287.

Barsotti G, Navalesi R, Giampietro O, et al. Effects of a vegetarian, supplemented diet on renal function, proteinuria, and glucose metabolism in patients with "overt" diabetic nephropathy and renal insufficiency. *Contrib Nephrol.* 1988;65: 87–94.

Bhathena SJ, Velasquez MT. Beneficial role of dietary phytoestrogens in obesity and diabetes. *Am J Clin Nutr.* 2002;76(6):1191–1201.

Bosch JP, Saccaggi A, Lauer A, et el. Renal functional reserve in humans. Effect of protein intake on glomerular filtration rate. *Am J Med.* 1983;75(6): 943–950.

Brouhard BH, LaGrone L. Effect of dietary protein restriction on functional renal reserve in diabetic nephropathy. *Am J Med.* 1990;89(4):427–431.

Campbell LV, Marmot PE, Dyer JA, et al. The high-monounsaturated fat diet as a practical alternative for NIDDM. *Diabetes Care.* 1994;17(3): 177–182.

Castelli WP. The triglyceride issue: A view from Framingham. *Am Heart J.* 1986;112(2):432–437.

Centers for Disease Control and Prevention (CDC). National diabetes fact sheet: General information and national estimates on diabetes in the United States, 2003. Atlanta, GA: U.S. Department of Human Services, Centers for Disease Control and Prevention; 2003. Available at: www.cdc. gov/diabetes/pubs/factsheet/htm. Accessed October 22, 2004.

Chandalia M, Garg A, Lutjohann D, et al. Beneficial effects of high dietary fiber intake in patients with type 2 diabetes mellitus. *N Engl J Med.* 2000;342(19):1392–1398.

Cohen D, Dodds R, Viberti G. Effect of protein restriction in insulin dependent diabetics at risk of nephropathy. *Br Med J.* 1987;294(6575):795–798.

Colditz GA, Manson JE, Stampfer MJ, et al. Diet and risk of clinical diabetes in women. *Am J Clin Nutr.* 1992;55(5):1018–1023.

Coulston AM, Hollenbeck CB, Swislocki AL, Reaven GM. Persistence of hypertriglyceridemic effect of low-fat high-carbohydrate diets in NIDDM patients. *Diabetes Care.* 1989;12(2):94–101.

Crane MG, Sample C. Regression of diabetic neuropathy on total vegetarian (vegan) diet. *J Nutr Med.* 1994;4:431–439.

D'Amico G, Gentile MG, Manna G, et al. Effect of vegetarian soy diet on hyperlipidaemia in nephrotic syndrome. *Lancet.* 1992;339(8802):1131–1134.

Dahlquist GG, Blom LG, Persson LA, et al. Dietary factors and the risk of developing insulin dependent diabetes in childhood. *Br Med J.* 1990; 300(6735):1302–1306.

Diabetes and Nutrition Study Group (DNSG), European Association for the Study of Diabetes (EASD). Recommendations for the nutritional management of patients with diabetes mellitus. *Diabetic Nutr Metab.* 1995;8:186–189.

Diabetes Control and Complications Trial Research Group. The effect of intensive treatment of diabetes on the development and progression of long-term complications in insulin-dependent diabetes mellitus. *N Engl J Med.* 1993;329(14): 977–986.

Edelman SV. Type II diabetes mellitus. *Adv Intern Med.* 1998;43:449–500.

El Nahas AM, Masters-Thomas AM, Brady SA, et al. Selective effect of low protein diets in chronic renal diseases. *Br Med J.* 1984;289(6455):1337–1341.

Evanoff GV, Thompson CS, Brown J, Weinman EJ. The effect of dietary protein restriction on the progression of diabetic nephropathy: A 12-month follow-up. *Arch Intern Med.* 1987;147(3):492–495.

Feskens EJ, van Dam RM. Dietary fat and the etiology of type 2 diabetes: An epidemiological perspective. *Nutr Metab Cardiovasc Dis.* 1999;9(2):87–95.

Feskens EJ, Virtanen S, Rasanen L, et al. Dietary factors determining diabetes and impaired glucose tolerance. *Diabetes Care.* 1995;18(8):1104–1112.

Ford ES, Mokdad AH. Fruit and vegetable consumption and diabetes mellitus incidence among U.S. adults. *Preven Med.* 2001;32(1):33–39.

Foster-Powell K, Holt SH, Brand-Miller JC. International table of glycemic index and glycemic load values: 2002. *Am J Clin Nutr.* 2002;76(1):5–56.

Franz MJ. The glycemic index: Not the most effective nutrition therapy intervention. *Diabetes Care.* 2003;26(8):2466–2468.

Franz MJ, Bantel JP, Beebe CA, et al. Evidence-based nutrition principles and recommendations for the treatment and prevention of diabetes and related complications. *Diabetes Care.* 2002;25(1):148–198.

Franz MJ, Horton ES, Bantle P, et al. Nutrition principles for the management of diabetes and related complications. *Diabetes Care.* 1994;17(5):490–518.

Fung TT, Hu FB, Pereira MA, et al. Whole-grain intake and the risk of type 2 diabetes: A prospective study in men. *Am J Clin Nutr.* 2002;76(3):535–540.

Garg A. High-monounsaturated-fat diets for patients with diabetes mellitus: A meta-analysis. *Am J Clin Nutr.* 1998;67(3, Suppl):577S–582S.

Garg A, Bantle JP, Henry RR, et al. Effects of varying carbohydrate content of diet in patients with non-insulin-dependent diabetes mellitus. *JAMA.* 1994;271(18):1421–1428.

Gear JS, Mann JI, Thorogood M, et al. Biochemical and haematological variables in vegetarians. *Br Med J.* 1980;280(6229):1415.

Gerhard GT, Ahmann A, Meeuws K, et al. Effects of a low-fat diet compared with those of a high-monounsaturated fat diet on body weight, plasma lipids and lipoproteins, and glycemic control in type 2 diabetes. *Am J Clin Nutr.* 2004;80(3):668–673.

Gross LS, Li L, Ford ES, Liu S. Increased consumption of refined carbohydrates and the epidemic of type 2 diabetes in the United States: An ecologic assessment. *Am J Clin Nutr.* 2004;79(5):774–779.

Grundy SM. The optimal ratio of fat-to-carbohydrate in the diet. *Ann Rev Nutr.* 1999;19:325–341.

Ha TK, Lean ME. Recommendations for the nutritional management of patients with diabetes mellitus. *Eur J Clin Nutr.* 1998;52(7):467–481.

Henry RR. Protein content of the diabetic diet. *Diabetes Care.* 1994;17(12):1502–1513.

Hollenbeck CB, Coulston AM, Reaven GM. Comparison of plasma glucose and insulin responses to mixed meals of high-, intermediate-, and low-glycemic potential. *Diabetes Care.* 1988;11(4):323–329.

Hu FB, van Dam R, Liu S. Diet and risk of type II diabetes: The role of types of fat and carbohydrate. *Diabetologia.* 2001;44(7):805–817.

Hua NW, Stoohs RA, Facchini FS. Low iron status and enhanced insulin sensitivity in lacto-ovo vegetarians. *Br J Nutr.* 2001;86(4):515–519.

Ihle BU, Becker GJ, Whitmore JA, et al. The effect of protein restriction on the progression of renal insufficiency. *N Engl J Med.* 1989;321(26):1773–1777.

James WP (Chair), Beaton G, Chung-Ming C, et al. for the World Health Organization (excerpted by editors of *Nutrition Review*). Diet, nutrition, and the prevention of chronic diseases: A report of the WHO Study Group on Diet, Nutrition and Prevention of Noncommunicable Diseases. *Nutr Rev.* 1991;49(10):291–301.

Jayagopal V, Albertazzi P, Kilpatrick ES, et al. Beneficial effects of soy phytoestrogen intake in postmenopausal women with type 2 diabetes. *Diabetes Care.* 2002;25(10):1709–1714.

Jenkins DJ, Kendall CW, Marchie A, et al. Type 2 diabetes and the vegetarian diet. *Am J Clin Nutr.* 2003;78(3, Suppl):610S–616S.

Jiang R, Ma J, Ascherio A, et al. Dietary iron intake and blood donations in relation to risk of type 2 diabetes in men: A prospective cohort study. *Am J Clin Nutr.* 2004;79(1):70-75.

Jibani MM, Bloodworth LL, Foden E, et al. Predominately vegetarian diet in patients with incipient and early clinical diabetic nephropathy: Effects on albumin excretion rate and nutritional status. *Diabetic Med.* 1991;8(10):949-953.

Jones DY, Judd JT, Taylor PR, et al. Influence of caloric contribution and saturation of dietary fat on plasma lipids in premenopausal women. *Am J Clin Nutr.* 1987;45(6):1451-1456.

Joslin E. *The Treatment of Diabetes Mellitus.* 4th ed. Philadelphia: Lea and Febiger; 1928.

Kawate R, Yamakido M, Nishimoto Y, et al. Diabetes mellitus and its vascular complications in Japanese migrants on the Island of Hawaii. *Diabetes Care.* 1979;2(2):161-170.

Kern PA. Lipid disorders in diabetes mellitus. *Mt Sinai J Med.* 1987;54(3):245-252.

King H, Rewers M. Diabetes in adults is now a Third World problem: The W.H.O. Ad Hoc Diabetes Reporting Group. *Bull WHO.* 1991;69(6):643-648.

Kontessis P, Jones S, Dodds R, et al. Renal, metabolic and hormonal responses to ingestion of animal and vegetable proteins. *Kidney Intl.* 1990;38(1):136-144.

Kontessis PA, Bossinakou I, Sarika L, et al. Renal, metabolic, and hormonal responses to proteins of different origin in normotensive, nonproteinuric type I diabetic patients. *Diabetes Care.* 1995;18(9):1233-1240.

Kris-Etherton P. Monounsaturated fatty acids and risk of cardiovascular disease. *Circulation.* 1999;100:1253-1258.

Levey AS, Adler S, Caggiula AW, et al. Effects of dietary protein restriction on the progression of advanced renal disease in the Modification of Diet in Renal Disease study. *Am J Kidney Dis.* 1996;27(5):652-663.

Lichtenstein AH, Schwab US. Relationship of dietary fat to glucose metabolism. *Atherosclerosis.* 2000;150(2):227-243.

Liese AD, Roach AK, Sparks KC, et al. Whole-grain intake and insulin sensitivity: The Insulin Resistance Atherosclerosis study. *Am J Clin Nutr.* 2003;78(5):965-971.

Liu S, Manson JE, Stampfer MJ, et al. A prospective study of whole-grain intake and risk of type 2 diabetes mellitus in US women. *Am J Public Health.* 2000;90(9):1409-1415.

Luscombe ND, Noakes M, Clifton PM. Diets high and low in glycemic index versus high monounsaturated fat diets: Effects on glucose and lipid metabolism in NIDDM. *Eur J Clin Nutr.* 1999;53(6):473-478.

Mann JI. Can dietary intervention produce long-term reduction in insulin resistance? *Br J Nutr.* 2000;83(1, Suppl):S169-S172.

Maschio G, Oldrizzi L, Tessitore N, et al. Early dietary protein and phosphorus restriction is effective in delaying progression of chronic renal failure. *Kidney Intl Suppl.* 1983;16:S273-S277.

Messina M, Messina V. Soyfoods, soybean isoflavones and bone health: A brief overview. *J Renal Nutr.* 2000;10(2):63-68.

Messina M, Messina V. *The Dietitian's Guide to Vegetarian Diets: Issues and Applications.* Gaithersburg, MD: Aspen Publishers; 1996.

Meyer KA, Kushi LH, Jacobs DR, et al. Carbohydrates, dietary fiber, and incident type 2 diabetes in older women. *Am J Clin Nutr.* 2000;71(4):921-930.

Meyer KA, Kushi LH, Jacobs DR, Folsom AR. Dietary fat and incidence of type 2 diabetes in older Iowa women. *Diabetes Care.* 2001;24(9):1528-1535.

Miller JC. Importance of glycemic index in diabetes. *Am J Clin Nutr.* 1994;59(3, Suppl):747S-752S.

Milne RM, Mann JL, Chisholm AW, Williams SM. Long-term comparison of three dietary prescriptions in the treatment of NIDDM. *Diabetes Care.* 1994;17(1):74-80.

Montonen J, Knekt P, Jarvinen R, et al. Whole-grain and fiber intake and the incidence of type 2 diabetes. *Am J Clin Nutr.* 2003;77(3):622-629.

Muntoni S, Cocco P, Aru G, et al. Nutritional factors and worldwide incidence of childhood type 1 diabetes. *Am J Clin Nutr.* 2000;71(6):1525-1529.

Nakamura H, Takasawa M, Kasahara S, et al. Effects of acute protein loads of different sources on renal function of patients with diabetic nephropathy. *Tohoku J Exper Med.* 1989;159(2):153–162.

Nicholson AS, Sklar M, Barnard ND, Gore S, Sullivan R, Browning S. Toward improved management of NIDDM: A randomized, controlled, pilot intervention using a low fat, vegetarian diet. *Preven Med.* 1999;29(2):87–91.

Nutrition Subcommittee, British Diabetic Association Professional Advisory Committee. Dietary recommendations for people with diabetes: An update for the 1990's. *Diabetic Med.* 1992;9: 189–202.

Parillo M, Riccardi G. Diet composition and the risk of type 2 diabetes: Epidemiological and clinical evidence. *Br J Nutr.* 2004;92(1):7–19.

Pedrini M, Levey A, Lau J, Chalmers T, Wang P. The effect of dietary protein restriction on the progression of diabetic and nondiabetic renal diseases: A meta-analysis. *Ann Intern Med.* 1996;124: 627–632.

Percheron C, Colette C, Astre C, Monnier L. Effects of moderate changes in protein intake on urinary albumin excretion in type I diabetic patients. *Nutrition.* 1995;11(4):345–349.

Pereira MA, Jacobs DR, Pins JJ, et al. Effect of whole grains on insulin sensitivity in overweight hyperinsulinemic adults. *Am J Clin Nutr.* 2002;75(5): 848–855.

Perez-Jimenez F, Lopez-Miranda J, Mata P. Protective effect of dietary monounsaturated fat on arteriosclerosis: Beyond cholesterol. *Atherosclerosis.* 2002;163(2):385–398.

Perlstein R, Willcox J, Hines C, Milosavljevic M. Glycemic index in diabetes management. *Aust J Nutr Diet.* 1997;54(2):57–63.

Primary Working Group, Centers for Disease Control and Prevention. Primary prevention of type 2 diabetes mellitus by lifestyle intervention: Implications for health policy. *Ann Intern Med.* 2004;140:951–957.

Reaven GM. How high the carbohydrate? *Diabetologia.* 1980;19(5):409–413.

Riccardi G, Rivellese AA. Effects of dietary fiber and carbohydrate on glucose and lipoprotein metabolism in diabetic patients. *Diabetes Care.* 1991; 14(12):1115–1125.

Riccardi G, Rivellese A, Pacioni D, et al. Separate influence of dietary carbohydrate and fibre on the metabolic control in diabetes. *Diabetologia.* 1984;26(2):116–121.

Rivellese A, Riccardi G, Giacco A, et al. Effect of dietary fibre on glucose control and serum lipoproteins in diabetic patients. *Lancet.* 1980;2(8192): 447–450.

Rivellese AA, Lilli S. Quality of dietary fatty acids, insulin sensitivity and type 2 diabetes. *Biomed Pharmacother.* 2003;57(2):84–87.

Rodriguez-Villar C, Manzanares JM, Casals E, et al. High-monounsaturated fat, olive oil-rich diet has effects similar to a high-carbohydrate diet on fasting and postprandial state and metabolic profiles of patients with type 2 diabetes. *Metabolism.* 2000;49(12):1511–1517.

Rodriguez-Villar C, Perez-Heras A, Mercade I, et al. Comparison of a high-carbohydrate and a high-monounsaturated fat, olive oil-rich diet on the susceptibility of LDL to oxidative modification in subjects with Type 2 diabetes mellitus. *Diabetic Med.* 2004;21(2):142–149.

Ros E. Dietary cis-monounsaturated fatty acids and metabolic control in type 2 diabetes. *Am J Clin Nutr.* 2003;78(3, Suppl):617S–625S.

Rosman JB, ter Wee PM, Meijer S, et al. Prospective randomised trial of early dietary protein restriction in chronic renal failure. *Lancet.* 1984;2(8415): 1291–1296.

Salmeron J, Hu FB, Manson JE, et al. Dietary fat intake and risk of type 2 diabetes in women. *Am J Clin Nutr.* 2001;73(6):1019–1026.

Schulze MB, Liu S, Rimm EB, et al. Glycemic index, glycemic load, and dietary fiber intake and incidence of type 2 diabetes in younger and middle-aged women. *Am J Clin Nutr.* 2004;80(2): 348–356.

Shils M, Olson J, Shike M, Ross A, eds. *Modern Nutrition in Health and Disease.* Philadelphia, PA: Lippincott/Williams and Wilkins; 1999.

Snehalatha C, Sivasankari S, Satyavani K, et al. Postprandial hypertriglyceridaemia in treated type 2 diabetic subjects—The role of dietary components. *Diabetes Res Clin. Pract.* 2000;48(1): 57–60.

Snowdon DA, Phillips RL. Does a vegetarian diet reduce the occurrence of diabetes? *Am J Public Health.* 1985;75(5):507-512.

Song Y, Manson JE, Buring JE, Liu S. A prospective study of red meat consumption and type 2 diabetes in middle-aged and elderly women. *Diabetes Care.* 2004;27(9):2108-2115.

Stevens J, Ahn K, Juhaeri P, et al. Dietary fiber intake and glycemic index and incidence of diabetes in African-American and white adults: The A.R.I.C. Study. *Diabetes Care.* 2002;25(10):1715-1721.

Steyn NP, Mann J, Bennett PH, et al. Diet, nutrition and the prevention of type 2 diabetes. *Public Health Nutr.* 2004;7(1A):147-165.

Stone NJ, Van Horn L. Therapeutic lifestyle change and Adult Treatment Panel III: Evidence then and now. *Curr Atheroscler Reps.* 2002;4(6):433-443.

Toeller M, Buyken A, Heitkamp G, et al. Protein intake and urinary albumin excretion rates in the EURODIAB IDDM Complications study. *Diabetologia.* 1997;40(10):1219-1226.

Trowell HC, Woodgreen MD. Dietary-fiber hypothesis of the etiology of diabetes mellitus. *Diabetes.* 1975;24(8):762-765.

Tsunehara CH, Leonetti DL, Fujimoto WY. Diet of second-generation Japanese-American men with and without non-insulin-dependent diabetes. *Am J Clin Nutr.* 1990;52(4):731-738.

van Dam R, Willett WC, Rimm EB, et al. Dietary fat and meat intake in relation to risk of type 2 diabetes in men. *Diabetes Care.* 2002;25(3):417-424.

Van Horn L. Fiber, lipids, and coronary heart disease. A statement for healthcare professionals from The Nutrition Committee, American Heart Association. *Circulation.* 1997:95(12):2701-2704.

Vessby B. Nutrition, lipids and diabetes mellitus. *Curr Opin Lipidol.* 1995;6(1):3-7.

Walker JD, Dodds RA, Bending J, et al. Restriction of dietary protein and progression of renal failure in diabetic nephropathy. *Lancet.* 1989;2(8677):1411-1415.

Walker KZ, O'Dea K, Nicholson GC, Muir JG. Dietary composition, body weight, and NIDDM: Comparison of high-fiber, high-carbohydrate, and modified-fat diets. *Diabetes Care.* 1995;18(3):401-403.

West KM, Kalbfleisch JM. Influence of nutritional factors on prevalence of diabetes. *Diabetes.* 1971;20(2):99-108.

Willett W, Manson J, Liu S. Glycemic index, glycemic load, and risk of type 2 diabetes. *Am J Clin Nutr.* 2002;76(1):274S-280S.

Wiseman ME, Hunt R, Goodwin A, et al. Dietary composition and renal function in healthy subjects. *Nephron.* 1987;46(1):37-42.

Wiseman MJ, Bognetti E, Dodds R, et al. Changes in renal function in response to protein restricted diet in type I (insulin-dependent) diabetic patients. *Diabetologia.* 1987;30(3):154-159.

Wolever TM. Metabolic effects of continuous feeding. *Metabolism.* 1990;39(9):947-951.

Zeller K, Whittaker E, Sullivan L, et al. Effect of restricting dietary protein on the progression of renal failure in patients with insulin-dependent diabetes mellitus. *N Engl J Med.* 1991;324(2):78-84.

16

Osteoporosis

John J. B. Anderson, PhD
Suzanne Havala Hobbs, DrPH, MS, RD

Introduction

This chapter summarizes the current published reports regarding the effects of vegetarian diets on bone health. Studies that have examined the bone health status of vegetarians and vegans are reviewed. Dietary factors that contribute to good bone health are also discussed. These dietary factors include protein, calcium, vitamin D, phosphorus, isoflavones and other phytoestrogens, and other minerals and vitamins. The chapter concludes with some practical recommendations for making appropriate dietary choices to assure good bone health.

Summary of the Scientific Literature

Studies of Bone Density in Vegetarians and Vegans

Early studies used single-photon absorptiometry (SPA) to measure bone mineral content (BMC) and bone mineral density (BMD) of the forearm bones. As measurement devices im-proved, data obtained using dual-energy X-ray absorptiometry (DXA) have become the standard for comparative bone studies. Many studies linking nutrient intakes with bone measurements (i.e., BMC and BMD) have been reported, but only a relatively small number of prospective studies have included information on vegetarians of any type (Reed, Tylavsky, & Anderson, 1994; Parsons et al., 1997; Barr et al., 1998).

Clinically diagnosed osteoporosis among vegetarians is considered to be similar to clinically diagnosed osteoporosis among omnivores. Measurements of BMC and BMD suggest similar patterns of early life development and then decay of the skeleton in late life in both vegetarians and omnivores (Garn, 1970).

Few data exist on skeletal measurements of vegans. Although strict vegetarians (vegans) might be considered at greater risk for osteoporosis than other vegetarians, because of the exclusion of dairy products, reports of measurements of BMC and BMD of adult vegans versus other types of vegetarians and omnivores remain inconclusive.

Early bone gain in prepubertal boys and girls may be critical for accumulating optimal bone mass, also known as *peak bone mass*, by about age 16 years for girls and later for boys. Adequate calcium intake seems to be most critical for optimal bone accrual (Parsons et al., 1997). So, vegetarian boys and girls must be doing reasonably well in their dietary intake of calcium, because they are accruing BMC similar to that of omnivorous adolescents, at least in the United States. In fact, a cross-sectional study of U.S. children consuming high fruit and vegetable intakes on a daily basis, compared to low consumers, showed beneficial effects on several bone parameters, including whole-body BMC and BMD (Tylavsky et al., 2004).

A vegetarian macrobiotic diet fed to young children in the Netherlands was found, at 9–15 years of age, to contribute to lower BMC measurements compared to control omnivores (Parsons et al., 1997). Such low BMC values have not been reported for vegetarian children in the United States.

Dietary Variables and Bone

Linkages between single dietary variables, such as calcium or isoflavones, and bone measurements have advanced our understanding of the potential benefits of vegetarian diets for bone health. This section attempts to explain how several individual nutrients may affect bone measurements—both positively and negatively. Keep in mind, however, that the overall benefits to bone may result more from a combination of these factors and a generally healthy lifestyle than from one or another of the individual nutrients alone. Also, short-term changes in dietary patterns are not likely to affect bone health, because of the slow turnover of bone tissue. Over the long term, however, dietary changes may have a large effect.

Protein

Bone tissue requires dietary protein for the synthesis of bone-specific proteins such as collagen and many cellular components. Amino acids from dietary sources, both plant and animal, are mixed in a random manner to make these bone proteins. Adverse effects typically occur when protein intake is not sufficient (<10% of total energy): growth ceases or continues at suboptimal rates. Conversely, excessive protein intake, especially from animal sources, may contribute to bone loss.

Animal proteins and plant proteins appear to have different effects on bone. Animal proteins contain fairly large amounts of sulfur in sulfur-containing amino acids and phosphorus bound to a few specific amino acids, especially in dairy proteins such as casein. The metabolism of these sulfur- and phosphate-containing amino acids generates inorganic acids that are excreted via the kidneys. As a consequence of this acidic environment, calcium ions are lost in the urine. When still circulating in blood, these inorganic acids also require buffering, or neutralizing, by bases from the skeleton. To achieve this neutralization, bone mineral is partially dissolved to release phosphate, a buffering agent. Calcium is released from bone along with phosphate. The net result of a high acid load is to increase losses of both BMC and BMD.

Acid generation resulting from the metabolism of sulfur- and phosphate-containing amino acids is greatly reduced in those who consume a vegetarian diet, compared to omnivores, because vegetarian diets contain less sulfur- and phosphate-containing amino acids. Vegetarians, in general, have less acidic urine (pH 6–8) than omnivores (pH <6). Strict vegetarians (vegans) have even higher urinary pH values, leaning toward the basic (pH > 7). This less acidic (or more basic) urine has long-term benefits for the skeleton: specifically, greater retention of mineral in bone (Barzel & Massey, 1998; Bushinsky, 1996) and potentially higher BMC and BMD (New et al., 2004), because there is less acid in the body that must be buffered by mineral removed from the skeleton.

Calcium and Vitamin D

Calcium and vitamin D are considered the most critical nutrients involved in bone development and maintenance. Adequate amounts of both nutrients are crucial to good bone health (Abrams & Stuff, 1994). Vitamin D, because of its stimulation of intestinal calcium absorption, increases the amount of calcium available for bone formation (Anderson & Toverud, 1993). Only a few prospective trials of the relationship between dietary calcium and bone in lacto-ovo vegetarians or vegans have been reported (Reed, Tylavsky, & Anderson, 1994; Parsons et al., 1997; Barr et al., 1998). Clearly, more investigations are needed on this linkage.

In lacto vegetarian diets, low intakes of calcium and vitamin D are unlikely, but deficits may exist if only limited amounts of milk and cheese are consumed. Intakes of both these nutrients are low in traditional vegan diets in the absence of fortification (calcium or vitamin D added to specific foods) or supplementation. Adult vegans who consumed calcium-enriched diets (e.g., calcium-fortified soy milk or calcium-fortified orange juice) and have reasonable calcium intakes (~800 mg/day) have been reported to have average bone measurements at five years of follow-up. Bone data of vegans were not different from mean values of lacto-ovo vegetarians or omnivores in this study, in which vitamin D intakes were presumed to be adequate (Reed, Tylavsky, & Anderson, 1994). Another prospective study, this one of premenopausal vegans, also found that

a long-term vegetarian diet with adequate calcium and vitamin D resulted in good bone measurements (Barr et al., 1998).

Table 16.1 summarizes the findings of the two prospective investigations (Reed, Tylavsky, & Anderson, 1994; Barr et al., 1998) that have examined the relationship between dietary calcium intake and bone health in adult women, plus a third investigation of children from the Netherlands who were raised on a macrobiotic vegan diet (Parsons et al., 1997). In contrast to previously published cross-sectional studies (Marsh et al., 1980; Tylavsky & Anderson, 1988; Hunt et al., 1989; Tesar et al., 1992), little or no skeletal benefits of dietary calcium (or diet as a whole) were found for vegetarians compared to omnivores. The cross-sectional studies, however, are now considered to have design flaws, including selection bias that cast doubt on the conclusions of the reports. Therefore, the focus here is on the prospective studies with more validity (listed in Table 16.1). In the prospective investigation of 49 lacto-ovo vegetarian (LOV) postmenopausal women, who were compared to 140 omnivorous postmenopausal women, bone loss measured as BMD over the 5-year period occurred at similar rates in each group, independent of dietary calcium intake (996 mg/d for omnivores and 733 mg/d for LOVs) (Reed, Tylavsky, & Anderson, 1994). In the study of a small number of premenopausal vegetarian and nonvegetarian women, dietary calcium intake did not seem to be a major determinant of BMD (Barr et al., 1998). In summary, the two prospective studies of adult women suggest that other variables, such as body weight and physical activity, may be more critical determinants of BMD than dietary calcium or other nutrients. Further research is needed on the relation of calcium intake to bone accrual by adolescent vegetarians, because only the one study (Parsons et al., 1997) has been done on boys and girls.

Table 16.1   Prospective Investigations of the Relationship between Calcium Intake Patterns and Bone in Vegetarians and Omnivores

Reference	Subjects	Ages	Duration	Bone Measurements	Conclusions
Reed, Tylavsky, & Anderson, 1994	U.S. LOVs vs. omnivores; postmenopausal females	> 60	5 years	Forearm BMD was same in both groups over 5-year period.	Dietary calcium had no effect on BMD.
Barr et al., 1998	Canadian women; vegetarian vs. nonvegetarian		13 months	Vertebral BMD remained the same in vegetarians, increased in nonvegetarians.	No effect of diet on BMD. Lower BMI of vegetarians key to lower BMD.
Parsons et al., 1997	Dutch babies; follow-up vs. control; boys and girls		9–15 years	Total body BMC and regional BMC.	Vegan* children had lower BMC. BMC was unrelated to dietary calcium, physical activity.

*Vegan = macrobiotic
Abbreviations:
   BMC = bone mineral content
   BMD = bone mineral density
   LOV = lacto-ovo vegetarian

Ratio of Calcium to Phosphorus in the Diet

The calcium-to-phosphorus (Ca:P) ratio in the diet has been examined in only a few studies. One group of researchers found that a low dietary Ca:P ratio results in a chronic elevation of parathyroid hormone (PTH), a hormone that contributes to bone loss; and an elevation, though less robust, in the active hormonal form of vitamin D, which improves calcium absorption (Calvo, Kumar, & Heath, 1990). The longest study was conducted for only 28 days, which makes it difficult to extrapolate to long-term losses in bone mass and density, because adaptation to the low Ca:P diet may occur.

Excessive consumption of dietary phosphorus, especially from cola-type beverages and foods with significant amounts of phosphorus additives, is considered to contribute to bone loss (Anderson et al., 2001). In the typical vegan diet, rich in cereal grains, much of the phosphorus is bound as phosphates to phytate, which makes the phosphorus much less bioavailable and, hence, improves the Ca:P ratio from a practical standpoint. Phosphates incorporated in dietary phospholipids in typical animal foods, in contrast, are digested and readily available for intestinal absorption; thus, these phosphate ions can disturb calcium homeostasis and increase PTH following a meal.

Other Minerals

Sodium is generally considered to exert adverse effects on calcium status. Excessive sodium intake is associated with increased loss of calcium in urine (Nordin et al., 1993). The diets of lacto-ovo vegetarians typically have less sodium (and more potassium) than the diets of omnivores (Tucker et al., 1999).

In contrast to sodium, dietary potassium, which is abundant in plant-based foods, has a positive influence on skeletal heath (New et al., 2000). Adequate potassium intake helps keep bone cells healthy by maintaining an adequate electrical charge differential across bone cell membranes. Excessive sodium intake tends to adversely affect both this charge differential and the intracellular functions of potassium. Dietary potassium also helps by neutralizing the acid generated from animal proteins containing amino acids with sulfur and phosphate. Additionally, high potassium intakes tend to decrease urinary calcium loss, whereas excessive dietary sodium intakes tend to increase urinary calcium loss. Vegetarian diets yield skeletal benefits by being low in acid-generating amino acids and by providing potassium.

Magnesium is found in large quantities in bone. About 60%–70% of all magnesium in the body is found in the skeleton, but its role in this tissue is not known except as an enzyme activator within bone cells. Magnesium is utilized by approximately 300 enzymes. The reason for the large amount of magnesium in bone may be simply that bone serves as a reservoir. Magnesium intake has been reported to be associated with greater BMD, especially of the hip, in elderly women and men (Tucker et al., 1999). Because vegetarian diets are typically much higher in magnesium than are nonvegetarian diets, magnesium-rich diets may protect against osteoporotic fractures.

Iron is important for bone health, in part because of its role in collagen formation, but relatively few human data on the role of this mineral in bone have been reported. Iron deficiencies may be critical for females, especially those involved in sports such as distance running. A case study of a lacto-ovo vegetarian university cross-country runner with stress fractures suggests that she had been consuming an iron-poor diet for several years (Anderson

et al., 1998). Whether her iron-deficiency anemia was directly or indirectly responsible for her stress fractures has not been established.

Soy Isoflavones and Other Phytoestrogens

The relation of soy isoflavones and other phytoestrogens to bone health has not been settled yet, but several studies suggest skeletal benefits of the isoflavones alone or the isoflavones together with soy protein. It has been known for almost two decades that the consumption of soy protein with isoflavones, compared to lactoalbumin, reduces the amount of calcium lost in the urine over several hours (up to 24 hours) following consumption (Anderson, Thomsen, & Christiansen, 1987). So, vegetarians who consume soy foods may lose less calcium in the urine than omnivores who consume meats and other animal foods.

Isoflavones, with or without soy protein, have also been shown to have bone-sparing effects in some (Alekel et al., 2000; Potter et al., 1998), but not all (Arjmandi & Smith, 2002) studies of peri- and postmenopausal women. One study of young women (20–25 years old) showed clearly that isoflavones had no effect on BMC or BMD (Anderson et al., 2002). Other perspectives on the isoflavone–bone relationship may be found in published reviews (Migliaccio & Anderson, 2003; Vincent & Fitzpatrick, 2000; Anthony, Anderson, & Alekel, 2003).

Vegetarians, in general, consume more isoflavones and phytoestrogens than nonvegetarians. This consumption pattern may be advantageous for bone health.

Vitamin K

Vitamin K has a beneficial effect on bone through its role in the production of a few proteins that, in addition to collagen, help make up the organic matrix of bone tissue. These matrix proteins assist in the normal mineralization of bone during formation of new bone tissue. In a prospective, randomized, controlled trial of early postmenopausal women (50–60 years of age), vitamin K decreased bone loss when supplemented along with calcium, vitamin D, magnesium, and zinc (Braam et al., 2004). Although frank deficiency of vitamin K has not resulted in major changes in bone tissue, optimal intakes of this fat-soluble vitamin help maintain bone, especially in the elder years. The bone structural changes resulting from vitamin K deficits are similar to those seen with vitamin D deficiency.

Vitamin K is provided almost entirely by plant sources. Intakes of vitamin K by vegetarians are greater than by omnivores.

Vitamin C

Vitamin C has long been known to be essential for the synthesis of collagen during new bone formation. These maturation reactions also require iron to produce the hydroxylysine and hydroxyproline residues that enhance the bending capability of the triple strands of mature collagen deposited as the major protein of the bone matrix. High intakes of vitamin C may contribute to greater BMD (Hall & Greendale, 1998). Further research is needed to corroborate this conclusion; we know, though, that vegetarians typically consume more vitamin C than do nonvegetarians.

Vitamin B12

A low concentration of plasma vitamin B12 (cobalamin) was found to be associated with low BMD in the Framingham osteoporosis study (Tucker et al., 2005). The important message of this report is that cobalamin may be critical for bone formation, and that low intakes may

place older adults at risk of osteoporotic fractures. This relatively new finding will have to be replicated in other investigations.

Dietary Fats

Free fatty acids in the small intestine can combine with calcium ions (and other minerals), thereby reducing calcium absorption by the gut. Also, omega-3 polyunsaturated fatty acids (PFAs) are now thought to improve bone formation and bone health during skeletal growth in early life, and also to help maintain bone in the adult years (Watkins et al., 2003; Reinwald et al., 2004).

The low-fat diets of vegetarians, especially vegans, are likely to result in fewer free fatty acids in the distal small intestine that can potentially reduce the intestinal absorption of calcium, magnesium, and other minerals. Vegans, however, typically have a lower intake of the bone-protecting omega-3 PFAs than do those who consume fish.

Lifestyle Factors That Influence Vegetarian Diets

Several lifestyle factors of vegetarians also may have positive or negative effects on bone health. Two of these are estrogen status and physical activity.

Estrogen status among premenopausal vegetarians, especially vegans, may be compromised by the high-fiber, high-plant-protein diet. The major reasons for lower serum estrogen concentrations and earlier menopause among strict vegetarians may be their lower lifetime fat intake, less fat storage, and limited conversion of androstenedione (an adrenal steroid) to estrogens in fat and other tissues (Anderson, 1999). Lower concentrations of circulating estrogens permit PTH to be more effective in increasing

Table 16.2 Major Dietary Factors Affecting Bone Health

Beneficial	Comment
Calcium	In DRI amounts; promotes PBM and suppresses PTH
Vitamin D	In DRI amounts; promotes Ca absorption and bone mineralization
Protein	In DRI amounts; promotes synthesis of bone proteins
Phosphorus	In DRI amounts; promotes bone mineral
Vitamin K	In DRI amounts; modifies bone matrix proteins
Magnesium	In DRI amounts; promotes bone cell functions
Potassium	In DRI amounts; promotes bone cell functions
Vitamin C	In DRI amounts; aids maturation of collagen
Energy	In DRI amounts; promotes PBM accrual and bone health

Adverse	Comment
Phosphorus	In excess; low Ca:P ratio increases PTH secretion and bone loss
Protein	In excess, especially animal protein; produces acid and bone loss
Sodium	In excess; proximal tubule (kidney) reabsorbs less Ca; Ca loss
Vitamin A	In excess; adversely alters bone tissue, especially hip; fracture
Calcium	Too little; results in low PBM development and maintenance
Vitamin D	Too little; lowers mineralization of bone
Protein	Too little; reduces synthesis of bone matrix proteins
Energy	Too little; reduces bone formation
Vitamin K	Too little; reduces maturation of matrix proteins
Vitamin C	Too little; reduces modification of collagen in bone tissue
Magnesium	Too little; reduces bone cell function and may contribute to loss
Potassium	Too little; reduces bone cell functions

Abbreviations:
Ca = calcium
DRI = Dietary Reference Intake
P = phosphorus (phosphate)
PBM = peak bone mass
PTH = parathyroid hormone

bone resorption and increases the fragility of the skeleton.

Physical activity itself is a strong promoter of bone health, assuming that nutritional intake is sufficient to meet all the nutrient needs of bone tissue. The major benefit of exercise is that gravitational forces that affect the muscle-bone linkages are potent stimulators of bone cells that promote new bone formation. Regular activity of practically all types, including gardening, walking, dancing, and sports, has modest protective effects on the skeleton (Kanders, Dempster, & Lindsay, 1988; Anderson, 2000). Regular exercise is a common feature of vegetarian lifestyles.

Summary

Many dietary factors influence bone development and maintenance. Table 16.2 summarizes several dietary variables in vegetarian diets that affect bone, either positively or negatively. Table 16.3 lists several foods that provide the nutrients critical for bone health. The benefits and disadvantages to bone health of a vegan diet are contrasted in Table 16.4. The totality of the vegetarian diet in the context of the environment of the individual is what determines health status. A well-balanced diet typically provides sufficient servings, according to the vegetarian food guide (Messina, Melina, & Mangels, 2003),

Table 16.3   Good Food Sources of Potassium, Magnesium, and Vitamins C, D, and K

Micronutrient	Food Sources
Potassium	Practically all fruits and vegetables
Magnesium	Fruits and vegetables, especially dark greens
Vitamin C	Fruits and vegetables
Vitamin D	Fortified cow's milk or soy milk
Vitamin K	Vegetables, especially dark greens

Table 16.4   The Benefits and Disadvantages to Bone Health of a Vegan Diet

Benefits
- Sufficient, yet marginal protein intake[*]
- Sufficient energy from macronutrients[*]
- Sufficient potassium[+]
- Sufficient magnesium[+]
- Sufficient vitamin K[+]
- Low sodium[*]

Disadvantages
- Low calcium intake and relatively low bioavailability of calcium in fortified soy milk
- Low vitamin D intake
- Low iron intake, especially lack of heme iron
- Low omega-3 (n-3) polyunsaturated fatty acids
- Low or limited intake of vitamin B12 (without supplementation)

[*]Less than in omnivores
[+]More than in omnivores

of all the bone-active nutrients, assuming that a vegan diet is fortified or supplemented with calcium and vitamin D. Other lifestyle factors are also important for both developing and maintaining bone.

Practical Aspects

Despite the low bioavailability of calcium from fortified soy milk compared to cow's milk (Heaney et al., 2000), soy milk is a practical non-dairy source of calcium from a quantitative perspective. Although the bioavailability is less, soy milk provides an almost equivalent amount of calcium compared to milk-based formulas. It is generally recommended that calcium-fortified soy milk be substituted for cow's milk on approximately a one-to-one basis.

Vegetarians may need to obtain calcium from dietary sources other than soy milk when, for instance, cost or soy allergy precludes consumption of soy milk in amounts that meet the recommendations for adequate calcium intake. Low amounts of calcium per serving exist in many other foods. The bioavailability of calcium from many greens and legumes is typically higher than for cow's milk, but these foods are often eaten in quantities insufficient to equal the amount of calcium present in the three to four daily servings of cow's milk currently recommended in the dietary guidelines.

The vegetarian food guide prepared by Messina and colleagues (Messina, Melina, & Mangels, 2003) provides examples of vegetarian foods in North America that contain fair or good amounts of calcium and other nutrients that support healthy bone development and maintenance. This food guide suggests that adequate intakes of calcium may be obtained from plant sources alone. The food guide recommends 8 servings per day of calcium-rich plant foods, especially calcium-fortified soy milk, for healthy adults (including pregnant and lactating women); 6 servings per day for children aged 4 to 8 years; and 10 servings per day for adolescents. Examples of rich plant sources of calcium include fortified fruit juice; figs; and leafy greens such as bok choy, broccoli, collards, kale, and Chinese cabbage; as well as fortified soy milk, tempeh, almonds, calcium-set tofu, cooked soybeans, soy nuts, and almond butter or sesame tahini.

Vegans need to be diligent about consuming calcium from a wide range of foods and in sufficient amounts to meet the Dietary Reference Intakes. Although it is presumed that nutrient requirements of vegetarians are no different from those of nonvegetarians, vegetarians may have some tradeoff protection from lower calcium intakes because they consume reduced amounts of animal protein and sodium, both of which increase urinary calcium losses.

Plant foods, which contain good amounts of potassium, magnesium, vitamin K, and vitamin C, should be consumed in sufficient amounts to develop and maintain good bone health. Fortified foods are the major sources of vitamin D for vegetarians, unless these individuals also consume a vitamin supplement. Toxicity of vitamin D occurs only at intakes much greater than current DRIs, so concerns about excessive consumption from fortified foods may no longer be warranted. Good amounts of these important nutrients for bone health are found in many foods (see Table 16.3).

Information is emerging that bone health may benefit from omega-3 fatty acids such as linolenic acid, EPA, and DHA. Plant foods that are rich sources of alpha-linolenic acid include flaxseed, walnuts, soybeans, and canola oil. There is only limited conversion of alpha-linolenic acid to EPA (5%–10%) and DHA (<5%); therefore, because the primary sources of EPA and DHA are fish and seafood, vegetarians may not be able to obtain adequate amounts of EPA and DHA. Eggs do provide a reasonable amount of DHA for lacto-ovo vegetarians, and about 10%–11% of DHA is retroconverted back to EPA. One would expect, therefore, that vegans (who do not consume eggs) would be at greater risk for DHA and EPA deficiency than lacto-ovo vegetarians and nonvegetarians. One report suggests, however, that vegans may have an enhanced efficiency of conversion from alpha-linolenic acid to EPA and DHA (Siscovick, Lemaitre, & Mozaffarian, 2003). More research is needed to determine the amounts that should be con-

sumed each day from foods and/or supplements. Unquestionably, food sources of omega-3 fatty acids are preferred, up to 3 g a day, but a supplement may be beneficial for those with documented cardiovascular disease. (The Food and Drug Administration has issued a qualified health claim for omega-3 fatty acids that is based on promising, though not definitive, research suggesting that these fatty acids reduce the risk of coronary heart disease.)

Limiting the consumption of heavily processed foods and foods with sodium salt additives is also considered to provide skeletal benefits, because of the more efficient renal reabsorption and, hence, conservation of calcium by the body when dietary sodium is lower (Massey & Whiting, 1996).

Of course, for best effects, healthy diets should be accompanied by healthy lifestyles. Physical activity is important to maintain good bone health. In addition, a nonsmoking lifestyle is very important, because smoking has adverse effects on the skeleton and may be an important risk factor for osteoporotic fractures. Certain drugs, such as corticosteroids, also are potent risk factors for osteoporosis.

Conclusion

This chapter provides background on the linkages between vegetarian eating practices and bone health. Many dietary factors remain important for the nutritional support of bone. They must be provided in optimal amounts for good bone development, bone health and maintenance during adult life, and fracture prevention during late life. The multifactorial nature of good bone health makes it difficult to identify the most critical determinants.

Published evidence now makes it abundantly clear that vegetarians can obtain sufficient amounts of all the nutrients that support normal age-specific bone measurements, with the possible exception that omega-3 PFAs may not be easily obtained in sufficient amounts. For greater assurance of nutrient adequacy, a once-per-day, age-specific, multinutrient supplement supplying not more than 100% of nutrient DRIs is recommended.

Though doubters may still exist, physical activity has now been established to be the single most robust contributor to bone development and maintenance throughout the life cycle.

Acknowledgments

The careful review of this manuscript by Martin Kohlmeier, MD, is appreciated. Also, assistance in preparing this manuscript by Agna Boass, PhD, is acknowledged. The support of and sharing of an unpublished manuscript by Bjorn Pettersson of Sweden, who reviewed data from practically all published bone studies of vegetarians, is appreciated.

References

Abrams SA, Stuff JE. Calcium metabolism in girls: Current dietary intakes lead to low rates of calcium absorption and retention during puberty. *Am J Clin Nutr.* 1994;60:739-743.

Alekel DL, St. Germain A, Peterson CT, et al. Isoflavone-rich soy protein isolate attenuates bone loss in the lumbar spine of perimenopausal women. *Am J Clin Nutr.* 2000;72:844-852.

Anderson JJB. The important role of physical activity in skeletal development: How exercise may counter low calcium intake. *Am J Clin Nutr.* 2000;71:1384-1386.

Anderson JJB. Plant-based diets and bone health: Nutritional implications. *Am J Clin Nutr.* 1999;70 (Suppl):539S-542S.

Anderson JJB, Chen XW, Boass A, et al. No effects on bone mineral content and bone mineral density in healthy, menstruating adult young women after one year. *J Am Coll Nutr.* 2002;21:388-393.

Anderson JJB, Sell ML, Garner SC, Calvo MS. Phosphorus. In: Bowman BA, Russell RM, eds. *Present Knowledge in Nutrition.* 8th ed. Washington, DC: ILSI Press; 2001:281-291.

Anderson JJB, Stender M, Rondano P, et al. Nutrition and bone in physical activity and sport. In: Wolinsky I, ed. *Nutrition in Exercise and Sport.* 3d ed. Boca Raton, FL: CRC Press; 1998:219-244.

Anderson JJB, Thomsen K, Christiansen C. High protein meals, insular hormones and urinary calcium excretion in human subjects. In: Christiansen C, Johansen JS, Riis BJ, eds. *Osteoporosis.* Vol. 1. Copenhagen: Osteopress ApS; 1987:240-244.

Anderson JJB, Toverud SU. Diet and vitamin D: A review with an emphasis on human function. *J Nutr Biochem.* 1993;5:58-65.

Anthony MS, Anderson JJB, Alekel L. Association between soy and/or isoflavones and bone: New evidence from epidemiologic studies. In: Gilani GS, Anderson JJB, eds. *Phytoestrogens and Health.* Champaign, IL: AOCS Press; 2003:331-340.

Arjmandi BH, Smith BJ. Soy isoflavones' osteoprotective role in postmenopausal women. *J Nutr Biochem.* 2002;13:130-137.

Barr SI, Prior JC, Janelle KC, Lentle BC. Spinal bone mineral density in premenopausal vegetarian and nonvegetarian women: Cross-sectional and prospective comparisons. *J Am Diet Assoc.* 1998;98:760-765.

Barzel US, Massey LK. Excess dietary protein can adversely affect bone. *J Nutr.* 1998;128:1051-1053.

Braam LA, Knapen MH, Geusens P, et al. Vitamin K$_1$ supplementation retards bone loss in postmenopausal women between 50 and 60 years of age. *Calcified Tissue Intl.* 2004;73:21-26.

Bushinsky DA. Metabolic alkalosis decreases bone calcium efflux by suppressing osteoclasts and stimulating osteoblasts. *Am J Physiol.* 1996;271:F216-F222.

Calvo MS, Kumar R, Heath H III. Persistently elevated parathyroid hormone secretion and action in young women after four weeks of ingesting high phosphorus low calcium diets. *J Clin Endocr Metab.* 1990;70:1334-1340.

Garn S. *The Earlier Gain and the Later Loss of Cortical Bone.* Boca Raton, FL: Charles C Thomas; 1970.

Hall SL, Greendale GA. The relation of dietary vitamin C intake to bone mineral density: Results from the PEPI study. *Calcified Tissue Intl.* 1998; 63:183–189.

Heaney RP, Dowell MS, Rafferty K, Bierman J. Bioavailability of the calcium in fortified soy imitation milk, with some observations on method. *Am J Clin Nutr.* 2000;71(5):1166–1169.

Hunt IF, Murphy NJ, Henderson C, et al. Bone mineral content in postmenopausal women: Comparison of omnivores and vegetarians. *Am J Clin Nutr.* 1989;50:517–523.

Kanders B, Dempster DW, Lindsay R. Interaction of calcium and physical activity of bone mass in young women. *J Bone Miner Res.* 1988;3:145–149.

Marsh AG, Sanchez TV, Mickelsen O, et al. Bone mineral mass in adult lacto-ovo-vegetarian and omnivorous women. *J Am Diet Assoc.* 1980;76: 148–151.

Massey LK, Whiting SJ. Dietary salt, urinary calcium, and bone loss: A review. *J Bone Miner Res.* 1996; 11:731–736.

Messina V, Melina V, Mangels AR. A new food guide for North American vegetarians. *J Am Diet Assoc.* 2003;103(6):771–775.

Migliaccio S, Anderson JJB. Isoflavones and skeletal health: Are they ready for clinical application? *Osteoporosis Intl.* 2003;14:361–368.

New SA, Macdonald HM, Campbell MK, et al. Positive association between net endogenous non-carbonic acid production (NEAP) and indexes of bone health in peri- and postmenopausal women. *Am J Clin Nutr.* 2004;79:131–138.

New SA, Robins SP, Campbell MK, et al. Dietary influences on bone mass and bone metabolism: Further evidence of a positive link between fruit and vegetable consumption and bone health? *Am J Clin Nutr.* 2000;71:142–151.

Nordin BEC, Need AG, Morris HA, Horowitz M. The nature and significance of the relationship between urinary sodium and urinary calcium in women. *J Nutr.* 1993;123:1615–1623.

Parsons TJ, van Dusseldorp MV, van der Vliet M, et al. Reduced bone mass in Dutch adolescents fed a macrobiotic diet early in life. *J Bone Miner Res.* 1997;12:1486–1494.

Potter SM, Baum JA, Teng H, et al. Soy protein and isoflavones: Their effects on blood lipids and bone density in postmenopausal women. *Am J Clin Nutr.* 1998;68(Suppl):1375S–1379S.

Reed JA, Tylavsky FA, Anderson JJB. Comparative changes in radial bone density of elderly female lactoovovegetarians and omnivores. *Am J Clin Nutr.* 1994;59(Suppl):1197S–2002S.

Reinwald S, Li Y, Moriguchi T, et al. Repletion with (n-3) fatty acids reverses bone structural deficits in (n-3)-deficient rats. *J Nutr.* 2004;134:388–394.

Siscovick DS, Lemaitre RN, Mozaffarian D. The fish story: A diet-heart hypothesis with clinical implications: n-3 polyunsaturated fatty acids, myocardial vulnerability, and sudden death. *Circulation.* 2003;107:2632–2634.

Tesar R, Notelovitz M, Shim E, Dauwell G, Brown J. Axial and peripheral bone density and nutrient intakes of postmenopausal vegetarian and omnivorous women. *Am J Clin Nutr.* 1992;56: 699–704.

Tucker KL, Hannan HT, Qiao N, et al. Low plasma vitamin B12 is associated with lower BMD: The Framingham Osteoporosis study. *J Bone Miner Res.* 2005;20:152–158.

Tucker KL, Hannan MT, Chen H, et al. Potassium and fruit and vegetables are associated with greater bone mineral density in elderly men and women. *Am J Clin Nutr.* 1999;69:727–736.

Tylavsky FA, Anderson JJB. Dietary factors in bone health of elderly lactoovovegetarian and omnivorous women. *Am J Clin Nutr.* 1988;48:842–849.

Tylavsky FA, Holliday K, Danish R, et al. Fruit and vegetable intake is an independent predictor of bone size in early-pubertal children. *Am J Clin Nutr.* 2004;79:311–317.

Vincent A, Fitzpatrick LA. Soy isoflavones: Are they useful in menopause? *Mayo Clin Proc.* 2000;75:1174–1184.

Watkins BA, Li Y, Lippman HE, Feng S. Modulatory effect of omega-3 polyunsaturated fatty acids on osteoblast function and bone metabolism. *Prostaglandins, Leukotrienes, Essential Fatty Acids.* 2003;68:387–398.

17

Gallbladder Disease, Diverticulitis, Appendicitis, Kidney Stones, and Kidney Failure

Valerie Kurtzhalts, MSN, APRN, BC
Peggy Carlson, MD

Introduction

This chapter investigates several diseases that are very prevalent in, and cause a significant amount of illness in, the United States. The first three are diseases of the digestive system: namely, gallbladder disease, diverticular disease, and appendicitis. We also discuss two common diseases of the kidneys: namely, kidney stones and kidney failure (chronic renal failure). In each case, we look at whether and how dietary factors and vegetarian diets can affect the incidence and/or progression of the disease.

Summary of the Scientific Literature

Gallbladder Disease

Gallbladder disease afflicts more than 20 million Americans, with approximately 1 million new cases diagnosed each year (Simon & Hudes, 1998; Tseng, Everhart, & Sandler, 1999). Gallstones account for more than 95% of gallbladder problems and result in more than 500,000

surgeries annually (National Institute of Diabetes and Digestive and Kidney Diseases [NIDDKD], 1993). In the United States, the cost attributable to gallstone disease and its complications has been estimated to be $6 billion to $8 billion yearly, representing approximately 1% of the national health care budget (Cotran, Kumar, & Collins, 1999).

The gallbladder is a pear-shaped sac located in the upper right quadrant of the abdominal cavity. It acts as a storage reservoir for bile received from the liver through the hepatic duct. The gallbladder itself is not necessary for biliary function, but bile, which is composed of water, cholesterol, lipids, bile salts, and bilirubin, is essential for the digestion and absorption of dietary fats. Bile is released, as needed, from the gallbladder through the common bile duct into the small intestine to aid in digestion. Gallstones can form from bile and accumulate in the gallbladder. Based on their composition, gallstones are classified as either cholesterol stones, pigment (bilirubin) stones, or amorphous stones (amorphous material, bile pigment, calcium, and protein) (Dowling, 2000). Choles-

250

terol stones are the most common type of gallstones in Western society. Increased biliary secretion of cholesterol from the liver, along with stasis and factors affecting cholesterol precipitation in the gallbladder, are thought to contribute to the formation of cholesterol stones (Tseng, Everhart, & Sandler, 1999).

When gallstones cause blockage of the duct leading out of the gallbladder, severe pain can result. Acute or chronic inflammation of the gallbladder is almost always associated with gallstones. Although not scientifically proven to cause cancer, gallstones are present in 60%–90% of the cases of carcinoma of the gallbladder, and it is presumed that the chronic irritation and trauma associated with gallstones may play a contributing role in cancer (Cotran, Kumar, & Collins, 1999).

The incidence of gallstones increases with age, and women are affected twice as often as men. Obesity has been identified as a major risk factor for the development of gallstones. Other risk factors include genetic predisposition, ethnicity, pregnancy, use of oral contraceptives or estrogen replacement, and rapid weight-loss diets.

Two studies have looked at the incidence of gallstones in vegetarians compared with nonvegetarians. Pixley et al. (1985) studied 762 women and found that 25% of the 632 nonvegetarians and 12% of the 130 vegetarians had gallstones visible on ultrasound or had previously had their gallbladders removed because of gallbladder disease. After controlling for two other known risk factors (body weight and age), the nonvegetarian women were found to have 1.9 times greater risk of developing gallstones compared to the vegetarian women. Kratzer et al. (1997) studied 1,116 blood donors with abdominal ultrasounds. Gallbladder disease (gallstones revealed by ultrasound or history of gallbladder removal) was found in 5.8% of the men and 6.8% of the women. Of the

48 vegetarians in the study, none were found to have gallstones.

One reason that vegetarians may have a lower incidence of gallstones is their generally lower body weight. Many studies have shown that obesity is strongly correlated with an increased risk of gallstone formation (Tseng, Everhart, & Sandler, 1999). Vegetarians are less likely to be overweight than meat eaters, and this fact may contribute to their lower risk of gallstones.

Dietary factors may be another reason for the lower incidence of gallstones among vegetarians. Diet has long been considered a potential risk factor for the development of gallstones. This conclusion is based partly on epidemiologic studies. Industrialized countries have a higher incidence of gallbladder disease than developing countries (Tseng, Everhart, & Sandler, 1999; Pixley & Mann, 1988; Smith & Gee, 1979; Burkitt & Tunstall, 1975). In addition, several studies have shown that among populations, as diets become more westernized, the risk for the development of gallstones increases (Tseng, Everhart, & Sandler, 1999; Smith & Gee, 1979; Burkitt & Tunstall, 1975).

Although epidemiologic studies and studies of vegetarians suggest that diet is implicated in the development of gallstones, the specific dietary factors that account for this effect have not yet been clearly elucidated. There are theoretical reasons why fiber might decrease the risk of gallstones. For instance, fiber decreases intestinal transport time; that is, it speeds up transport of material through the intestine. One effect of this decreased transport time is decreased absorption of cholesterol (the primary component of gallstones) and deoxycholic acid (a bile acid that has been linked to increased gallstone formation) (Dowling, 2000). It has been suggested that decreased transport times may lower intestinal pH, which may in turn decrease the absorption of deoxycholic acid (Dowling, 2000). Faster transport time may also decrease the time available for bacteria to produce deoxycholic acid (Tseng, Everhart, & Sandler, 1999; Dowling, 2000; VanBerge-Henegouwen, Portincasa, & vanErpecum, 1997; Hayes, Livingston, & Trautwein, 1992). Many studies have, in fact, found lower incidences of gallstones among those consuming higher-fiber diets; however, some studies have not shown such a relationship, and any clear association between dietary fiber and gallstone formation remains elusive (Tseng, Everhart, & Sandler, 1999; VanBerge-Henegouwen, Portincasa, & vanErpecum, 1997; Hayes, Livingston, & Trautwein, 1992; Bennett & Cerda, 1996).

Because most gallstones are composed primarily of cholesterol, it has been hypothesized that increased cholesterol intake might contribute to increased gallstone formation. However, the results of studies on this point have been inconsistent, and no correlation has been proven (Tseng, Everhart, & Sandler, 1999; Hayes, Livingston, & Trautwein, 1992). Also, studies of the relationship between total dietary fat and gallstone formation have been inconsistent, and have provided little evidence of an association (Tseng, Everhart, & Sandler, 1999; Hayes, Livingston, & Trautwein, 1992). Studies on specific types of dietary fat (saturated, monounsaturated, and polyunsaturated fats) have, likewise, not produced convincing evidence for a role of fat in gallstone formation (Tseng, Everhart, & Sandler, 1999). Some studies have shown protective effects for vegetables, vegetable fat, vegetable protein, or fiber from vegetables; however, other studies have not (Tseng, Everhart, & Sandler, 1999; Hayes, Livingston, & Trautwein, 1992). Although some studies have found associations between gallstones and the consumption of meat, animal fat, and animal protein, others have not found such an association (Tseng, Everhart, & Sandler, 1999).

Diverticular Disease and Appendicitis

Diverticular Disease

Diverticular disease affects 2 million Americans and is associated with increasing age, occurring in 50% of the adult population over the age of 60 (Cotran, Kumar, & Collins, 1999). Some 300,000 new cases are diagnosed each year (NIDDKD, 1995). Most people with diverticular disease remain asymptomatic, with 20% eventually developing symptoms such as abdominal pain or bleeding. These problems account for 440,000 hospitalizations and 2 million doctor visits annually (NIDDKD, 1995).

Diverticular disease can be congenital, but it is most often acquired. It can occur in numerous locations along the digestive tract. Most commonly, diverticulosis affects the colon and is characterized by multiple small outpouchings of the colonic mucosa through weak spots along the colon wall. These pouches, called *diverticula*, can become infected or inflamed, a condition referred to as *diverticulitis*.

Although found worldwide, diverticular disease is particularly a disease of Western industrialized countries where the diet is typically low in fiber (Cheskin & Lamport, 1995). Diverticular disease was not prevalent in this country until the early 1900s, when processed foods, composed of refined, low-fiber flour, were first introduced. Diverticular disease is rarely found in countries where people consume a high-fiber plant diet, and at this time a low-fiber diet is generally accepted as a predisposing factor for this disease.

Doctors have identified two main factors in the development of diverticulae. The first is a localized weakness in the colonic wall, and the second is increased pressure within the colon itself (Cotran, Kumar, & Collins, 1999). With a high-fiber diet, the volume and bulk of stool are increased. This increases the diameter of the colon, which, in turn, lowers the pressure in the colon. Also, with a high-fiber diet, stools are softer and intestinal transit time is less, which decreases the constipation and straining commonly associated with diverticular disease. Additionally, dietary fiber is degraded to short-chain fatty acids, which appear to play a role in maintaining colon health.

Research studies support the important role that dietary fiber plays in preventing diverticular disease, and have suggested that the risk of symptomatic diverticular disease is even higher when a low-fiber diet also includes large amounts of fat or red meat (Aldoori et al., 1994). In the Health Professionals Follow-up Study of 47,888 men, total dietary fiber was inversely associated with the risk of diverticular disease. The risk was even greater for men on a diet high in red meat and low in fiber. Men on a diet high in red meat and low in fiber were three times more likely to develop diverticulosis (Aldoori et al., 1994). A study from Greece compared people who frequently consumed vegetables, but rarely ate meat, with people who frequently consumed meat but rarely ate vegetables. The researchers found that the risk of developing diverticular disease was almost 50-fold higher for the meat eaters (Manousos et al., 1985). Also, in Asians meat consumption has been associated with right-sided diverticulosis (Lin et al., 2000). It has been theorized that dietary intake of red meat may play a role in promoting the growth of bacteria that precipitate the production of substances that weaken the colonic wall (Messina & Messina, 1996).

Vegetarians do consume significantly more fiber than meat eaters, with an average intake almost twice that of nonvegetarians. This may contribute to a lower risk of diverticular disease for vegetarians. Gear compared vegetarians (mean dietary fiber intake 41.5g/day) to non-

vegetarians (mean dietary fiber intake 21.4 g/day) and found that the incidence of diverticular disease was 33% among nonvegetarians, but only 12% among vegetarians (Gear et al., 1979).

Appendicitis

Another common problem involving the lower portion of the digestive tract is inflammation of the appendix, known as *acute appendicitis*. This disease affects 1 in 500 people; it occurs in all age groups, but is most common in adolescents and young adults. In 50%–80% of the cases, acute appendicitis is associated with an obstruction at the opening of the appendix, which precipitates a series of events that eventually leads to tissue death and infection. If untreated, the appendix may rupture. The most common cause of obstruction is a *fecalith*, which is a hard mass of stool. Other, less common causes are gallstones, tumors, and intestinal worms.

Research has been done to try to determine the factors associated with acute appendicitis and identify any possible preventive measures. Studies have yielded conflicting results, and there is still a great deal of uncertainty in the identification of specific precipitating factors (Jones et al., 1985). Acute appendicitis rarely occurs in traditional Third World populations, raising the question of a dietary factor. Several studies support this correlation of diet with appendicitis. One study found a greater prevalence of both appendicitis and fecaliths in people living in a developed country (Canada) than in those living in developing countries (in Africa). The study also found an increased prevalence of fecaliths in those with appendicitis as compared to those without. The authors concluded that the data support the theory that a lower-fiber diet, typical in developed societies, leads to increased fecalith formation and, therefore, also to an increased risk of appendicitis (Jones et al., 1985). Other studies have suggested a protective effect against appendicitis for green vegetables and tomatoes (Barker, Morris, & Nelson, 1986); a decreased risk of appendicitis in children aged 7 to 18 with an increased intake of fiber from whole-grain foods (Brender et al., 1985); and a 50% lower risk of requiring an emergency appendectomy among those consuming a vegetarian diet compared to those consuming a nonvegetarian diet (Appleby et al., 1995).

Kidney Stones

Kidney stones are exactly what their name suggests. They are small (usually about 2–10 mm), hard aggregates of minerals and organic compounds that form in the kidney. They can pass out of the kidney into the ureter, the narrow tube that connects the kidney to the bladder. Symptoms occur if the stones become stuck in the ureter and prevent urine from passing from the kidney into the bladder. The resultant increase in pressure due to the blockage of urine causes pain, which can be quite severe. Most kidney stones eventually pass through the ureter and out of the body on their own. However, some stones—usually the larger ones—must be either removed surgically or broken up in order to pass. In the United States, about 12% of men and 5% of women will have a kidney stone at some time in their life (Curhan, 1999).

Based on their composition, kidney stones are classified into three main types. The most common kidney stones (85%) are composed of calcium: either calcium oxalate, calcium phosphate, or a combination of the two (Saklayen, 1997). A smaller percentage of stones are composed of magnesium ammonium phosphate (6%–20%), uric acid (6%–17%), or cystine

(0.5%–3%) (Saklayen, 1997). In general, most individuals who develop kidney stones have, in their urine, higher concentrations of substances that contribute to kidney stone formation (calcium, oxalate, uric acid) and a lower concentrations of substances known to impede kidney stone formation (citrate, magnesium, pyrophosphate, many organic compounds) (Saklayen, 1997; Martini & Wood, 2000).

Epidemiologic studies suggest that environmental, particularly dietary, factors can increase one's risk of developing kidney stones. As societies become more affluent or industrialized and diets become more Westernized, the incidence of kidney stones appears to increase (Robertson et al., 1979; Hess, 2002).

Few studies have looked at the incidence of kidney stones among vegetarians. Robertson surveyed 2,592 vegetarians in the United Kingdom and found that the incidence of kidney stones among this group was only 40%–60% of that predicted for a similar group of age-, sex-, and social-class-matched members of the general population (Robertson, Peacock, & Marshall, 1982). In another study, Robertson calculated the risk of kidney stone formation from the amounts of urinary calcium, oxalate, and uric acid in the urine of vegetarians compared with nonvegetarians. He found lower urinary calcium, oxalate, and uric acid in the vegetarians. He concluded that the overall relative probability of forming stones was considerably lower in the vegetarian group (Robertson et al., 1979).

Although many dietary factors have been hypothesized to affect the risk of kidney stone formation, the three that have gained the most scientific support are protein, potassium, and fluids. Several studies have shown that those who consume greater amounts of dietary protein are at greater risk for the development of kidney stones (Giannini et al., 1999). There are several possible explanations for this effect of protein. High protein intake is associated with increased urinary excretion of calcium (Giannini et al., 1999; Kerstetter & Allen, 1990). Dietary protein increases the filtration rate of the kidneys, which, in turn, increases urinary calcium excretion (Martini & Wood, 2000; Kerstetter & Allen, 1990). The mild metabolic acidosis caused by excessive protein intake (especially intake of sulfur amino acid-rich proteins) may stimulate calcium reabsorption from bone, thereby leading to increased calcium in the urine (Robertson et al., 1979; Giannini et al., 1999). Also, a more acidic urine, found in those with increased protein intake, inhibits the reabsorption of calcium in the kidney and increases the reabsorption of citrate (an inhibitor of kidney stone formation) in the kidney, leading to increased amounts of calcium and decreased amounts of citrate in the urine (Martini & Wood, 2000; Giannini et al., 1999). Additionally, high protein intake also leads to increased uric acid in the urine (Giannini et al., 1999). Increased uric acid in the urine not only increases the incidence of uric acid stones, but also increases the incidence of calcium stones, perhaps by serving as a nidus for calcium stone formation or by interfering with inhibitors of calcium stone formation (Robertson, Peacock, & Hodgkinson, 1979; Fellstrom et al., 1983).

It appears that animal protein, rather than plant protein, is the primary protein responsible for increasing the risk of kidney stones (Hess, 2002). In the Health Professionals Follow-up Study, a 4-year study of 45,619 men, intake of animal protein was directly associated with an increased risk of stone formation (Curhan et al., 1993). In his study of 85 men who had a history of kidney stones, Robertson found that recurrent stone formers had significantly higher intakes of total protein than normal individuals, and this difference was almost entirely attributable to a higher intake of animal protein (Robertson et al., 1979). In another study, conducted in England, Robertson also found a marked cor-

relation between the incidence of kidney stones and the consumption of animal protein (Robertson, Peacock, & Hodgkinson, 1979). Conversely, in populations with a relatively high intake of vegetable protein compared with animal protein, there appears to be a lower incidence of kidney stones (Robertson et al., 1979). Martini studied 77 calcium stone formers and found that, in comparison to a group of controls, the intake of animal protein was higher in the stone patients; however, plant protein intake in the two groups was similar (Martini et al., 1993).

Animal protein intake increases the urinary excretion of uric acid and calcium, and lowers urinary citrate excretion, all of which predispose a person to the formation of calcium stones (Robertson et al., 1979; Fellstrom et al., 1983; Curhan et al., 1993; Breslau et al., 1988; Giannini et al., 1999). As compared to vegetable protein, animal protein has greater amounts of sulfur-containing amino acids (Breslau et al., 1988), which, as mentioned earlier, increase urinary calcium. Additionally, animal proteins have higher purine content, which, because purines are metabolized to uric acid, leads to greater urinary uric acid concentrations (Breslau et al., 1988). Differing results have been obtained regarding urinary oxalate, with some studies showing increased amounts of urinary oxalate with greater animal protein consumption and other studies showing increased amounts with greater vegetable protein consumption (Robertson et al., 1979; Breslau et al., 1988; Brockis, Levitt, & Cruthers, 1982).

Breslau studied 15 people during periods when they were placed on diets that contained vegetable protein, vegetable and egg protein, and then animal protein. As the animal-protein content of the diet increased, urinary calcium and uric acid were increased and urinary citrate excretion was reduced. However, urinary oxalate was higher on the vegetarian diet (Breslau et al., 1988). A study of 30 omnivores and 30 vegetarians found that increased animal protein consumption resulted in increased urinary calcium and uric acid (Brockis, Levitt, & Cruthers, 1982).

Increasing one's consumption of fluids can decrease one's risk of kidney stones (Hess, 2002; Jaeger, 1994; Meschi et al., 2004). Increasing fluids can reduce the concentration of all kidney stone-forming salts and may also improve the urinary clearance of crystals (Meschi et al., 2004).

Studies have also suggested that those individuals with greater dietary potassium have a decreased risk of kidney stones (Curhan & Curhan, 1994). Higher potassium intake can decrease calcium and increase citrate in the urine (Meschi et al., 2004).

Hess et al. (1994) found that lower intake of vegetable fibers leads to lower urinary citrate excretion. Urinary citrate protects against calcium stones because it reduces urinary supersaturation by complexing with calcium. It also inhibits growth and aggregation of calcium oxalate and calcium phosphate crystals (Hess, 2002). Therefore, vegetable intake may protect against kidney stones.

Keeping weight under control can also decrease the incidence of stone formation. As body mass index (BMI) increases from normal to more than 32 kg/m^2, the risk of stone formation increases from 7.1% to 9.8% in men and from 2.5% to 4.4% in women (Meschi et al., 2004). In both the Nurses' Health Study and the Health Professionals Follow-up Study, the prevalence and incidence of kidney stone disease were directly associated with weight and BMI (Curhan et al., 1998). As body weight increases, urinary excretion of oxalate and uric acid also increases (Curhan et al., 1998).

Perhaps somewhat surprisingly, studies have shown that those with higher intakes of dietary calcium actually have a lower risk of develop-

ing kidney stones. In the Health Professionals Follow-up Study, men in the highest quintile of dietary calcium intake had a 34% lower risk of kidney stone formation than those in the lowest quintile (Curhan et al., 1993). In the Nurses' Health Study of 91,731 female nurses, women in the highest quintile of dietary calcium intake had a 35% lower risk of stone formation than women in the lowest quintile (Curhan et al., 1997). Other studies have also suggested this relationship (Robertson, Peacock, & Marshall, 1982). As most stones are composed of calcium, this would seem intuitively backward; however, greater calcium intake means more calcium in the intestine, where it can then bind with oxalate, decreasing the amount of oxalate in the body (Hess, 2002; Meschi et al., 2004). Oxalate is one of the main ingredients in one of the most common types of kidney stones (calcium oxalate). It may be that small decreases in oxalate have a greater impact on decreasing the risk of stone formation than small increases in calcium intake (Martini & Wood, 2000).

Studies suggest that dietary sodium may also influence the incidence of kidney stones. Excessive sodium intake is associated with increased calcium excretion. Increased sodium intake may, therefore, increase kidney stone formation (Martini & Wood, 2000; Jaeger, 1994; Meschi et al., 2004).

The reasons behind the apparent decreased risk of kidney stone formation in vegetarians may be multiple. One might be the vegetarians' lower intake of protein, particularly their lower intake of animal protein. One way in which decreased protein intake may affect the risk of kidney stones is by decreasing urine acidity. Further support of this hypothesis came from a study of 20 South African males, each of whom was placed on 5 different diets for 4 days. The study found that while a subject was on a vegetarian diet, his urinary pH was less acidic (Rodgers & Lewandowski, 2002). Other factors that may be responsible for the lower risk of kidney stones among vegetarians are decreased obesity and increased dietary potassium and vegetable fiber intake.

Despite the fact that many studies have investigated the effect of diet on kidney stone formation, there is a paucity of studies regarding the effect of diet modification on the risk of recurrence of kidney stone formation in kidney stone patients. Hiatt investigated the risk of recurrent kidney stone formation in those on a low-animal-protein, high-fiber diet compared with those on a control diet, and found, contrary to expectations, that after 4.5 years, those on the low-protein diet had a greater risk of recurrence of kidney stone (Hiatt et al., 1996). This study conflicts with epidemiologic associations between protein intake and stone formation, and some have noted severe limitations with this study (Martini & Wood, 2000; Hess, 2002). A more recent study compared a low-calcium diet with a diet consisting of normal calcium intake, low intake of animal protein and salt, and high potassium intake in a group of 60 men with a history of kidney stones. The researchers found that after 5 years, 38.3% of those on the low-calcium intake had kidney stone recurrences, compared to 20% in the alternative dietary group (Meschi et al., 2004).

Kidney Failure (Chronic Renal Failure)

The kidneys are vital, complex organs that perform a variety of necessary functions in the body. These functions include filtration and excretion of waste products; regulation of water and salt balances; maintenance of acid balance in the blood; and release of hormones that regulate blood pressure, red cell production in the bones, and calcium maintenance. When problems occur with the kidneys, the health conse-

quences can be serious and sometimes life-threatening.

Approximately 3.5 million people are affected by conditions that impair kidney function or cause permanent kidney failure (NIDDKD, 1998). Chronic illnesses, such as diabetes, heart disease, and high blood pressure, or inherited diseases, such as polycystic kidney disease, can lead to kidney failure. Other causes include poisons, medications, and trauma. Acute renal failure (ARF) occurs quickly, often as a result of trauma or chemical injury. Chronic renal failure (CRF) happens more slowly. In end-stage renal disease (ESRD), the kidneys are permanently damaged, with almost complete or complete loss of function. People with ESRD are dependent on either dialysis or kidney transplantation to survive.

Doctors and researchers use several laboratory measurements to determine the degree of kidney damage caused by disease or injury. Creatinine, a byproduct of normal muscle breakdown, is often measured comparatively in the blood and urine, to reveal how well the kidneys are filtering. The resulting measurement, called *creatinine clearance*, best reflects the filtering ability of the kidneys, commonly referred to as the *glomerular filtration rate (GFR)*. Other indicators of poor kidney function include the presence of protein in the urine, and an increase in blood urea nitrogen (BUN), a waste product of protein use in cells.

In the end stages of kidney disease, several waste products, many of them the result of protein metabolism, accumulate in the body and can cause symptoms such as nausea, vomiting, and itching. Those with severe kidney disease are encouraged to consume a low-protein diet to help ameliorate these symptoms.

Low-protein diets can not only help decrease the symptoms of ESRD, but they can also help decrease the progression of kidney disease. Research has shown that the GFR and the renal plasma flow (blood flow) increase in correlation with the amount of dietary protein ingested. In other words, protein in the diet increases the workload of the kidneys. It is felt that the increased GFR and renal plasma flow that accompany a high protein intake increase the pressure gradient within the kidney, resulting in kidney damage. Many studies have shown that, for those with kidney disease, dietary protein restriction can limit the progression of their kidney disease (Henry, 1994; Zeller, 1991; Wiseman et al., 1987; Percheron et al., 1995; Maschio et al., 1983; Ihle et al., 1989; Rosman et al., 1984; El Nahas et al., 1984; Levey et al., 1996; Alvestrand, Ahlberg, & Bergstrom, 1983; Barsotti, Ciardella et al., 1988; Zeller et al., 1991; Walker et al., 1989; Evanoff et al., 1987; American Diabetes Association, 1999; Brouhard & LaGrone, 1990; Cohen, Dodds, & Viberti, 1987).

There is considerable evidence that not all proteins are harmful to the kidneys. Plant proteins, including soy protein, do not appear to have the deleterious effects on the kidney that are seen with animal proteins. Current research indicates that soy protein, when substituted for animal protein, tends to lower GFR and renal blood flow (Kontessis et al., 1990; Nakamura et al., 1989; Kontessis et al., 1995). In the EURODIAB IDDM Complications study of 2,696 diabetics, increased excretion of urinary protein (specifically increased albumin excretion, which can be a sign of kidney damage) was correlated with intakes of total protein and animal protein, but not vegetable protein (Toeller et al., 1997).

Several studies have suggested that a vegetarian diet may be beneficial in terms of kidney function. Lower levels of GFR and urinary albumin excretion have been described in vegans and lacto vegetarians compared with omnivores (Kontessis et al., 1990; Wiseman et al., 1987; Bosch et al., 1983). Jibani found that in those who consumed a near-vegetarian diet, there was decreased albumin (protein) excretion, although it could not be determined if this was due to a reduction in animal protein or to the lower total protein content of the vegetarian diet (Jibani et al., 1991). A vegetarian diet in which soy protein replaced all animal protein was shown to decrease urinary protein loss in patients with nephrotic kidney disease; in this case, though, it should be noted that the vegetarian diet also contained less overall protein (D'Amico et al., 1992). In another study, a vegetarian diet was found to decrease the progression of kidney disease in eight diabetics (Barsotti, Navalesi et al., 1988). Kontessis et al. (1990) found that when individuals with diabetes were placed on a near-vegetarian diet, GFR and renal plasma flow were lower than in those consuming a nonvegetarian diet containing a similar amount of protein.

Further work is needed to establish whether those with kidney disease can consume a diet higher in protein if that protein comes from vegetable sources rather than animal sources (Shils et al., 1999). Some have suggested that perhaps a diet substituting soy protein for animal protein could be used as an alternative to a low-animal-protein diet in the treatment of kidney failure (Anderson et al., 1998). Those with kidney failure should be cognizant of the higher potassium and phosphorus content of soy foods and monitor these levels appropriately (Messina & Messina, 2000). Low-nitrogen, low-phosphorus vegetarian and vegan diets are well tolerated by patients with chronic renal failure (Barsotti et al., 1996; Soroka et al., 1998).

The benefits of a vegetarian diet in the management of kidney disease are not confined to reduced disease progression and reduced symptoms of kidney disease. Such a diet may afford additional benefit in protecting against other health problems associated with kidney disease. Compared with the general public, those with end-stage renal disease have a disproportionately greater risk of many diseases, including high blood pressure, coronary artery disease, diverticular disease, gallstones, and constipation. Vegetarian diets have been shown to help reduce the risk of these diseases.

Practical Aspects

Studies indicate that vegetarians have a lower incidence of diverticular disease, and that the primary reason for this appears to be the higher fiber content of a vegetarian diet. Therefore, vegetarians should eat a diet high in fiber to best decrease their risk of this disease. Evidence from the few studies that have been done also suggests that vegetarians have a lower incidence of appendicitis, and that a high-fiber diet may be an important factor in this case also.

Preliminary evidence suggests that vegetarians have lower incidences of gallbladder disease and kidney stones. In both of these cases, science is in an early stage in its investigation into which dietary factors affect the development of these diseases, so it is difficult to make precise dietary recommendations for vegetarians. For gallbladder disease, one factor that may be important is a high-fiber diet. In the case of kidney stones, low consumption of animal protein, as well as adequate intakes of potassium and fluids, may be beneficial.

In regard to kidney failure (chronic renal failure), the role of a vegetarian diet has yet to be clearly elucidated. Evidence is overwhelming that a high-protein diet is detrimental to the progression of kidney failure. Initial studies suggest that plant protein may not have the detrimental effect of animal protein. Therefore, persons with kidney disease may want to decrease or eliminate their intake of animal protein. Very preliminary evidence also suggests that vegetarian diets may slow the progression of kidney disease. A well-balanced vegetarian diet will reduce the incidence of many diseases for which those with existing kidney disease find themselves at increased risk, such as high blood pressure and coronary artery disease. It is crucial that those with kidney failure have their diet closely monitored by a physician.

Conclusion

Early evidence indicates that vegetarians have a lower risk of gallstones than nonvegetarians. The exact dietary factors that influence the development of gallstones have yet to be clearly elucidated. Dietary fiber and the lower body weights of vegetarians may contribute to their lower risk of gallstones.

Vegetarians have a lower incidence of diverticular disease. This is most likely due in large part to their higher fiber intake. Meat consumption may also play a role in diverticular disease.

Although few studies have been done, it appears that vegetarians may have a lower incidence of appendicitis. The exact dietary factors to which this can be attributed have not been clarified, but again fiber may play an important role.

Few studies have looked at the incidence of kidney stones among vegetarians, but the available evidence suggests that vegetarians are at lower risk. The exact aspects of diet that are involved in the development of kidney stones have not yet been clearly identified. Most evidence suggests that dietary protein, especially animal protein, may increase one's risk for the development of kidney stones. Vegetarian diets tend to have a lower protein content, and specifically a lower animal protein content, than nonvegetarian diets, and this may partly explain the apparent decreased risk of kidney stones seen among vegetarians. A lower incidence of obesity and a higher intake of potassium may also help prevent the development of kidney stones among vegetarians.

Kidney disease (chronic renal failure) is a complex and serious illness. The interactions of dietary factors in the development, progression, and treatment of this disease are, likewise, complex. Science is only starting to elucidate the role that diet plays in this disease, but the evidence is fairly clear that a high-protein diet is detrimental to the progression of kidney disease. Preliminary studies indicate that this detrimental effect may be true of animal protein, but not of plant protein. Only a very few studies have been done on the effects of vegetarian diets on kidney function and on kidney disease; however, those that have been conducted do suggest beneficial effects. These effects may be due to the lower protein—specifically the lower animal protein—content of a vegetarian diet, but other factors may also be involved. Vegetarian diets may also be useful to those with kidney disease because of the lower risk such diets afford for several diseases, such as high blood pressure and heart disease, which are prevalent among those with kidney disease. It is important that those with kidney disease have their diets closely monitored by a physician, as there are many dietary factors that must be carefully controlled by those whose kidneys are functioning poorly.

References

Aldoori WH, Giovannucci EL, Rimm EB, et al. A prospective study of diet and the risk of symptomatic diverticular disease in men. *Am J Clin Nutr.* Nov 1994;60(5):757-764.

Alvestrand A, Ahlberg M, Bergstrom J. Retardation of the progression of renal insufficiency in patients treated with low-protein diets. *Kidney Intl Suppl.* 1983;24(Suppl 16):S268-S272.

American Diabetes Association. Diabetic nephropathy. *Diabetes Care.* 1999;22(Suppl 1):S66-S69.

Anderson JW, Blake JE, Turner J, Smith B. Effects of soy protein on renal function and proteinuria in patients with type 2 diabetes. *Am J Clin Nutr.* 1998;68(6, Suppl):1347S-1353S.

Appleby P, Thorogood M, McPherson K, Mann J. Emergency appendicectomy and meat consumption in the UK. *J Epidemiol & Community Health.* 1995;49(6):594-596.

Barker DJ, Morris J, Nelson M. Vegetable consumption and acute appendicitis in 59 areas in England and Wales. *Br Med J* (clinical research ed.). 1986; 292(6525):927-930.

Barsotti G, Ciardella F, Morelli A, et al. Nutritional treatment of renal failure in type 1 diabetic nephropathy. *Clin Nephrol.* 1988;29(6):280-287.

Barsotti G, Morelli E, Cupisti A, et al. A low-nitrogen low-phosphorus vegan diet for patients with chronic renal failure. *Nephron.* 1996:74(2):390-394.

Barsotti G, Navalesi R, Giampietro O, et al. Effects of a vegetarian, supplemented diet on renal function, proteinuria, and glucose metabolism in patients with "overt" diabetic nephropathy and renal insufficiency. *Contrib Nephrol.* 1988;65:87-94.

Bennett WB, Cerda JJ. Dietary fiber: Fact and fiction. *Dig Discuss.* 1996;14(1):43-58.

Bosch JP, Saccaggi A, Lauer A, et al. Renal functional reserve in humans: Effect of protein intake on glomerular filtration rate. *Am J Med.* 1983;75(6): 943-950.

Brender JD, Weiss NS, Koepsell TD, Marcuse EF. Fiber intake and childhood appendicitis. *Am J Public Health.* 1985;75(4):399-400.

Breslau NA, Brinkley L, Hill KO, Pak CY. Relationship of animal protein-rich diet to kidney stone formations and calcium metabolism. *J Clin Endocr Metab.* 1988;66(1):140-146.

Brockis J, Levitt AJ, Cruthers SM. The effects of vegetable and animal protein diets on calcium, urate and oxalate excretion. *Br J Urol.* 1982;54(6): 590-593.

Brouhard BH, LaGrone L. Effect of dietary protein restriction on functional renal reserve in diabetic nephropathy. *Am J Med.* 1990;89(4):427-431.

Burkitt D, Tunstall M. Gall-stones: Geographical and chronological features. *J Trop Med Hygiene.* 1975;78(6):140-144.

Cheskin LJ, Lamport RD. Diverticular disease. Epidemiology and pharmacological treatment. *Drugs & Aging.* 1995;6(1):55–63.

Cohen D, Dodds R, Viberti G. Effect of protein restriction in insulin dependent diabetics at risk of nephropathy. *Br Med J.* 1987;294(6575):795–798.

Cotran RS, Kumar V, Collins T. *Robbins Pathologic Basis of Disease.* 6th ed. Philadelphia: W. B. Saunders; 1999.

Curhan G, Willett WC, Speizer FE, et al. Comparison of dietary calcium with supplemental calcium and other nutrients as factors affecting the risk for kidney stones in women. *Ann Intern Med.* 1997;126(7):497–504.

Curhan GC. Epidemiologic evidence for the role of oxalate in idiopathic nephrolithiasis. *J Endourol.* 1999;13(9):629–631.

Curhan GC, Curhan SG. Dietary factors and kidney stone formation. *Compr Ther.* 1994;20(9):485–489.

Curhan GC, Willett WC, Rimm EB, et al. Body size and risk of kidney stones. *J Am Soc Nephrol.* 1998;9(9):1645–1652.

Curhan GC, Willett WC, Rimm EB, Stampher MJ. A prospective study of dietary calcium and other nutrients and the risk of symptomatic kidney stones. *N Engl J Med.* 1993(12);328:833–838.

D'Amico G, Gentile MG, Manna G, et al. Effect of vegetarian soy diet on hyperlipidaemia in nephrotic syndrome. *Lancet.* 1992;339(8802):1131–1134.

Dowling R. Review: Pathogenesis of gallstones. *Aliment Pharmacol Ther.* 2000:14(Suppl 2):39–47.

El Nahas AM, Masters-Thomas AM, Brady SA, et al. Selective effect of low protein diets in chronic renal diseases. *Br Med J.* 1984;289(6455):1337–1341.

Evanoff GV, Thompson CS, Brown J, Weinman EJ. The effect of dietary protein restriction on the progression of diabetic nephropathy: A 12-month follow-up. *Arch Intern Med.* 1987;147(3):492–495.

Fellstrom B, Danielson BG, Karlstrom B, et al. The influence of a high dietary intake of purine-rich animal protein on urinary urate excretion and supersaturation in renal stone disease. *Clin Sci.* (London). 1983:64(4):399–405.

Gear JS, Ware A, Fursdon P, et al. Symptomless diverticular disease and intake of dietary fibre. *Lancet.* 1979;1(8115):511–514.

Giannini S, Nobile M, Sartori L, et al. Acute effects of moderate dietary protein restriction in patients with idiopathic hypercalciuria and calcium nephrolithiasis. *Am J Clin Nutr.* 1999;69(2):267–271.

Hayes KC, Livingston A, Trautwein E. Dietary impact on biliary lipids and gallstones. *Ann Rev Nutr.* 1992;12:299–326.

Henry RR. Protein content of the diabetic diet. *Diabetes Care.* 1994;17(12):1502–1513.

Hess B. Nutritional aspects of stone disease. *Endocr Metab Clin N Am.* 2002;31(4):1017–1030.

Hess B, Michel R, Takkinen R, et al. Risk factors for low urinary citrate in calcium nephrolithiasis: Low vegetable fibre intake and low urine volume to be added to the list. *Nephrol Dial Transplant.* 1994;9(6):642–649.

Hiatt RA, Ettinger B, Caan B, et al. Randomized controlled trial of a low animal protein, high fiber diet in the prevention of recurrent calcium oxalate kidney stones. *Am J Epidemiol.* 1996;144(1):25–33.

Ihle BU, Becker GJ, Whitmore JA, et al. The effect of protein restriction on the progression of renal insufficiency. *N Engl J Med.* 1989;321(26):1773–1777.

Jaeger P. Prevention of recurrent calcium stones: Diet versus drugs. *Miner Electrolyte Metab.* 1994;20(6):410–413.

Jibani MM, Bloodworth LL, Foden E, et al. Predominately vegetarian diet in patients with incipient and early clinical diabetic nephropathy: Effects on albumin excretion rate and nutritional status. *Diabetic Med.* 1991;8(10):949–953.

Jones BA, Demetriades D, Segal I, Burkitt DP. The prevalence of appendiceal fecaliths in patients with and without appendicitis. A comparative study from Canada and South Africa. *Ann Surg.* 1985;202(1):80–82.

Kerstetter JE, Allen KH. Dietary protein increases urinary calcium. *J Nutr.* 1990;120(1):134–136.

Kontessis P, Jones S, Dodds R, et al. Renal, metabolic and hormonal responses to ingestion of animal and vegetable proteins. *Kidney Intl.* 1990;38(1):136–144.

Kontessis PA, Bossinakou I, Sarika L, et al. Renal, metabolic, and hormonal responses to proteins of different origin in normotensive, nonproteinuric type I diabetic patients. *Diabetes Care.* 1995; 18(9):1233-1240.

Kratzer W, Kachele V, Mason RA, et al. Gallstone prevalence in relation to smoking, alcohol, coffee consumption, and nutrition: The Ulm Gallstone study. *Scand J Gastroenterol.* 1997;32(9): 953-958.

Levey AS, Adler S, Caggiula AW, et al. Effects of dietary protein restriction on the progression of advanced renal disease in the Modification of Diet in Renal Disease study. *Am J Kidney Dis.* 1996; 27(5):652-663.

Lin OS, Soon MS, Wu SS, et al. Dietary habits and right-sided colonic diverticulosis. *Dis Colon Rectum.* 2000;43(10):1412-1418.

Manousos O, Day NE, Tzonou A, et al. Diet and other factors in the aetiology of diverticulosis: An epidemiological study in Greece. *Gut.* 1985;26(6): 544-549.

Martini L, Heilberg IP, Cuppari L, et al. Dietary habits of calcium stone formers. *Braz J Med Biol Res.* 1993;26(8):805-812.

Martini LA, Wood R. Should dietary calcium and protein be restricted in patients with nephrolithiasis? *Nutr Rev.* 2000;58(4):111-117.

Maschio G, Oldrizzi L, Tessitore N, et al. Early dietary protein and phosphorus restriction is effective in delaying progression of chronic renal failure. *Kidney Intl Suppl.* 1983;16:S273-S277.

Meschi T, Schianchi T, Ridolo E, et al. Body weight, diet and water intake in preventing stone disease. *Urol Intl.* 2004;72(Suppl 1):29-33.

Messina M, Messina V. Soyfoods, soybean isoflavones and bone health: A brief overview. *J Renal Nutr.* 2000;10(2):63-68.

Messina M, Messina V. *The Dietitian's Guide to Vegetarian Diets: Issues and Applications.* Gaithersburg, MD: Aspen Publishers; 1996.

Nakamura H, Takasawa M, Kasahara S, et al. Effects of acute protein loads of different sources on renal function of patients with diabetic nephropathy. *Tohoku J Exper Med.* 1989;159(2):153-162.

National Institute of Diabetes and Digestive and Kidney Diseases (NIDDKD). *Kidney and Urologic Diseases Statistics for the United States.* NIH Publication No. 99-3895. Washington, DC: National Institute of Health, U.S. Public Health Service; Aug 1998.

National Institute of Diabetes and Digestive and Kidney Diseases. *Digestive Diseases Statistics.* NIH Publication No. 95-3873. Washington, DC: National Institutes of Health, U.S. Public Health Service; Feb 1995.

National Institute of Diabetes and Digestive and Kidney Diseases. *Gallstones.* NIH Publication No. 95-2897. Washington, DC: National Institutes of Health, U.S. Public Health Service; Mar 1993.

Percheron C, Colette C, Astre C, Monnier L. Effects of moderate changes in protein intake on urinary albumin excretion in type I diabetic patients. *Nutrition.* 1995;11(4):345-349.

Pixley F, Mann J. Dietary factors in the aetiology of gall stones: A case control study. *Gut.* 1988;29(11): 1511-1515.

Pixley F, Wilson D, McPherson K, Mann J. Effect of vegetarianism on development of gall stones in women. *Br Med J.* 1985;291(6487):11-12.

Robertson W, Peacock M, Marshall D. Prevalence of urinary stone disease in vegetarians. *Eur Urol.* 1982;8(6):334-339.

Robertson WG, Peacock M, Heyburn J, et al. Should recurrent calcium oxalate stone formers become vegetarians? *Br J Urol.* 1979;51(6):427-431.

Robertson WG, Peacock M, Hodgkinson A. Dietary changes and the incidence of urinary calculi in the U.K. between 1958 and 1976. *J Chronic Dis.* 1979;32(6):469-476.

Rodgers AL, Lewandowski S. Effects of 5 different diets on urinary risk factors for calcium oxalate kidney stone formation: Evidence of different renal handling mechanisms in different race groups. *J Urol.* 2002;168(3):931-936.

Rosman JB, ter Wee PM, Meijer S, et al. Prospective randomised trial of early dietary protein restriction in chronic renal failure. *Lancet.* 1984;2(8415): 1291-1296.

Saklayen MG. Medical management of nephrolithiasis. *Med Clin N Am.* 1997;81(3):785-799.

Shils M, Olson J, Shike M, Ross A, eds. *Modern Nutrition in Health and Disease.* Philadelphia, PA: Lippincott/Williams and Wilkins; 1999.

Simon J, Hudes ES. Serum ascorbic acid and other correlates of gallbladder disease among U.S. adults. *Am J Public Health.* 1998;88(8):1208–1212.

Smith DA, Gee MI. A dietary survey to determine the relationship between diet and cholelithiasis. *Am J Clin Nutr.* 1979;32(17):1519–1526.

Soroka N, Silverberg DS, Greemland M, et al. Comparison of a vegetable-based (soya) and an animal-based low-protein diet in predialysis chronic renal failure patients. *Nephron.* 1998;79(2):173–180.

Toeller M, Buyken A, Heitkamp G, et al. Protein intake and urinary albumin excretion rates in the EURODIAB IDDM Complications study. *Diabetologia.* 1997;40(10):1219–1226.

Tseng M, Everhart JM, Sandler RS. Dietary intake and gallbladder disease: A review. *Public Health Nutr.* 1999;2(2):161–172.

VanBerge-Henegouwen GP, Portincasa P, vanErpecum KJ. Effect of lactulose and fiber-rich diets on bile in relation to gallstone disease: An update. *Scand J Gastroenterol.* 1997;222(Suppl):68–71.

Walker JD, Bending JJ, Dodds RA, et al. Restriction of dietary protein and progression of renal failure in diabetic nephropathy. *Lancet.* 1989; 2(8677): 1411–1415. Erratum in *Lancet.* 1989;2(8678–8679):1540.

Wiseman MJ, Bognetti E, Dodds R, et al. Changes in renal function in response to protein restricted diet in type I (insulin-dependent) diabetic patients. *Diabetologia.* 1987;30(3):154–159.

Wiseman ME, Hunt R, Goodwin A, et al. Dietary composition and renal function in healthy subjects. *Nephron.* 1987;46(1):37–42.

Zeller K. Low-protein diets in renal disease. *Diabetes Care.* 1991;14(9):856–866.

Zeller K, Whittaker E, Sullivan L, et al. Effect of restricting dietary protein on the progression of renal failure in patients with insulin-dependent diabetes mellitus. *N Engl J Med.* 1991;324(2): 78–84.

18

Vegetarian Diets and Children

Jeanene Fogli, MS, RD, LDN
Carol M. Meerschaert, RD, LDN

Introduction

A commissioned survey indicates that 2% of 6- to 17-year-old children and adolescents in the United States are vegetarians, and around 0.5% of this age group are vegan (Vegetarian Resource Group, 2001). Many are children of vegetarian parents; others chose a vegetarian lifestyle based on preferences or ethical concerns.

All diets for children must be appropriately planned to meet the nutrient needs of the growing child. The American Dietetic Association indicates that vegetarian and vegan children have growth similar to nonvegetarian children and adequate intake of all required nutrients when their diets are planned well (Mangels, Messina, & Melina, 2003).

Summary of the Scientific Literature

Calories

Adequate caloric intake is essential to the growth of all children. Most children, who have high nutrient needs and small stomachs, need both meals and snacks to fulfill nutrient and calorie needs. The 2005 *Dietary Guidelines for Americans,* which are intended to represent recommendations appropriate for children over the age of two, support vegetarian diets for children (Dietary Guidelines Advisory Committee, 2004): "Vegetarian diets can be consistent with the *Dietary Guidelines for Americans,* and meet Recommended Dietary Allowances for nutrients" (U.S. Department of Agriculture, 2000).

The physical bulk of the diet should be considered when choosing foods for a vegetarian child. The bulk of the diet can easily be reduced so that the young child does not feel full before adequate caloric intake has been achieved. One way to decrease bulk is to provide several small meals during the day and offer snacks as needed to meet calorie needs. Also, whole grains can be mixed with refined grains to lessen the bulk of the diet. Table 18.1 lists nutrient sources appropriate for vegan and lacto-ovo vegetarian diets.

Protein

Protein needs can be met easily if vegetarian children eat a variety of plant foods and have

Table 18.1   Vegetarian and Vegan Sources of Nutrients of Concern for Children

Nutrient	Acceptable Sources for Vegan Diets	Additional Foods Acceptable for Lacto-Ovo Vegetarian Diets
Protein	Whole grains, legumes, and soy-based or wheat-based (gluten) meat analogs. Grains can provide a great deal of protein, as several servings are eaten each day.	Dairy and eggs
Calcium	Fortified soy, rice, or other "milks"; fortified juices, such as apple (usually only 100 mg of calcium/serving), orange, and cranberry juice; dark-green low-oxalate vegetables (kale, collard greens).	Cow's milk, goat's milk, other dairy products, supplements derived from dairy products
Iron	Breast milk, iron-fortified infant formula, some soy milk (such as Pacific brand), soy products, legumes, whole grains, dried fruits, fortified breakfast cereal, food cooked in cast-iron pans. Encourage vitamin C sources at each meal for optimal iron absorption.	
Riboflavin	Fortified soy milk, legumes, grains, vegetables.	Cow's milk
Vitamin B12	B12-fortified soy milk, Red Star brand Vegetarian Support Formula nutritional yeast, fortified breakfast cereals, fortified meat analogs, vitamin supplements.	Dairy and eggs
Zinc	Nuts, legumes, wheat germ.	Dairy and eggs

an adequate intake of calories. Proteins are synthesized by the body from foods that contain the appropriate essential amino acids. These amino acids need not be taken within the context of the same meal, but can be consumed at various times throughout the day; for example, at different meals during the day or during snacks (Young & Pellett, 1994). Consuming a variety of protein-containing foods helps ensure that vegetarian children have adequate intake of all essential amino acids.

The Recommended Dietary Allowance (RDA) is the average intake required to meet the nutritional needs of 97% of the population at a given age. The protein needs for children of various ages are higher than those of adults, because of the increased demands of growth (Food and Nutrition Board [FNB], 2002a). The RDAs for protein are listed in Table 18.2. One should note that they differ based on the amount of growth taking place during that life stage.

Table 18.2   Protein Requirements by Age

Age Range	Protein Requirement
1–3 years	1.10 grams/kg body weight per day or 13 grams/day
4–9 years	0.95 grams/kg body weight per day or 19 grams/day
10–13 years	0.95 grams/kg body weight per day or 34 grams/day
14–18 years	0.85 grams/kg body weight per day or 52 grams/day

Although vegetarian diets tend to be lower in total protein, protein needs can easily be met with a healthful vegetarian diet. Protein intake in both lacto-ovo vegetarians and vegans appears to be adequate. Diets of vegetarian children, whether lacto-ovo or vegan, generally meet or exceed recommendations for protein (Messina, Mangels, & Messina, 2004). The frequency and variety of meals for children assist

Table 18.3   Comparison of Two Vegetarian Breakfasts for a School-Aged Child

Ovo-Lacto Vegetarian	Vegan
1 scrambled egg	1 cup cooked millet with 1 Tbsp. blackstrap molasses
1 slice whole-wheat toast	1 slice whole-wheat toast with 2 Tbsp. peanut butter
1 tsp. margarine	1 cup apple juice
8 oz. 1% milk	
TOTAL	TOTAL
17 g protein	18 g protein
14 g fat	19 g fat
1.7 mg iron	6.5 mg iron
353 mg calcium	219 mg calcium

in providing the complement of amino acids needed for protein synthesis.

When assessing the protein intake of a child who follows a vegetarian diet, it is important to examine all the protein in the diet, not just protein from concentrated sources. Vegetarian children may get a significant amount of their protein from grains and vegetables simply because of the large number of servings eaten per day. Table 18.3 illustrates this point.

Calcium

Osteoporosis prevention appears to be enhanced by achieving maximum bone mass in the first years of life. Recommended intake of calcium for children ages 1 through 3 years is 500mg/day, for ages 4 through 8 years is 800mg/day, and in adolescence (ages 13–18 years) is 1,300 mg/day (FNB, 1997). Dietary intake data from the Continuing Survey of Food Intake of Individuals indicates that the intake of calcium by all children is significantly lower than the recommended amount (Nusser et al., 1996). This is a concern for all children; consistent, adequate intake is important.

Currently, the major source of calcium in the U.S. food supply is dairy, which supplies more than 70% of dietary calcium (Center for Nutrition Policy and Promotion [CNPP], 1996). Milk is an excellent source of calcium, providing 300 mg of calcium per cup. Other vegetarian sources of calcium for children include calcium-fortified juices, waffles, and cereals; calcium-fortified soy and rice beverages; tofu; and blackstrap molasses. There are also several low-oxalate green vegetables that are high in absorbable calcium, such as bok choy and collard greens.

Calcium requirements can also be met through the use of calcium supplements. There are chewable, liquid, and powdered calcium supplements that can be used for children who cannot or will not swallow pills. Powdered calcium, nonfat dry cow's milk, and calcium-fortified soy milk powders can all be "hidden" in recipes such as for hot cereal, muffins, pancakes, and lentil loaf, to boost the calcium content for children whose intake is still falling below the recommendations.

Iron

Iron-deficiency anemia is the most common childhood nutritional problem in both vegetarian and nonvegetarian children, with higher risks being seen in female and African American children (FNB, 2002c; Ganji, Hampl, & Betts, 2003). Although meat contains heme iron that is better absorbed than the non-heme iron found in plant foods, iron-deficiency anemia is no more likely to occur in vegetarian than nonvegetarian children (Messina, Mangels, & Messina, 2004). In young children, iron deficiency is associated with behavioral problems and reduced cognitive performance that may not be fully reversible by iron replacement (FNB, 2002b).

Good iron sources for vegetarian children include whole or enriched grains and grain products, iron-fortified cereals, legumes, and green leafy vegetables. Consuming foods rich in vitamin C at the same meal enhances non-heme iron absorption.

Vitamin B12

Lacto-ovo vegetarians obtain dietary B12 from eggs and dairy products. Vegans consume no animal products, so they must consume vitamin B12-fortified foods or supplements. Several foods popular with children are fortified with a vegetarian (nonanimal-derived) vitamin B12, such as breakfast cereals (Total), Red Star brand Vegetarian Support Formula nutritional yeast, meat analogs, and some soy milks. Therefore, all vegetarian children should be able to find an acceptable source of vitamin B12. There are also several chewable vegetarian vitamins that include B12, including Hero Nutritional's Yummi Bears, Pioneer Chewable Vitamin/Mineral for Adults and Children, and American Health Chewy Bears Multi-Vitamins.

Most reports of dietary B12 deficiency in the literature with regard to vegetarian children concern people following a macrobiotic diet (Messina, Mangels, & Messina, 2004). Some foods commonly included in a macrobiotic diet, such

as tempeh (a cultured whole soybean product), sea vegetables (kelp, kombu, arame), miso (a fermented soybean paste), algae, and spirulina had previously been reported to contain vitamin B12. The current thinking, however, is that much of this is actually B12 analogs, which may interfere with active vitamin B12 absorption (Cousins, 1996).

Because a B12 deficiency poses a risk of permanent neurological damage, it is critical to ensure a reliable source of this essential vitamin. The RDA for vitamin B12 is 0.9 micrograms (µg)/day for 1- to 3-year-olds, 1.2 µg/day for 4- to 8-year-olds, 1.8 µg/day for boys 9–18 years old, and 2.4 µg/day for girls 9–18 years old (O'Connell et al., 1989).

Zinc

Little information is available on the zinc content of diets of vegetarian children (Messina, Mangels, & Messina, 2004). Zinc from breast milk is better absorbed than zinc found in infant formula, probably because of the presence of zinc-binding proteins in human milk (Ryan, 1997). Vegetarian children should include a variety of zinc-rich foods in their diets, such as whole-grain pasta, wheat germ, fortified cereals, cheese, legumes, and peanut butter. The recommended intake of zinc for infants is 3 mg/day for children aged 7 months to 3 years, and 5 mg/day for 4- to 8-year-olds. The recommended intake differs by gender as children age. It is 8 mg/day for 9- to 13-year-olds, and then 11 mg/day for 14- to 18-year-old boys, and 9 mg/day for 14- to 18-year-old girls (Ganji, Hampl, & Betts, 2003). This recommended amount can be reached with whole grain and cereal intake. National surveys indicate that most children easily meet their zinc needs with these foods, because vegetarians and omnivores have similar sources (CNPP, 1996).

Diet for Infancy

All infants begin life as vegetarians, as meat is generally not introduced into the diet until the latter half of the first year of life. Breastfeeding is the recommended feeding method for all infants. Breastfeeding rates among vegetarians are much higher than in the general population; breastfeeding rates among vegetarians above 95% have been reported (Sanders & Reddy, 1994). In the United States, only 20% of infants in the general population are still being breast-fed at 6 months of age (Dewey et al., 1992), but studies examining vegan children showed that most were breast-fed well into the second year of life (Kuczmarski et al., 2000). The growth pattern of breast-fed children is similar to that of non-breast-fed children during the first six months of life, and is slightly slower thereafter. This may be due to the extended time of breastfeeding alone (Specker et al., 1988). Because most vegetarian infants are breast-fed, growth should be assessed using tools designed for infants consistent with the feeding method chosen by the parents. The latest growth charts are designed to assess breast-fed and formula-fed infants separately and can be used to track growth accordingly (Hergenrather et al., 1981).

The milk produced by vegetarian mothers is nutritionally adequate, and breast-fed infants of well-nourished vegetarian mothers grow and develop normally (Messina, Mangels, & Messina, 2004). There are few data on the growth of nonmacrobiotic vegan infants (Messina, Mangels, & Messina, 2004). Current research indicates that only newly absorbed vitamin B12 (as opposed to that stored in the mother's body) is passed through the breast milk. Nursing mothers must thus establish and maintain good dietary sources of B12 throughout the nursing period (Committee on Nutrition, 1983). The zinc content of breast milk is not sufficient for the second six months; therefore, foods containing zinc should be introduced during that time (Ganji, Hampl, & Betts, 2003).

A 1981 report published in the *New England Journal of Medicine* noted that milk from vegetarian mothers had fewer pesticide residues than milk from mothers in the general population (Skinner et al., 1997). Vegetarian infants who are not breast-fed should receive appropriate cow's milk-based infant formula or soy-based infant formula. Soy or other "milks" are not a substitute for infant formula. Soy formulas are acceptable to most vegan families and support normal growth in infants (Mangels & Messina, 2001). Infant nutritional needs can easily be met by adequate breastfeeding or formula feeding.

Toddlers

Vegetarian toddlers should be expected to have the same nutritional concerns as omnivore toddlers: namely, a dislike of vegetables, "picky" eating habits, and food jags (when children choose one food for a period of time and then move on to another single food item or food group) (Sabaté et al., 1991). Commercial, full-fat, fortified soy milk, or cow's milk, can be used as a primary beverage starting at age one year or older for a child who is growing normally and is eating a variety of foods (Tayter & Stanek, 1989). Foods that are rich in energy and nutrients, such as legume spreads, tofu, and mashed avocado, should be used when the infant is being weaned. Dietary fat should not be restricted in children younger than two years. A vegetarian diet planned in accord with current dietary recommendations can meet the nutritional needs of toddlers and preschoolers and aid in the establishment of lifelong healthy eating patterns (Dietary Guidelines Advisory Committee, 2004; U.S. Department of Agriculture, 2000). Young children need more than just three meals a day, though. Nutritious snacks can add significantly to the nutrient intake of the vegetarian child.

School-Aged Children

Many school-aged children have been eating a vegetarian diet from birth. However, it is becoming more common for children as young as seven or eight years old to choose such a diet for themselves.

A common misconception is that vegetarian children will have poor growth. Studies of Seventh-Day Adventist children, who mostly follow a lacto-ovo vegetarian diet, show that they are slightly taller than omnivores (Sanders & Manning, 1992). Other studies of lacto-ovo vegetarian children have shown growth rates that match or exceed normal (Messina, Mangels, & Messina, 2004; Messina & Mangels, 2001).

Most studies of vegan children in the United States have been done on children following a macrobiotic diet. One exception is the FARM study. The FARM is a vegan community in Tennessee. A sample of 404 children, vegan from birth, were slightly shorter than controls at age 1 to 3, and were comparable in height at age 10 (Sanders & Reddy, 1994). Studies of British vegan (nonmacrobiotic) children showed that they were taller than controls and a bit lighter (Messina & Mangels, 2001).

The average protein intake of vegetarian children generally meets the RDA; however, vegetarian children may consume less protein than omnivores (Food and Nutrition Service, 2001). Vegan children may have protein needs that are slightly higher than those of other vegetarians and omnivores, because of differences in protein quality from plants, but their needs can be met when a variety of plant foods is consumed regularly (FNB, 2002a; Sabaté et al., 1991).

The USDA's National School Lunch Program does allow nonmeat protein products to be used, but few public schools regularly feature vegetarian menu items (O'Connor et al., 1987). The protein content of school lunches without the meat item is therefore not adequate for vegetarians. Some children prefer not to have the school lunch if it is served with the meat on the tray. It is recommended that children who are vegetarian bring foods from home to supplement what they receive in a school lunch, or pack a complete meal.

Adolescents

Few data are available on the eating habits and growth of vegetarian adolescents, although studies suggest that there is little difference between vegetarians and nonvegetarians (Perry et al., 2001). Some professionals have suggested that eliminating food groups, as one would when adopting a vegetarian diet, may be a first step leading to eating disorders. Some health professionals have noted that vegetarian diets are somewhat more common among teens with eating disorders than in the general adolescent population (Janelle & Barr, 1995; Donovan & Gibson, 1995). Of course, this does not imply that all teenagers who adopt a vegetarian diet are exhibiting or at high risk of an eating disorder; however, parents of all teens should be aware of behaviors consistent with disordered eating (Perry et al., 2002).

Vegetarian diets can offer nutritional advantages to teenagers. Vegetarian teens are reported to consume more fiber, folate, vitamin A, and vitamin C than nonvegetarians because they eat more fruits and vegetables and fewer sweets (Messina & Burke, 1997; Rosenbloom, 2000). Nutrients that may fall short in their diets include calcium, vitamin D, iron, zinc, and vitamin B12.

Table 18.4 Meal Planning Guidelines for Vegetarian Children

Food Group	1–4 Years	5–6 Years	7–12 Years	13–18 Years
Grains	4 servings	6 servings	7 servings	10 servings
Leafy green vegetables	2–4 tsp.	1/4 cup	1 serving	1–2 servings
Other vegetables	1/4–1/2 cup	1/4–1/2 cup	3 servings	3 servings
Fruits	3/4–1½ cups	1–2 cups	2 servings	4 servings
Legumes	1/4–1/2 cup	1/2–1 cup	2 servings	2 servings
Nuts and seeds	1–2 Tbsp.	1–2 Tbsp.	1 serving	1 serving
Milk (breast milk, soy, or cow)	3 cups	3 cups	3 cups	3 cups
Fats	3 tsp.	4 tsp.	5 tsp.	4 tsp.

Source: Adapted from Messina M, Messina V. *The Dietitian's Guide to Vegetarian Diets: Issues and Applications.* Gaithersburg, MD: Aspen Publishers; 1996.

Athletes

Vegetarian diets can meet the needs of the child athlete. Protein needs may be elevated because training increases amino acid metabolism, but vegetarian diets that meet energy needs and include good sources of protein (e.g., soy foods, legumes) can provide adequate protein without use of special foods or supplements (Rosenbloom, 2000).

All children who participate in sports should consume carbohydrates soon after vigorous exercise, to replete glycogen stores, and should be certain to eat when they are hungry to replace calories burned during athletics (Rosenbloom, 2000).

Practical Aspects

Many of the same dietary concerns apply to both the vegetarian and the omnivorous child. Parents should be aware of their children's intake of various types of foods. Vegetarian children should be encouraged to consume an adequate amount of calories and protein, while meeting all their nutrient needs by eating a variety of fruits and vegetables daily.

Table 18.4 contains meal planning guidelines for the appropriate amounts of nutrients, arranged by age. Table 18.5 contrasts sample menus, with intake amounts, for a 5-year-old and a 13-year-old.

Caloric Intake

Be sure the diet has sufficient caloric density so that the child does not feel full before energy needs are met. High-fat foods should not be overly restricted, and children should be encouraged to eat several small meals and snacks daily.

To reduce bulk, replace servings of whole grains with refined grains (while maintaining healthy intake of fiber). Some dried fruits and vegetables and cooked fruits can also be substituted for fresh raw fruits and vegetables.

To add calories:

- Add fruit to hot and cold cereal.
- Add dry milk to pancakes and baked goods.
- Add seeds and nuts to cereal or trail mix.
- Add nut butters, hummus, butter, and whole-milk yogurt to the diet.

Table 18.5 Sample Menus for 5-Year-Old and 13-Year-Old Vegan Children

	5-Year-Old	13-Year-Old
Breakfast		
Oatmeal	1 cup	1 cup
Raisins	1 tsp.	2 tsp.
Orange juice	1 cup	1 cup
Whole-wheat bagel	none	one
Almond butter	none	2 Tbsp.
Lunch		
Peanut butter and banana		
sandwich on whole wheat	1 each	1 each
Hummus	3 Tbsp.	4 Tbsp.
Baby carrots	9 each	12 each
Fortified soy milk	1 cup	1 cup
Molasses cookie	none	one
Dinner		
Creamy green soup		
(made with collard greens)	1 cup	1 cup
Crackers	6 each	6 each
Tofu cutlet with gravy	4 oz.	4 oz.
Baked potato	none	one medium
Fortified soy milk	1 cup	1 cup
Snacks		
Almonds	1 Tbsp.	3 Tbsp.
Figs	1/4 cup	1/4 cup
Crackers, whole wheat	none	6
Totals:		
Calories	1,515	2,673
Protein (g)	50	81
Fat (g)	44	88
Vitamin C (mg)	156	188
Iron (mg)	12.6	22.6
Calcium (mg)	894	1,294

Calcium

Most children do not consume enough calcium. Vegetarian children get calcium from breast milk; dairy products; calcium-fortified juices, waffles, and cereals; calcium-fortified soy and rice beverages; low-oxalate vegetables like collard greens and bok choy; and blackstrap molasses. In addition, baked goods made with either cow's milk or fortified soy milk contribute significant amounts of calcium to the child's diet. For chil-

dren with a low dietary intake of calcium, a supplement may be desired. Liquid, chewable, and dissolvable supplements flavored to appeal to children are commercially available.

Vitamin D

In southern climates, sunshine can promote the body's production of vitamin D year-round. In northern states, there is not adequate sunshine in the winter to allow the body to produce vitamin D. Vitamin D synthesis is poorer in dark-skinned persons, and can be blocked by sunscreen; therefore, a dietary source is recommended for all children. Fluid cow's milk, fortified soy or rice milk, fortified breakfast cereals and orange juice, or a vitamin supplement can be used as a vitamin D source.

Iron

Iron-deficiency anemia is a common nutritional problem in all children. Look for a good source of dietary iron, such as whole grains, beans, or dried fruits. Vitamin C enhances non-heme iron absorption. Drinking citrus juice with a sandwich on whole-grain bread or adding orange slices to a spinach salad will improve iron absorption.

Vitamin B12

If the child is vegan, be sure there is an adequate source of vitamin B12 in the diet. Red Star brand Nutritional Yeast Vegetarian Support Formula, fortified "milks," meat analogs, and some breakfast cereals are good vegan vitamin B12 sources. Most children's multivitamins contain vitamin B12.

Protein

If caloric intake is adequate and the child is not eating an excessive amount of empty-calorie foods, protein intake will most likely be adequate. The frequency of meals in a young child's diet greatly assists in providing a variety of amino acids to be available for protein synthesis throughout the day. Legumes, grains, soy products, meat analogs, nut butters, dairy prod-

ucts, and eggs are all concentrated protein sources. Vegetarian children may get a significant amount of their protein requirement from the large amounts of grains and vegetables eaten per day. Numerous meat alternatives, including hot dogs, sausages, and "chicken" nuggets, are available at most grocery stores.

Fat

Concern about total dietary fat and saturated fat has led many families to use nonfat or low-fat dairy products. Infants get adequate fat and protein from breast milk or infant formula. Toddlers need an adequate fat intake for proper growth and for many, using whole-fat dairy products achieves this goal. In contrast, some families who use dairy products find it more convenient to purchase only reduced-fat or nonfat dairy products and see to it that young children get fat from other foods. Full-fat soy milk is generally recommended for young children. Low-fat soy milk and rice milk contain low levels of fat and protein. If these products are used, parents must be sure that children are getting adequate fat and protein from other dietary sources. Breastfeeding a child through the second year of life helps ensure adequate fat and protein intake as well.

Picky Eaters

Raising a child on a vegetarian diet does not guarantee that the child will like all vegetables. Toddlers are notorious for strong food preferences, and vegetarian toddlers are no exception. Parents can use the same techniques as for omnivore children. Vegetarian teens are still teens, and therefore common teen eating habits are to be expected. Foods with low nutrient density, such as french fries and nondairy desserts, may be chosen over green leafy vegetables. Assessing a child's diet over the course of a week or a month gives a more accurate dietary picture than simply looking at the intake during one or two days. Children commonly go on food jags, eating several servings of one food for a few days and refusing anything else. Over time, children with adequate guidance and a variety of healthy food choices will balance their diets.

Substitution Chart

There is no one food that a child *has* to eat, but there are nutrients that they *have* to get. This substitution section will help find a way to get the needed nutrition without having to consume disliked foods or foods to which the child may be allergic.

Calcium

- *Sources:* Fortified rice or soy milk, greens (collard, mustard, turnip, kale), broccoli, tahini, figs, almonds, calcium-precipitated tofu, calcium-fortified orange juice, calcium-fortified cereals and waffles, blackstrap molasses, supplements.
- *Suggestions:* Make the milk into shakes; add milk to pancakes and other foods. Sneak powdered calcium supplements or powdered soy milk into baked goods and pancakes. Try chocolate, strawberry, and vanilla soy, rice, and cow's milk.

Vitamin D

- *Sources:* Fortified rice or soymilk and orange juice, breakfast cereals, vitamin supplements.

- *Suggestions:* Hide the milk in baked goods, soups, and so on. Get sunshine (about 15 minutes per day)!

Protein

- *Sources:* Soy milk, grains, nut butters, nuts and seeds, dairy products, meat analogs, eggs, beans, high-protein vegetables like broccoli and peas.
- *Suggestions:* Hide beans by mashing them and adding them to soup. Use refried beans or hummus as a spread instead of mayo or mustard. Try dips and sauces. Add tofu crumbles to tomato sauce for pasta.

Iron

- *Sources:* Beans, soy milk, iron-fortified breads, cereals, dried fruits, green leafy vegetables, vitamin supplements with iron.
- *Suggestions:* Provide a vitamin C-rich food with every meal. Add dry fruit to cereal; add citrus to a green salad; drink citrus juice with all meals.

Fiber

- *Sources:* Beans, whole-grain cereals, dried fruits, vegetables, fruits.
- *Suggestions:* Use a mixture of white and whole-wheat flour when making baked goods. Encourage children to eat a variety of fruits and vegetables daily.

Vitamin C

- *Sources:* Citrus fruit, strawberries, melon, vegetables (green peppers, potatoes, hot peppers).
- *Suggestions:* Mix strawberry or orange juice into pancakes and drinks. Freeze fruit juice into juice pops.

Vitamin A

- *Sources:* Orange vegetables (carrots, winter squash); fruits (red grapefruit, orange juice).
- *Suggestions:* Hide veggie juice in fruit juice. Try carrot juice mixed with apple juice. Try pumpkin pancakes or muffins. Add veggies to soup.

Conclusion

Vegetarian diets can easily meet the nutritional needs of the growing child. Most of the nutritional concerns and issues that vegetarian families have are exactly the same as for all other families. The scientific literature shows a positive relationship between vegetarian diets and reduced risk of several chronic diseases and conditions, including obesity, coronary artery disease, hypertension, diabetes mellitus, and some types of cancer (Dietary Guidelines Advisory Committee, 2004; U.S. Department of Agriculture, 2000). If children maintain a vegetarian diet throughout their lives, they are at a decreased risk of these chronic diseases.

Meal Planning for Those in "Mixed" (Vegetarian and Nonvegetarian) Families

1. Serve meals that each person assembles himself or herself (chef salad served salad-bar style, tacos, etc.).
2. Revise dishes currently made with meat. It can be easy to assemble a small non-meat lasagna alongside a meat-containing one. Chili, pizza, bean soup, and pasta sauce can all be made without meat or with meat analogs.
3. Serve meatless favorites that the entire family enjoys several times a week. Typi-

cal meals include cheese pizza, vegetable soup with sandwiches, and bean burritos.
4. Many dishes, such as vegetable and grain casseroles, can serve as the entree for the vegetarian and a side dish for the omnivores.

References

Center for Nutrition Policy and Promotion (CNPP), U.S. Department of Agriculture (USDA). *Nutrient Content of the US Food Supply, 1990-1994: Preliminary Data.* Washington, DC: USDA; 1996.

Committee on Nutrition, Academy of Pediatrics. Soy protein formulas: Recommendations for use in infant feeding. *Pediatrics.* 1983;359-363.

Cousins RJ. Zinc. In: Ziegler EE, Filer LJ Jr, eds. *Present Knowledge in Nutrition.* 7th ed. Washington, DC: ILSI Press; 1996:293-306.

Dewey KG, Heinig MJ, Nommsen LA, Peerson JM, Lonnerdal B. Growth of breast-fed and formula-fed infants from 0 to 18 months: The DARLING study. *Pediatrics.* Jun 1992;89(6, Pt 1):1035-1041.

Dietary Guidelines Advisory Committee, U.S. Department of Health and Human Services. *The Report of the Dietary Guidelines Advisory Committee on Dietary Guidelines for Americans, 2005.* 2004. Available at http://www.health.gov/dietary guidelines/dga2005/report/. Accessed July 7, 2007.

Donovan UM, Gibson RS. Iron and zinc status of young women aged 14 to 19 years consuming vegetarian and omnivorous diets. *J Am Coll Nutr.* 1995;14:463-472.

Food and Nutrition Board (FNB), Institute of Medicine. *Dietary Reference Intakes for Energy, Carbohydrate, Fiber, Fat, Fatty Acids, Cholesterol, Protein, and Amino Acids (Macronutrients).* Washington, DC: National Academy Press; 2002a.

Food and Nutrition Board, Institute of Medicine. *Dietary Reference Intakes for Thiamin, Riboflavin, Niacin, Vitamin B6, Folate, Vitamin B12, Pantothenic Acid, Biotin, and Choline.* Washington, DC: National Academy Press; 2002b.

Food and Nutrition Board, Institute of Medicine. *Dietary Reference Intakes for Vitamin A, Vitamin K, Arsenic, Boron, Chromium, Copper, Iodine, Iron, Manganese, Molybdenum, Nickel, Silicon, Vanadium, and Zinc.* Washington, DC: National Academy Press; 2002c.

Food and Nutrition Board, Institute of Medicine. *Dietary Reference Intakes for Calcium, Phosphorus, Magnesium, Vitamin D, and Fluoride.* Washington, DC: National Academy Press; 1997.

Food and Nutrition Service, U.S. Department of Agriculture. Menu planning in the National School Lunch Program. Sept 2001. Available at http://www.fns.usda.gov/cnd/menu/menu.planning.approaches.for.lunches.doc. Accessed July 6, 2007.

Ganji V, Hampl JS, Betts NM. Race-, gender- and age-specific differences in dietary micronutrient intakes of US children. *Intl J Food Sci Nutr.* Nov 2003;54(6):485-490.

Hergenrather J, Hlady G, Wallace B, Savage E. Pollutants in breast milk of vegetarians [letter]. *N Engl J Med.* 1981;304:792.

Janelle KC, Barr SI. Nutrient intakes and eating behavior scores of vegetarian and nonvegetarian women. *J Am Diet Assoc.* 1995;95:180-189.

Kuczmarski RJ, Ogden CL, Grummer-Strawn LM, et al. CDC growth charts: United States. *Adv Data.* Jun 2000;8(314):1-27.

Mangels AR, Messina V. Considerations in planning vegan diets: Infants. *J Am Diet Assoc.* 2001;101:670-677.

Mangels AR, Messina V, Melina V. Position of the American Dietetic Association and Dietitians of Canada: Vegetarian diets. *J Am Diet Assoc.* 2003;103(6):748-765.

Messina V, Mangels AR. Considerations in planning vegan diets: Children. *J Am Diet Assoc.* 2001;101:661-669.

Messina V, Mangels R, Messina M. *The Dietitian's Guide to Vegetarian Diets: Issues and Applications.* 2d ed. Sudbury, MA: Jones and Bartlett Publishers; 2004.

Messina VL, Burke KI. Position of The American Dietetic Association: Vegetarian diets. *J Am Diet Assoc.* 1997;97:1317-1321.

Nusser SM, Carriquiry AL, Dodd KW, Fuller WA. A semiparametric transformations approach to estimating usual daily intake distributions. *J Am Statis Assoc.* 1996;91:1440-1449.

O'Connell JM, Dibley MJ, Sierra J, Wallace B, Marks JS, Yip R. Growth of vegetarian children: The Farm study. *Pediatrics.* 1989;84:475-481.

O'Connor MA, Touyz SW, Dunn SM, Beumont PJ. Vegetarianism in anorexia nervosa? A review of 116 consecutive cases. *Med J Aust.* 1987;147(11-12):540-542.

Perry CL, McGuire MT, Neumark-Sztainer D, Story M. Adolescent vegetarians. How well do their dietary patterns meet the Healthy People 2010 objectives? *Arch Pediatr Adolesc Med.* 2002;156:431-437.

Perry CL, McGuire MT, Newmark-Sztainer D, Story M. Characteristics of vegetarian adolescents in a multiethnic urban population. *J Adolesc Health.* 2001;29:406-416.

Rosenbloom CA. *Sports Nutrition: A Guide for Professionals Working with Active People.* 3d ed. Chicago: American Dietetic Association; 2000.

Ryan AS. The resurgence of breastfeeding in the United States. *Pediatrics.* 1997;99:E12.

Sabaté J, Linsted KD, Harris RD, Sanchez A. Attained height of lacto-ovo vegetarian children and adolescents. *Eur J Clin Nutr.* 1991;45:51-58.

Sanders TAB, Manning J. The growth and development of vegan children. *J Hum Nutr Diet.* 1992;5:11-21.

Sanders TAB, Reddy S. Vegetarian diets and children. *Am J Clin Nutr.* 1994;59 (Suppl):1176S-1181S.

Skinner JD, Carruth BR, Hoouck KS, et al. Longitudinal study of nutrient and food intake of infants aged 2 to 24 months. *J Am Diet Assoc.* 1997;97:496-504.

Specker BL, Miller D, Norman EJ, Greene T, Hayes KC. Increased urinary methylmalonic acid excretion in breast-fed infants of vegetarian mothers and identification of an acceptable dietary source of vitamin B12. *Am J Clin Nutr.* 1988;47:89-92.

Tayter MS, Stanek KL. Anthropometric and dietary assessment of omnivore and lacto-ovo-vegetarian children. *J Am Diet Assoc.* 1989;89:1661-1663.

U.S. Department of Agriculture. *Dietary Guidelines for Americans*. 5th ed. Washington, DC: Government Printing Office; 2000.

The Vegetarian Resource Group. How many teens are vegetarian? How many kids don't eat meat? *Vegetarian Journal*. Jan/Feb 2001. Available at: http://www.vrg.org/journal/vj2001jan/2001 janteen.htm. Accessed July 6, 2007.

Young VR, Pellett PL. Plant proteins in relation to human protein and amino acid nutrition. *Am J Clin Nutr*. 1994; 59(Suppl):1203S–1212S.

19

Pregnancy and Lactation

Reed Mangels, PhD, RD, FADA

Introduction

Pregnancy is a time of increased nutritional needs, both to support the rapidly growing fetus and to allow for the changes occurring in the pregnant woman's body. Throughout pregnancy, recommended intakes of many vitamins and minerals are higher than for the nonpregnant state. For example, the recommendations for both folic acid and iron are about 50 percent higher in pregnancy (Food and Nutrition Board [FNB], 1998; FNB, 2002b). During lactation, nutritional needs are similar to those in pregnancy, to allow milk synthesis and to meet maternal needs. These increased nutrient needs during pregnancy and lactation can be met by a vegetarian diet (Mangels, Messina, & Melina, 2003). Special considerations during pregnancy and lactation, which are discussed in this chapter, include energy needs and intakes of protein, omega-3 fatty acids, calcium, vitamin D, iron, iodine, and vitamin B12. The role of nutrition in some complications of pregnancy is also discussed. The effect of a vegetarian diet on milk composition is described.

Summary of the Scientific Literature

Pregnancy

Weight Gain

Weight gain in pregnancy, especially during the second and third trimesters, plays an important role in the fetus's growth. Low weight gain in pregnancy is associated with an increased risk of having an infant who is small for gestational age and who is thus at risk for impaired neurobehavioral development (Subcommittee on Nutritional Status and Weight Gain During Pregnancy [SNS], 1990). Infant mortality is also higher in infants who are small for gestational age and whose mothers have low weight gain. Low weight gain may also be associated with an increased risk of preterm delivery (SNS, 1990).

Vegetarians as a group tend to be leaner than nonvegetarians, with vegans having a lower body mass index (measure of fatness) than other vegetarians (Spencer et al., 2003). However, weight gain of pregnant vegetarians, both lacto-ovo and vegan, has been reported to be adequate (King, Stein, & Doyle, 1981; Carter, Furman, & Hutcheson, 1987; Ward et al., 1988). Birth weights of infants of vegetarian women have frequently been shown to be similar to those of infants of nonvegetarians and to birth weight norms (King, Stein, & Doyle, 1981; Ward et al., 1988; O'Connell et al., 1989; Dwyer et al., 1980; Thomas & Ellis, 1977; Abu-Assal & Craig, 1984; Drake, Reddy, & Davies, 1998; Lakin, Haggarty, & Abramovich, 1998). In some cases, however, birth weights of infants born to vegan women were slightly lower than of infants with nonvegetarian mothers (Sanders & Reddy, 1992); infant health and neurobehavioral status were not reported. Low birth weights have been seen in infants of macrobiotic women in the Netherlands (Dagnelie et al., 1988; Dagnelie et al., 1989) and Hindu vegetarians (McFadyen et al., 1984). These low weights have been attributed to low maternal weight gain and lower maternal intakes of energy, iron, folate, or vitamin B12 (Dagnelie et al., 1988; Dagnelie et al., 1989; McFadyen et al., 1984).

Current weight-gain recommendations (SNS, 1990) are applicable to vegetarians. These call for a 25- to 35-pound gain for women who are of average weight prior to pregnancy. Women who were underweight prior to pregnancy should gain 28–40 pounds. Overweight women should gain 15–25 pounds. Adolescents may need to gain 30–45 pounds. A general trend is to have little weight gain (around 2 to 4 pounds) for the first 12 weeks. Then, in the second and third trimesters, a weight gain of a pound to a pound and a half a week is common.

Extra dietary energy is required to meet the weight-gain recommendations for pregnancy. The total energy cost of a pregnancy is estimated to be around 80,000 calories over the 280 days of pregnancy (SNS, 1990; Prentice & Goldberg, 2000). Assuming that caloric intake does not increase during the first month of pregnancy, an additional 340 calories per day in the second trimester and 452 calories per day in the third trimester should meet energy needs (FNB, 2002a).

Protein

Protein needs increase during pregnancy to support the expansion of blood volume and growth of maternal tissue, as well as growth of the fetus and placenta (SNS, 1990). Current recommendations for protein in pregnancy call for an increase of 25 grams of protein per day, for a total of 71 grams per day of protein in the second and third trimesters (FNB, 2002a) for the average woman.

Omega-3 Fatty Acids

Docosahexaenoic acid (DHA) is a long-chain omega-3 fatty acid present in all cells of the body, and found in especially high concentrations in the brain and retina. Higher intakes of DHA during pregnancy have been associated with improvements in gestational length, infant visual function, and development of the nervous system (McCann & Ames, 2005; Williams & Burdge, 2006; Jensen, 2006; Cheatham, Colombo, & Carlson, 2006). There are few sources of this fatty acid in the vegetarian and vegan diet. Infants of vegetarian mothers have been reported to have lower cord levels of DHA than do infants of nonvegetarians (Lakin, Haggarty, & Abramovich, 1998; Reddy, Sanders, & Obeid, 1994). DHA can be synthesized from linolenic acid or obtained from a vegetarian DHA supplement derived from microalgae (Conquer & Holub, 1996). The rate of production of DHA from linolenic acid is quite low (Williams & Burdge, 2006), so DHA supplements or use of foods fortified with DHA are frequently recommended in pregnancy.

Iron

Iron needs in pregnancy are much higher than usual because of the increase in the amount of the mother's blood and because of blood formed for the fetus. Despite compensatory mechanisms such as cessation of menstruation and increased iron absorption, the iron requirement of pregnancy is quite high, so the diet must be especially rich in iron. Iron supplements of 30 milligrams (mg) daily during the second and third trimesters, along with an iron-rich diet, are commonly recommended for both vegetarian and nonvegetarian women (Centers for Disease Control and Prevention, 1998). Additional iron may be needed in the case of iron deficiency.

Iron-deficiency anemia is not uncommon during pregnancy, in both vegetarians and nonvegetarians. Several studies of pregnant vegetarians have suggested that dietary iron intakes were close to recommended levels (Finley, Dewey et al., 1985), although Drake et al. found that iron supplements were needed to meet iron recommendations for lacto-ovo vegetarians, fish eaters, and meat eaters (Drake, Reddy, & Davies, 1998). All pregnant women, including vegetarians, should be checked for iron-deficiency anemia and consider supplementation if they are unable to meet their needs through diet alone.

Calcium and Vitamin D

Calcium is needed in pregnancy for synthesis of fetal bones and teeth. Approximately 25 to 30 grams of calcium are transferred to the fetus, primarily in the third trimester (SNS, 1990). Historically, women have been advised to substantially increase their calcium intake during pregnancy in order to meet the fetus's needs without compromising maternal bone. However, pregnant women appear to adapt to increased

needs by increasing calcium absorption, resulting in a generally positive calcium balance during pregnancy (Prentice, 2000; FNB, 1997). The Institute of Medicine concluded that as long as calcium intake prior to pregnancy was adequate for maximizing bone accretion, dietary calcium need not be increased during pregnancy (FNB, 1997). The calcium recommendation for pregnant women age 19 and older is 1,000 milligrams a day (FNB, 1997). Adolescents appear to have an increased need for calcium to support their own bone development (Chan et al., 1987); thus, current recommendations for pregnant adolescents under the age of 19 call for 1,300 milligrams of calcium daily (FNB, 1997).

Calcium intakes of lacto-ovo vegetarian women are often close to levels recommended for pregnancy, whereas calcium intakes of vegan women are generally lower (Messina, Mangels, & Messina, 2004). Pregnant women whose diets do not contain adequate calcium should add calcium-rich foods to the diet or use supplemental calcium (SNS, 1990). This appears to be especially important in adolescents.

Vitamin D plays an important role in maintenance of maternal calcium status. Its role in placental transport of calcium is not clear, nor is its role in fetal vitamin D status. Vitamin D status of vegetarians can vary based on sunlight exposure and dietary choices (Webb, Kline, & Holick, 1988; Matsuoka et al., 1987; Dent & Gupta, 1975; Maxwell et al., 1981). Generally, regular use of vitamin D-fortified cow's milk can meet vitamin D requirements. Fortified foods, such as some cereals and some brands of soy milk, are another way to meet vitamin D needs. The Institute of Medicine recommends that a vitamin D supplement of 10 micrograms (400 IU) daily be taken by pregnant vegans who live at northern latitudes in the winter and by those with minimal exposure to sunlight (SNS, 1990).

Iodine

Iodine may be low in vegetarian diets, especially if iodized salt is not selected (Remer, Neubert, & Manz, 1999; Krajcovicova-Kudlackova et al., 2003). Iodine plays a key role in brain development (FNB, 2002b), so iodine deficiency in pregnancy should be avoided. Regular use of iodized salt at the table and in cooking will generally provide adequate amounts of iodine. Women who do not use iodized salt can obtain iodine from a supplement. Not all prenatal supplements contain iodine, so it is important to check the nutrient label. Sea vegetables are another possible source of iodine, but their content is variable (Teas et al., 2004), and, if excessive, can lead to problems in infants (Nishiyama et al., 2004).

Vitamin B12

Vitamin B12 is needed during pregnancy for normal cell division and protein synthesis. Vitamin B12 is a concern only for vegetarians who use few or no dairy products or eggs or who are unable to adequately absorb vitamin B12. It appears that maternal stores of vitamin B12 may not be available to the fetus (Lubby et al., 1958) and that the maternal diet or supplements should supply vitamin B12 to avoid deficiency in the infant. The recommended level of vitamin B12 in pregnancy is 2.6 micrograms per day (FNB, 1998). Pregnant vegans who have not been including reliable sources of vitamin B12 in their diets (fortified foods or supplements) may consider having their blood vitamin B12 levels checked.

Zinc

The recommended intake of zinc increases by 38% during pregnancy (FNB, 2002b). Many women in the United States have difficulty meeting the RDA for zinc during pregnancy. Several studies have examined vegetarians' zinc status during pregnancy. One found that although vegetarians' diets were slightly lower in zinc than those of nonvegetarians, the vegetarians' blood and urine zinc levels were similar to those of nonvegetarians (King, Stein, & Doyle, 1981). In another study, vegetarians' zinc intakes were found to be similar to those of nonvegetarians (Abu-Assal & Craig, 1984). Because zinc status is difficult to assess, and zinc plays important roles in both growth and development and reduction of risk of complications of labor and delivery (Jameson, 1993; Caulfield et al., 1998), pregnant vegetarians should emphasize good food sources of zinc.

Zinc supplements are another option. Supplemental zinc is recommended when more than 30 milligrams of iron are used per day (SNS, 1990), because iron in large doses appears to depress plasma zinc in pregnancy (Dawson, Albers, & McGanity, 1989).

Vegetarian Diets and Complications of Pregnancy

One study examined the rate of preeclampsia, a potentially serious problem in pregnancy, in a community of vegans in Tennessee between 1977 and 1982. Of 775 vegan pregnancies, there was only one case of preeclampsia (Carter, Furman, & Hutcheson, 1987). This is a much lower rate than that seen in the general population.

Although no research has examined vegetarian diets in pregnant women with diabetes, it is clear that adequate vegetarian diets can be planned to meet the needs of both pregnancy and diabetes. Careful attention and individualization based on diet history, glycemic responses, weight changes, and individual preferences are essential for a successful outcome

(Fagen, King, & Erick, 1995). There are no studies of the incidence of gestational diabetes in vegetarians compared to nonvegetarians.

Vegetarian Nutrition during Lactation

More vegetarian women tend to breastfeed, and to continue breastfeeding for a longer time, than do nonvegetarians (O'Connell et al., 1989; Sanders, 1988). Several studies have shown that growth of infants of lactating vegetarians is normal (Mangels, Messina, & Melina, 2003). The reported poor growth of 4- to 6-month-old infants of macrobiotic women was apparently due to intakes of breast milk as low as 350 mL per day (Dagnelie et al., 1989). This low intake could have been due to early weaning, inadequate nursing, or inadequate maternal diet.

Milk Composition

The nutrient content of breast milk is affected by maternal diet. Milk from vegetarians who are well nourished is expected to be similar to milk from well-nourished nonvegetarians (Finley, 1985). This is true of most nutrients. A significant difference is seen in milk fatty acid composition, however. Vegetarians have higher milk concentrations of polyunsaturated fatty acids derived from dietary vegetable fat and lower concentrations of fatty acids derived from animal fat (Sanders & Reddy, 1992; Specker, Wey, & Miller, 1987; Finley, Lonnerdal et al., 1985). These differences do not appear to affect infant health.

DHA levels have been shown to be lower in the breast milk of vegan women compared to both lacto-ovo vegetarians and omnivores. Mean percentages of DHA in milk from vegans, lacto-ovo vegetarians, and nonvegetarians were 0.14%, 0.30%, and 0.37%, respectively (Sanders &

Reddy, 1992). Studies of neuronal functioning and visual acuity suggest that consumption of DHA may provide some advantage for infants (Uauy et al., 1996; Jensen, 2006; Cheatham, Colombo, & Carlson, 2006). DHA derived from microalgae, when used by lactating women, has been shown to be effective in increasing the level of DHA in their infants' blood (Jensen et al., 2005).

One important difference between breast milk of vegetarian and nonvegetarian women is its contaminant concentration. Studies of vegetarians show lower levels of pesticides, such as hexachlorobenzene, chlordane, and hepatachlor, and industrial byproducts, such as polychlorinated biphenyls (PCBs), in their breast milk (Dagnelie et al., 1992; Hergenrather et al., 1981). This is apparently due to vegetarians' avoidance of meat products. Levels of contaminants in breast milk would be expected to be lowest in vegans, and at least one study has found that maternal intakes of meat and dairy products have a large influence on milk levels of dieldrin and PCBs (Dagnelie et al., 1992).

Studies of lactating women suggest that their dietary calcium intake has little effect on the calcium content of their milk (Prentice et al., 1995; Kalkwarf et al., 1996). Despite losing close to 200 milligrams daily in breast milk, women's calcium absorption does not appear to increase during lactation (FNB, 1997; Specker, 1994; Ritchie et al., 1998). There is some decrease in urinary calcium losses, and calcium is mobilized from the mother's bones to supply calcium for breast milk (Prentice, 2000; FNB, 1997). Increasing dietary calcium cannot prevent this loss of calcium from the bones. Because dietary calcium does not appear to prevent the loss of calcium from the mother's bones, calcium recommendations are not increased for lactating women (FNB, 1997). Calcium intakes of vegetarians are variable; many studies have found that lacto-ovo vegetarian women do consume the recommended 1,000 mg or more of calcium daily, whereas vegan women seldom reach this level without supplementation or use of calcium-fortified foods (Messina, Mangels, & Messina, 2004).

Breast-milk vitamin D content varies with maternal diet and sun exposure (Prentice et al., 1995; Specker et al., 1985), but is normally quite low. Adequate vitamin D, either from diet or sun exposure, is important during lactation to maintain maternal calcium status and prevent bone demineralization. Vitamin D supplements are recommended for women who avoid vitamin D-fortified foods and who have limited sunlight exposure (Subcommittee on Nutrition During Lactation, 1991). Because of the low levels of vitamin D in breast milk, infants who do not have adequate sun exposure should receive a supplement of 200 IU per day of vitamin D, beginning within the first 2 months. Thirty minutes of sunlight exposure per week while wearing only a diaper, or two hours per week while fully clothed without a hat, appear to maintain adequate vitamin D levels in light-skinned infants in moderate climates (Specker et al., 1985). Dark-skinned infants and those who live at northern latitudes may be at risk of vitamin D deficiency, however, and vitamin D supplementation is advised in these cases.

Studies have reported low plasma vitamin B12 levels in macrobiotic lactating women (Specker et al., 1987) and their infants (Specker et al., 1990), low maternal milk vitamin B12 levels in these women (Dagnelie et al., 1989; Specker et al., 1990), and elevated urinary methylmalonic acid (an indicator of vitamin B12 deficiency) in macrobiotic women (Specker et al., 1985) and their infants (Specker et al., 1987; Specker et al., 1990). Some studies suggest that vitamin B12 from maternal stores is not available to the breastfed infant (Specker et al., 1987), though not all research supports this (Specker

et al., 1990). It is important that vegan women who are breastfeeding include regular vitamin B12 supplements or fortified foods in their diets, or that breastfed infants receive vitamin B12 supplements. With the exception of vitamin B12, guidelines for supplementation of vegan infants are the same as for omnivore infants.

Practical Aspects

Weight Gain in Pregnancy

Women who were underweight prior to pregnancy or who are having difficulty gaining weight in pregnancy may need to use concentrated sources of calories and nutrients. These foods include milkshakes (soy milk or cow's milk blended with fruit and tofu or yogurt), nuts and nut butters, dried fruits, soy products, and bean dips. Small, frequent meals and snacks can help to increase food intake.

Protein

If a woman's diet is varied and contains good protein sources, such as soy products, beans, and grains, or dairy products and eggs, and weight gain is appropriate, it is likely that the increased protein needs of pregnancy will be met. Many women get the extra protein they need simply by eating more of the foods they usually eat. As an example, 10–15 grams of protein can be added by adding 2 cups of soy milk or 9 ounces of tofu or 3 ounces of tempeh or 1½ bagels to the usual diet.

Omega-3 Fatty Acids

Omega-3 fatty acids can be synthesized, to a limited extent, from linolenic acid. Good sources of linolenic acid include ground flaxseed, flax-seed oil, canola oil, and soy products (Mangels, Messina, & Melina, 2003). Limiting dietary linoleic acid (corn oil, safflower oil, sunflower oil) and trans fatty acids (partially hydrogenated fats) can enhance DHA production (Brenner & Peluffo, 1969; Innis & King, 1999). During pregnancy and lactation, because of increased omega-3 fatty acid requirements, a direct source of DHA should be considered. These sources include DHA supplements derived from micro-algae and foods that have been enriched with microalgae-derived DHA, such as soy milk, energy bars, yogurt, and veggie burgers.

Iron

Even when iron supplements are used, pregnant vegetarians should choose high-iron foods, such as whole grains, dried beans, tofu, and green leafy vegetables, daily. Iron supplements should not be taken at the same time as calcium supplements, and should be taken between meals to maximize absorption (SNS, 1990).

Calcium and Vitamin D

Some plant-based calcium sources that are well absorbed are calcium-fortified soy milk and orange juice; soybeans; dark green leafy vegetables, such as collard greens, kale, and turnip greens; and calcium-precipitated tofu. Food sources of vitamin D for vegetarians include vitamin D-fortified breakfast cereals, vitamin D-fortified cow's milk, and vitamin D-fortified soy milk and rice milk. Ergocalciferol, or vitamin D2, is made on a commercial scale from yeast and is used to fortify some foods.

Iodine

Three-quarters of a teaspoon of iodized salt, used in cooking and at the table, will meet the iodine recommendations for pregnancy. If iodized salt is not used, an iodine supplement may be needed. Some, but not all, prenatal supplements contain iodine.

Vitamin B12

Foods that have been fortified with vitamin B12 include some cereals, some soy milks, and Red Star Vegetarian Support Formula nutritional yeast. Foods that have traditionally been proposed as good sources of vitamin B12, such as tempeh, sea vegetables, and algae, have been shown to be unreliable and, thus, inappropriate sources (Specker et al., 1987; Herbert, 1988). In addition, these foods may contain vitamin B12 analogs (substances that mimic vitamin B12 but that actually block vitamin B12 absorption).

Nausea and Vomiting

Nausea and vomiting, also called morning sickness, are a concern of many pregnant women, vegetarians included. Many women are repulsed by foods that used to make up the bulk of their diet, such as salads, dried beans, and soy milk. These aversions are extremely common in early pregnancy and are believed to be due to a heightened sense of smell, possibly because of hormonal changes (Erick, 1994). Eating low-fat, high-carbohydrate foods that are digested more quickly; eating often; avoiding foods with strong smells; and eating healthful foods that are tolerated are some coping mechanisms that may help during this time. The health care provider should be contacted if a pregnant

Table 19.1 Food Guide for Pregnant and Lactating Vegetarians

Food Group	Number of Servings
Grains	6 or more, pregnancy or lactation (a serving is 1 slice of bread or ½ cup cooked cereal, grain, or pasta, or ¾ to 1 cup ready-to-eat cereal)
Legumes, nuts, and other protein-rich foods	7 or more, pregnancy; 8 or more, lactation (a serving is ½ cup cooked beans, tofu, tempeh, or TVP; or 1 ounce of meat analog; or 2 Tbsp. nut or seed butter; or ½ cup fortified soy milk, ½ cup cow's milk, or ½ cup yogurt)
Vegetables	4 or more, pregnancy and lactation (a serving is ½ cup cooked or 1 cup raw vegetables)
Fruits	2 or more, pregnancy and lactation (a serving is ½ cup canned fruit or juice or 1 medium fruit)
Calcium-rich foods	8 or more, pregnancy and lactation (a serving is ½ cup calcium-fortified juice or soy milk; 1 cup cooked bok choy, collards, Chinese cabbage, kale, mustard greens, or okra; ½ cup milk or yogurt; ½ cup calcium-set tofu; ¾ oz. cheese; 1 oz. calcium-fortified cereal)
Fats	2 or more, pregnancy and lactation (a serving is 1 tsp. oil or margarine)

Note: These guidelines show the minimum number of servings recommended. Many women will need more calories to support adequate weight gain in pregnancy and weight maintenance during lactation. In this case, additional servings of foods can be added and fats such as oil and salad dressing used to increase calories.

Regular sources of vitamin B12 and omega-3 fatty acids should be used.

Source: Adapted from *Journal of the American Dietetic Association*, volume 103, appearing as Messina V, Melina V, Mangels AR. A new food guide for North American vegetarians. *J Am Diet Assoc.* 2003;103:771–775, with permission from The American Dietetic Association.

woman is unable to eat or to drink adequate amounts of fluids for 24 hours.

Diet Guides

A number of food guides have been developed for pregnant and lactating vegetarians. Table 19.1 reproduces part of one such guide (Messina, Melina, & Mangels, 2003).

Conclusion

A vegetarian diet planned in accord with current dietary recommendations can easily meet the nutritional needs of pregnancy and lac-

tation (Mangels, Messina, & Melina, 2003). Potential benefits of a vegetarian diet in pregnancy and lactation include a possibly reduced risk of preeclampsia, a complication of pregnancy (Carter, Furman, & Hutcheson, 1987); and lower levels of environmental contaminants in breast milk (Dagnelie et al., 1992; Hergenrather et al., 1981).

References

Abu-Assal MJ, Craig WJ. The zinc status of pregnant women. *Nutr Rep Intl.* 1984;29:485–494.

Brenner RR, Peluffo RO. Regulation of unsaturated fatty acid biosynthesis. *Biochim Biophys Acta.* 1969;176:471–479.

Carter JP, Furman T, Hutcheson HR. Preeclampsia and reproductive performance in a community of vegans. *South Med J.* 1987;80:692–697.

Caulfield LE, Zavaleta N, Shankar AN, et al. Potential contribution of maternal zinc supplementation during pregnancy to maternal and child survival. *Am J Clin Nutr.* 1998;68(Suppl):499S–508S.

Centers for Disease Control and Prevention. Recommendations to prevent and control iron deficiency in the United States. *MMWR.* 1998;47(RR-3):1–29.

Chan GM, McMurry M, Westover K, et al. Effects of increased dietary calcium intake upon the calcium and bone mineral status of lactating adolescent and adult women. *Am J Clin Nutr.* 1987;46:319–323.

Cheatham CL, Colombo J, Carlson SE. n-3 fatty acids and cognitive and visual acuity development: Methodologic and conceptual considerations. *Am J Clin Nutr.* 2006;83(Suppl):1458S–1466S.

Conquer JA, Holub BJ. Supplementation with an algae source of docosahexaenoic acid increases (n-3) fatty acid status and alters selected risk factors for heart disease in vegetarian subjects. *J Nutr.* 1996;126:3032–3039.

Dagnelie PC, van Staveren WA, Roos AH, et al. Nutrients and contaminants in human milk from mothers on macrobiotic and omnivorous diets. *Eur J Clin Nutr.* 1992;46:355–366.

Dagnelie PC, van Staveren WA, van Klaveren JD, Burema J. Do children on macrobiotic diets show catch-up growth? *Eur J Clin Nutr.* 1988;42:1007–1016.

Dagnelie PC, van Staveren WA, Vergote FJVRA, et al. Nutritional status of infants aged 4 to 18 months on macrobiotic diets and matched omnivorous control infants: A population-based mixed-longitudinal study. II. Growth and psychomotor development. *Eur J Clin Nutr.* 1989;43:325–338.

Dawson EB, Albers J, McGanity WJ. Serum zinc changes due to iron supplementation in teen-age pregnancy. *Am J Clin Nutr.* 1989;50:848–852.

Dent CE, Gupta MM. Plasma 25-hydroxyvitamin-D levels during pregnancy and in vegetarian and nonvegetarian Asians. *Lancet.* 1975;2:1057–1060.

Drake R, Reddy S, Davies J. Nutrient intake during pregnancy and pregnancy outcome of lacto-ovo-vegetarians, fish-eaters and nonvegetarians. *Veg Nutr.* 1998;2:45–52.

Dwyer JT, Andrew EM, Valadian I, Reed RB. Size, obesity, and leanness in vegetarian preschool children. *J Am Diet Assoc.* 1980;77:434–439.

Erick M. Hyperolfaction as a factor in hyperemesis gravidarum: Considerations for nutritional management. *Persp Appl Nutr.* 1994;2:3–9.

Fagen C, King JD, Erick M. Nutrition management in women with gestational diabetes mellitus: A review by ADA's Diabetes Care and Education dietetic practice group. *J Am Diet Assoc.* 1995;95:460–467.

Finley DA. Effects of vegetarian diets upon the composition of human milk. In: Hamosh M, Goldman AS, eds. *Human Lactation 2. Maternal and Environmental Factors.* New York: Plenum Press; 1986.

Finley DA, Dewey KG, Lonnerdal B, Grivetti LE. Food choices of vegetarians and nonvegetarians during pregnancy and lactation. *J Am Diet Assoc.* 1985;85:678–685.

Finley DA, Lonnerdal B, Dewey KG, Grivetti LE. Breast milk composition: Fat content and fatty acid composition in vegetarians and nonvegetarians. *Am J Clin Nutr.* 1985;41:787–800.

Food and Nutrition Board (FNB), Institute of Medicine. *Dietary Reference Intakes for Energy, Carbohydrate, Fiber, Fat, Fatty Acids, Cholesterol, Protein, and Amino Acids (Macronutrients).* Washington, DC: National Academy Press; 2002a.

Food and Nutrition Board, Institute of Medicine. *Dietary Reference Intakes for Vitamin A, Vitamin K, Arsenic, Boron, Chromium, Copper, Iodine, Iron, Manganese, Molybdenum, Nickel, Silicon, Vanadium, and Zinc.* Washington, DC: National Academy Press; 2002b.

Food and Nutrition Board, Institute of Medicine. *Dietary Reference Intakes for Thiamin, Riboflavin, Niacin, Vitamin B6, Folate, Vitamin B12, Pantothenic Acid, Biotin, and Choline.* Washington, DC: National Academy Press; 1998.

Food and Nutrition Board, Institute of Medicine. *Dietary Reference Intakes for Calcium, Phosphorus, Magnesium, Vitamin D, and Fluoride.* Washington, DC: National Academy Press; 1997.

Herbert V. Vitamin B-12: Plant sources, requirements, and assay. *Am J Clin Nutr.* 1988;48:852–858.

Hergenrather J, Hlady G, Wallace B, Savage E. Pollutants in breast milk of vegetarians [letter]. *N Engl J Med.* 1981;304:792.

Innis SM, King DJ, trans. Fatty acids in human milk are inversely associated with concentrations of essential all-cis n-6 and n-3 fatty acids and determine trans, but not n-6 and n-3, fatty acids in plasma lipids of breast-fed infants. *Am J Clin Nutr.* 1999;70:383–390.

Jameson S. Zinc status in pregnancy: The effect of zinc therapy on perinatal mortality, prematurity, and placental ablation. *Ann NY Acad Sci.* 1993;678:178–192.

Jensen CL. Effects of n-3 fatty acids during pregnancy and lactation. *Am J Clin Nutr.* 2006;83(Suppl):1452S–1457S.

Jensen CL, Voigt RG, Prager TC, et al. Effects of maternal docosahexaenoic acid on visual function and neurodevelopment in breastfed term infants. *Am J Clin Nutr.* 2005;82:125–132.

Kalkwarf HJ, Specker BL, Heubi JE, et al. Intestinal calcium absorption of women during lactation and after weaning. *Am J Clin Nutr.* 1996;63:526–531.

King JC, Stein T, Doyle M. Effect of vegetarianism on the zinc status of pregnant women. *Am J Clin Nutr.* 1981;34:1049–1055.

Krajcovicova-Kudlackova M, Buckova K, Klimes I, Sebokova E. Iodine deficiency in vegetarians and vegans. *Ann Nutr Metab.* 2003;47(5):183–185.

Lakin V, Haggarty P, Abramovich DR. Dietary intake and tissue concentrations of fatty acids in omnivore, vegetarian, and diabetic pregnancy. *Prostaglandins, Leukotrienes, Essential Fatty Acids.* 1998;58:209–220.

Lubby AL, Cooperman JM, Donnfeld AM, et al. Observations on transfer of vitamin B-12 from mother to fetus and newborn. *Am J Dis Child.* 1958;96:532–533.

Mangels AR, Messina V, Melina V. Position of the American Dietetic Association and Dietitians of Canada: Vegetarian diets. *J Am Diet Assoc.* 2003;103(6):748–765.

Matsuoka LY, Ide L, Wortsman J, et al. Sunscreen suppresses cutaneous vitamin D synthesis. *J Clin Endocr Metab.* 1987;64:1165–1168.

Maxwell JD, Ang L, Brooke OG, Brown IRF. Vitamin D supplements enhance weight gain and nutritional status in pregnant Asians. *Br J Obstet Gyn.* 1981;88:987–991.

McCann JC, Ames BN. Is docosahexaenoic acid, an n-3 long-chain polyunsaturated fatty acid, required for development of normal brain function? An overview of evidence from cognitive and behavioral tests in humans and animals. *Am J Clin Nutr.* 2005;82:281–295.

McFadyen IR, Campbell-Brown M, Abraham R, North WRS, Haines AP. Factors affecting birthweights in Hindus, Moslems, and Europeans. *Br J Obstet Gyn.* 1984;91:968–972.

Messina V, Mangels R, Messina M. *The Dietitian's Guide to Vegetarian Diets: Issues and Applications.* 2d ed. Sudbury, MA: Jones and Bartlett Publishers; 2004.

Messina V, Melina V, Mangels AR. A new food guide for North American vegetarians. *J Am Diet Assoc.* 2003;103(6):771–775.

Nishiyama S, Mikeda T, Okada T, Nakamura K, Kotani T, Hishinuma A. Transient hypothyroidism or persistent hyperthyrotropinemia in neonates born to mothers with excessive iodine intake. *Thyroid.* 2004;14:1077–1083.

O'Connell JM, Dibley MJ, Sierra J, Wallace B, Marks JS, Yip R. Growth of vegetarian children: The Farm study. *Pediatrics.* 1989;84:475–481.

Prentice A. Maternal calcium metabolism and bone mineral status. *Am J Clin Nutr.* 2000;71(Suppl):1312S–1316S.

Prentice A, Jarjou LM, Cole TJ, et al. Calcium requirements of lactating Gambian mothers: Effects of a calcium supplement on breastmilk calcium concentration, maternal bone mineral content, and urinary calcium excretion. *Am J Clin Nutr.* 1995;62:58–67.

Prentice AM, Goldberg GR. Energy adaptations in human pregnancy: Limits and long-term consequences. *Am J Clin Nutr.* 2000;71:1226S–1232S.

Reddy S, Sanders TAB, Obeid O. The influence of maternal vegetarian diet on essential fatty acid status of the newborn. *Eur J Clin Nutr.* 1994;48:358–368.

Remer T, Neubert A, Manz F. Increased risk of iodine deficiency with vegetarian nutrition *Br J Nutr.* 1999;81(1):45–49.

Ritchie LD, Fung EB, Halloran BP, et al. A longitudinal study of calcium homeostasis during human pregnancy and lactation and after resumption of menses. *Am J Clin Nutr.* 1998;67:693–701.

Sanders TAB. Growth and development of British vegan children. *Am J Clin Nutr.* 1988;48:822–825.

Sanders TAB, Reddy S. The influence of a vegetarian diet on the fatty acid composition of human milk and the essential fatty acid status of the infant. *J Pediatr.* 1992:120(4, Pt 2):S71–S77.

Specker BL. Do North American women need supplemental vitamin D during pregnancy or lactation? *Am J Clin Nutr.* 1994;59(Suppl):484S–491S.

Specker BL, Black A, Allen L, Morrow F. Vitamin B-12: Low milk concentrations are related to low serum concentrations in vegetarian women and to methylmalonic aciduria in their infants. *Am J Clin Nutr.* 1990;52:1073–1076.

Specker BL, Miller D, Norman EJ, Greene T, Hayes KC. Increased urinary methylmalonic acid excretion in breast-fed infants of vegetarian mothers and identification of an acceptable dietary source of vitamin B12. *Am J Clin Nutr.* 1987;47:89–92.

Specker BL, Valanis B, Hertzberg V, Edwards N, Tsang RC. Sunshine exposure and serum-25-hydroxy-vitamin D concentrations in exclusively breast-fed infants. *J Pediatr.* 1985;107:372–376.

Specker BL, Wey HE, Miller D. Differences in fatty acid composition of human milk in vegetarian and nonvegetarian women: Long-term effect of diet. *J Pediatr Gastr Nutr.* 1987;6:764–768.

Spencer EA, Appleby PN, Davey GK, Key TJ. Diet and body mass index in 38,000 EPIC-Oxford meat-eaters, fish-eaters, vegetarians and vegans. *Intl J Obes Related Metab Disord.* 2003;27:728–734.

Subcommittee on Nutrition During Lactation, Institute of Medicine. *Nutrition during Lactation.* Washington, DC: National Academy Press; 1991.

Subcommittee on Nutritional Status and Weight Gain During Pregnancy (SNS), Institute of Medicine. *Nutrition during Pregnancy.* Washington, DC: National Academy Press; 1990.

Teas J, Pino S, Critchley A, Braverman LE. Variability of iodine content in common commercially available edible seaweeds. *Thyroid.* 2004;14(10):836–841.

Thomas J, Ellis FR. The health of vegans during pregnancy. *Proc Nutr Soc.* 1977;36:46A.

Uauy R, Peirano P, Hoffman D, et al. Role of essential fatty acids in the function of the developing nervous system. *Lipids.* 1996;3:S167–S176.

Ward RJ, Abraham R, McFadyen IR, et al. Assessment of trace metal intake and status in a Gujerati pregnant Asian population and their influence of the outcome of pregnancy. *Br J Obstet Gyn.* 1988;95:676–682.

Webb AR, Kline L, Holick MF. Influence of season and latitude on the cutaneous synthesis of vitamin D3: Exposure to winter sunlight in Boston and Edmonton will not promote vitamin D3 synthesis in human skin. *J Clin Endocr Metab.* 1988;67:373–378.

Williams CM, Burdge G. Long-chain n-3 PUFA: Plant v. marine sources. *Proc Nutr Soc.* 2006;65:42–50.

20

Optimal Nutrition for Active Vegetarians and Vegetarian Athletes

D. Enette Larson-Meyer, PhD, RD, FACSM
Mary Helen Niemeyer, MD, MPH, FAAFP

Introduction

The best diet for athletes is one that obtains the bulk of the energy from carbohydrate, and is also adequate in total energy, protein, fat, vitamins, minerals, and fluid. Most experts agree that vegetarian diets can both meet the needs of all athletes—from the casual and recreational athlete to the world-class competitor (American College of Sports Medicine [ACSM], American Dietetic Association, and Dietitians of Canada, 2000; Williams, 1995; Maughan, 2002; Mangels, Messina, & Melina, 2003; International Center for Sports Nutrition, 1997)—and provide health benefits in the prevention and treatment of certain diseases (ACSM, 2000; Mangels, Messina, & Melina, 2003). Quite interestingly, the diets of the early Greek and Roman Olympian athletes were nearly vegetarian, consisting mostly of cereals, fruits, vegetables, legumes, and wine diluted with water (Grandjean, 1997). Currently, many active and well-known, top-level athletes follow vegetarian diets, including French Olympic figure skater Surya Bonaly, powerlifter Bill Manetti, Heisman Trophy football player Desmond Howard, and tennis champion Martina Navratilova (Messina & Messina, 1996).

Like most athletes, vegetarian athletes are likely to benefit from education on food choices. This chapter reviews the current literature related to sports nutrition and vegetarian diets, and discusses how the casual exerciser and the competitive athlete can best choose a vegetarian diet that will provide adequate nutrition for optimal training, peak performance, and good health. Specifically, this chapter reviews the energy, micronutrient, vitamin, mineral, and fluid requirements of the active vegetarian and vegetarian athlete and provides tips for maintaining nutrition and hydration status during heavy training and competition. The chapter also discusses supplements of interest to vegetarian athletes, weight reduction for athletes, the special nutritional concerns of the female vegetarian athlete, and the potential benefits of a vegetarian diet for athletic performance.

Summary of the Scientific Literature

Overview of Energy Utilization during Exercise

The mobilization of body fuels into energy is a complex process. It is modulated primarily by exercise intensity and duration, but also by training status and nutritional intake (Hargreaves, 2000). During exercise, the immediate source of energy is the disruption of high-energy phosphate bonds of adenosine triphosphate (ATP) and creatine phosphate (CP), which are found in all cells (Hargreaves, 2000; McArdle, Katch, & Katch, 1999). Existing ATP and CP in muscle cells are expended within seconds of exercise initiation and must be regenerated from energy stored within the chemical bonds of carbohydrate, fat, and protein. CP and muscle glycogen (the starch-like form in which carbohydrate is stored) are the main fuels for high-intensity exercise of short duration, where performance capacity is limited by lactate accumulation and muscle-cell acidosis (byproducts of the rapid reaction that generates energy from carbohydrate, commonly called "fast" or "anaerobic" glycolysis). Oxidation of glucose, glycogen, and free fatty acids (from adipose tissue and muscle triglyceride stores) supplies the energy needed for exercise lasting longer than about two minutes; the relative contribution of fat increases with longer duration or lower intensity of muscular work (Hargreaves, 2000; McArdle, Katch, & Katch, 1999; Romijn et al., 1993; Romijn et al., 2000). Muscle and liver glycogen and muscle triglycerides may be almost completely depleted in exercise lasting longer than about two to three hours. Under these conditions, glucose made from amino acids (via gluconeogenesis) and adipose-tissue triglycerides serve as the major source of fuel, but cannot be used rapidly enough to support moderate to intense bouts of exercise (McArdle, Katch, & Katch,

1999). The contribution of protein as a fuel during exercise is minimal—between 5%–10% of total needs—but increases in latter stages of exhaustive exercise when amino acids are converted to glucose.

Requirements for Energy and Energy-Generating Nutrients

Energy

Daily energy or calorie needs vary considerably among individual athletes and depend on the athlete's body size, body composition, gender, training regimen, and general activity pattern. The energy needs of an athlete, measured by doubly labeled water (a state-of-the-art technique that allows measurement of energy expenditure outside the laboratory), are shown to vary from about 2,600 kcal per day in female swimmers to about 8,500 kcal per day in male cyclists participating in the Tour de France bicycle race (Goran, 1995). The energy requirements of smaller or less active individuals may be slightly less. Vegetarianism does not necessarily affect energy needs, although it is interesting to note that resting energy expenditure (REE) has been shown to be approximately 11% higher in vegetarians compared to nonvegetarians (Toth & Poehlman, 1994). Researchers have hypothesized that this is due to the habitual high-carbohydrate composition of the vegetarian diet, in combination with increased basal activity of the sympathetic nervous system (Toth & Poehlman, 1994). REE is also acutely elevated for several hours after vigorous exercise (Borsheim & Bahr, 2003).

Daily energy needs or total daily energy expenditure (DEE) can be approximated using several different published methods (Manore & Thompson, 2000). The easiest is to directly estimate DEE using an activity factor that best

Table 20.1 Estimation of Daily Energy Needs by Factorial Methods

- Obtain weight in kilograms (weight in pounds divided by 2.2).
- Directly estimate daily energy expenditure (DEE) by multiplying weight in kilograms by the appropriate energy expenditure factor below (kcal/kilogram/day).

Category	Energy Expenditure (kcal/kilogram/day)
Moderate Activity	
Men	41
Women	37
Heavy Activity	
Men	50
Women	44
Exceptional Activity	
Men	58
Women	51

Source: Adapted from Manore & Thompson, 2000.

describes the athlete's physical activity patterns (including training and nontraining) (see Table 20.1; Manore & Thompson, 2000). For active and athletic individuals, the activity factors are classified categorically as moderate, heavy, or exceptional. Another method is to estimate the individual components of DEE, including the REE, the energy expenditure required during training (TEE) and during nontraining (NTEE) activities, and the energy required to digest and metabolize food (called the thermic effect of food, TEF) (see Table 20.2). Although somewhat cumbersome, estimation of DEE from its components accounts for more variation in activity patterns and is preferred for athletes who are either interested in their energy needs or struggling to lose, maintain, or gain body weight. It should be noted, however, that all methods are still estimates and are associated with some degree of error.

Meeting energy needs should be the first nutritional priority for all athletes. Energy balance is achieved when caloric intake (the sum of energy from food, fluids, and supplements consumed) equals DEE. Although some athletes may need to tilt the energy balance one way or the other to gain or lose body mass, it is particularly important that athletes maintain adequate energy intake during periods of intense aerobic and/or strength training to permit adequate tissue repair and remodeling. Sufficient energy consumption is important for maximizing the effect of training, maintaining body mass, and maintaining good health. Inadequate energy intake can result in loss of muscle mass, menstrual cycle dysfunction, loss of or failure to gain bone density, and an increased risk of injury, illness, and fatigue (ACSM, 2000).

Some active vegetarians may have trouble meeting energy needs (Grandjean, 1987). This may be due to excessively high energy requirements, food choices that are bulky or too high in fiber, or hectic schedules that do not allow adequate time to eat. Striving to eat 6–8 meals/snacks per day and doing adequate planning ("brown-bag" lunches, snacks packed in the gym bag or kept in a desk drawer, etc.) may help remedy this situation. When appropriate, athletes can increase energy intake and decrease fiber by consuming 1/3 to 1/2 of their cereal/grain servings from refined rather than whole-grain sources and by replacing some high-fiber fruit/vegetable servings with juice servings. Active vegetarians may find the Vegetarian Food Guide Pyramid (Messina, Melina, & Mangels, 2003) (see Figure 20.1) to be a helpful tool for meeting their energy needs and maintaining a sound, healthful vegetarian diet. Individuals who exercise regularly will need to eat toward the upper number of servings (or in some cases more) on the food guide pyramid, however, to meet the increased energy needs of that exercise and training. More detailed eating plans for

Table 20.2 Calculation of Daily Energy Needs

Energy Expenditure	Formula	Example: Female college soccer player who practices for 90 minutes and weight-trains for 30 minutes.	Example: Male recreational runner who works as a musician and runs 35 miles per week (average of 43 min/day at a 7-mph pace).
Resting energy expenditure (REE)	REE = 22 × Fat-Free Mass (kg)	Weight = 60 kg Body fat = 20% (lean body weight = 48 kg) 22 × 48 = 1,056 kcal	Weight = 75 kg Body fat =16% (lean body weight = 63 kg) 22 × 63 = 1,386 kcal
Energy expenditure during nontraining physical activity (NTEE)	Light activity = 1.3 × REE Moderate activity = 1.5 × REE Heavy activity = 1.5 × REE	Assume light occupational activity (student): 0.3 × 1,056 kcal = 317 kcal	Assume moderate occupational activity (stands, moves, loads/unloads equipment regularly, some sitting): 0.5 × 1,386 kcal = 693 kcal
Energy expenditure during training (TEE)	Refer to physical activities charts (found in many nutrition or exercise physiology texts)	A 60-kg athlete uses ~8.0 kcal/min. for soccer practice & 6.8 kcal/min. for weight training: 8.0 kcal/min. × 90 min. = 720 kcal 6.8 kcal/min. × 30 min. = 204 kcal	A 75-kg male uses ~14.1 kcal/min when running at a steady 7.0-mph pace: 14.1 × 43 min = 606 kcal
Total daily energy expenditure (DEE)	DEE = REE + NTEE + TEE	1,056 + 317 +720 + 204 = ~2,297 kcal/day	1,386 + 693 + 606 = ~2,685 kcal/day
Thermic effect of food (TEF)	Add an additional 6%–10% to DEE to account for TEF	2,297 × 1.06 = 2,435 kcal/day 2,297 × 1.10 = 2,527 kcal/day	2,685 × 1.06 = 2,846 kcal/day 2,685 × 1.10 = 2,953 kcal/day

Note: The Cunningham equation for estimating REE (147) has been shown to more closely estimate the actual REE of endurance-trained men and women (149) than other available equations..

Figure 20.1   Vegetarian Food Guide Pyramid

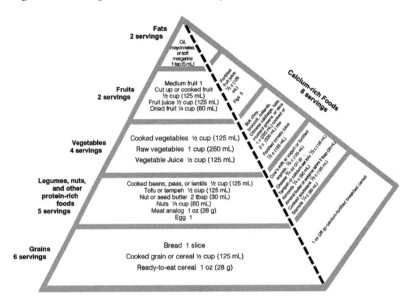

Source: Reprinted from Messina V, Melina V, Mangels AR. A new food guide for North American vegetarians. *J Am Diet Assoc.* 2003;103(6):771–775, with permission from the American Dietetic Association.

vegetarian and vegan athletes have also been developed by Messina and Messina (1996) and Houtkooper (1992). Sample menus for a 3,000-kcal vegetarian diet and a 4,600-kcal vegan diet are presented in Table 20.3. (Refer to Chapter 22 for more information on planning vegetarian diets in general.)

Carbohydrate

Carbohydrates should make up the bulk of the vegetarian athlete's diet. Although carbohydrate, fat, and to a lesser extent protein are all used to fuel physical activity, carbohydrate is the only fuel that can sustain the moderate- to high-level activity required in most sports and athletic endeavors, and also be used by the brain and central nervous system. Carbohydrate stores, which are found in muscle and the liver as glycogen, are limited and become depleted during the prolonged (longer than about 90 minutes) and intense intermittent activities (stop-and-go running; intense court play; brisk, difficult-terrain hiking, etc.) common in training, competition, and some outdoor recreational activities. Depleted liver and muscle glycogen stores correlate with low blood sugar (liver glycogen is a reservoir for blood sugar during exercise) and muscle- and whole-body fatigue, respectively; this depleted state is described in some athletic circles as "hitting the wall" or "bonking."

Diets high in carbohydrate are important because they maintain muscle and liver glycogen stores (Casey et al., 2000; Bergstrom et al., 1967; Nilsson & Hultman, 1973; Goforth et al., 2003) and optimize performance during both prolonged, moderate-intensity exercise (e.g., distance running and cycling) (Spencer, Yan, & Katz, 1991; O'Keeffe et al., 1989; Brewer, Williams, & Patton, 1988; Coggan & Swanson, 1992) and intermittent high-intensity exercise (Pizza et al.,

Table 20.3   Sample Vegetarian/Vegan Menus

Sample 3,000-Calorie Vegetarian Menu	Sample 4,500-Calorie Vegan Menu
Breakfast	
1 cup raisin bran	1½ cups raisin bran
1 cup skim milk	1 cup fortified soy milk
2 slices mixed-grain toast	3 slices mixed-grain toast
2 tsp. low-trans fat margarine	3 tsp. low-trans fat margarine
medium banana	medium banana
8 oz. fruit juice	8 oz. fruit juice
Lunch	
veggie whole-wheat pita stuffed with shredded spinach, sliced tomato, 2 oz. feta cheese & 2 tsp. olive oil	tofu salad on a 4-oz. hoagie roll (1 cup firm tofu, 2 tsp. mustard, 2 tsp. soy mayonnaise, lettuce, tomato)
large apple	large apple
2 small oatmeal cookies	3 small oatmeal cookies
	8 oz. carrot juice
Snack	
sesame seed bagel	sesame seed bagel
1 Tbsp. peanut butter & 1 Tbsp. jam	1 Tbsp. peanut butter & 1 Tbsp. jam
	1 cup fortified soy milk
Dinner	
lentil spaghetti sauce (1 cup cooked lentils, ½ onion, 1½ cup canned tomatoes, & 1 Tbsp. olive oil)	lentil spaghetti sauce (1 cup cooked lentils, ½ onion, 1½ cup canned tomatoes, & 1 Tbsp. olive oil)
3 oz. dry pasta, cooked	4 oz. dry pasta, cooked
1 Tbsp. parmesan cheese	
2 (1-oz.) slices french bread dipped in 1 Tbsp. olive oil	3 (1-oz.) slices french bread dipped in 2 Tbsp. olive oil
1 cup steamed broccoli	1½ cups steamed collards
Snack	
1 cup fruit-flavored yogurt	1 cup fruit sorbet
	1 oz. toasted almonds
3,066 kcal:	**4,626 kcal:**
469 g carbohydrate, 106 g protein, 85 g fat	705 g carbohydrate, 146 g protein, 136 g fat
61% carbohydrate, 14% protein, 25% fat	61% carbohydrate, 13% protein, 26% fat
1,600 mg calcium, 29 mg iron, 14 mg zinc	1,100 mg calcium, 60 mg iron, 15 mg zinc

Note: Assumes that grain products are made from enriched flour.

1995; Larson et al., 1994), such as sprinting at the end of an endurance segment or intermittent bouts of exercise (Hargreaves et al., 1984; Sugiura & Kobayashi, 1998). Thus, for many athletes this translates into a longer playing (or exercising) time before fatigue and faster sprinting potential at the end of a game or race. Also of interest is the inherent ability of carbohydrate (compared to fat) to delay the onset of fatigue by preserving the energy state of exercising muscle (i.e., the phosphorylation potential or ratio of CP to its breakdown product, inorganic phosphate) (Larson et al., 1994). This biochemical influence is likely related to the ability of carbohydrate to rapidly generate more energy per mole of oxygen consumed.

The current recommendation by the American College of Sports Medicine, the American Dietetic Association, and the Dietitians of Canada is that athletes and active individuals consume 6 to 10 grams of carbohydrate per kilogram of body mass daily (ACSM, 2000), rather than focusing on a certain percentage of calories coming from carbohydrate. Athletes with higher energy demands, such as collegiate, serious recreational, or elite-level athletes in heavy training, should strive for the upper range of close to 9 to 10 grams per kilogram of body mass per day (4 to 4.5 grams/pound). Conversely, female athletes and those participating at a level that demands less training (e.g., at the recreational, club, or secondary school level) may require only 6 to 7 grams of carbohydrate per kilogram of body mass (2.7 to 3.2 grams/pound). A general understanding of the carbohydrate content of foods and beverages (Table 20.4), combined with information provided on the food label (which in the United States lists the carbohydrate content of most foods in grams per serving), should help athletes meet their recommended carbohydrate intake.

Knowledge of carbohydrate sources is also useful in assuring adequate carbohydrate intake before, during, and after exercise. Occasionally counting carbohydrate intake at a meal, snack, or over the course of a day may assist athletes in meeting these guidelines. This activity is particularly useful when compared with a training log or feedback from a coach, and should help the athlete make the connection between carbohydrate intake and performance. For example, an athlete may notice that low carbohydrate intake on a particular day was associated with lightheadedness or "dead" legs after training.

Protein

Dietary protein provides the amino acid building blocks that form the structural basis of muscle tissue and enzymes, and can also serve as a source of energy during exercise. In general, the protein needs of athletes are higher than those of inactive individuals and vary according to the type of activity and the level of training. Protein needs of active vegetarians who perform light to moderate activity several times a week are very likely met by the Recommended Dietary Allowance (RDA) of 0.8 grams per kilogram of body mass; protein requirements of athletes who are training more vigorously may be considerably higher than the RDA. The protein recommendations for endurance athletes are estimated to be 1.2 to 1.4 grams per kilogram of body weight per day, whereas those for resistance- and strength-trained athletes may be as high as 1.6 to 1.7 grams per kilogram of body mass per day (ACSM, 2000). The rationale for the additional protein during training is based on the need to repair exercise-induced microdamage to muscle fibers, the small use of protein for fuel during exercise, and the need for additional protein to support muscle development. Although studies have not yet addressed the specific needs of vegetarian athletes, several experts have suggested that vegetarians may need to consume about 10% more protein than omnivores, to account for the lower digestibility of plant compared to animal proteins (National Research Council, 1989). Accordingly, the protein requirements of endurance, resistance-, and strength-trained vegetarian athletes (based on the aforementioned recommendations for athletes) would be about 1.3 to 1.8 grams per kilogram of body mass (ACSM, 2000).

Vegetarian athletes can easily achieve adequate protein intake providing their diet is adequate in energy and contains a variety of plant-based protein foods. The once-prevalent

Table 20.4   Approximate Carbohydrate Content of Selected Foods and Beverages

Food	Portion	Carbohydrate (grams)
Bagel	2–3 oz.	30–45
Bread, sliced	1 slice	15
Breakfast cereal, cold	1/3–1/2 cup (varies)	15–20
Breakfast cereal, hot	1/2 cup	15
Bun or English muffin	1 whole	30
Corn	1/2 cup	15
Fluid replacement beverage	1 cup	15–19
Fruit, all	1/2 cup	15
Orange, peach, pear	medium	15
apple or banana	large	30
fruit, dried	1/3–1/2 cup	60
Fruit juice and lemonade	1 cup	30–45
Jam, jelly, honey, syrup	1 Tbsp.	15
Legumes (pinto, kidney, garbanzo, etc.)	1/3 cup	15
Milk	1 cup	12
Pancake	5-inch, thin	15
Pasta, cooked	1/2 cup	15
Potato, mashed	1/2 cup	15
Potato, baked	1 medium	30
Rice	1/3 cup	15
Roll	1 small (1 oz.)	15
Soda	12 oz.	40–45
Sports bar	1 bar	40–60
Sugar	1 tsp.	4
Vegetables (nonstarchy)	1/2 cup	6
Vegetables (starchy)	1/2 cup	15
Yogurt, fruited	1 cup	40–45

Developed based on the Diabetic Exchange List for Meal Planning, 1995 (American Diabetes Association and the American Dietetic Association. *Exchange Lists for Meal Planning.* Alexandria, VA: American Diabetes Association Inc.; 2003).

belief that vegetarians need to eat specific combinations of plant proteins in the same meal has been dispelled (at least for adults) (Young & Pellett, 1994) and replaced with the recommendation simply to consume a variety of plant-based, protein-rich foods over the course of a day (Mangels, Messina, & Melina, 2003; Young & Pellett, 1994). Plant-based, protein-rich foods include legumes, soy products, grains, nuts, and seeds; these are listed in Table 20.5 along with the protein content of commercially available and lacto-ovo vegetarian protein sources.

Although surveys have found that most athletes consume adequate protein (Messina & Messina, 1996; Manore & Thompson, 2000), this list (along with information on food labels) can be used by athletes concerned about their dietary protein. Athletes who tend to lack in protein are those who focus too much on carbohydrates or who consume too little food in general. Athletes who are concerned about their protein intake should strive to add between one and three servings of protein-rich vegetarian foods to their regular meals or snacks. For

Table 20.5 Approximate Protein Content of Selected Foods and Beverages

Food	Portion	Protein (grams)
Bread, grains, rice, pasta	serving	2–3
Cheese, medium and hard	1 oz.	7
Cheese, cottage	1/4 cup	8
Egg, whole	1 large	7
Legumes (most beans and peas)	1/2 cup cooked	7
Milk, all	1 cup	8
Nuts, most	2 Tbsp.	7
Peanut butter	2 Tbsp.	7
Tofu, firm	1 cup	20
Tofu, soft	1 cup	10
Vegetables, most	1/2 cup cooked	2–3
Vegetarian "burgers"	1 patty	6–16
Vegetarian "burger" crumbles	1/2 cup	7–11
Vegetarian "chicken" patty/nuggets	1 serving	7–15
Vegetarian "dogs"	1 dog	9–12
Yogurt, all	1 cup	8

Note: Studies in humans have found that isolated soy protein is comparable in quality to that of animal proteins (Young, 1991; Gausseres et al., 1997).

example, add soy milk to a fruit snack, lentils to spaghetti sauce, tofu to a stir-fry, or garbanzo beans to a salad.

Fat

Fat is a necessary component of the diet, providing essential components of cell membranes, essential fatty acids, and associated nutrients such as vitamins E, A, and D. Dietary fat should make up the remainder of energy intake after the athlete's carbohydrate and protein needs have been met. The latest sports nutrition consensus from the American College of Sports Medicine, the American Dietetic Association, and the Dietitians of Canada is that the athlete's diet should contain approximately 20%–25% of total energy from fat. However, athletes with high energy needs can still meet their carbohydrate and protein requirements on a diet that provides 30%–35% or more of energy from

fat (ACSM, 2000). For example, a 70-kilogram athlete expending 5,000 kcal can meet carbohydrate and protein needs on a diet that provides about 35% of the energy from fat:

- 70 kilograms × 10 g carbohydrate/kilogram = 700 g or 2,800 kcal from carbohydrate
- 70 kilograms × 1.4 g protein/kilogram = 98 g or 392 kcal from protein
- 5,000 kcal (total) – 2,800 kcal from carbohydrate + 392 kcal from protein = 1,808 kcal from fat
- 1,808 kcal from fat/5,000 total kcal × 100 = 36.2% of kcal from fat

In all cases, however, it is recommended that athletes select foods that are high in mono- and polyunsaturated fatty acids, including omega-3 fatty acids, and limit foods with saturated and trans fatty acids. Food sources that contain mono- and polyunsaturated fatty acids include nuts, seeds, nut butters, tahini, avocados, olives, olive oil, sesame oil, and canola oil. Walnuts, flaxseed, flaxseed oil, canola oil, and hemp oil (as well as fatty fish) are particularly good sources of omega-3 fatty acids and are thought to reduce inflammation and lower the risk for many age-related diseases (Grimble & Tappia, 1998). Foods that contain saturated and trans fatty acids include full-fat dairy products, butter, and many processed bakery items, snacks, and fast-food products. Indeed, the Vegetarian Food Guide Pyramid (Figure 20.1) emphasizes the importance of fat intake and specifies that a minimum of two servings of fat per day be consumed from fat-rich plant foods (Messina, Melina, & Mangels, 2003).

The vegetarian athlete should understand that the diet should be adequate in fat and not be either too low in total fat or too high in saturated or processed fats. Studies have noted that diets too low in fat (in which fat constitutes less than 15% of the total daily energy consumed) may compromise immune function (Venkatraman & Pendergast, 1998; Venkatraman et al., 1997), elevate serum triglycerides (Brown & Cox, 1998; Larson-Meyer, Hunter, & Newcomer, 2002), contribute to exercise-induced amenorrhea (Crist & Hill, 1990; Deuster et al., 1986; Laughlin & Yen, 1996), and possibly impair performance (Muoio et al., 1994) by reducing the fat stored within the muscle cell (Decombaz et al., 2001; Larson-Meyer, Hunter, & Newcomer, 2002) that is crucial for supplying free fatty acids to skeletal muscle during prolonged exercise of moderate to high intensity (65%–80% of maximal oxygen uptake) (Romijn et al., 1993; Romijn et al., 2000). It is a misconception that energy-balanced diets that contain dietary fat promote weight gain or increase adiposity or obesity. It is true, though, that diets too high in saturated and trans fat sources have been linked to increased risk of heart disease (Sacks & Katan, 2002; Hu & Willett, 2002).

Requirements for Vitamins and Minerals

Vitamins and minerals, though not energy sources themselves, play important roles in energy production, musculoskeletal health, and immune function. They also assist in protecting body cells and tissues (including skeletal muscle) from oxidative damage, and assist in the building and repair of muscle tissue following exercise. Most athletes can meet their need for vitamins and minerals by consuming a diet that provides adequate energy and consists of a variety of wholesome foods (i.e., similar to that suggested by the Vegetarian Food Guide Pyramid). Because of hectic training and work/school schedules, however, athletes may be prone to make poor food choices, resulting in deficient intake of many vitamins and minerals. Surveys of various groups of athletes have suggested that intakes of iron, calcium, and zinc are often insufficient (ACSM, 2000), particularly among female athletes (Manore, 1999); research in vegetarian and vegan populations in general have found that their vitamin B12, vitamin D, riboflavin, and iodine status may also occasionally be compromised (Mangels, Messina, & Melina, 2003). Although food choice is important, the athletes at greatest risk for poor vitamin and mineral status are those who restrict energy intake, employ severe weight-loss practices, or consume excessive quantities of processed foods (Manore & Thompson, 2000; Williams, 1999).

Because it is always preferable to improve nutritional status through better food choices, the following subsections briefly discuss the minerals and vitamins that may be low in the diets of active vegetarians and vegetarian athletes. In certain cases, a multivitamin and mineral supplement may be needed to improve overall micronutrient status.

Calcium

Calcium, the most abundant mineral in the body, is necessary for bone formation, muscle contraction, and nerve impulse transmission. Regular exercise has not been shown to increase calcium requirements above that of the general population. Thus, adult vegetarian athletes should strive for the recommended intake of 1,000 mg of calcium per day, and those under the age of 18 should strive for 1,300 mg per day. Evidence suggests that amenorrheic athletes (those not experiencing a menstrual cycle for at least 3 months) may require an intake of 1,500 mg per day to retain calcium balance (Heaney, Recker, & Saville, 1978). Low calcium intake has been associated with an increased risk of stress fractures (Myburgh et al., 1990) and decreased bone density, particularly in amenorrheic athletes (Wolman et al., 1992).

Male athletes, and female athletes with regular menstrual periods, can meet calcium requirements by including several servings of dairy products or eight servings of calcium-containing plant foods daily. The Vegetarian Food Guide Pyramid (Figure 20.1) can be a useful guide for vegetarians striving to meet their calcium needs (Messina, Melina, & Mangels, 2003). Plant foods that are rich in absorbable calcium include low-oxalate green leafy vegetables (collard, mustard, and turnip greens), tofu (set with calcium), fortified soy and rice milks, textured vegetable protein, tahini, certain legumes, fortified orange juice, almonds, and blackstrap molasses. Research has suggested that calcium absorption from most of these foods is as good as or better than from milk (Weaver & Plawecki, 1994; Weaver, Proulx, & Heaney, 1999; Heaney et al., 2000). However, the calcium in fortified soy milk, most legumes, nuts, and seeds is absorbed slightly less well. Foods with a high oxalate or phytate content (including rhubarb, spinach, Swiss chard, and beet greens) are not good sources of easily absorbed calcium.

Although it is certainly possible to maintain calcium balance on a plant-based diet in a Western lifestyle (Mangels, Messina, & Melina, 2003; Weaver, Proulx, & Heaney, 1999; Kohlenberg-Mueller & Raschka, 2003), some active vegetarians may find it more convenient to use fortified foods or calcium supplements to help meet their calcium requirements. Calcium carbonate and calcium citrate are well-absorbed sources used in supplements; calcium carbonate is generally less expensive. Recent studies have noted that long-term supplementation with calcium carbonate does not compromise iron status in iron-replete adults (Minihane & Fairweather-Tait, 1998) (as was once thought), but that it is best to take calcium supplements several hours after a meal (for example, at bedtime) rather than with meals (Hallberg, 1998). Because vitamin D is also required for adequate calcium absorption, regulation of serum calcium levels, and promotion of bone health, a calcium supplement that also contains vitamin D is advised if the athlete is at risk for low-vitamin D status. Those at risk for compromised vitamin D status include athletes with low intakes of fortified foods or supplements; limited sun exposure (especially in northern climates); and/or chronic, diligent use of sunscreen (Holick, 2004). Poor vitamin D status may manifest in compromised calcium balance, altered inflammation and immune function, and unexplained muscle pain (Tangpricha et al., 2004; Holick, 2004). Foods that are fortified with vitamin D include certain brands of soy and rice milks, breakfast cereals, and margarines, as well as cow's milk (Mangels, Messina, & Melina, 2003). Vegetarians are cautioned, however, because the animal form of the vitamin, vitamin D3 (cholecalciferol), is thought to be utilized with greater efficiency than the vegetarian form, D2 (ergocalciferol) (Trang et al., 1998).

Iron

The major function of iron in the body is the formation of compounds essential to the transport and utilization of oxygen, which include hemoglobin in blood, myoglobin in muscle, and enzymes in the energy-generating pathways. Iron deficiency, with or without anemia, can compromise athletic performance and adaptation to aerobic training (Hinton et al., 2000; Brownlie et al., 2004). All athletes, and female athletes in particular, are at risk of iron-depletion and iron-deficiency anemia (Fogelholm, 1995).

Iron deficiency may occur because of increased iron loss, decreased iron intake, or decreased iron absorption. Studies have found that iron loss is increased in some athletes due to gastrointestinal bleeding (Robertson, Maughan, & Davidson, 1987) (potentially stemming from the regular use of anti-inflammatory medications; Davies, 1995), heavy sweating (Waller & Haymes, 1996), red blood cell destruction from the stress of repetitive foot strikes in running and jumping (Eichner, 1985), and/or menstrual bleeding (Malczewska, Raczynski, & Stupnicki, 2000). Studies have also found that iron intake tends to be inadequate in athletes who restrict food intake or make poor food choices (Eichner, 1992). Quite interestingly, surveys have reported that although vegetarian athletes (Snyder, Dvorak, & Roepke, 1989) and nonathletes (Messina & Messina, 1996; Craig, 1994) alike typically have iron intakes that are similar to those of their nonvegetarian counterparts, the vegetarians tend to have lower iron status. The lower iron status in vegetarians is most likely due to consumption of iron in a form that is less well absorbed. Iron is found in both animal and plant foods, but the form found in most animal foods (heme iron) is more bioavailable (15%–35% absorption) than the elemental iron found in plant foods (2%–20% absorption) (Craig, 1994).

In most cases, vegetarian athletes can achieve normal iron status by educating themselves on the plant sources of iron and the factors that enhance and interfere with iron absorption. The approximate iron content of selected iron-rich plant foods is presented in Chapter 5 (Table 5.3). Iron absorption from plant sources can be enhanced by consumption of vitamin C-containing foods (citrus fruit or juice, tomatoes, melon, etc.) and inhibited by excessive intake of tea, coffee, milk, or soda. For example, an athlete who consumes milk or tea with a bean burrito or lentil soup at lunch could replace the beverage with citrus fruit juice to enhance the absorption of iron from that meal. Vegetarian athletes concerned about their iron status may want to take a multivitamin and mineral supplement containing iron. Athletes should not, however, take iron supplements alone unless prescribed or monitored by their physicians. The physician can find out whether iron status is compromised by checking the athlete's serum ferritin level or serum iron-binding capacity. Hemoglobin, hematocrit, and red blood cell levels are not good indicators of iron status in endurance athletes (Schumacher et al., 2002). These markers are often lower than the normal range in endurance-trained individuals because of expanded plasma volume. The physician can also ensure that the athlete is not at risk of an iron-overload disease called *hemochromatosis* (Herbert, 1992).

Zinc

Zinc is a component of many enzymes in the body, including those involved in protein synthesis, DNA synthesis, reproductive function, and immune function. Several of these enzymes are also involved in the major pathways of energy metabolism, including lactate dehydrogenase, which is important for the lactic acid energy system. Little is known regarding the zinc requirements of vegetarian athletes. There is some concern, however, that vegetarian athletes may be a group prone to poor zinc status. Concern is raised by the reported altered zinc status in athletes during heavy training (Lukaski, 1995; Micheletti, Rossi, & Rufini, 2001), coupled with the reported low zinc intake of athletes in general (ACSM, 2000; Micheletti, Rossi, & Rufini, 2001) and, possibly, vegetarians in particular (Hunt, 2003). Absorption of this mineral from plant-based diets is somewhat lower than from meat-containing diets, because of the higher phytate concentrations in plant foods (Hunt, 2003) and the lower intake of animal foods that tend to enhance zinc absorption (Hunt, 2003). A study from the U.S. Department of Agriculture found that nonathletic women were able to maintain normal zinc status on a lacto-ovo vegetarian diet containing legumes and whole grains, even though the diet was lower in total zinc and higher in phytate and fiber than the control meat-containing diet (Hunt, Matthys, & Johnson, 1998). The researchers recommended that vegetarians strive to consume legumes and whole grain on a regular basis, which is also a wise suggestion for active vegetarians and athletes in heavy training.

In addition to legumes and whole-grain products, other plant sources of zinc include hard cheeses, fortified cereals, nuts, soy, and commercially available vegetarian products (Mangels, Messina, & Melina, 2003). Although more research is needed, published studies have found that zinc supplementation does not influence zinc levels during training (Manore et al., 1993; Singh, Moses, & Deuster, 1992) and appears to have no benefit for athletic performance (Singh, Moses, & Deuster, 1992). This may be because

serum zinc is not a good marker of zinc status (see Chapter 8 for further information).

Iodine

The body's main use of iodine is as a component of thyroid hormone. Thyroid hormone is an important regulator of energy metabolism and protein synthesis. Iodine status is not generally a concern for athletes living in industrial countries, due to iodine fortification of table salt. Recent studies in nonathletic adults, however, have found that vegetarians may be at increased risk of iodine deficiency (Krajcovicova-Kudlackova et al., 2003; Remer, Neubert, & Manz, 1999; Lightowler & Davies, 1998). One study in nonathletic adults found that one-fourth of the vegetarians and 80% of the vegans suffered from iodine deficiency, compared to 9% of those on a mixed diet (Krajcovicova-Kudlackova et al., 2003). The higher prevalence of iodine deficiency among vegetarians might be due to the consumption of plant foods (Krajcovicova-Kudlackova et al., 2003) grown in soil with low iodine levels (Remer, Neubert, & Manz, 1999), limited consumption of cow's milk (Lightowler & Davies, 1998), limited intake of fish or sea products (Krajcovicova-Kudlackova et al., 2003), and reduced iodine intake from iodized salt (Krajcovicova-Kudlackova et al., 2003; Remer, Neubert, & Manz, 1999). In contrast, vegetarians who consume a lot of sea vegetables may have more than adequate intakes of iodine (Mangels, Messina, & Melina, 2003). Vegetarian athletes can ensure adequate iodine status by consuming half a teaspoon of iodized salt daily (Mangels, Messina, & Melina, 2003).

B Vitamins

The B-complex vitamins consist of a set of several vitamins that in general assist in the release of energy from carbohydrate, fat, and protein. Some of the B-complex vitamins—folate, vitamin B6, and riboflavin—are frequently low in the diets of some female athletes (Manore, 1999; Woolf & Manore, 2006). The dietary requirement for each B vitamin is determined individually. For thiamine (B1), riboflavin (B2), and niacin (B3), recommendations are proportional to energy intake and are apparently not altered by increased training or physical exertion (out of proportion to increased energy needs). For pyridoxine (B6), requirements are based on protein intake. For folate and B12, needs are considered similar to the dietary requirement of sedentary individuals and are apparently not altered by increased training or physical exertion. Active individuals who restrict their energy intake or make poor dietary choices are at greatest risk of poor thiamine, riboflavin, and vitamin B6 status (Manore, 2000). Depending on food choice, vegetarian diets can easily meet the requirements for most of the B vitamins (see Chapter 9). Riboflavin (Grandjean, 1987) and B12, however, are potential exceptions, as both vitamins are of special interest to athletes and intake of both tends to be low in vegetarian diets containing little to no dairy or animal products.

Riboflavin is important for the formation of enzymes known as *flavoproteins*, which are involved in production of energy from carbohydrate and fats. Several studies have suggested that riboflavin needs are increased in individuals who begin an exercise program (Belko, 1987; Soares et al., 1993), which may include athletes who suddenly increase their training volume. Although riboflavin is widely distributed in foods, major sources include milk, other dairy products, meat, and eggs. An 8-ounce glass of milk, for example, contains 20% of the RDA for riboflavin. Although the few studies of riboflavin intake of vegans have indicated that intakes are generally at or above the recom-

mended level (Messina & Messina, 1996), athletes who consume little to no dairy need to make an effort to regularly consume riboflavin-containing plant foods. Good plant sources of riboflavin include whole-grain and fortified breads and cereals, beans, peas, lentils, tofu, nuts, seeds, tahini, bananas, asparagus, figs, dark-green leafy vegetables, avocados, and most sea vegetables (seaweed, kombu, arame, sulse).

Vitamin B12 has been of interest in the athletic community for years. In fact, injections of B12 are popular with some athletes, trainers, and coaches because of the belief that the vitamin will increase energy and enhance endurance performance. The major function of B12 is as part of an enzyme complex (coenzyme) that is essential in the synthesis of DNA and red blood cells, and in the formation of the protective myelin sheath around nerve fibers. Although there is some conjecture that athletes may have increased B12 requirements due to their higher turnover of red blood cells, research has not proven this to be true (Messina & Messina, 1996). In the absence of actual deficiency, studies have not supported any benefit of B12 injections (Than et al., 1978) or of high-dose B12 supplementation with a multivitamin (Singh, Moses, & Deuster, 1992).

Vitamin B12 is of interest to vegan populations because the active form of this vitamin (cobalamin) is found exclusively in animal products (Herrmann & Geisel, 2002). Thus, vegan athletes need to regularly consume B12-fortified foods, such as Red Star brand nutritional yeast, soy milk, breakfast cereals, and meat analogs that are B12 fortified (e.g., vegetarian burgers and hot dogs). Nori and chlorella seaweeds are not a reliable source of bioavailable B12 (Rauma et al., 1995). Because of the irreversible neurological damage that can occur with vitamin B12 deficiency, it is recommended that vegans have their B12 status monitored regularly by their physicians (Herrmann & Geisel, 2002). The typical symptoms of B12 deficiency (usually apparent in the red blood cells) can be masked by high intake of folate, another B vitamin found abundantly in plant foods. Vegetarian athletes who consume dairy products and/or eggs are at little risk of vitamin B12 deficiency (Mangels, Messina, & Melina, 2003; Herrmann & Geisel, 2002).

Nutritional Supplements

Numerous nutritional supplements that claim to enhance sports performance are used by athletes of all levels, including vegetarian athletes. Research into these performance enhancers is constantly evolving, but for the most part has revealed few supplements (apart from carbohydrate-containing agents) that have proven effective in well-controlled studies (McNaughton, Dalton, & Palmer, 1999; Applegate, 1999; Branch, 2003). Full discussion of performance-enhancing aids can be found elsewhere (McNaughton, Dalton, & Palmer, 1999; Applegate, 1999; Juhn, 2003; Steen & Coleman, 1999) and is beyond the scope of this chapter, but a quick overview of those of particular interest to vegetarian athletes—protein, creatine, carnitine, and caffeine—is included here. As a general rule, however, the vegetarian athlete should not consider supplements in lieu of following a good sports diet.

Protein

As discussed earlier in this chapter, the protein needs of vegetarian and vegan athletes can be met by diet alone. For convenience, protein-containing nutrition beverages (e.g., Go, Boost, soy protein-isolate drinks) or protein bars (e.g., Genisoy) can be used occasionally to supplement the diet. These products, however, are not necessary and should never be considered replacements for food. Research has confirmed that protein or amino acid supplements consumed in excess of daily needs do not improve performance or stimulate greater muscle gain (Kreider, Miriel, & Bertun, 1993; Nikawa et al., 2002). Although several investigators are currently exploring whether consumption of certain individual proteins (isolated soy protein, or casein or whey isolates from milk) (Nikawa et al., 2002; Boirie et al., 1997; Dangin et al., 2001) is likely to promote greater gains in lean tissue, convincing evidence in humans is not yet available and also ignores the way protein is typically consumed—in a mixed meal from whole foods. One recent study, however, found that soy protein did not result in as much muscle protein accretion following resistance training as did milk protein containing similar energy and nitrogen contents (Wilkinson et al., 2007), but these findings deserve further investigation.

Creatine

Most of the creatine found in the body is in skeletal muscle, where it exists primarily as CP (Balsom, Soderlund, & Ekblom, 1994). As described earlier, CP is an important storage form of energy that buffers ATP and thus serves to maintain the bioenergetic state of exercising muscle. A large number of studies conducted since the early 1990s have found that oral creatine supplementation is effective in increasing body mass (by 1–2 kilograms) and performance in high-intensity, short-duration exercise tasks, including strength training and repetitive cycling or sprinting (Branch, 2003; Juhn, 2003; Juhn & Tarnopolsky, 1998; Terjung et al., 2000). Supplementation does not, however, appear to enhance performance during swimming or endurance running (Branch, 2003; Juhn, 2003; Juhn & Tarnopolsky, 1998; Terjung et al., 2000). The average dietary intake of creatine is about 2 g per day in meat eaters (Balsom, Soderlund,

& Ekblom, 1994), but is negligible in vegetarians because it is found primarily in muscle (animal) tissue. Even though creatine can be made in the body from three amino acids (glycine, arginine, and methionine) (Balsom, Soderlund, & Ekblom, 1994), the creatine levels in blood (Delanghe et al., 1989; Shomrat, Weinstein, & Katz, 2000) and skeletal muscle (Harris, Soderlund, & Hultman, 1992; Lukaszuk et al., 2002; Burke et al., 2003) were found to be lower in both vegetarians and nonvegetarians following an experimental vegetarian diet than in nonvegetarians consuming a typical meat-containing diet. Several (Shomrat, Weinstein, & Katz, 2000; Burke et al., 2003), but not all, studies (Clarys, Zinzen, & Hebbelinck, 1997) have also reported that vegetarians respond better to oral creatine supplementation than do nonvegetarians. In these studies, vegetarians were found to experience greater increases than nonvegetarians in skeletal muscle CP, total creatine, lean tissue mass, and work performance during weight training (Burke et al., 2003) and anaerobic bicycle performance (Shomrat, Weinstein, & Katz, 2000). Thus, there is some support for the idea that vegetarian athletes in particular may benefit from creatine supplementation. Creatine supplementation is not associated with any short-term safety issues, but its long-term safety is not known (Terjung et al., 2000). Creatine is reportedly not synthesized from animal derivatives, but it may be wise to check with the manufacturer.

Carnitine

Carnitine plays a central role in the metabolism of fat by transporting fatty acids from the outer part of the cell into the mitochondria where the fatty acids are used for energy (Brass, 2000). Dietary carnitine comes from meats and dairy products, but not from plant foods. Like creatine, blood levels of carnitine have been found to be lower in vegetarians (Delanghe et al., 1989), despite the body's ability to make it from amino acids (lysine and methionine) in the liver (Rebouche & Chenard, 1991). Not surprisingly, carnitine has been targeted as a potential "fat burner" and endurance performance enhancer. Clinical studies, however, have not found that carnitine supplementation increases fat utilization at rest or during exercise, improves exercise performance, or promotes body fat loss (Brass, 2000; Dyck, 2000). Nevertheless, vegetarian athletes may be a target of aggressive marketing by supplement companies.

Caffeine

Caffeine is probably the most casually and widely used sports-enhancing supplement, because of its availability and social acceptance (Paluska, 2003). Caffeine (or its sister derivatives theophylline and theobromine) occurs naturally in specific foods, including coffee, tea, and chocolate; it is also added to soda, sports bars and gels, and some medications (Applegate, 1999; Graham, 2001). Caffeine is thought to improve performance both by acting as a central nervous system stimulant (affecting perception of effort, warding off drowsiness, increasing alertness) and by facilitating force production in the muscle. Well-controlled laboratory studies have found that caffeine (3–13 mg/kilogram of body mass) taken 1 hour prior to or during exercise improves endurance performance by prolonging time to exhaustion (Clarkson, 1993; Graham & Spriet, 1996) and improving time-trial performance (Cox et al., 2002). Studies demonstrating a benefit of caffeine on shorter, more intense events are less abundant, but also suggest a potential ergogenic potential (Paluska, 2003). Thus, vegetarian athletes who enjoy coffee, tea, or other caffeinated beverages may find it beneficial to consume them in the pre-event meal (although there is some suggestion that caffeine from supplements may be more effective; Graham, 2001). Habitual intake does not appear to diminish caffeine's ergogenic properties (Paluska, 2003; Graham, 2001). There is no evidence to suggest that caffeine leads to dehydration or electrolyte imbalance during exercise (Armstrong, 2002).

Nutrition before, during, and after Exercise

Before Exercise

The meal before a competition or exercise session should provide adequate carbohydrate and fluid, and prevent both hunger and gastrointestinal distress. Studies have shown that consuming between 1 and 5 g of carbohydrate per kilogram of body mass, 1 to 4 hours before endurance exercise, has the potential to improve endurance performance by as much as 14% (Coyle et al., 1992). It is also thought to benefit stop-and-go events of higher intensity. Based on these findings, general guidelines are to consume 1 to 2 grams of carbohydrate per kilogram of body mass between 1 and 2 hours before exercise or 3 to 4 grams of carbohydrate per kilogram approximately 4 hours before exercise. For example, a 90-kilogram athlete who eats breakfast 90 minutes before exercising should strive to consume between 90 and 180 grams of carbohydrate in the pre-event meal. (Refer to Table 20.4 and the food label to assist in calculating the carbohydrate content of specific foods.) Within these guidelines, athletes should select familiar, well-tolerated, high-carbohydrate foods that are low in sodium, fat, simple sugars, fiber, and excess spice. Some studies have suggested a performance benefit to consuming foods with a low rather than high glycemic index (for example, lentils or bran cereal rather than mashed potatoes or corn flakes), as they may provide a slower-release source of glucose during exercise (Siu & Wong, 2004). In addition, the American College of Sports Medicine recommends drinking 1.5 to 2.5 cups of fluid (400–600 ml) 2 to 3 hours before exercise (ACSM, 2000; ACSM, 1996). Guidelines for special circumstances, such as nausea and rebound hypoglycemia (low blood sugar), are presented in Box 20.1.

During Exercise

Carbohydrate ingestion at a rate of between 30–75 grams/hour has been shown to benefit performance during moderate-intensity endurance exercise (running, cycling, and cross-country skiing events lasting longer than 2 hours) (Coggan & Swanson, 1992) and during intermittent, high-intensity activities of shorter duration (soccer, court play, and repetitive sprinting) (Below et al., 1995; Ball et al., 1995; Nicholas et al., 1995). It is speculated that carbohydrate intake during exercise benefits performance by preventing low blood sugar and preserving carbohydrate utilization in the latter part of exercise when liver and muscle glycogen stores become depleted.

Consumption of fluids during exercise is key to preventing dehydration. Dehydration can drastically impair performance and can also have serious health consequences. To prevent dehydration, the American College of Sports Medicine recommends that athletes drink enough fluid during exercise to replace whatever is lost through sweating (ACSM, 1996). See Box 20.2 for information on calculating sweat rate and determining personal fluid requirements. A typical sweat rate is between 800 and 1,500 milliliters per hour, and is even higher during exercise in a hot and humid environment. Ingestion of a sports drink containing the recommended concentration of 6%–8% carbohy-

Box 20.1 Special Concerns for Pre-Event Meals

Nausea Pre-event emotional tension or anxiety may delay digestive time and contribute to nausea and even vomiting before a practice or competition. Research has suggested that liquid meals are more easily tolerated and digested under these conditions. Specifically, the athlete who gets pre-exercise nausea should attempt to consume 1 to 2 liquid supplements or shakes as tolerated. A few soda crackers or a piece of dry toast are also options. Water should also be consumed as tolerated.

"Low Blood Sugar" Although rare, some athletes experience a condition called "rebound hypoglycemia" (low blood sugar) during exercise when carbohydrate foods are consumed within 20 to 60 minutes of exercise. Symptoms specifically associated with low blood sugar include lightheadedness, fatigue, tiredness, and shakiness. In this instance, the pre-event meal should be consumed 90–120 minutes before exercise and consist mostly of low-glycemic-index, carbohydrate-containing foods. If necessary, 1–2 cups of a carbohydrate-containing fluid replacement beverage can be consumed 5–10 minutes before exercise.

Hunger Fluid replacement beverages or "sports drinks" consumed 10 minutes before exercise (practice or conditioning) may delay feelings of hunger and have benefits similar to carbohydrate consumption during exercise. These beverages are readily absorbed and appear in the bloodstream within 5–10 minutes of ingestion. When consumed in this fashion, fluid replacement beverages do not contribute to rebound hypoglycemia.

drate by volume (grams carbohydrate/mL of fluid) (ACSM, 2000; Gisolfi et al., 1992) can simultaneously meet carbohydrate and fluid needs. Alternatively, natural sources of carbohydrate, including diluted fruit juices (4 ounces of juice in 4 ounces of water = 6% solution), low-sodium vegetable juices such as carrot juice (7% solution), and honey or solid foods work equally well, providing that solid foods are ingested with water (Neufer et al., 1987; van der Brug et al., 1995; Coleman, 1994; Lugo et al., 1993; Robergs et al., 1998; Lancaster et al., 2001) and are easily digestible. The guideline is to consume approximately 8 ounces (240 mL) of water with every 15 g of carbohydrate ingested as a solid food—in effect, producing a 6% solution. A pinch of table salt can also be added to juices or low-sodium solids as necessary for events lasting longer than three to four hours (Gisolfi & Duchman, 1992).

After Exercise

Glycogen stores can be completely depleted at the end of a hard practice or workout. Consumption of carbohydrate within 20–30 minutes after exercise is essential for replenishing muscle glycogen stores and enhancing muscle recovery and muscle protein synthesis (Tipton et al., 2001; Levenhagen et al., 2001; Miller et al., 2003; Roy et al., 1997; Roy et al., 2002). Although earlier studies indicated that muscle glycogen could be replenished within 24 hours (providing the post-exercise intake and overall diet is high in carbohydrate) (Williams, 1999), more recent studies have determined that the rate of muscle glycogen replenishment is increased by selecting foods with a high glycemic index (Burke, Collier, & Hargreaves, 1993; Jozsi et al., 1996) or those containing both carbohydrate and protein (about 1 g protein to

Box 20.2   Estimating Sweat Rate and Fluid Requirements during Exercise

- Determine nude body mass in kilograms (after using the restroom). Scale must be accurate to 0.1 kg or 0.1 pound.
- Perform regular exercise or training for 1 hour without consuming any fluids (can also perform exercise for 30 minutes and multiply answer by 2).
- Towel off and determine nude body mass.
- Subtract post-exercise body mass from pre-exercise body mass.
- Body mass loss is directly proportional to fluid loss: 1 kilogram = 1 liter (or 1 pound = 2 cups).

Example:
An athlete weighs 80.5 kilograms before exercise and 79.6 kilograms after exercising for 1 hour.

- 80.5 − 79.6 = 0.9 kilogram
- 0.9 kilogram = 0.9 liters or 900 mL
- Sweat rate = 900 mL/hour

If this athlete replaces sweat loss by consuming a 6% fluid replacement beverage, he or she will consume 54 grams of carbohydrate/hour; 54 grams of carbohydrate is within the recommended intake of 30–60 grams/hour.

3 g carbohydrate) (Ivy et al., 2002). Because low muscle glycogen stores can impair subsequent performance, an increased rate of glycogen replacement is important to athletes performing multiple workouts or events within a 24- to 48-hour period. The current recommendation to replace muscle glycogen and ensure rapid recovery is to consume 1.5 grams of carbohydrate per kilogram of body mass within the first 30 minutes after exercise, and again every 2 hours over a 4- to 6-hour period (ACSM, 2000). Because hard exercise and competition often impair appetite, it may be easier for the athlete to consume a beverage or snack containing carbohydrate and protein immediately after exercise and consume a mixed meal containing carbohydrates, protein, and fat a few hours later.

To replace lost body fluids, athletes should consume at least 1 liter (preferably closer to 1.5 liters) of fluid for every kilogram of body mass lost during exercise (2 cups for every

pound lost) (ACSM, 1996; Shirreffs et al., 1996), and make an effort to include sodium and potassium in the recovery meal(s) (Maughan, Leiper, & Shirreffs, 1996). Although vegetarians are likely to choose foods containing ample potassium (e.g., fruits, vegetables), some may intentionally or unintentionally avoid sodium-containing foods. Sodium intake can be of concern during periods of heavy training in athletes who avoid salt or processed foods, because the typical sweat loss is about 690 mg of sodium per hour (Gisolfi & Duchman, 1992). Thus, more liberal intakes of sodium are often appropriate in the athletic population.

Special Concerns for the Vegetarian Athlete Requiring Weight Reduction

Certain individual athletes may be predisposed to weight gain, because of genetic factors or environmental influences (overeating, sedentary lifestyle when not training). Athletes appear to be particularly prone to weight gain during the freshman year of college, or after taking a new job, getting married, having children, or going through menopause. Although the reasons for weight gain vary, and may be different from individual to individual, an underlying imbalance between energy expenditure and energy intake is almost always noted. For example, freshman team athletes commonly gain weight during their first year because they play less during games or matches, yet eat as much as their junior and senior teammates. Adult athletes often gain weight because real-life responsibilities either decrease the time they can spend exercising and/or produce an environment that encourages overeating.

When weight reduction is required, weight loss should be accomplished slowly and not during the competitive season (ACSM, 2000). The general recommendation is to consume a well-balanced diet (discussed earlier) that is approximately 500 to no more than 1,000 kcal/day less than required (ACSM, 2000; Jakicic et al., 2001). This should promote weight loss of 1 to 2 pounds/week. Weight reduction in athletes, however, can be somewhat problematic, because the diminished energy intake can compromise exercise performance and nutrient intake (ACSM, 2000). Consultation with a registered dietitian trained in sports nutrition can help athletes at all levels maintain a healthful diet while reducing total energy intake to promote gradual weight loss. For example, the athlete should be instructed to consume carbohydrates on the lower range and protein on the higher range recommended for athletes, and to reduce dietary fat intake to no less than 20% of energy intake (as discussed earlier). These recommendations, however, may vary slightly by sport and individual tolerances.

By no means should an athlete attempt to follow any of the restrictive low-carbohydrate diets (such as the Adkins, South Beach, or "Mayo Clinic" diets) that are popular among some individuals (Manore, 1999). Low-carbohydrate diets are contraindicated for athletic training and performance. On a similar note, athletes should not attempt to maintain unrealistic body weight (ACSM, 2000), defined as body weight that cannot be maintained without drastic eating or exercise habits.

Special Concerns for the Female Vegetarian Athlete

Female athletes who are driven to excel in their chosen sports may be at risk of developing disorders of the "female athlete triad": disordered eating, amenorrhea, and osteoporosis (Manore, 1999; West, 1998; Beals & Manore, 2002; Nieman, 1988). Disordered eating is common among women due to the pressure to succeed in sports by achieving or maintaining an unrealistically low body weight through food restriction and strenuous and/or prolonged exercise. Several studies have also noted that disordered eating behaviors tend to be more prevalent among vegetarians (O'Connor et al., 1987; Huse & Lucas, 1984; Neumark-Sztainer et al., 1997), which most experts believe is because vegetarianism is seen as a socially acceptable way to reduce energy and fat intake. In addition, exercising women experience more amenorrhea than their sedentary counterparts; the prevalence of this problem is reported to be between 1%–44% among athletic women (Loucks, 2001). Amenorrhea is most common among distance runners, gymnasts, and ballerinas, but is also found in cyclists, rowers, swimmers, and team sport athletes.

The mechanism responsible for disruption of normal menstrual (reproductive) function is unknown, but evidence favoring inadequate energy availability (i.e., energy requirements more than energy intake, called the *energy drain hypothesis*), rather than stress or overly lean body composition, is continuing to accumulate (Loucks, 2003). Several studies involving predominately endurance runners have found that amenorrheic athletes report reduced intake of total energy (Kaiserauer et al., 1989; Nelson et al., 1986), protein (Kaiserauer et al., 1989; Nelson et al., 1986), fat (Deuster et al., 1986; Kaiserauer et al., 1989), and zinc (Deuster et al., 1986), and higher intakes of fiber (Deuster et al., 1986; Lloyd et al., 1987) and vitamin A than their teammates with normal menstruation cycles.

Although there is some indication that menstrual-cycle disturbances may be higher in vegetarians (Barr, 1999) and vegetarian athletes (Kaiserauer et al., 1989; Brooks et al., 1984), these findings are not consistently reported (Barr, 1999; Slavin, Lutter, & Cushman, 1984) and can be explained by study design issues (Barr, 1999). For instance, studies commonly define *vegetarians* as individuals having a "low-meat diet," not necessarily a truly vegetarian diet (Kaiserauer et al., 1989; Brooks et al., 1984), and may also attract a biased sample of vegetarians. For example, those with menstrual-cycle disturbances may be more likely to volunteer for a study on menstrual-cycle disturbances (Barr, 1999). Nonetheless, female vegetarian athletes should understand that loss of the menstrual cycle is unhealthy and is not a normal part of training. The low circulating estrogen levels associated with loss of monthly cycles can predispose athletes to reduced bone density, premature osteoporosis, and increased risk of stress fractures or other overuse injuries. An athlete experiencing amenorrhea should see her team or personal physician for a thorough evaluation.

Potential Benefits of Vegetarian Diet

As noted in various chapters in this book, vegetarian diets may have many health advantages over the typical American diet. Whether such a diet can potentially affect training or sports performance has not been fully explored. Although a handful of studies in the early 1900s investigated the value of vegetarian diet as a means of increasing physical capacity, most of these studies were not adequately designed (based on today's standards), and in a few cases may have resulted in the answer the investigators or the athletes desired: namely, that a vegan or vegetarian diet was superior to a meat-containing diet (see Nieman, 1988, for a review of the literature). Indeed, in his interpretation of these studies, Nieman (1988) suggested that the superior performance of some of the early vegetarian athletes is possibly explained both by their motivation to demonstrate excellence and by their high carbohydrate intake. More recent and better controlled cross-sectional studies have found that vegetarian men and women have aerobic or anaerobic capacities similar to those of their equally trained meat-eating counterparts (Hanne, Dlin, & Rotstein, 1986), and also perform similarly when challenged to a 1,000-km endurance run (Eisinger et al., 1994). Another study found that endurance performance was not altered in male omnivorous athletes placed on a lacto-ovo vegetarian diet, compared to a meat-rich macronutrient-controlled diet, for 6 weeks (Richter et al., 1991; Raben et al., 1992), although total testosterone was found to decrease slightly in those on the vegetarian diet (Raben et al., 1992). The authors speculated that the decrease in testosterone was most likely temporary and related to the high-fiber intake (98 g vs. 47 g) with the vegetarian diet. Thus, available evidence supports neither a beneficial nor a detrimental effect of a vegetarian diet on physical performance capacity.

More recent research, however, suggests that a potential advantage of a plant-based diet may be its content of antioxidant vitamins and phytochemicals. Athletes following a vegetarian diet may be more likely to have higher intakes of the antioxidant vitamins (vitamin C, vitamin E, and beta-carotene) and other phytochemicals, as is true of vegetarian diets in general (Krajcovicova-Kudlackova et al., 2003; Rauma & Mykkanen, 2000). Muscular exercise promotes the production of free radicals and other reactive oxygen species in the working muscle that are thought to be responsible for exercise-induced protein oxidation, and contribute to muscle fatigue (Powers et al., 2004). Several reviews have summarized the current knowledge of the potential benefits of antioxidant supplements for protection against free radical production and lipid peroxidation (Powers et al., 2004; Kanter, 1995; Clarkson, 1995; Urso & Clarkson, 2003). In brief, supplementation with antioxidants appears to reduce lipid peroxidation, but has not been shown to enhance exercise performance. Research is needed to determine whether a plant-based diet naturally high in antioxidants and phytochemicals would enhance recovery, prevent injury, and attenuate the oxidative damage that occurs with heavy training.

Practical Aspects

- Vegetarian diets can easily meet the nutrition needs of all athletes, from the casual and recreational athlete to the elite athlete.
- A good sports diet obtains the bulk of calories from carbohydrate-rich grains, fruits, and vegetables, and contains several servings of protein-rich foods, calcium-containing plant or dairy foods, nuts, and vegetable oils.
- An athlete's energy requirements can vary from 2,000 to more than 6,000 kcal per day, depending on body size, gender, age, and training and nontraining physical activity. There is some evidence that vegetarians may have higher energy requirements than their nonvegetarian teammates.
- Carbohydrates are the main energy source for high-intensity exercise. In general, vegetarian athletes should consume about 6–10 grams of carbohydrate per kilogram of body mass per day. Before, during, and after exercise, food selections should include adequate amounts of easily digested, high-carbohydrate foods.
- Fat is used primarily during prolonged exercise of moderate intensity and during low-level activity. In general, dietary fat should contribute about 20%–25% of energy, but may be higher in athletes with higher energy needs.
- Protein needs of athletes can easily be met on a vegetarian diet, providing that energy intake is also adequate. Athletes concerned about meeting their protein requirements should select more protein-rich foods, such as legumes and soy products. Protein in the post-exercise meal may enhance recovery.
- Vegetarian athletes should take care to select foods rich in calcium, iron, zinc, riboflavin, and B12, and to ensure that their iron and vitamin D status is normal. A multivitamin and mineral supplement is usually necessary only if the athlete is restricting energy intake or making poor food choices.
- Nutritional supplements should not be used in lieu of good food choices. Certain supplements of interest to competitive

vegetarian athletes include protein, creatine, and caffeine.

- Active vegetarians should ensure that they consume plenty of fluids before, during, and after exercise.
- When weight or body fat reduction is required in adult athletes, weight loss should be accomplished slowly, and not during a competitive season. Athletes desiring weight or body fat loss should consume a well-balanced vegetarian diet that is 500 to 1,000 kcal/day less than required.
- Female vegetarians who maintain adequate energy intake are at no greater risk of amenorrhea or poor bone health than are nonvegetarians. Some female athletes may report being vegetarian to mask an eating disorder.
- Available evidence supports neither a beneficial nor detrimental effect of a vegetarian diet on physical performance capacity. More research is needed to determine if diets rich in antioxidants reduce muscle fatigue or improve recovery.

Conclusion

Athletes at all levels of performance can meet their energy and nutrient needs on a vegetarian diet that contains a variety of plant foods, including grain products, fruits, vegetables, protein-rich plant foods, and (if desired) dairy products and eggs. Depending upon food preferences, eating patterns, and exercise intensity, however, the diet of some athletes may be lacking in certain key nutrients, including total energy, carbohydrate, protein, fat, calcium, vitamin D, iron, zinc, iodine, riboflavin, and vitamin B12. In these cases, athletes can generally improve nutrient status and maybe even performance by consistently making an effort to select foods containing the nutrient(s) they

lack. Although research strongly suggests that a plant-based diet may offer many health benefits to athletes and nonathletes alike, there is little evidence to suggest that vegetarian diets per se are better than omnivorous diets for improving athletic training and performance.

References

American College of Sports Medicine. Position stand: Exercise and fluid replacement. *Med Sci Sports Exer.* 1996;28(1):i–vi.

American College of Sports Medicine, American Dietetic Association, and Dietitians of Canada. Nutrition and athletic performance: Joint position statement. *Med Sci Sports Exer.* 2000;32(12): 2130–2145.

American Diabetes Association and the American Dietetic Association. *Exchange Lists for Meal Planning.* Alexandria, VA: American Diabetes Association Inc.; 2003.

Applegate E. Effective nutritional ergogenic aids. *Intl J Sport Nutr.* 1999;9(2):229–239.

Armstrong LE. Caffeine, body fluid-electrolyte balance, and exercise performance. *Intl J Sport Nutr Exer Metab.* 2002;12(2):189–206.

Ball TC, Headley SA, Vanderburgh PM, Smith JC. Periodic carbohydrate replacement during 50 min of high-intensity cycling improves subsequent sprint performance. *Intl J Sport Nutr.* 1995;5(2): 151–158.

Balsom P, Soderlund K, Ekblom B. Creatine in humans with special reference to creatine supplementation. *Sports Med.* 1994;18(4):268–280.

Barr SI. Vegetarianism and menstrual cycle disturbances: Is there an association? *Am J Clin Nutr.* 1999;70(3, Suppl):549S–554S.

Beals KA, Manore MM. Disorders of the female athlete triad among collegiate athletes. *Intl J Sport Nutr Exer Metab.* 2002;12(3):281–293.

Belko A. Vitamins and exercise—An update. *Med Sci Sports Exer.* 1987;19(5):S191–S196.

Below P, Mora-Rodriguez R, Gonzalez AJ, Coyle E. Fluid and carbohydrate ingestion independently improve performance during 1 hr of intense exercise. *Med Sci Sports Exer.* 1995;27(2):200–210.

Bergstrom J, Hermansen L, Hultman E, Saltin B. Diet, muscle glycogen and physical performance. *Acta Physiol Scand.* 1967;71:140–150.

Boirie Y, Dangin M, Gachon P, Vasson MP, Maubois JL, Beaufrere B. Slow and fast dietary proteins differently modulate postprandial protein accretion. Proc Natl Acad Sci USA. 1997;94(26):14930–14935.

Borsheim E, Bahr R. Effect of exercise intensity, duration and mode on post-exercise oxygen consumption. *Sports Med.* 2003;33(14):1037–1060.

Branch JD. Effect of creatine supplementation on body composition and performance: A meta-analysis. *Intl J Sport Nutr.* 2003;13(2):198–226.

Brass EP. Supplemental carnitine and exercise. *Am J Clin Nutr.* 2000;72(2, Suppl):618S–623S.

Brewer J, Williams C, Patton A. The influence of high carbohydrate diets on endurance running performance. *Eur J Appl Physiol.* 1988;57:698–706.

Brooks S, Sanborn C, Albrecht B, Wagner W. Diet in athletic amenorrhoea [letter]. *Lancet.* 1984;2:559–560.

Brown RC, Cox CM. Effects of high fat versus high carbohydrate diets on plasma lipids and lipoproteins in endurance athletes. *Med Sci Sports Exer.* 1998;30(12):1677–1683.

Brownlie T, Utermohlen V, Hinton PS, Haas JD. Tissue iron deficiency without anemia impairs adaptation in endurance capacity after aerobic training in previously untrained women. *Am J Clin Nutr.* 2004;79(3):437–443.

Burke DG, Chilibeck PD, Parise G, Candow DG, Mahoney D, Tarnopolsky M. Effect of creatine and weight training on muscle creatine and performance in vegetarians. *Med Sci Sports Exer.* 2003;35(11):1946–1955.

Burke L, Collier G, Hargreaves M. Muscle glycogen storage after prolonged exercise: Effect of the glycemic index of carbohydrate feedings. *J Appl Physiol.* 1993;75(2):1019–1023.

Casey A, Mann R, Banister K, et al. Effect of carbohydrate ingestion on glycogen resynthesis in human liver and skeletal muscle, measured by (13)C MRS. *Am J Physiol Endocr Metab.* 2000;278(1):E65–75.

Clarkson P. Antioxidants and physical performance. *Crit Rev Food Sci Nutr.* 1995;35(1&2):131–141.

Clarkson PM. Nutritional ergogenic aids: Caffeine. *Intl J Sport Nutr.* 1993;3(1):103–111.

Clarys P, Zinzen E, Hebbelinck M. The effect of oral creatine supplementation on torque production in a vegetarian and non-vegetarian population: A double blind study. *Veg Nutr.* 1997;1:100–105.

Coggan AR, Swanson SC. Nutritional manipulations before and during endurance exercise: Effects on performance. *Med Sci Sports Exer.* 1992;24(4):S331–S335.

Coleman E. Update on carbohydrate: Solid versus liquid. *Intl J Sport Nutr.* 1994;4(2):80–88.

Cox GR, Desbrow B, Montgomery PG, et al. Effect of different protocols of caffeine intake on metabolism and endurance performance. *J Appl Physiol.* 2002;93(3):990–999.

Coyle E, Coggan A, Davis J, Sherman W. Current thoughts and practical considerations concerning substrate utilization during exercise. *Sports Sci Exch.* 1992;Spring(7):1–4.

Craig W. Iron status of vegetarians. *Am J Clin Nutr.* 1994;59(Suppl):1233S–1237S.

Crist DM, Hill JM. Diet and insulinlike growth factor I in relation to body composition in women with exercise-induced hypothalamic amenorrhea. *J Am Coll Nutr.* 1990;9(3):200–204.

Dangin M, Boirie Y, Garcia-Rodenas C, et al. The digestion rate of protein is an independent regulating factor of postprandial protein retention. *Am J Physiol Endocr Metab.* 2001;280(2):E340–E348.

Davies NM. Toxicity of nonsteroidal anti-inflammatory drugs in the large intestine. *Dis Colon Rectum.* 1995;38(12):1311–1321.

Decombaz J, Schmitt B, Ith M, et al. Postexercise fat intake repletes intramyocellular lipids but no faster in trained than in sedentary subjects. *Am J Physiol Regul Integr Comp Physiol.* 2001;281(3):R760–R769.

Delanghe J, De Slypere J-P, De Buyzere M, Robbrecht J, Wieme R, Vermeulen A. Normal reference values for creatine, creatinine, and carnitine are lower in vegetarians. *Clin Chem.* 1989;35:1802–1803.

Deuster PA, Kyle SB, Moser PB, Vigersky RA, Singh A, Schoomaker EB. Nutritional intakes and status of highly trained amenorrheic and eumenorrheic women runners. *Fertility Sterility.* 1986;46(4): 636-643.

Dyck DJ. Dietary fat intake, supplements, and weight loss. *Can J Appl Physiol.* 2000;25(6):495-523.

Eichner E. Sports anemia, iron supplements, and blood doping. *Med Sci Sports Exer.* 1992;1992 (Suppl 9):S315-S318.

Eichner E. Runner's macrocytosis: A clue to foot-strike hemolysis. *Am J Med.* 1985;78:321-325.

Eisinger M, Plath M, Jung L, Leitzmann C. Nutrient intake of endurance runners with ovo-lacto-vegetarian diet and regular western diet. *Zuitschrift fur Emahrungswissenschaft.* 1994;33(3): 217-229.

Fogelholm M. Indicators of vitamin and mineral status in athletes' blood: A review. *Intl J Sport Nutr.* 1995;5(4):267-284.

Gausseres N, Catala I, Mahe S, et al. Whole-body protein turnover in humans fed a soy protein-rich vegetable diet. *Eur J Clin Nutr.* 1997;51(5): 308-311.

Gisolfi C, Duchman S. Guidelines for optimal replacement beverages for different athletic events. *Med Sci Sports Exer.* 1992;24(6):679-687.

Gisolfi CV, Summers RW, Schedl HP, Bleiler TL. Intestinal water absorption from selected carbohydrate solutions in humans. *J Appl Physiol.* 1992; 73(5):2142-2150.

Goforth HW Jr, Laurent D, Prusaczyk WK, Schneider KE, Petersen KF, Shulman GI. Effects of depletion exercise and light training on muscle glycogen supercompensation in men. *Am J Physiol.* 2003; 285(6):E1304-E1311.

Goran M. Variation in total energy expenditure in humans. *Obes Res.* 1995;3(1):59-66.

Graham EE, Spriet LL. Caffeine and exercise performance. *Gatorade Sports Sci Exch.* 1996;9(1).

Graham TE. Caffeine and exercise: Metabolism, endurance and performance. *Sports Med.* 2001; 31(11):785-807.

Grandjean A. The vegetarian athlete. *Physician & Sportsmedicine.* 1987;15(5):191-194.

Grandjean AC. Diets of elite athletes: Has the discipline of sports nutrition made an impact? *J Nutr.* 1997;127(5, Suppl):874S-877S.

Grimble, RF, Tappia, PS. Modulation of pro-inflammatory cytokine biology by unsaturated fatty acids. *Z Ernahrungswiss.* 1998;37(Suppl 1):57-65.

Hallberg L. Does calcium interfere with iron absorption? [editorial]. *Am J Clin Nutr.* 1998;68:3-4.

Hanne N, Dlin R, Rotstein A. Physical fitness, anthropometric and metabolic parameters in vegetarian athletes. *J Sports Med Phys Fitness.* 1986;26(2): 180-185.

Hargreaves M. Skeletal muscle metabolism during exercise in humans. *Clin Exp Pharmacol Physiol.* 2000;27(3):225-228.

Hargreaves M, Costill D, Coggan A, Fink W, Nishibata I. Effect of carbohydrate feedings on muscle glycogen utilization and exercise performance. *Med Sci Sports Exer.* 1984;16(3):219-222.

Harris RC, Soderlund K, Hultman E. Elevation of creatine in resting and exercised muscle of normal subjects by creatine supplementation. *Clin Sci.* 1992;83:367-374.

Heaney R, Recker R, Saville P. Menopausal changes in calcium balance performance. *J Lab Clin Med.* 1978;92:953-962.

Heaney RP, Dowell MS, Rafferty K, Bierman J. Bioavailability of the calcium in fortified soy imitation milk, with some observations on method. *Am J Clin Nutr.* 2000;71(5):1166-1169.

Herbert V. Everyone should be tested for iron disorders. *J Am Diet Assoc.* 1992;92(12):1502-1509.

Herrmann W, Geisel J. Vegetarian lifestyle and monitoring of vitamin B-12 status. *Clin Chim Acta.* 2002;326(1-2):47-59.

Hinton PS, Giordano C, Brownlie T, Haas JD. Iron supplementation improves endurance after training in iron-depleted, nonanemic women. *J Appl Physiol.* 2000;88(3):1103-1111.

Holick MF. Sunlight and vitamin D for bone health and prevention of autoimmune diseases, cancers, and cardiovascular disease. *Am J Clin Nutr.* 2004; 80:1678S-1688S.

Houtkooper L. Food selection for endurance sports. *Med Sci Sports Exer.* 1992;24(9):S349-S359.

Hu FB, Willett WC. Optimal diets for prevention of coronary heart disease. *JAMA.* 2002;288(20):2569-2578.

Hunt JR, Matthys LA, Johnson LK. Zinc absorption, mineral balance, and blood lipids in women consuming controlled lacto-ovo-vegetarian and omnivorous diets for 8 wks. *Am J Clin Nutr.* 1998; 67:421–430.

Hunt JR. Bioavailability of iron, zinc, and other trace minerals from vegetarian diets. *Am J Clin Nutr.* 2003;78(3, Suppl):633S–639S.

Huse DM, Lucas AR. Dietary patterns in anorexia nervosa. *Am J Clin Nutr.* 1984;40:251–254.

International Center for Sports Nutrition. Vegetarian diets. *Olympic Coach.* 1997;Winter.

Ivy JL, Goforth HW Jr, Damon BM, McCauley TR, Parsons EC, Price TB. Early postexercise muscle glycogen recovery is enhanced with a carbohydrate-protein supplement. *J Appl Physiol.* 2002;93(4):1337–1344.

Jakicic JM, Clark K, Coleman E, et al. American College of Sports Medicine position stand: Appropriate intervention strategies for weight loss and prevention of weight regain for adults. *Med Sci Sports Exer.* 2001;33(12):2145–2156.

Jozsi AC, Trappe TA, Starling RD, et al. The influence of starch structure on glycogen resynthesis and subsequent cycling performance. *Intl J Sports Med.* 1996;17(5):373–378.

Juhn M. Popular sports supplements and ergogenic aids. *Sports Med.* 2003;33(12):921–939.

Juhn MS, Tarnopolsky M. Oral creatine supplementation and athletic performance: A critical review. *Clin J Sport Med.* 1998;8(4):286–297.

Kaiserauer S, Snyder A, Sleeper M, Zierath J. Nutritional, physiological, and menstrual status of distance runners. *Med Sci Sports Exer.* 1989;21:120–125.

Kanter M. Free radicals and exercise: Effects of nutritional antioxidant supplementation. *Exer Sport Sci Rev.* 1995;12:375–397.

Kohlenberg-Mueller K, Raschka L. Calcium balance in young adults on a vegan and lactovegetarian diet. *J Bone Miner Metab.* 2003;21(1):28–33.

Krajcovicova-Kudlackova M, Buckova K, Klimes I, Sebokova E. Iodine deficiency in vegetarians and vegans. *Ann Nutr Metab.* 2003;47(5):183–185

Krajcovicova-Kudlackova M, Ursinyova M, Blazicek P, et al. Free radical disease prevention and nutrition. *Bratisl Lek Listy* 2003;104(2):64–68.

Kreider R, Miriel V, Bertun E. Amino acid supplementation and exercise performance: Analysis of the proposed ergogenic value. *Sports Med.* 1993;16(3): 190–209.

Lancaster S, Kreider RB, Rasmussen C, et al. Effects of honey supplementation on glucose, insulin, and endurance cycling performance. *FASEB J.* 2001;15(Suppl):LB315.

Larson DE, Hesslink RL, Hrovat MI, Fishman RS, Systrom DM. Dietary effects on exercising muscle metabolism and performance by ^{31}P-MRS. *J Appl Physiol.* 1994;77(3):1108–1115.

Larson-Meyer DE, Hunter GR, Newcomer BR. Influence of endurance running and recovery diet on intramyocellular lipid content in women: A ^{1}H-NMR study. *Am J Physiol.* 2002;282:E95–E106.

Laughlin GA, Yen SS. Nutritional and endocrine-metabolic aberrations in amenorrheic athletes. *J Clin Endocr Metab.* 1996;81:4301–4309.

Levenhagen DK, Gresham JD, Carlson MG, Maron DJ, Borel MJ, Flakoll PJ. Postexercise nutrient intake timing in humans is critical to recovery of leg glucose and protein homeostasis. *Am J Physiol Endocr Metab.* 2001;280(6):E982–E993.

Lightowler HJ, Davies GJ. Iodine intake and iodine deficiency in vegans as assessed by the duplicate-portion technique and urinary iodine excretion. *Br J Nutr.* 1998;80(6):529–535.

Lloyd T, Buchanen J, Bitzer S, Waldman C, Myers C, Ford B. Interrelationship of diet, athletic activity, menstrual status, and bone density in collegiate women. *Am J Clin Nutr.* 1987;46:681–684.

Loucks AB. Energy availability, not body fatness, regulates reproductive function in women. *Exer Sport Sci Rev.* 2003;31(3):144–148.

Loucks AB. Physical health of the female athlete: Observations, effects, and causes of reproductive disorders. *Can J Appl Physiol.* 2001;26(Suppl): S176–S185.

Lugo M, Sherman WM, Wimer GS, Garleb K. Metabolic responses when different forms of carbohydrate energy are consumed during cycling. *Intl J Sport Nutr.* 1993;3(4):398–407.

Lukaski H. Micronutrients (magnesium, zinc, and copper): Are mineral supplements needed for athletes? *Intl J Sport Nutr.* 1995;5(Suppl):S74–S83.

Lukaszuk JM, Robertson RJ, Arch JE, et al. Effect of creatine supplementation and a lacto-ovo-vegetarian diet on muscle creatine concentration. *Intl J Sport Nutr.* 2002;12(3):336–348.

Malczewska J, Raczynski G, Stupnicki R. Iron status in female endurance athletes and in non-athletes. *Intl J Sport Nutr.* 2000;10(3):260–276.

Mangels AR, Messina V, Melina V. Position of the American Dietetic Association and Dietitians of Canada: Vegetarian diets. *J Am Diet Assoc.* 2003;103(6):748–765.

Manore M. Low carbohydrate diets back in the news. *ACSM's Health & Fitness J.* 1999;3(5):41.

Manore M, Helleksen J, Merkel J, Skinner J. Longitudinal changes in zinc status in untrained men: Effects of two different 12-week exercise training programs and zinc supplementation. *J Am Diet Assoc.* 1993;93(10):1165–1168.

Manore M, Thompson J. *Sport Nutrition for Health and Performance.* Champaign, IL: Human Kinetics; 2000.

Manore MM. Effect of physical activity on thiamine, riboflavin, and vitamin B-6 requirements. *Am J Clin Nutr.* 2000;72(2, Suppl):598S–606S.

Manore MM. Nutritional needs of the female athlete. *Clin Sports Med.* 1999;18(3):549–563.

Maughan R. The athlete's diet: Nutritional goals and dietary strategies. *Proc Nutr Soc.* 2002;61(1):87–96.

Maughan R, Leiper J, Shirreffs S. Restoration of fluid balance after exercise-induced dehydration: Effects of food and fluid intake. *Eur J Appl Physiol.* 1996;73:317–325.

McArdle W, Katch F, Katch V. *Sports and Exercise Nutrition.* Baltimore: Lippincott/Williams & Wilkins, 1999.

McNaughton L, Dalton B, Palmer G. Sodium bicarbonate can be used as an ergogenic aid in high-intensity, competitive cycle ergometry of 1 hr duration. *Eur J Appl Physiol.* 1999;80:64–69.

Messina V, Melina V, Mangels AR. A new food guide for North American vegetarians. *J Am Diet Assoc.* 2003;103(6):771–775.

Messina M, Messina V. *The Dietitian's Guide to Vegetarian Diets: Issues and Applications.* Gaithersburg, MD: Aspen Publishers; 1996.

Micheletti A, Rossi R, Rufini S. Zinc status in athletes: Relation to diet and exercise. *Sports Med.* 2001;31(8):577–582.

Miller SL, Tipton KD, Chinkes DL, Wolf SE, Wolfe RR. Independent and combined effects of amino acids and glucose after resistance exercise. *Med Sci Sports Exer.* 2003;35(3):449–455.

Minihane A, Fairweather-Tait S. Effect of calcium supplementation on daily nonheme-iron absorption and long-term iron status. *Am J Clin Nutr.* 1998;68:96–102.

Muoio DM, Leddy JJ, Horvath PJ, Awad AB, Pendergast DR. Effect of dietary fat on metabolic adjustments to maximal VO_2 and endurance in runners. *Med Sci Sports Exer.* 1994;26(1):81–88.

Myburgh K, Hutchins J, Fataar A, Hough S, Noakes T. Low bone density is an etiologic factor for stress fractures in athletes. *Ann Intern Med.* 1990;113:754–759.

National Research Council. *Recommended Dietary Allowances.* 10th ed. Washington, DC: National Academy Press; 1989.

Nelson M, Fisher E, Catsos P, Meredith C, Turksoy R, Evans W. Diet and bone status in amenorrheic runners. *Am J Clin Nutr.* 1986;43:910–916.

Neufer P, Costill D, Flynn M, Kirwan J, Mitchell J, Houmard J. Improvements in exercise performance: Effects of carbohydrate feedings and diet. *J Appl Physiol.* 1987;62(3):983–988.

Neumark-Sztainer D, Story M, Resnick MD, Blum RW. Adolescent vegetarians. A behavioral profile of a school-based population in Minnesota. *Arch Pediatr Adolesc Med.* 1997;151:833–838.

Nicholas C, Williams C, Phillips G, Nowitz A. Influence of ingesting a carbohydrate-electrolyte solution on endurance capacity during intermittent, high intensity shuttle running. *J Sports Sci.* 1995;13(4):283–290.

Nieman D. Vegetarian dietary practices and endurance performance. *Am J Clin Nutr.* 1988;48:754–761.

Nikawa T, Ikemoto M, Sakai T, et al. Effects of a soy protein diet on exercise-induced muscle protein catabolism in rats. *Nutrition.* 2002;18(6):490–495.

Nilsson L, Hultman E. Liver glycogen in man—The effect of total starvation or a carbohydrate-poor diet followed by carbohydrate refeeding. *Scand J Clin Lab Investig.* 1973;32:325–330.

O'Connor MA, Touyz SW, Dunn SM, Beumont PJ. Vegetarianism in anorexia nervosa? A review of 116 consecutive cases. *Med J Aust.* 1987;147 (11-12):540-542.

O'Keeffe K, Keith R, Wilson G, Blessing D. Dietary carbohydrate intake and endurance exercise performance of trained female cyclists. *Nutr Res.* 1989;9:819-830.

Paluska SA. Caffeine and exercise. *Curr Sports Med Reps.* 2003;2(4):213-219.

Pizza F, Flynn M, Duscha B, Holden J, Kubitz E. A carbohydrate loading regimen improves high intensity, short duration exercise performance. *Intl J Sport Nutr.* 1995;5(2):110-116.

Powers SK, DeRuisseau KC, Quindry J, Hamilton KL. Dietary antioxidants and exercise. *J Sports Sci.* 2004;22(1):81-94.

Raben A, Kiens B, Richter EA, et al. Serum sex hormones and endurance performance after a lacto-ovo vegetarian and a mixed diet. *Med Sci Sports Exer.* 1992;24(11):1290-1297.

Rauma A, Torronen R, Hanninen O, Mykkanen H. Vitamin B-12 status of long-term adherents of a strict uncooked vegan diet ("living food diet") is compromised. *J Nutr.* 1995;125(10):2511-2515.

Rauma AL, Mykkanen H. Antioxidant status in vegetarians versus omnivores. *Nutrition.* 2000;16(2): 111-119.

Rebouche C, Chenard C. Metabolic fate of dietary carnitine in human adults: Identification and quantification of urinary and fecal metabolites. *J Nutr.* 1991;121:539-546.

Remer T, Neubert A, Manz F. Increased risk of iodine deficiency with vegetarian nutrition. *Br J Nutr.* 1999;81(1):45-49.

Richter EA, Kiens B, Raben A, Tvede N, Pedersen BK. Immune parameters in male athletes after a lacto-ovo vegetarian diet and a mixed Western diet. *Med Sci Sports Exer.* 1991;23(5):517-521.

Robergs RA, McMinn SB, Mermier C, Leadbetter GR, Ruby B, Quinn C. Blood glucose and glucoregulatory hormone responses to solid and liquid carbohydrate ingestion during exercise. *Intl J Sport Nutr.* 1998;8(1):70-83.

Robertson J, Maughan R, Davidson R. Faecal blood loss in response to exercise. *Br Med J.* 1987;295: 303-305.

Romijn JA, Coyle EF, Sidossis LS, Rosenblatt J, Wolfe RR. Substrate metabolism during different exercise intensities in endurance-trained women. *J Appl Physiol.* 2000;88(5):1707-1714.

Romijn JA, Coyle EF, Sidossis LS, et al. Regulation of endogenous fat and carbohydrate metabolism in relation to exercise intensity and duration. *Am J Physiol Endocr Metab.* 1993;265(28):E380-E391.

Roy B, Tarnopolsky M, MacDougall J, Fowles J, Yarasheski K. Effect of glucose supplement after resistance training on protein metabolism. *Clin J Sport Med.* 1997;8(1):70.

Roy BD, Luttmer K, Bosman MJ, Tarnopolsky MA. The influence of post-exercise macronutrient intake on energy balance and protein metabolism in active females participating in endurance training. *Intl J Sport Nutr.* 2002;12(2):172-188.

Sacks FM, Katan M. Randomized clinical trials on the effects of dietary fat and carbohydrate on plasma lipoproteins and cardiovascular disease. *Am J Med.* 2002;113(Suppl 9B):13S-24S.

Schumacher YO, Schmid A, Grathwohl D, Bultermann D, Berg A. Hematological indices and iron status in athletes of various sports and performances. *Med Sci Sports Exer.* 2002;34(5):869-875.

Shirreffs SM, Taylor AJ, Leiper JB, Maughan RJ. Post-exercise rehydration in man: Effects of volume consumed and drink sodium content. *Med Sci Sports Exer.* 1996;28(10):1260-1271.

Shomrat A, Weinstein Y, Katz A. Effect of creatine feeding on maximal exercise performance in vegetarians. *Eur J Appl Physiol.* 2000;82(4):321-325.

Singh A, Moses F, Deuster P. Chronic multivitamin-mineral supplementation does not enhance physical performance. *Med Sci Sports Exer.* 1992;24: 726-732.

Siu PM, Wong SH. Use of the glycemic index: Effects on feeding patterns and exercise performance. *J Physiol Anthropol Appl Human Sci.* 2004; 23(1):1-6.

Slavin J, Lutter J, Cushman S. Amenorrhea in vegetarian athletes [letter] *Lancet.* 1984;1984(1):1474-1475.

Snyder A, Dvorak L, Roepke J. Influence of dietary iron source on measures of iron status among female runners. *Med Sci Sports Exer.* 1989;21(1): 7-10.

Soares M, Satyanarayana K, Bamji M, Jacob C, Ramana Y, Rao S. The effect of exercise on the riboflavin status of adult men. *Br J Nutr.* 1993;69(2):541-551.

Spencer M, Yan Z, Katz A. Carbohydrate supplementation attenuates IMP accumulation in human muscle during prolonged exercise. *Am J Physiol.* 1991;261(Cell Physiol 30):C71-C76.

Steen SN, Coleman E. Selected ergogenic aids used by athletes. *Nutr Clin Pract.* 1999;14:287-295.

Sugiura K, Kobayashi K. Effect of carbohydrate ingestion on sprint performance following continuous and intermittent exercise. *Med Sci Sports Exer.* 1998;30(11):1624-1630.

Tangpricha V, Turner A, Spina C, Decastro S, Chen TC, Holick MF. Tanning is associated with optimal vitamin D status (serum 25-hydroxyvitamin D concentration) and higher bone mineral density. *Am J Clin Nutr.* 2004;80:1645-1649.

Terjung RL, Clarkson P, Eichner ER, et al. American College of Sports Medicine roundtable: The physiological and health effects of oral creatine supplementation. *Med Sci Sports Exer.* 2000;32(3):706-717.

Than T-M, May M-W, Aug K-S, Mya-Tu M. The effect of vitamin B12 on physical performance capacity. *Br J Nutr.* 1978;40:269-273.

Thompson J, Manore M. Predicted and measured resting metabolic rate of male and female endurance athletes. *Journal of The American Dietetic Association.* 96:30-34, 1996.

Tipton KD, Rasmussen BB, Miller SL, et al. Timing of amino acid-carbohydrate ingestion alters anabolic response of muscle to resistance exercise. *Am J Physiol Endocr Metab.* 2001;281(2):E197-E206.

Toth MJ, Poehlman, ET. Sympathetic nervous system activity and resting metabolic rate in vegetarians. *Metabolism.* 1994;43(5):621-625.

Trang HM, Cole DE, Rubin LA, Pierratos A, Siu S, Vieth R. Evidence that vitamin D3 increases serum 25-hydroxyvitamin D more efficiently than does vitamin D2. *Am J Clin Nutr.* 1998;68:854-858.

Urso ML, Clarkson PM. Oxidative stress, exercise, and antioxidant supplementation. *Toxicology.* 2003;189(1-2):41-54.

van der Brug GE, Peters HP, Hardeman MR, Schep G, Mosterd WL. Hemorheological response to prolonged exercise—No effects of different kinds of feedings. *Intl J Sports Med.* 1995;16(4):231-237.

Venkatraman JT, Pendergast D. Effects of the level of dietary fat intake and endurance exercise on plasma cytokines in runners. *Med Sci Sports Exer.* 1998;30(8):1198-1204.

Venkatraman JT, Rowland JA, Denardin E, Horvath PJ, Pendergast D. Influence of the level of dietary lipid intake and maximal exercise on the immune status in runners. *Med Sci Sports Exer.* 1997; 29(3):333-344.

Waller M, Haymes E. The effects of heat and exercise on sweat iron loss. *Med Sci Sports Exer.* 1996; 28(2):197-203.

Weaver C, Plawecki K. Dietary calcium: Adequacy of a vegetarian diet. *Am J Clin Nutr.* 1994;59 (Suppl):1238S-1241S.

Weaver CM, Proulx WR, Heaney R. Choices for achieving adequate dietary calcium with a vegetarian diet. *Am J Clin Nutr.* 1999;70(3,Suppl): 543S-548S.

West RV. The female athlete. The triad of disordered eating, amenorrhoea and osteoporosis. *Sports Med.* 1998;26(2):63-71.

Wilkinson SB, Tarnopolsky MA, Macdonald MJ, Macdonald JR, Armstrong D, Phillips SM. Consumption of fluid skim milk promotes greater muscle protein accretion after resistance exercise than does consumption of an isonitrogenous and isoenergetic soy-protein beverage. *Am J Clin Nutr.* 2007;85:1031-1040.

Williams C. Macronutrients and performance. *J Sports Sci.* 1995;13(Spec No):S1-10.

Williams MH. Nutrition for Health, Fitness and Sport. 5th ed. Boston: McGraw-Hill; 1999.

Wolman R, Clark P, McNally E, Harries M, Reeve J. Dietary calcium as a statistical determinant of trabecular bone density in amenorrhoeic and oestrogen-replete athletes. *Bone Miner.* 1992;17: 415-423.

Woolf K, Manore MM. B-vitamins and exercise: does exercise alter requirements? *Intl J Sport Nutr Exerc Metab.* 2006;16:453-484.

Young V. Soy protein in relation to human protein and amino acid nutrition. *J Am Diet Assoc.* 1991;91:828-835.

Young VR, Pellett PL. Plant proteins in relation to human protein and amino acid nutrition. *Am J Clin Nutr.* 1994;59(Suppl):1203S-1212S.

21

Environmental and Food Safety Aspects of Vegetarian Diets

Carl V. Phillips, MPP, PhD
Simon K. Emms, PhD
Erin L. Kraker, MS, REHS

Introduction

The primary focus of this book is the personal health implications of choosing a vegetarian diet. However, your dietary choices, arguably more than any other consumer decision, have consequences for others also. Choosing to consume or avoid animal-based foods affects the well-being of animals used for food or food production, a topic beyond the scope of this book but covered well in several recent works (Regan, 2003; Scully, 2002) and many important works from previous decades. Good starting points for the latter include Mason and Singer's (1980) visceral book, the philosophical tour de force by Regan (1983), and the compelling but widely overlooked book by Midgley (1998). These issues are sometimes referred to as the ethical side of vegetarianism, but they do not address another major set of ethical issues associated with choosing vegetarianism: the impact of animal foods on the environment.

Vegetarianism and the environment is a topic similar in scope to vegetarianism and health, so a single chapter can provide only a brief overview of the many important factors in this issue. However, the core message of this chapter can be summarized in a few words: Among practical actions that most Westerners can take to help the environment, moving toward a more vegetarian diet offers the most benefit.

The vast majority of people in the United States, Canada, the United Kingdom, and other places where this book is likely to be available consider themselves environmentalists or express concern about the environment. Depending on how the question is phrased and which population is polled, survey results regularly find that more than 50%, and sometimes as much as 90%, of the population agree with pro-environmental statements. Most educated people are aware that Western standards of living take a huge toll on the environment. What they may not know is that reducing the consumption of animal foods is one of the few things they personally can do to make a substantial reduction in their environmental impact. (Reducing use of motorized transport by the same proportion would have a similar impact, but is unlikely to be practical for most people. Achieving similar benefits by reducing the use of other consumable goods and ownership of durable goods would require such huge reductions as to be virtually impossible for most individuals.)

Many people choose to indulge in unhealthy consumption of animal foods, which from the perspective of their own health should be seen as a legitimate choice (assuming they are well-informed about the health implications). After all, we all make potentially injurious choices every day. What is striking, though, is how often people who otherwise try to have a positive impact on the world casually say, "I'll have the steak, with the calamari appetizer." Few people seem to realize that one such meal incurs environmental costs that probably exceed a year's worth of environmental benefits from their habit of carefully sorting recyclables.

Types of Animal Food Production

To fully understand the environmental impacts of eating animals, it is necessary to recognize three basic types of animal food production:

1. *Intensive production* involves raising animals at high densities, and importing their feed from elsewhere. These production facilities consist of various forms of feedlots (most often defined as any animal agriculture operation so concentrated that foliage cannot grow, but usually used to refer to operations that substantially exceed that threshold). These include concentrated outdoor pens for "finishing" cows, giant indoor hog factories, battery chicken buildings where the animals are stacked like books in a library, many types of aquaculture ("fish farming"), and other facilities.
2. *Nonintensive production* consists largely of grazing animals (mostly cattle, with lesser numbers of sheep and other species)

on rangeland, at lower densities and with less importation of feed, as the animals find much or all of their food themselves. It also includes some forms of shellfish aquaculture.
3. *Harvesting* involves the collection of wild species from their native habitat (not to be confused with use of the term to describe the collection of grain crops from agricultural land). Industrial fishing is by far the most important type of animal harvesting, but other examples include deer and duck hunting.

Each of these forms of production has negative environmental impacts, though the exact effects vary among the production methods.

A Variety of Environmental Impacts

Food production is not the clean, environmentally harmonious process that Americans are told about in grade school. It has environmental impacts similar to those of other heavy industries, including consumption of water resources and petrochemicals, pollution of the air and water, and damage to natural areas and habitats; as well as impacts not usually caused by other industries, including the intentional reduction of biodiversity and the use of massive amounts of land (with the resulting loss of natural habitat, sources of natural pollution reduction, and recreational land). Both plant and animal agriculture have these effects, but animal food production is the dirtiest and most resource-intensive agricultural sector.

The equation is simple: Intensive agriculture (which produces most of the animal foods consumed in rich countries) requires several kilograms of plant food to be grown for each kilogram of animal food produced; grazing, even when it occurs in areas that could not be used to produce plant food for human consumption, still uses huge amounts of land. Other impacts are direct products of the animals themselves, such as methane production in the intestines and from manure, which leads to global warming. Still other effects are due to modern production methods, such as antibiotic overuse, manure disposal problems, and the local water pollution, stench, and insect infestations caused by extremely concentrated facilities. The negative environmental impacts of producing animal foods include almost every major modern environmental concern.

To summarize, compared to equivalent amounts of plant food, producing animal food through feedlots, grazing, fishing, or other means:

- Uses more land for crops and grazing, leading to the destruction or degradation of native ecosystems, particularly forests and grasslands.
- Overtaxes marine and other aquatic ecosystems.
- Uses more water, petroleum, and capital as inputs.
- Pollutes both groundwater and surface water, leading to a variety of ecological and human health problems.
- Uses more pesticides.
- Creates major waste disposal problems.
- Plays a major role in global warming.
- Has locally undesirable side effects, such as odor and insects near animal production facilities.
- Provides a breeding ground for human pathogens and accelerates the evolution of antibiotic-resistant microbes.

The variety of impacts may make it difficult to appreciate the importance of their total magnitude. Negative consequences of our actions are often presented as quite specific: printing a document from your computer contributes to deforestation, moving to a new suburb con-

tributes to loss of wildlife habitat, and spraying pesticides on the lawn pollutes rivers. But animal agriculture does all of these—and to a much greater extent—and more.

For a variety of ethical reasons, many concerned consumers avoid some products (beef because of the impacts of grazing on habitats; certain fish because they are endangered; pork and eggs because of the particularly nasty treatment of animals in their production), but remain unaware of the impacts of other animal foods. To fully understand the breadth and magnitude of the impacts, we must consider each production method and its particular impacts.

Summary of the Scientific Literature

Unfortunately, there is little in the way of accurate, relatively unbiased, big-picture presentation of information on vegetarianism and the environment. Most of the environmental impacts have been closely studied, but they are largely treated as unrelated problems. This lack of a comprehensive summary is not terribly surprising, given how complicated even one of the previously mentioned impacts is. Listing the environmental impacts of animal agriculture (and thus the environmental benefits of avoiding animal foods) is relatively straightforward, and many such lists are available. Quantifying those impacts is considerably more difficult, and to our knowledge no one has come close to providing a comprehensive answer to the pertinent question: How much more damage to the environment does someone eating a Western meat-centered diet do compared to someone eating a Western vegetarian diet?

The fierce politics surrounding agriculture, ecology, and public health combine with those surrounding dietary choice, further challenging readers who seek honest reporting. As with the health impacts of a vegetarian diet, the environmental impacts of Western animal agriculture generate a wide collection of propaganda, half-truths, and out-and-out lies by both the advocates of animal agriculture as currently practiced and the advocates of vegetarianism. Unfortunately, unlike information about nutrition, for which there are some balanced, authoritative, comprehensive sources, information about environmental impacts is spotty and almost impossible to divorce from politics. This is particularly true for the effects of growing feed crops (probably the biggest environmental impact of modern Western animal agriculture); other environmental impacts are better documented.

Although there have been a few attempts at serious research to provide a holistic view of the environmental impacts of animal agriculture, the most widely read summaries tend to be overstated and based on a Malthusian premise (the notion that we will shortly be exhausting our resources and suffer a cataclysm, which has repeatedly been proved inaccurate and ignores certain fundamentals of economics), or have been outright inaccurate. The former category includes the widely cited works of Pimentel (e.g., Pimentel & Pimentel, 1996) and the World Watch Institute (e.g., Brown, Flavin, & French, 1998), and some popular books on vegetarianism (e.g., Marcus, 1997). The latter includes Robbins's best-selling book on vegetarianism (1987). This is most unfortunate, because the unvarnished truth about the environmental impacts of animal agriculture is quite impressive, but is much less likely to be believed when it is bundled with claims that can easily be shown to be false or speculative.

A great deal of information is available from the U.S. Department of Agriculture (USDA), particularly the Economic Research Service (see the USDA and ERS websites), and from publications in the academic literature on agriculture and agricultural economics. Unfortunately, that literature is not terribly accessible to the average reader. As difficult as it is for laypersons to correctly interpret daily newspaper articles drawn from the health science literature, the agricultural literature may be more difficult still, as most of it is very specific and oriented toward professionals in the field. Moreover, the USDA and state agriculture departments, their counterparts in most other countries, and most professors at schools of agriculture see their primary mission as supporting (or even promoting) the existing agriculture industries. So, even though their raw data are generally reliable, their focus and conclusions tend to play down the huge environmental impacts. Perhaps the closest thing to an exception is the *Generic Environmental Impact Statement on Animal Agriculture* (Johnson, 2001) carried out by the state of Minnesota, which contains chapters on various topics written by professors at the University of Minnesota in 2000 and 2001 (including the first author of this chapter). This provides a fairly comprehensive summary of various impacts (though the emphasis is on feedlots), but some reading between the lines of the pro-industry bias is still required.

Mainstream environmental groups—not biased toward the food industry, though also not inclined to overstate the benefits of going vegetarian—offer good, readable summaries on some issues, particularly effluent from feedlots and the resulting water and air pollution (Sierra Club, 1999; Hopper, 2002; Marks, 2001). Unfortunately, environmental groups have considerably less to say about cropland use and other impacts of animal agriculture.

Those wanting more information about any specific topic—land use, ecosystem degradation, environmental health, and so on—can find an extensive scientific literature. Most of it, however, has a narrow focus on particular technical goals for reducing environmental impacts, and says nothing about the big picture. Moreover, the literature that explores how animal agriculture could be made cleaner seldom acknowledges the option of simply reducing consumption, and thus does not present estimates of the benefits of going vegetarian; it is usually necessary to extract numbers from the literature and do additional calculations.

Impacts of Intensive Farming Operations

Intensive farming operations, called *concentrated animal feeding operations* (CAFOs) by those who want to avoid the more common term *feedlot*, create environmental impacts through both inputs and outputs. The latter are easier to study and appreciate (millions of tons of pig manure make a potent argument), though the former deserve more attention.

Land, Water, and Energy Use

The biggest environmental problem with using animals to produce food on a large scale is that it is not very efficient. Even with intensive production methods, where animals are confined, bred, and drugged to make production more efficient, we still lose the vast majority of the inputs. When you look at most farmland, you see plants growing, and probably think of plant-food production. However, a huge proportion of those plants represent feed for livestock rather than people; in the United States, up to 10 times as much corn (and more than twice as much of all grains and beans combined) is used in intensive animal agriculture as is eaten by people. (These are the authors' estimates based on USDA data [Baker, Chambers, & Allen, 2004]. These numbers are necessarily fuzzy due to ambiguities about how to count exports, highly processed food ingredients such as corn sugars, uses where the mass of the plants is divided between sectors, and other uses that do

not fall clearly into the category of either feed or human food.) When you look out across agricultural land, though, you should not think "cornfield"; instead, think "hog field" (or "chicken field," etc.), because that is what is being produced more often than not. The use of so much cropland for feedlot animals causes the loss of native habitats, soil erosion, reductions in biodiversity, and the loss of recreational land and waterways. Crop production also consumes irrigation water, energy, and petrochemical fertilizers, and produces runoff that pollutes surface water.

It is difficult to summarize the total environmental impact of feed crops, even when one adds up the impacts of inputs, land use, and effluent. But because crops produced for human consumption have similar impacts, it is easier, and probably more enlightening, to estimate how much *more* impact animal foods have than direct human consumption of the plant foods. Over the last few decades, studies have typically estimated that animal foods require three to ten times as much crop production as an equivalent amount of plant food. For example, Church's 1991 analysis estimated it takes seven pounds of corn and soy to produce one pound of pork. More recent summaries usually cite lower ratios, reflecting a trend toward technology that provides greater efficiency.

The estimate of feed conversion efficiency that appears to be most frequently used at the time of this writing is a ratio of 1.4 to 1 (originally estimated by the industry group, Council for Agricultural Science and Technology [CAST]). This number is a misleading underestimate, but its repetition by industry apologists makes it a good starting point, and it can be corrected for obvious flaws to provide a fairly convincing estimate (though it is worth noting that even if the number is completely accurate, it still represents a substantially greater impact of animal foods compared to plant foods).

First, the ratio is expressed in terms of protein content of the plant and animal foods. However, because animal flesh, eggs, and milk contain a higher portion of total energy (calories), in the form of protein, than do the plants that are fed to them (typically several times as much), the ratio of plant-food energy (not to mention micronutrients) to animal-food energy is larger. (As an aside, the habit of measuring the total quantity of food in terms of protein is difficult to explain, given that no modern society has ever had foodways that were protein constrained. For all practical purposes, everyone who is not starving gets plenty of protein, so total food energy (calories) is the proper measure of quantity. Whatever the origin of the protein fixation, the incentives for animal food industries (with their substantial influence over government and other organizations that deal with nutrition) to perpetuate the myth of protein supremacy are obvious.

Second, plants grown for animal feed are optimized for the animals, not people, so it is disingenuous to simply measure how much human food could be produced from the same plants. The right measure is how much human staple food could be produced by the same quantity of land, water, petroleum, and other inputs.

Third, the ratio is based on global production of all animal foods, and includes huge numbers of grazing ruminants in the developed and developing world. These animals consume wild-growing plants of almost no food value to humans, and so have little relevance to the efficiency of feeding operations. Averaging them in is like trying to claim that there is practically no pollution from oil leaks by calculating the average amount spilled by all businesses rather than by oil companies. The environmental impacts from grazing are quite different, though no less substantial, and are discussed later in this chapter. Correcting for these factors (particularly the first and last) yields an estimate in the range of 5 to 1.

Other methods for calculating this ratio based on other sources—all of which will be inexact due to ambiguity about what to count and imperfect data—yield results in the same range. Some results are as low as about 3 to 1, but no realistic estimate comes out much lower (especially if we avoid averaging intensive animal production with grazing).

It is worth remembering that even this level of efficiency, particularly the "improvements" made over the past two decades, comes at the cost of treating animals like machines, killing them as soon as their maximum growth (or high-volume egg laying or lactation) ends, and doing nothing to keep them comfortable, let alone happy, unless doing so also increases feed conversion rates. Treating the animals better (as most people would demand if they knew about the conditions the animals suffer) while still trying to produce such huge quantities of animal food would further decrease efficiency and thus increase the environmental impacts.

The use of land to grow feed crops means that it is not available for other uses, including natural habitat. It is difficult to quantify exactly how much habitat loss should be blamed on particular agricultural practices. Roughly speaking, of course, if a production process requires five times as much crop production, it uses five times as much cropland. It is extremely difficult, however, to estimate how much of the extra production comes in the form of more intensive growing methods (using more petrochemicals and water on the same land), and how much comes from leaving less land for other uses. It is also extremely difficult to estimate how much loss of unmanaged land (including deforestation, discussed more in relation to grazing, later in this chapter) should be attributed to Western tastes for meat (as opposed to such things as impoverished people trying to eke out a living). Nonetheless, animal agriculture clearly plays a huge role in removing land from natural uses, and deserves much of the blame for habitat and ecosystem destruction that is typically assigned to logging, industrial activity, and suburban sprawl.

In fairness, it should be noted that some animals can eat waste plant matter (for example, stalks left over from plant-food production) and other food that people cannot or will not consume. Thus, so long as animals were fed mostly such waste, and were not so concentrated as to create a waste disposal or overgrazing problem, animal foods could be produced in environmentally friendly ways. This observation is relevant to small farms, particularly in the developing world, but has little relevance to the large industrial food production operations that are the sources of almost all animal foods in North America and most of the developed world. Environmentally friendly animal food production methods probably could not supply the large quantity of animal foods currently consumed in the developed world and, in any case, are not how production is carried out. (They are, however, frequently invoked by those who would distract us from the huge environmental impacts and animal suffering resulting from large-scale animal food production, in an often-successful attempt to pretend that their animal factories are just large small farms.)

Beyond the ratio of crops to animal food, a few estimates of the resource consumption impacts of intensive agriculture are telling. American beef production, despite taking advantage of nonirrigated plants on grazing land, consumes more than 400 gallons of piped water per pound of beef produced. (This estimate is from an industry-sponsored study from more than a decade ago [Beckett & Oltjen, 1995],

which was done in response to the clearly exaggerated numbers often quoted by some vegetarian advocates. Though the analysis is necessarily imperfect, it appears to be basically valid and is clearly a much better estimate than the numbers five or ten times as high that are occasionally found in some pro-vegetarian literature. As a higher portion of cattle weight gain takes place in feedlots rather than grazing land, the average water consumption will increase, though 400–500 gallons per pound probably remains a good estimate.)

Other animal food production uses less water, but still many times as much as production of staple plant foods (grains and beans), and more than growing most fruits and vegetables. In most western states, livestock agriculture consumes one-third of all irrigation water (roughly five times as much as is consumed by all household uses combined); this includes areas using water from dwindling aquifers.

Estimating total petrochemical use (mainly fertilizer and energy) is quite difficult, but most such usage is from the growing and processing of feed crops. Relatively little energy is used for the animals themselves, thanks to the horrid efficiencies of factory farms. Thus, the ratio of petrochemical use by animal foods versus plant foods can be estimated as a bit more than the feed conversion ratio.

Aquaculture as Intensive Farming

Many people think of fish and other seafood as a benign alternative to terrestrial animal food, and many people who are otherwise vegetarian continue to eat seafood. To the extent that people are aware of environmental problems, overharvesting of wild species (discussed later) is their main concern. Thus, it is worth emphasizing two things at the start of any discussion of the environmental impacts of eating seafood.

First, consuming seafood is at least as environmentally unfriendly as consuming land animals, and arguably worse for many types of seafood. Second, many forms of aquaculture (fish farming) that produce seafood for Western consumers are extremely harmful to natural environments, rather than the benign solution to overharvesting of natural populations that they are often perceived as being. A substantial fraction of seafood found in Western markets is produced by intensive forms of aquaculture, which place demands on the environment similar to those of raising land animals in feedlots. An excellent review of the environmental impacts of aquaculture is provided by Naylor et al. (2000), and much of the information here was obtained from that source and the references contained in it. A less technical overview of the same topic is provided by Naylor et al. (2001), obtainable from the Ecological Society of America.

Just as most of the environmental impacts of feedlots come from the growing of feed crops, production of the feed needed for aquaculture causes tremendous environmental harm. Fish and shrimp raised intensively are fed artificial foods because they live at densities that are too high to be supported by the natural foods present in their ponds or holding tanks. The composition of this feed depends on the species being reared, but carnivorous species, such as salmon, trout, marine shrimp, and many marine fish, are fed a diet containing 30%-70% fish protein and fish oil (Naylor et al., 2000). The aquaculture industry uses approximately 10 million metric tons of fish each year (more than 10% of the total worldwide catch of 89-96 million metric tons) to produce the food eaten by farmed species, with 2.5 to 5 kg of wild-caught fish typically being needed to produce 1 kg of farmed carnivorous fish or shrimp (Naylor et al., 2000; Food and Agriculture Department, 2002; Weber, 2003). As the aquaculture industry

expands, in response to increasing demand and the collapse of natural marine fisheries, the harvesting of wild fish (typically small pelagic [open-ocean living] species like sardines and anchovies that have low commercial value in the West) to produce fish meal is likely to further undermine marine ecosystems and affect the abundance and distribution of large, predatory fish, marine mammals, and sea birds. Such effects have already been documented in Norway and Peru (see references in Naylor et al., 2000). In addition, the fish ground up into fish meal to provide Western consumers with cheap salmon and shrimp are often an important food source for coastal, subsistence communities in the developing world (see references in Naylor et al., 2000).

In some parts of the world, aquaculture is also responsible for widespread destruction of native ecosystems. For example, a large fraction (the actual number is very hard to determine, but information in Cascorbi [2004] suggests that it is likely to be at least 20%-30%, and possibly much more) of the shrimp purchased in the United States is supplied by fish farms in southeast Asia, where shrimp and milkfish farming is responsible for the destruction of mangrove forests and other coastal ecosystems to provide land for holding ponds. Mangrove forests act as nurseries for juvenile coral reef fish (Mumby et al., 2004), are essential habitat for some species, and protect coral reefs and seagrass beds from damage due to sediment runoff and excessive nutrient input from nearby agricultural land. They also help to protect coastal environments generally from flooding and wind damage caused by storms, hurricanes, and typhoons (Naylor et al., 2000). Aquaculture ponds are also created by flooding coastal rice fields with salt water, thereby permanently damaging the soil, reducing the amount of land available for rice production, and causing violent conflict between local farmers and members of the aquaculture industry (McQuaid, 1996; Goldenberg, 1997; Primavera, 1997; Cooley, 1999). Moreover, because shrimp are frequently raised at extremely high densities, diseases are a constant threat (despite high input of antibiotics), and most farms have to be abandoned after only a few years, necessitating further environmental destruction as new operations are set up elsewhere.

In theory, and to some extent in practice, raising herbivorous or omnivorous species, such as tilapia, carp, and catfish, is much less harmful to the marine environment, because the diets of these fish consist mostly of soybean, cottonseed, and peanut meal, and—for small-scale operations (family farm ponds, which exist mostly in east Asia)—of manure and other nonhuman-food sources. However, in actual operation, fish meal and fish oil constitute 10%–15% of the diet even for these species, and farmers often use more fish meal than is necessary, either because they imperfectly understand the dietary needs of their stock or as a deliberate strategy to increase weight gain (Naylor et al., 2000). Conversion inefficiencies mean that approximately 2 kilograms of feed are needed to produce 1 kilogram of these types of fish (Naylor et al., 2000).

The aquaculture industry also contributes to the spread of fish diseases to new parts of the world when farmed species are raised away from their natural habitats or when they are raised at such high densities in their natural habitats that diseases develop into epidemics that spread out of control. Such effects have been documented in Atlantic salmon populations in Europe and shrimp populations in Texas (see references in Naylor et al., 2000). (The spread of exotic diseases from imported food species to native populations also occurs with terrestrial animals, but on land the damage has pretty much been done, and few native populations exist that have not already survived the impacts of exotic imports.)

Scientists have also become increasingly concerned by what might be called genetic pollution: the harm done to natural populations when farmed species escape and interbreed with wild relatives. In Atlantic salmon, farmed fish have been bred to have a high growth rate for commercial reasons, but a side effect of this artificial selection is that their survival rate when they escape is only 2% that of wild individuals. Hybrids between wild and farmed individuals have much lower embryonic survival, adult longevity, and adult return rates to the spawning grounds. The number of escapes each year may approach 2 million, so it is feared that the Atlantic salmon, already endangered by pollution and overfishing, may be driven extinct by the high mortality rates of farmed-wild hybrids (McGinnity et al., 2003).

Pollution from Effluent

Although both plant and animal agriculture pollute the environment, animal production is particularly harmful because of the amount of cropland needed to produce animal feed and because of the large amounts of manure produced on feedlots, particularly hog farms and chicken batteries. Water draining from croplands typically contains high concentrations of fertilizer (mostly compounds of nitrogen and phosphorus), and when this runoff reaches natural water bodies it encourages the excessive growth of algae and other aquatic plants. When these die and decompose, oxygen levels in the water drop, jeopardizing the health of both freshwater and marine ecosystems. For example, the enormous "dead zone" that develops in the Gulf of Mexico each year is recognized as being caused by excessive nitrogen input from agricultural land in the Mississippi drainage, and it should be kept in mind that a large portion of crop fields upstream are dedicated to animal feed, not human plant foods. Howarth et al. (2000) provide an excellent summary of the effects of nutrient pollution on coastal ecosystems. High levels of nitrogen compounds in drinking water are an environmental health problem and can be a serious threat to infants (Nowlin, 1997; Webb & Archer, 1994). For example, more than 15% of rural wells in the U.S. Midwest exceed the U.S. drinking water standard for nitrate contamination (Jackson, 1998). Similarly, increased crop production increases pesticide runoff and drinking water pollution. As an example of all this, "hog fields" (that is, corn crops) consume about 40% of the country's nitrogen fertilizer (Hallberg, 1989)—much of which damages the unmanaged ecosystems it finds its way into (Socolow, 1999)—along with about half the herbicides and insecticides applied to all crops (Conservation Foundation, 1986).

Manure and other waste from animal-processing facilities are additional major sources of water pollution. They also create terrible local environmental problems, such as insect densities normally seen only in horror movies, and 150 volatile compounds that produce odors and potentially hazardous gases (Thomas, 1996). Many large feedlots produce waste that is equivalent to the sewage from a small or even medium-sized city, but they lack the sewage treatment that such a city would have. Instead, much of this manure is poured into lagoons, where it leaches into the groundwater or spills into surface water (Harkin, 1997).

Relative to the inputs of intensive animal agriculture (land, water, and energy uses), which account for most of its environmental impacts, a great deal has been written in the environmental and popular press about its unwanted outputs. This can be explained by a combination of politics—everyone hates manure runoff, but feedcrop farming is considered a local economic benefit and a way to preserve the farming lifestyle (a perception that is largely incorrect in the era of industrial agriculture, but this topic is beyond the present scope)—and the relative ease of measuring the effluent and communicating its implications. Thus, readers seeking more details about this impact will have no difficulty finding information.

Manure, in its role as fertilizer, is typically portrayed as a valuable renewable resource. Such a claim is disingenuous, however, as the net loss in nutrients belies the claim of renewability. Even if all manure were applied as fertilizer (rather than outgassing, leaching from holding facilities, or being otherwise disposed of), food for feeding an animal would still use more fertilizer than is produced by the animal. At best, we can call manure a useful byproduct that makes an inefficient system slightly less inefficient. The net loss is exacerbated because the nutrients in manure are a poor match for what crops need (Eng, 1996), and it is overapplied in some areas to reduce transport costs (Cummings, 1998). Additionally, "natural" does not mean clean. Manure fertilizer concentrates heavy metals and other elements in the land, particularly phosphorus, sodium, potassium, copper, and zinc (Thu, 1996).

The impact of animal agriculture on our air is subtler than its effects on land and water, but is nonetheless significant. Methane production by livestock (ruminants create a huge amount of methane when they digest the cellulose in their forage) and animal waste (particularly storage lagoons) is a major contribution to greenhouse gas production (Energy Information Administration, 2003). The contribution of the world's animal agriculture to global warming is roughly the same as all U.S. fossil fuel use, which most people think of as the worst offender. Much, and sometimes most, of the nitrogen in storage lagoons changes from liquid to ammonia gas and escapes into the atmosphere (Hoag, Roka, & Zering, 1993; Midwest Plan Service, 1985). The gaseous ammonia is stripped from the atmosphere by rain, and the resulting acid deposition (acid rain) can substantially damage natural habitats. Once again, animal agriculture contributes to environmental injuries that are usually blamed entirely on other dirty industries.

Many forms of intensive aquaculture have polluting effects similar to those of intensive animal agriculture. Effluent from these operations contains high concentrations of uneaten food, fish feces and urine, fish scales and slime, sediments, and antibiotics needed to control disease spread, all of which are typically released into nearby aquatic ecosystems. Large quantities of food and feces accumulating around fish holding pens in coastal waters can interfere with the natural processes of nutrient recycling, and nitrogenous waste products can increase to such concentrations that they are toxic to marine organisms, including the fish and shrimp being farmed. Not surprisingly, such pollution is particularly severe in regions where the aquaculture industry is widespread, and also where the effluent discharges into shallow or enclosed water bodies. Naylor et al. (2000) provide numerous references on all these effects.

Foodborne Illness and Chemical Contamination of Foods

In addition to contributing to heart disease and other chronic ailments (as detailed in other chapters of this book), animal foods are responsible for a large portion of human infectious disease. Intensive agriculture contributes to foodborne disease because of the huge pathogen load in feces (whether stored in lagoons or spread as fertilizer) and in large numbers of animals living in close quarters. Meat and eggs provide fertile media for growing pathogens, which is especially problematic when feces come into contact with carcasses, as they do in high-volume slaughter operations. Because

the pathogens generated by animal food production spread to water supplies and other foods (including vegetarian foods), this is an environmental health problem rather than just a personal matter such as nutrition.

Although the proximate source of a foodborne illness case or outbreak is a plant food roughly as often as it is an animal food (meaning that the risk of foodborne disease is probably not substantially different for vegetarians and nonvegetarians), the pathogens in plant food often come from animal agriculture or cross-contamination from animal food. Plant foods are contaminated by manure, poor human hygiene, and sometimes wildlife, as well as being cross-contaminated by infected animal foods in restaurants and other facilities that handle both. Moreover, and unfortunately for the vegetarian, the animal foods are often then well-cooked, killing the pathogens, while the contaminated plant foods are not. For example, although chicken and eggs have a very high rate of contamination, they are generally cooked thoroughly, so it is plant foods like alfalfa sprouts (frequently contaminated by manure as seeds and always served raw) that food safety experts most often recommend that people avoid entirely. It is probably the case that keeping your kitchen free of meat and eggs (as opposed to not eating them, per se) will dramatically reduce your risk of foodborne disease.

Antibiotics are used extensively in animal agriculture. Primarily, they are fed to healthy animals as a growth promoter rather than as medicine, because (for reasons not fully understood) they make the animals gain weight faster and with a higher feed-conversion ratio. Such use has long been suspected to lead to human pathogens with antibiotic resistance, and for several specific antibiotic-pathogen combinations the evidence for the connection is fairly conclusive. The more an antibiotic is used (for whatever purpose), the more pathogens evolve to be resistant to it. This is particularly true for subtherapeutic doses like the feed supplements, which allow colonies of pathogens to survive exposure while favoring the evolution of resistant strains. When huge quantities of antibiotics are used to promote livestock growth (more than half of the total antibiotic use in the United States is for this purpose), they work less well for curing diseases in humans or other animals. Infections that resist antibiotics that previously could cure them are now extremely common and sometimes deadly.

With swine flu getting so much press in the 1970s and bird flu generating attention at the time of this writing, there is a clear message that intensive animal agriculture contributes to human diseases. Unfortunately, the labeling of these two particular strains obscures the fact that most influenza strains and some other human diseases incubate in agricultural animals. Without large-scale animal agriculture, these diseases—which kill tens of thousands of Americans in a typical year and millions worldwide when there is a particularly bad outbreak—would be dramatically reduced. Other modern scourges have been traced to the harvesting of animals for food and the transmission of infectious agents from them to humans (e.g., SARS apparently resulted from the harvesting and eating of wild species in China, specifically the raccoon-like animal called the civet cat; HIV originated from a simian (monkey) virus and most likely was transmitted to humans through the harvesting of African primates for food sometime in the 20th century).

Manure runoff, in addition to its ecological impacts, results in contamination of both surface water and groundwater by organisms that cause human disease (Bitton & Harvey, 1992). Contamination risks include the emergence of highly toxic algae like the dinoflagellate *Pfiesteria piseida*, as well as such less exotic scourges as coliform bacteria, *Cryptosporidium*, and *Giardia*.

Chemical (nonbiological) contamination presents a different food safety issue. Other than occasional strange cases, the biggest concern is heavy metal bioaccumulation (where chemicals from an animal's many meals are concentrated in its flesh), particularly mercury contamination of certain fish (which, needless to say, should be avoided for health reasons). Animals also bioaccumulate (and thus concentrate in their flesh or milk) other potentially harmful chemicals that naturally occur in plants or are introduced as agricultural chemicals or industrial pollutants (e.g., dioxins and PCBs). However, animals also metabolize some naturally occurring or introduced chemicals in their feed, reducing exposure compared to eating plant foods, so there is a tradeoff.

Of the exposures unique to animal foods, the most talked about is bovine spongiform encephalopathy (BSE or mad cow disease), which vegetarians avoid by not eating products from cows and certain other animals. However, we know little about that disease and so cannot be sure how much risk reduction results from eating vegetarian. (At the extreme, it is theoretically possible that some people are genetically predisposed to catch the disease from just a few molecules of the protein that apparently causes it, so even dedicated vegans may be as much at risk as other people, since complete avoidance of all animal food products is virtually impossible.) Moreover, it is not clear how widespread the human manifestation of the disease is or could be. It has affected a nontrivial number of people in the United Kingdom, though far fewer than the alarmists (including certain vegetarian advocates) were suggesting 5 or 10 years ago.

Hormones that are fed to livestock can be found in animal foods to some extent. A tiny fraction of these hormones are not fully digested in the human stomach and enter the bloodstream of the people who eat those foods. However, the health implications (if any) of this are poorly understood. The exogenous hormones fed to agricultural animals are not much different from hormones that the animals produce themselves, and which therefore are found naturally in animal foods. Although these hormones have not been definitively linked to human disease, they are suspected of not being entirely harmless in some cases.

Unlike the nutritional implications of dietary choice, these health impacts have implications for everyone, making them environmental and ethical concerns rather than just personal ones. Vegetarians cannot avoid these health risks, but choosing a vegetarian diet contributes to reducing them. The effect is not as simple and direct as other benefits: for example, one chicken not eaten is a chicken that never suffers confinement, does not consume grain, and does not produce manure, but the spread of an infectious disease is rarely affected by small reductions in animal density. A population of 99,999 chickens is just as likely to perpetuate an epidemic as a population of 100,000. In addition, a Western vegetarian is unlikely to reduce animal agriculture in Asia (where most of the global infectious agents incubate) or stop the harvesting of infected game. However, there is still a positive contribution from avoiding animal foods.

Impacts of Grazing

Although grazing animals are reared at much lower densities than occurs in intensive feeding operations, and although both feed inputs and polluting outputs are lower, grazing can have substantial environmental impacts. These effects depend on the type of land used and the densities at which the grazing animals are raised. In the United States, cattle for beef production are grazed over large areas of the arid

Western plains (areas commonly known as *rangelands*) and for the dairy industry in the Northeast and parts of the northern Midwest. With 55% of the total land area of the United States classified as rangeland, forage land, or pasture (USDA Agricultural Research Service, 2003), and 85% of the 307 million acres of federal land in the West being grazed by domestic livestock for at least part of the year (CAST, 1996), the potential impact of grazing practices on the landscape of this country is enormous.

In the West, grazing occurs mostly on grasslands and shrublands that form the natural ecological communities in this part of the country. Indeed, some make the case that cattle are now important substitutes for the large herds of native herbivores (bison, elk, pronghorn, and mule deer) that were once an integral component of these ecosystems. However, this argument falls apart if cattle are raised at such high densities that they overgraze the native plant communities, damage the soil, and trample riparian (streamside) and other wetland habitat to obtain drinking water. This argument also ignores a sad part of the environmental legacy of animal agriculture: the fact that the destruction of North America's native grazing mammal populations was largely due to the fencing of their rangelands for ranching in the 19th century. It is generally agreed that overgrazing caused substantial damage to Western rangelands in the late 19th century (USDA Natural Resources Conservation Service, 1996; CAST, 1996), but their current state of health is a matter of debate. Perhaps not surprisingly, organizations with links to the cattle-ranching industry have tended to see rangelands as being in good health. For example, in 1996 the Council for Agricultural Science and Technology claimed that "United States rangelands, with some exceptions, are now in their best condition this century" (CAST, 1996). In contrast, some conservation organizations see many of these regions as badly overgrazed, with major reform of grazing practices being necessary to restore them to their former health (Armour, Duff, & Elmore, 1991; Wildlife Society, *Wildlife Policy Statement*; Sierra Club, *Federal Public Lands*).

The past few years have seen something of a convergence of perspectives. Agricultural scientists (if not yet ranchers themselves) have increasingly recognized that management of grazing lands must take into account the impact of livestock on soil and water quality, native biodiversity, invasive weeds, and riparian and wetland communities (CAST, 2002), and some conservation organizations such as the Nature Conservancy are starting to see cattle grazing as an important habitat management tool. Not surprisingly, none of these groups is considering the question from a vegetarian perspective: What would happen if there were no cattle ranching for food production? Undoubtedly, if cattle were managed solely as bison substitutes, to maintain and restore native ecosystems, grazing practices would differ substantially from what they are today, though there seems little reason even to consider the implications of such a radical change in the short run.

Unlike beef cattle in the West, dairy cattle that graze in the Northeastern states and upper Midwest are not living within natural grassland communities, but on pastures created by clearing of native deciduous woodland. Thus, from an ecological perspective, the question is not whether native ecosystems are being damaged by overgrazing, but whether it would be beneficial to abandon these pasturelands and allow woodlands to replace them once again. Before the start of European settlement in 1620, the eastern United States was covered by approximately 2.5 million square kilometers of forest. By 1872, coverage had been reduced by around 50%, and most of the forest that remained had been cut at some time in the past. Since then,

at least half the lost forest has returned, so that today coverage is about 75% of that during presettlement times (Pimm, 2001). This is an average, of course: Forests are still largely absent from most agriculturally productive lowlands, coverage varies from state to state, and in many regions forest habitat is highly fragmented. Allowing dairy pastures to revert to forest could, by increasing total forest area and reducing fragmentation, contribute substantially to the biodiversity and the population densities of many plants and animals native to the eastern United States.

There is also a huge amount of cattle grazing throughout the rest of the world, both for local consumption and for export to the United States and other countries. Imports to the United States (mostly for processing as ground beef) have risen steadily since 1997 and from 2000–2003 exceeded 3,000 million pounds per year (Economic Research Service). Most of this meat is obtained from grass-fed (i.e., rangeland and pasture) cattle, so the grazing practices in countries that export beef to the United States should be an important issue for U.S. consumers concerned about the environment. Taking 2002 as a typical year (trade in 2003 was distorted by the BSE scare in Canada), Australia and Canada each contributed about 35% to total beef imports, followed by New Zealand (19%), and Brazil (6%), with Central America, Argentina, and Uruguay making up the final 5%. That same year, the United States imported around 1.7 million live cattle from Canada (mainly for slaughter) and another 800,000 from Mexico (mainly for fattening on U.S. feedlots before slaughter) (Economic Research Service).

Assessing the total ecological impact of U.S. beef and cattle imports is obviously extremely complicated, depending as it does on the types of land being grazed and the grazing practices employed by numerous countries. However, the following generalizations can be made.

1. In countries where cattle are raised on native grasslands (principally Canada, Australia, Argentina, and Uruguay, but also parts of New Zealand, Brazil, and Mexico), the same considerations as those discussed for U.S. rangelands apply (i.e., are grazing densities so high as to disrupt normal ecosystem functioning and cause declining biodiversity in natural or semi-natural dryland habitats?). Given that overgrazing has degraded around 35 million square km of the Earth's 46 million square km of dry land (Pimm, 2001), the answer to this question for many regions is almost certainly yes.

2. In countries where cattle are raised on pastures that were once forest (most of Central America and parts of New Zealand, Brazil, and Mexico), we need to consider the potential advantages of removing cattle and allowing these pastures to revert to native forests. Even more so than for dairy pasture in the United States, these advantages are likely to be substantial. They encompass not only the restoration and maintenance of native biodiversity, but also the provision of important ecosystem functions such as nutrient and soil retention and, in some parts of the world such as Central America, prevention of the flooding and landslides that kill many people and cause tremendous damage to human infrastructure.

3. It is potentially very misleading to use the volume of beef exports to the United States as an index of the amount of environmental damage done by cattle ranching in individual countries. For example, although imports from Brazil are only one-sixth of those from Canada or Australia, government-subsidized cattle ranching in Brazil has been a major factor driving Am-azonian deforestation (Moran et al., 1994). Given the enormous biodiversity of the Amazon rainforest, habitat destruction here is likely to cause far more species extinctions than overgrazing in Canada or Australia. An even more extreme example (at least to date) is Costa Rica, a tiny Central American country that contributes an equally tiny amount to total U.S. beef imports. Beef cattle production in Costa Rica accelerated rapidly in the 1960s, and in the 1980s Costa Rica ranked in the top 10 countries worldwide in terms of percentage loss of its native forests. By 1983, the country had lost more than 80% of its forest cover, with most of the deforestation being driven by the demand for cattle pasture, and most of the meat produced being exported to the United States to make ground beef and pet food (Boucher et al., 1983; Hartshorn, 1992).

In summary, on a worldwide scale, overgrazing damages soil systems by compaction, erosion, and loss of nutrients, and native plant communities have become substantially degraded both by the direct effects of grazers and by the invasion of nonnative weed species in disturbed habitats. In some parts of the globe, severe overgrazing has turned potentially productive ecosystems into deserts. In other regions, grazing lands have been created by the destruction of large tracts of native forest. Increased water runoff and erosion from damaged lands can cause nutrient and sediment pollution of lakes, rivers, and streams, and high concentrations of cattle around water sources can degrade riparian ecosystems by damaging the vegetation, trampling and eroding streambeds, and destroying fish habitats. A highly readable account of many of these impacts can be found in Pimm (2001).

Impacts of Harvesting

Fishing

Industrial-scale fishing is increasingly recognized as a highly destructive way of providing food. There is a large and increasing volume of literature on the environmental impacts of the global fishing industry, including an excellent summary by Pauly et al. (2002). Other good, readable accounts of some of these impacts have been written by Pauly et al. (2000) and Hutchings and Reynolds (2004). The website of the Monterey Bay Aquarium provides detailed analyses of the environmental impacts of harvesting and fish farming for many individual species of seafood.

Although the oceans were once thought to contain a nearly inexhaustible supply of fish, the increasing technological sophistication of industrial fishing has repeatedly caused the serious depletion of exploited populations, sometimes driving them to the point of regional or global extinction (Cook, Sinclair, & Stefánsson, 1997; Pitcher, 1998; Casey & Myers, 1998; Hutchings, 2000). These declines have been particularly severe for the large predatory fish preferred by Western consumers, including bottom-dwelling species, such as codfishes and flatfishes, on coastal shelves; and pelagic species, such as tuna and swordfish, in the open ocean. In 13 major ecological regions throughout the globe, industrial fishing has caused the biomass of these species to decline by an average of 80% within 15 years of the start of harvesting, and it has been estimated that 90% of the world's large predatory fish have been lost since preindustrial times (Myers & Worm, 2003). Worldwide fish catch has been declining by about 0.7 million metric tons per year since the late 1980s (Pauly et al., 2002); the trend was revealed only after it was discovered that the People's Republic of China had been systemat-

ically overreporting its catches (Watson & Pauly, 2001). The vast majority of currently harvested populations are either being fully exploited or overexploited (FAO Fisheries Department, 2002). More worrying still is the fact that most fish populations seem to recover very slowly after overexploitation (Hutchings, 2000); some species may be in terminal decline (Pitcher, 1998; Casey & Myers, 1998). When preferred species have been fished to commercial extinction, other species, typically those at a lower trophic level, then start to be exploited. This trend, commonly termed "fishing down the food web," can cause catches to increase at first, but eventually they begin to decline again (Pauly et al., 1998). Not only does this practice appear to be an unsustainable way of providing food for people, it may also be undermining global marine ecosystems and changing the structure of their communities in a variety of unpredictable ways (Pauly et al., 2002). Some of these changes, such as periodic blooms of toxic algae, can be harmful both to other marine creatures and to human health (Van Dolah, Roelke, & Greene, 2001).

The harm done by industrial fishing is not restricted to overexploitation of target species alone. Bottom trawling and dredging damage or destroy ocean-floor ecosystems (Norse & Watling, 1999), including only recently discovered cold-water coral reefs (Hall-Spencer, Allain, & Fosså, 2002); undermine coastal food webs by reducing the productivity of bottom-dwelling organisms at basal trophic levels; and even lower juvenile survival rates of the species that are being commercially exploited (see references in Pauly et al., 2002). The wholesale destruction caused by commercial trawling is hidden from view tens or hundreds of meters beneath the ocean surface, but photographs (Schiermeier, 2002) show that it can reasonably be compared to the clear-cutting of forests that promotes widespread public outrage (Watling & Norse, 1998).

Drift-netting, purse-seining, and long-lining all catch and kill many nontarget species, including whales and dolphins, marine turtles, and sea birds. Marine mammals and birds that depend on fish that are overexploited by humans may suffer drastic declines in abundance, or even direct persecution because they are regarded as competitors for harvested species.

Some forms of aquaculture are effectively harvesting systems, because the fish and shrimp that are raised are caught as fry from the wild rather than being bred in captivity. As with other forms of fishing, fry harvesting can result in overexploitation of wild populations and excessive by-catch of unwanted species that are harmed or killed in the process. In the case of giant tiger shrimp, a popular luxury seafood item throughout the United States that is produced by the aquaculture industry of India and Bangladesh, up to 160 unwanted fry of fish and other shrimp are discarded for every tiger shrimp fry that is collected (see references in Naylor et al., 2000).

Other Harvesting

Other harvesting, specifically hunting, contributes a trivial portion of the animal food consumed in the industrialized world, and the environmental impacts are minimal. Indeed, hunting probably has net positive impacts, given that hunters (particularly those who shoot migratory birds) actively advocate for habitat preservation. However, habitats that support deer and game birds are not necessarily fully functioning ecosystems, and may be quite unnatural, so the positive impacts should not be overstated. In particular, efforts to intentionally maintain large deer populations (which are then hunted in the name of population control) do little to improve the ecology or natural resources of environments where the deer live.

Practical Aspects

Most of us are concerned about ecosystem destruction, fuel and water use, pollution, and environmental health. The huge environmental benefits of a vegetarian diet, despite being difficult to quantify, should not be ignored. Avoiding meat consumption has a direct and proportional effect. Every bite of plant food you eat instead of animal food is that much less animal agriculture that is needed. Though we cannot quantify very precisely, there is little doubt that nothing else can reduce your impact so much without dramatically changing your lifestyle. Avoidance of animal food dwarfs the combined benefits of recycling, turning down your thermostat, installing low-flow shower-heads, and keeping your yard natural.

Certain opponents of modern lifestyles and their environmental impacts call for massive changes in how we live, finding little value in small steps toward environmental protection. It is indeed true that virtually no one from the societies that will likely provide most of the readers of this book—middle- and upper-class residents of the United States, Canada, the United Kingdom, and other rich countries—has room to be smug about how lightly they tread on the environment. The fact of the matter is that few of us are willing to live like peasants. For those of us who would like to do what we can, but still live basically as we currently do, there is no better place to start than by reducing our consumption of animal foods.

In theory, animal agriculture need not be so destructive. Small-scale animal operations allow nonintensive grazing and the feeding of silage (the parts of plants not edible by humans) to a few animals, while the manure is applied to the fields to provide needed fertilizer. Small "sustainable agriculture" operations sell meat and other animal products produced in relatively environmentally friendly ways, and represent a partial improvement over conventionally produced animal products. Still, even most sustainable operations use some feed grain (with the resulting feed-conversion inefficiency), and in any case it is not the source of food you find in the grocery store.

However, those motivated to avoid animal foods for reasons other than the environment will find little or no advantage from sustainable operations. The animals in sustainable operations are likely to be treated better (merely by not being in concentrated facilities), but conditions vary (even explicit claims like "free range" often mean a lot less than they imply), and the animals' last minutes of life may or may not be better. Moreover, unlike most consumer goods (including mass-produced food), where another unit will be produced for each unit you buy, the total production of "sustainable" food appears to be substantially constrained by the limited number of people willing to devote their land, labor, and lifestyle to producing it. Thus, unfortunately, when you buy sustainably produced (humanely raised, free-range, etc.) animal foods, you may be encouraging the production of more of the same to some extent, but you are also consuming a limited resource, taking it from another consumer who would have bought it. Simple economics tells us that the marginal consumer you crowd out of the market will buy conventionally produced food instead, and thus the net impact of buying the sustainable animal food product is quite similar to what it would have been if you had bought the conventionally produced product.

Conclusion

Most people's understanding of nutrition falls into a one-food-one-nutrient mythology: vitamin C comes from orange juice; potassium comes from bananas; protein comes from meat (a notion that ignores the ample protein in beans, vegetables, and other plant foods, and is a nontrivial part of the resistance to vegetarianism). Similar misconceptions apply to environmental degradation, where the perception is that forests are destroyed by logging, air is polluted by cars and smokestacks, and water is polluted by petrochemical spills. When something is nonspecific in its effects (e.g., tomatoes are great sources of both vitamin C and potassium; animal agriculture injures land, air, and water in dozens of ways), those effects are typically not recognized. This is even more true when the pathways are complicated (animal agriculture contributes to global warming through waste products, deforestation, and energy use, and damages rivers because of crop farming, manure runoff, and overgrazing) and the exact effects are not well or easily measured. It is little wonder that most people do not realize how dirty animal agriculture is.

A vegetarian diet is not an environmental panacea. All but the most frugal Westerners, even vegetarians, consume a great deal of resources in their foodways. Just as vegetarian and nonvegetarian diets can be more or less healthful, they can be more or less environmentally friendly—and the worst vegetarian choices are clearly worse than the best nonvegetarian choices for both nutrition and the environment (e.g., importing off-season produce uses a lot more resources than raising and butchering your own chickens). As a general rule, though, when you choose plant foods instead of animal foods, you reduce your impact on the environment, typically by half, three-quarters, or more, depending on how you measure it. The total environmental benefit of eating a vegetarian diet (or close to it) rather than a meat-centered diet is likely greater that the sum of every other environmentally friendly action you will take in your life.

Acknowledgment

An earlier version of part of this material, authored by the third and first authors of this chapter, appeared in the *Loma Linda University Nutrition and Health Letter.* See Lees & Phillips, 1999.

References

Armour CL, Duff DA, Elmore W. American Fisheries Society Policy Statement #23: Effects of livestock grazing on riparian stream ecosystems. *Fisheries.* 1991;16(1):7–11.

Baker A, Chambers W, Allen E. *Feed Situation and Outlook Yearbook.* USDA Economic Research Service; Apr 2004. Available at: usda.mannlib.cornell.edu/reports/erssor/field/fds-bby/fds2004.pdf. Accessed March 21, 2005.

Beckett JL, Oltjen JW. Role of ruminant livestock in sustainable agricultural systems. *J Animal Sci.* 1995;74:1406–1409.

Bitton G, Harvey W. Transport of pathogens through soils and aquifers. *J Envir Microbiology.* 1992;5:103–124.

Boucher DH, Hansen M, Risch S, et al. Agriculture. In: Janzen DH, ed. *Costa Rican Natural History.* Chicago, IL: University of Chicago Press; 1983:66–73.

Brown LR, Flavin C, French H. *State of the World 1998.* Washington, DC: Worldwatch Institute; 1998.

Cascorbi A. Seafood report: Shrimp. Vol. 3. Farm-raised shrimp worldwide overview. *Monterey Bay Aquarium Seafood Watch.* 2004. Available at: http://www.mbayaq.org/cr/seafoodwatch.asp. Accessed February 24, 2005.

Casey JM, Myers RA. Near extinction of a large, widely distributed fish. *Science.* 1998;281:690–692.

Church DC. *Livestock Feeds and Feeding.* Englewood Cliffs, NJ: Prentice Hall; 1991.

Conservation Foundation. *Agriculture and the Environment in a Changing World Economy.* Washington, DC: The Conservation Foundation; 1986.

Cook RM, Sinclair A, Stefánsson G. Potential collapse of North Sea cod stocks. *Nature.* 1997;385:521–522.

Cooley DR. Mangroves, aquaculture and coastal communities: Applying cultural models to coastal zone management. *Culture & Agriculture.* 1999;21(2):13–18.

Council for Agricultural Science and Technology. Available at: http://www.cast-science.org. Accessed January 10, 2005.

Council for Agricultural Science and Technology (CAST). *Issue Paper 22: Environmental Impacts of Livestock on U.S. Grazing Lands.* Ames, IA: CAST; 2002.

Council for Agricultural Science and Technology. *Report 129: Grazing on Public Lands.* Ames, IA: CAST; 1996.

Cummings D. Environmental impacts of large animal production. Report for United States Department of Agriculture Center for Emerging Issues; 1998.

Economic Research Service, U.S. Department of Agriculture. Available at: http://ers.usda.gov. Accessed February 15, 2005.

Energy Information Administration, U.S. Department of Energy. Emissions of greenhouse gasses in the United States 2003. Available at: http://www.eia.doe.gov/oiaf/1605/ggrpt/methane.html. Accessed February 15, 2005.

Eng K. Nutrition, manure, environment do not equal a simple equation. *Feedstuffs.* October 21, 1996; 68(44):11–12.

FAO Fisheries Department. *The State of World Fisheries and Aquaculture (SOFIA).* 2002. Available at: http://www.fao.org/sof/sofia/index_en.htm. Accessed March 21, 2005.

Food and Agriculture Department (FAD), United Nations Fisheries Department. The state of world fisheries and aquaculture (SOFIA). Rome; 2002. Available at: http://www.fao.org/sof/sofia/index_en.htm. Accessed January 30, 2005.

Goldenberg S. King prawn rules in a poison sea. *Observer* (London). May 18, 1997.

Hall-Spencer J, Allain V, and Fosså JH. Trawling damage to Northeast Atlantic ancient coral reefs. *Proc Royal Soc London Series B269.* 2002:507–511.

Hallberg G. Nitrate in ground water in the United States. In: Follett RF, ed. *Nitrogen Management and Ground Water Protection.* Amsterdam: Elsevier Science Publishers; 1989.

Harkin T, ed. *An Overview of Animal Waste Pollution in America: Environmental Risks of Livestock and Poultry Production.* Compiled by the Minority Staff of the U.S. Senate Committee on Agriculture, Nutrition, and Forestry. Washington, DC: GPO; Dec 1997.

Hartshorn GS. Forest loss and future options in Central America. In: Hagen, JM III, Johnston DW, eds. *Ecology and Conservation of Neotropical Migrant Landbirds.* Washington, DC: Smithsonian Institute Press; 1992:13-19.

Hoag DL, Roka FM, Zering KD. Are manure nutrients an economic resource or waste? In: *Proceedings of the Conference of Agricultural Research to Protect Water Quality.* Minneapolis, MN: Soil and Water Conservation Society; 1993.

Hopper R. *Going to Market: The Cost of Industrialized Agriculture.* St. Paul, MN: Izaak Walton League of America; Jan 2002.

Howarth R, Anderson J, Cloern C, et al. Nutrient pollution of coastal rivers, bays and seas. *Issues in Ecology.* 2000;No. 7. Washington, DC: Ecological Society of America.

Hutchings JA. Collapse and recovery of marine fishes. *Nature.* 2000;406:882-885.

Hutchings JA, Reynolds JD. Marine fish population collapses: Consequences for recovery and extinction risk. *Bioscience.* 2004;54:297-309.

Jackson LL. Large scale swine production and water quality. In: Thu KM, Durenberger EP, eds. *Pigs, Orofits and Rural Communities.* Albany, NY: SUNY Press; 1998.

Johnson G. *Generic Environmental Impact Statement on Animal Agriculture: Public Review Draft.* Minnesota Planning Environmental Quality Board; Aug 2001. Available at: http://www.eqb.state.mn.us/resource.html?Id=1232. Accessed February 10, 2005.

Lees EL, Phillips CV. Dietary choice: It affects the planet's health too. *Loma Linda Univ Nutr Health Letter.* 1999. Available at: http://www.llu.edu/llu/vegetarian/diet.htm. Accessed March 14, 2005.

Marcus E. *Vegan: The New Ethics of Eating.* Ithaca, NY: McBooks Press; 1997.

Marks R. *Cesspools of Shame.* New York: Natural Resources Defense Council; July 2001.

Mason J, Singer P. *Animal Factories.* New York: Crown; 1980 (rev ed.: Three Rivers Press; 1990).

McGinnity P, Prodöhl P, Ferguson R, et al. Fitness reduction and potential extinction of wild populations of Atlantic salmon, *Salmor salar,* as a result of interactions with escaped farm salmon. *Proc Royal Soc London.* Series B, 2003;270:2443-2450.

McQuaid J. Thailand transformed by shrimp boom. *Times Picayune* (New Orleans, LA). Mar 28, 1996.

Midgley M. *Animals and Why They Matter.* Athens, GA: University of Georgia Press; 1998.

Midwest Plan Service. *Livestock Waste Facilities Handbook.* 2d ed. Ames, IA: Iowa State University; 1985.

Monterey Bay Aquarium. Available at: http://www.mbayaq.org/. Accessed February 16, 2005.

Moran EF, Brondizio E, Mausel P, et al. Integrating Amazonian vegetation, land use, and satellite data. *Bioscience.* 1994;44:329-338.

Mumby PJ, Edwards AJ, Arias-Gonzalez JE, et al. Mangroves enhance the biomass of coral reef fish communities in the Caribbean. *Nature.* 2004;427:533-536.

Myers RA, Worm B. Rapid worldwide depletion of predatory fish communities. *Nature.* 2003;423:280-283.

Naylor RL, Goldburg RJ, Primavera JH, et al. Effect of aquaculture on world fish supplies. *Nature.* 2000;405(6790):1017-1024.

Naylor RL, Goldburg RJ, Primavera JH, et al. Effects of aquaculture on world fish supplies. *Issues in Ecology.* 2001; No. 8. Washington, DC: Ecological Society of America.

Norse EA, Watling L. Impacts of mobile fishing gear: The biodiversity perspective. In: *American Fisheries Society Symposium.* 1999;22:31-40.

Nowlin M. Environmental implications of livestock production. *J Soil Water Conservation.* 1997;52:314-317.

Pauly D, Christensen V, Dalsgaard J, et al. Fishing down marine food webs. *Science.* 1998;279:860-863.

Pauly D, Christensen V, Froese R, et al. Fishing down aquatic food webs. *Am Sci.* 2000;88:46–51.

Pauly D, Christensen V, Guénette S, et al. Towards sustainability in world fisheries. *Nature.* 2002; 418:689–695.

Pimentel D, Pimentel M. *Food, Energy and Society.* Boulder, CO: University of Colorado Press; 1996.

Pimm SL. *The World According to Pimm: A Scientist Audits the Earth.* New York: McGraw-Hill; 2001.

Pitcher TJ. A cover story: Fisheries may drive stocks to extinction. *Rev Fish Biol Fisheries.* 1998;8: 367–370.

Primavera JH. Socio-economic impacts of shrimp culture. *Aquaculture Res.* 1997;28:815–827.

Regan T. *Empty Cages: Facing the Challenge of Animal Rights.* Lanham, MD: Rowman & Littlefield; 2003.

Regan T. *The Case for Animal Rights.* University of California Press; 1983.

Robbins J. *Diet for a New America: How Your Food Choices Affect Your Health, Happiness and the Future of Life on Earth.* Walpole, NH: Stillpoint Publishing; 1987.

Schiermeier Q. How many more fish in the sea? *Nature.* 2002;419:662–665.

Scully M. *Dominion: The Power of Man, the Suffering of Animals, and the Call to Mercy.* New York: St Martin's Press; 2002.

Sierra Club. *Corporate Hogs at the Public Trough.* San Francisco, CA: Sierra Club; 1999.

Sierra Club. *Federal Public Lands Grazing Policy.* Available at: http://www.sierraclub.org/policy/conservation/grazing.asp. Accessed February 18, 2005.

Socolow R. Nitrogen management and the future of food: Lessons from the management of energy and carbon. *Proc Natl Acad Sci.* 1999;96(11): 6001–6008.

Thomas ED. All about odors. In: *Animal Agriculture and the Environment: Nutrients, Pathogens and Community Relations.* Proceedings of the Animal Agriculture and the Environment and North American Conference; 1996:214–219.

Thu K, ed. *Understanding the Impacts of Large-Scale Swine Production: Proceedings from an Interdisciplinary Scientific Workshop.* Iowa City, IA: University of Iowa; 1996.

U.S. Department of Agriculture. Available at: www.usda.gov/wps/portal/usdahome. Accessed January 30, 2005.

USDA Agricultural Research Service. *Rangeland, Pasture, and Forages National Program Annual Report.* 2003. Available at: http://www.ars.usda.gov/research/programs/programs.htm?NP_CODE=205. Accessed February 19, 2005.

USDA Natural Resources Conservation Service. *Rangeland Health: RCA Issue Brief #10.* 1996. Available at: http://www.nrcs.usda.gov/technical/land/pubs/ib10text.html. Accessed March 10, 2005.

Van Dolah FM, Roelke DL, Greene RM. Health and ecological impacts of harmful algal blooms: Risk assessment needs. *Hum Ecol Risk Assess.* 2001; 7:1329–1345.

Watling L, Norse EA. Disturbance of the seabed by mobile fishing gear: A comparison to forest clear-cutting. *Conserv Biol.* 1998;12:1180.

Watson R, Pauly D. Systematic distortions in world fisheries catch trends. *Nature.* 2001;414:534–536.

Webb J, Archer JR. Pollution of soils and watercourses by wastes from livestock production systems. In: Dewi AP, Axford RF, Fayez M, et al., eds. *Pollution in Livestock Production Systems.* Wallingford, UK: CAB International; 1994.

Weber ML. What price farmed fish: A review of the environmental and social costs of farming carnivorous fish. *Seaweb Aquaculture Clearinghouse.* 2003. Available at: http://www.seaweb.org/resources/sac/. Accessed February 2, 2005.

The Wildlife Society. *Wildlife Policy Statement—Livestock Grazing on Federal Rangelands in the Western United States.* Available at: http://www.wildlife.org/policy/index.cfm?tname=policystatements&statement=ps27. Accessed January 15, 2005.

22

Planning Nutritious Vegetarian Diets

Cheryl Sullivan, MA, RD

Introduction

The basic rule for planning a vegetarian diet is fairly simple: Eat a wide variety of plant foods. Tying down the specifics is a little more complicated. General public health recommendations, such as the USDA Food Guide Pyramid (United States Department of Agriculture, 1996), may suggest legumes as an option in the "meat" group, but such recommendations are not adequate guides for vegetarians—and certainly not for vegans. These guidelines are designed for a population that regularly consumes meat and dairy products, and the research on which they are based is conducted primarily on omnivores. Furthermore, the huge economic impact of food consumption patterns makes such recommendations vulnerable to the influence of various food industries. One result is that American guidelines recommend daily consumption of dairy products, when in fact they are not a necessary part of the diet at all.

The importance of adopting adequate guidelines specifically for vegetarians is underscored by the fact that the number of new vegetarians is growing rapidly. Most of them have no experience selecting food for a plant-based diet and cannot rely on the basic eating patterns they learned growing up as omnivores; they need clear and simple guidelines to help them make good food choices.

Summary of the Scientific Literature

Food Guides

There is no single correct way to plan a vegetarian diet. Lifestyle, food traditions and availability, ethnicity, and personal taste all influence food choices. Nonetheless, following basic guidelines can help ensure that all nutritional needs are met, especially in a country where most people are unfamiliar with vegetarian eating. Numerous plans have been developed to answer this need for easy-to-use food guides for vegetarians. These plans group foods with similar nutrient composition, thereby offering a range of choices that will meet particular nutritional requirements.

Figure 22.1 Vegetarian Food Guide Pyramid

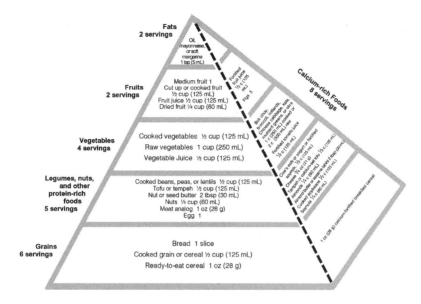

Source: Reprinted from Messina V, Melina V, Mangels AR. A new food guide for North American vegetarians. *J Am Diet Assoc.* 2003;103(6):771–775, with permission from the American Dietetic Association.

One of the most common approaches to designing vegetarian guidelines is to modify the familiar USDA Food Guide Pyramid to omit meat (and sometimes dairy) and to include a wider range of vegetarian food choices. Most plans place grains at the base of the pyramid, followed by vegetables and fruits, although there is some variability in the recommended number of servings, serving size, and the particular content of each group. The pyramid representation has advantages, in that people are familiar with it and it provides a clear visual guide, but in some cases it has the potential to confuse consumers. The top portion of the USDA Food Guide Pyramid, for example, represents foods to eat sparingly; in contrast, some vegetarian pyramids use the top to indicate foods that are essential for vegans or all vegetarians. Among the more prominent guidelines are the following.

Food Guide for North American Vegetarians

The Food Guide for North American Vegetarians (Messina, Melina, & Mangels, 2003) was designed to fit the familiar pyramid format (or the Canadian rainbow), with the notable exception that it omits a separate dairy group and instead visually presents a wide range of calcium choices for each food group (Figure 22.1). Working up from the base of the pyramid, recommendations are for a minimum of six servings of grains, five of protein-rich foods, four of vegetables, two of fruits, and two of fats. Eight servings daily should be chosen from the calcium-rich foods, but these may be double-counted in the appropriate food groups (e.g., one cup of cooked broccoli counts as one calcium serving and also as two half-cup servings of vegetables). By expanding calcium choices

Figure 22.2   Tips for Meal Planning

- Choose a wide variety of foods.
- The number of servings in each group is for minimum daily intakes.Choose more foods from any of the groups to meet energy needs.
- A serving from the calcium-rich food group provides approximately 10% of adult daily requirements. Choose eight or more servings per day.These also count toward servings from the other food groups in the guide. For example, ½ cup (125 mL) of fortified fruit juice counts as a calcium-rich food and also counts toward servings from the fruit group.
- Include 2 servings every day of foods that supply n-3 fats.Foods rich in n-3 fats are found in the legumes/ nuts group and in the fats group.A serving is 1 teaspoon (5 mL) of flaxseed oil, 3 teaspoons (15 mL) of canola or soybean oil, 1 tablespoon (15 mL) of ground flaxseed, or ¼ cup (60 mL) of walnuts. Olive and canola oils are the best choices for cooking to balance the fats in your diet.
- Servings of nuts and seeds may be used in place of servings from the fats group.
- Be sure to get adequate vitamin D from daily sun exposure or through fortified foods or supplements. Cow's milk and some brands of soy milk and breakfast cereals are fortified with vitamin D.
- Include at least three good food sources of vitamin B12 in your diet every day.These include 1 table-spoon (15 mL) of Red Star Vegetarian Support Formula nutritional yeast, 1 cup (250 mL) of fortified soy milk, ½ cup (125 mL) of cow's milk, ¾ cup (185 mL) of yogurt, 1 large egg, 1 ounce (28 g) of fortified breakfast cereal, and/or 1½ oz (42 g) of fortified meat analog. If you don't eat these foods regularly (at least 3 servings per day), take a daily vitamin B12 supplement of 5 to 10 micrograms (μg) or a weekly B12 supplement of 2,000 μg.
- If you include sweets or alcohol in your diet,consume these foods in moderation. Get most of your daily calories from the foods in the Vegetarian Food Guide.

Source: Reprinted from Messina V, Melina V, Mangels AR. A new food guide for North American vegetarians. *J Amer Diet Assoc.* 2003;103:771-775, with permission from the American Dietetic Association.

beyond dairy products or fortified nondairy drinks,this guide emphasizes eating from a wide range of healthful plant foods. Vegans as well as lacto vegetarians can easily use this pyramid, along with its accompanying meal planning tips (Figure 22.2), to assist in making good food choices.

New York Medical College Vegetarian Pyramid

The New York Medical College Vegetarian Pyramid (1994) has some unusual features.The grains group at the base of the pyramid also includes starchy vegetables, such as corn and peas, although otherwise the grains, vegetable, and fruit groups are similar to those in other guidelines. A more substantial difference is that the "meat and fish substitutes" group has serving sizes that are twice as large as commonly recommended. This could potentially lead to high intakes of fat or cholesterol for a person who frequently chooses a serving of one-half cup nuts or two eggs. To meet the needs of vegans, the "dairy and dairy substitutes" group includes fortified soy milk, but the tip of the pyramid also makes specific recommendations for vegans to consume vegetable oil (for calories and essential fatty acids), blackstrap molasses (for iron and calcium), and fortified brewer's yeast (for riboflavin and vitamin B12) on a daily basis.Though these foods are nutritious choices,eating these particular foods is not the only way to obtain those nutrients.Vegetarians may also object to viewing their nutritious plant-based choices as "substitutes" for meat and dairy.

The New Becoming Vegetarian Food Guide

The New Becoming Vegetarian Food Guide (Melina & Davis, 2003), an updated version of *Becoming Vegetarian* (Melina, Davis, & Harrison, 1995), offers another food guide in the pyramid format, although the shape does not suit these recommendations well. For example, a larger number of servings of calcium-rich foods is placed above a smaller number of servings of vegetables. The base of the pyramid is 6 to 11 servings of grains, followed by at least 3 servings of vegetables and 2 or more servings of fruit. The "Milks and Alternates" group recommends six to eight servings of high-calcium foods, including plant foods that are naturally high in calcium, as well as fortified foods and dairy products (serving sizes of dairy products are half what they are on the USDA Food Guide Pyramid, to fit with the greater number of recommended servings). The two to three recommended servings of beans and alternates include legumes, tofu, vegetarian meat analogs, nuts, seeds, eggs, and soy milk. The tip of the pyramid includes one to two servings of foods that provide omega-3 fatty acids, and mentions vitamins D and B12. The accompanying text helps to clarify the details, which are not always obvious from the pyramid presentation alone. Exercise and adequate hydration are also visually represented next to the pyramid.

The Vegetarian Way Food Guide

Lacto vegetarians, vegans, and even macrobiotic vegetarians can all use the Vegetarian Way Food Guide (Messina & Messina, 1996, pp. 238-241), which is in chart rather than pyramid form. The minimum number of servings for some groups is larger than in most other guides: eight from the grains group; four from vegetables, including one serving of leafy greens; and three from

fruits. The dairy group is omitted altogether, as it is not a dietary essential. Lower-fat cow's milk is included with fortified nondairy milks, legumes, nuts, and seeds in a group of foods that provide protein and calcium. Five servings a day from this group are recommended, and calcium-rich foods from other groups are highlighted. Two or three servings of fat are recommended, but this guide suggests limiting processed snack foods as well as other foods high in saturated fat, cholesterol, and sugar.

The Traditional Healthy Vegetarian Diet Pyramid

The Traditional Healthy Vegetarian Diet Pyramid, designed and published by the Oldways Preservation & Exchange Trust in conjunction with the Harvard School of Public Health (1998), is one of several traditional diets Oldways has placed into the currently popular pyramid model. The pyramid, which includes physical activity at the base, recommends foods for consumption at each meal (fruits, vegetables, whole grains, and legumes), foods to be eaten every day (nuts and seeds; egg whites, soy milk, or dairy; plant oils), and foods to be consumed occasionally or in small quantities (eggs and sweets). The plan in many ways exemplifies the basic vegetarian rule of eating a wide variety of plant foods, and is appealing in its simplicity. However, its lack of specified serving sizes does not provide adequate guidance in a country where food is abundant, and the recommended eating pattern would be a big adjustment for most Americans.

Other Vegetarian Food Guides

Other vegetarian guidelines have been developed to serve a variety of needs. Before the development of the popular pyramid models, authors of vegetarian cookbooks would often create their own nutrition guides. The most extensive of these was in *Laurel's Kitchen* (Robertson, Flinders, & Godfrey, 1976), one of the most popular vegetarian handbooks of the 1970s and 1980s. Their final guidelines, in *The New Laurel's Kitchen* (Robertson, Flinders, & Ruppenthal, 1986), were based on whole grains and vegetables, completed with "super vegetables" (dark leafy greens, edible-pod peas, brussels sprouts, broccoli, asparagus, lima beans, peas) and legumes or dairy, and filled out with a variety of whole foods. The more recent food guides described earlier have largely superseded these earlier guidelines.

Currently, vegetarian dietary guidelines are also being devised to prevent or alleviate specific medical conditions. Dean Ornish's "Reversal Diet" for heart disease (Ornish, 1990), which is a very-low-fat, whole-foods vegetarian diet, is one of these.

Supplements

Plant foods provide a wealth of nutrients necessary for good health: vitamins, minerals, fiber, and an array of protective phytochemicals. We are just beginning to learn about the health value of many of the components in plants, so we are far from understanding which components are active, what they do, how they interact with each other, how much is optimal for humans, and so forth. We are a long way from being able to package the total value of a plant food into a pill or powder. Whenever possible, dietary needs should be met from food.

Vitamin and mineral supplements are no more essential for vegetarians who eat a well-balanced diet than for omnivores. Vitamin B12, which cannot be obtained from plant foods, appears to be the one exception. Vegans must consume a fortified food or a supplement to meet their B12 requirement. In addition, current recommendations from the Food and Nutrition Board of the Institute of Medicine are that all Americans over the age of 50 take supplementary B12 to compensate for age-related malabsorption of foodbound B12 (Food and Nutrition Board, 1998).

There are circumstances, however, in which supplementation is appropriate. Although a well-planned diet can provide all the needed nutrients (except for vitamin B12), many American vegetarians regularly consume highly processed foods and must rely on the limited vegetarian fare available when eating away from home. For these people, or anyone whose diet is less than optimal, supplementation may be a good idea. It will not change such a diet into a perfect one, but it will provide a margin of error. Some vegetarian food guides recommend a daily multivitamin-mineral supplement for this reason (Ornish, 1990). Supplements of specific nutrients, such as calcium, should be taken if food choices do not provide sufficient intake.

Some foods are highly concentrated sources of nutrients and can be viewed as supplemental foods when taken regularly for their nutritive value. Nutritional yeast that has been grown on a culture rich in cobalamin or riboflavin is one such food; blackstrap molasses (for iron and calcium) and flaxseed oil (for omega-3 fatty acids) are others that are sometimes recommended for vegetarians (New York Medical College, 1994). These are certainly nutritious additions to the diet, but are not essential foods in and of themselves because these nutrients can be obtained elsewhere.

Practical Aspects

Not only do vegetarians need a food guide, they need to know how to use it. New vegetarians are often at a loss when it comes to putting together a meal. The traditional method of planning dinner around the meat does not apply anymore, and it may be hard to think of anything other than a peanut butter sandwich for lunch. In addition, vegetarian staples such as tofu are unfamiliar to many people. To help vegetarians get a variety of nutritious foods in a convenient and familiar way, many food guides come with meal plans and even recipes.

As long as a variety of foods is consumed over the course of a day, what goes together in a particular meal is not usually of major consequence. The main exception to this is that a good source of vitamin C should be consumed when eating iron-rich foods, to increase iron absorption. Many vegetarians still believe that they must eat complementary proteins at the same time to get "complete" protein, and structure their meals accordingly. Although this is certainly acceptable, it is not necessary for every meal to have a perfect balance of essential amino acids, as long as a variety of foods is chosen over the course of the day.

It is also not necessary to completely abandon customary meal patterns when adopting a vegetarian diet. Familiar dishes like pizza and pasta are often already meatless, and can easily be adapted to a vegetarian diet. There are also many commercially prepared meat analogs, such as vegetarian burgers or meatless burger crumbles, that can be substituted in place of meat products. These strategies can ease the transition, which may make a difference in long-term adherence to a vegetarian diet. (For suggestions on making a transition to a vegetarian diet, see Vegetarian Nutrition Dietetic Practice Group, 2001.) A gradual transition will also give the body a chance to adapt to new foods. A good vegetarian diet is likely to be higher in fiber than an omnivorous diet and it may initially cause some discomfort—and embarrassment—for new vegetarians who make big changes too quickly.

Vegetarians must remember that there is more to a nutritious vegetarian diet than simply avoiding meat; they must choose a wholesome variety of plant foods. Otherwise, it is very possible to have a vegetarian junk-food diet. The abundance and easy availability of highly processed foods make it easy to take in too many calories but not enough nutrients. Like other Americans, vegetarians need to be careful not to overeat.

Finding one's way in a meat-and-dairy world may require some adjustments, especially for vegans. There are new foods to cook at home, new choices to make when dining out, and social obstacles to confront when eating with friends and family. Several books are available that deal with both the practical and nutritional issues of following a vegetarian diet (e.g., Messina & Messina, 1996; Melina & Davis, 2003; Havala, 2001), and vegetarians should consider purchasing one.

Conclusion

Planning a well-balanced vegetarian diet is no harder than planning a meat-based diet. This does not mean that vegetarians can simply drop meat from their diet and be on their way. In a country with so much processed convenience food available, and so many pressures to eat, it takes real commitment to follow a nutritious eating plan. Vegans will have to pay especially close attention to their food choices. Although many studies show that vegetarians have reduced rates of disease, these health benefits will probably not extend to those eating a meatless diet of highly processed, low-nutrient foods. Choosing a varied diet based on whole plant foods may make the difference.

References

Food and Nutrition Board, Institute of Medicine. *Dietary Reference Intakes for Thiamin, Riboflavin, Niacin, Vitamin B6, Folate, Vitamin B12, Pantothenic Acid, Biotin, and Choline.* Washington, DC: National Academy Press; 1998. Available at:http://books.nap.edu/openbook/0309065542/html/index.html. Accessed October 19, 2004.

Havala S. *Being Vegetarian for Dummies.* New York: Hungry Minds; 2001.

Melina V, Davis B. *The New Becoming Vegetarian: The Essential Guide to a Healthy Vegetarian Diet.* Summertown, TN: Healthy Living Publications; 2003.

Melina V, Davis B, Harrison V. *Becoming Vegetarian: The Complete Guide to Adopting a Healthy Vegetarian Diet.* Summertown, TN: Book Publishing; 1995.

Messina V, Melina V, Mangels AR. A new food guide for North American vegetarians. *J Am Diet Assoc.* 2003;103(6):771-775. Available at: http://www.eatright.org/Public/NutritionInformation/92_17086.cfm. Accessed October 19, 2004.

Messina VM, Messina M. *The Vegetarian Way.* New York: Three Rivers Press; 1996.

New York Medical College. *New York Medical College Vegetarian Pyramid.* Valhallah, NY: New York Medical College; 1994.

Oldways Preservation & Exchange Trust. *The Official Traditional Healthy Vegetarian Diet Pyramid.* Cambridge, MA; 1998. Available at: http://www.oldwayspt.org/pyramids/veg/p_veg.html. Accessed October 19, 2004.

Ornish D. *Dr. Dean Ornish's Program for Reversing Heart Disease.* New York: Ballantine Books; 1990. Available at: http://my.webmd.com/content/pages/9/3068_9408.htm. Accessed October 19, 2004.

Robertson L, Flinders C, Godfrey B. *Laurel's Kitchen: A Handbook for Vegetarian Cookery & Nutrition.* Berkeley, CA: Nilgiri Press; 1976.

Robertson L, Flinders C, Ruppenthal B. *The New Laurel's Kitchen: A Handbook for Vegetarian Cookery & Nutrition.* Berkeley, CA: Ten Speed Press; 1986.

United States Department of Agriculture. *The Food Guide Pyramid: A Guide to Daily Food Choices.* 1992, updated 1996. Available at: http://www.nal.usda.gov/fnic/Fpyr/pyramid.html. Accessed October 19, 2004.

Vegetarian Nutrition Dietetic Practice Group, American Dietetic Association. *Making the Change to a Vegetarian Diet.* Fact Sheet; 2001. Available for order at: http://www.vegetariannutrition.net/fact_sheets.htm.

23

Conclusion: Summary of Protective Factors

Virginia Messina, MPH, RD
Peggy Carlson, MD

Although there is abundant evidence that vegetarians have lower risks for some chronic diseases than nonvegetarians, and that vegans may have even lower risk, it is not always easy to determine how much of this is due to diet and how much to an overall healthy lifestyle. It has been suggested that vegetarians enjoy better health simply because they embrace a range of health-promoting habits. Vegetarians may be more likely to exercise (although we do not know this for certain) and less likely to smoke than nonvegetarians; this may affect health as much as differences in diet. There is, however, ample evidence that diet is a major contributing factor to the good health enjoyed by vegetarians.

Science and attitudes toward diet have converged somewhat over the years as vegetarian diets have gained respect (and even some praise) from science and garnered acceptance (and even thanks) from the public. In the past, dietary deficiencies were more prevalent, and science wanted to know if vegetarian diets could be healthful. Hundreds of studies have been done, so we now know that well-balanced vegetarian diets are healthy. When chronic diseases with a link to dietary excess began eroding health (heart disease, cancer, stroke, obesity, diabetes), science wanted to know if vegetarian diets might be healthier than the typical omnivorous diet. A few hundred studies blossomed into a few thousand studies, and the answer is coming back yes. Vegetarian diets offer health-protective, and in some cases such as heart disease, health-improving, benefits. With this knowledge about the health benefits of a vegetarian diet is coming a change in attitude, as more people are choosing vegetarian diets to protect and promote health.

With any diet, one must follow guidelines to ensure that all needed nutrients are consumed and that unnecessary or even harmful foods are avoided. A vegetarian diet is no different in that respect. Such things as too many calories or too much junk food and saturated fat can be an issue for some vegetarians. Those consuming vegetarian diets also face some unique differences from other diets. Vitamin B12 is a prime example. Vitamin B12 is lacking in today's plant foods, but is amply present in animal foods. Therefore, vegans, who by definition eat no animal products, should recognize the need to include vitamin B12-fortified foods or vitamin B12 supplements in their diet. Other nutrients that may require special attention by some vegetarians include calcium, zinc, and the omega-3, long-chain polyunsaturated fatty acids. Again, all of these nutrients can be easily obtained from appropriate nonanimal sources.

Although those who consume vegetarian diets do need to be cognizant of certain areas, to ensure that their diet is complete, science is beginning to find that there are even greater challenges in designing a meat-based diet that is complete. These challenges remain largely unrecognized by much of the public. This lack of awareness is leading to poor diet choices and an epidemic of resultant diseases. One thinks of the typical Western diet as being a diet of excess: too many calories, too much saturated fat and cholesterol, too many refined-grain products, too much meat, and too many high-fat dairy products. However, it may be that the Western diet is, equally importantly, a diet of deficiency: too few fruits and vegetables, whole grains, vitamins, phytochemicals, antioxidants, unsaturated fats, and high-fiber foods.

No one magic bullet has been found to explain the health benefits of a vegetarian diet. It is even likely that not all the potential magic bullets have been considered—or even discovered! More likely is that there is not one magic bullet, but rather a team of bullets that work together to defend against disease.

Vegetarian diets differ from nonvegetarian diets in one obvious way: no meat (and, in the case of vegan diets, no animal products at all). However, science has shown that vegetarian diets are really different in many other ways as well. Some of these differences we know quite a lot about; other differences are only now becoming apparent and attracting scientific study. It is clear that many of these differences may be powerful influences on health.

Factors in Vegetarian Diets That Are Protective

Fiber

Vegetarians consume approximately two to three times as much fiber as omnivores. High intakes of soluble fiber reduce cholesterol levels and help to regulate blood sugar levels. High intakes of fiber may be associated with reduced risks of colon cancer, diverticulitis, diabetes, and appendicitis.

Antioxidants

Antioxidants are found in a wide range of plant foods. Whole grains, nuts, legumes, fruits and vegetables, and even vegetable oils all contribute antioxidants to the diet. Antioxidants protect cells from damage by free radicals. They may protect against the damaging oxidative effects on LDL cholesterol that promote atherosclerosis. Research suggests that they may also play a key role in guarding against cellular damage that can initiate cancer. Science is just beginning to unravel the many potential benefits that antioxidants may have for health. Vegetarians have higher intakes than omnivores of many of the prime antioxidants, such as vitamin C, vitamin E, carotenoids, and many of the phytochemicals with antioxidant properties.

Phytochemicals

Phytochemicals are little powerhouse chemicals found in a wide range of plant foods. Thousands of phytochemicals have been identified to date. They have a wide spectrum of possible health-protective properties. Undoubtedly, science has yet even to scratch the surface of their possible benefits. In addition to serving as anti-oxidants, phytochemicals have other properties that fight cancer, lower cholesterol, decrease blood clotting, and decrease inflammation. Phytochemicals with an estrogen-like structure—the phytoestrogens—may also be important in health. Vegetarians, because of their greater consumption of plant foods, will typically have higher intakes of many phytochemicals.

Unsaturated Fats (Monounsaturated and Polyunsaturated Fats)

Although fats have gotten a bad reputation, many of their harmful properties can be attributed to saturated, not unsaturated, fats. When unsaturated fats replace saturated fats in the diet, they decrease cholesterol and may increase good cholesterol (HDL cholesterol). Some unsaturated fats may lower blood pressure, decrease blood clotting, and decrease the susceptibility of LDL cholesterol to oxidative damage. Unsaturated fats may protect against illnesses such as heart disease and diabetes. Vegetarians tend to consume more unsaturated fats than do omnivores.

Potassium

A greater intake of potassium has been associated with lower risks of high blood pressure, stroke, and kidney stones. Vegetarians tend to consume more potassium than nonvegetarians.

Fruits and Vegetables

An increase in fruit and vegetable intake has been associated with a lower risk of several chronic diseases. Fruit and vegetable consump-

tion has been associated in some studies with lower risk of coronary artery (heart) disease, some cancers, diabetes, high blood pressure, and stroke. These health-protective effects of fruits and vegetables may be attributable to one or more of their components, including fiber, antioxidants, phytochemicals, and vitamins.

Vegetarian Diets May Be More Healthful Because of Lower Intakes of These Factors

Saturated Fat

The saturated type of fat, found in many foods, but at the highest level in meats and full-fat dairy products, is the greatest determinant of elevated blood cholesterol levels. Saturated fat has been linked to an increased risk of heart disease, and there are ongoing studies to determine whether it is also linked to other chronic diseases, such as stroke, diabetes, and some cancers.

Cholesterol

Dietary cholesterol raises blood cholesterol levels, although it has a lesser impact than saturated fat. Elevated serum cholesterol increases the risk of coronary artery disease. Lacto-ovo vegetarian diets tend to be low in cholesterol, and vegan diets, because they contain no animal products, have no cholesterol.

Meat

There is no unequivocal evidence linking consumption of meat, in and of itself, to any chronic disease. Some studies have shown a possible link with diabetes, diverticular disease, and some cancers, including colon cancer. Meat also contributes saturated fat and cholesterol to the diet, while taking the place of more healthful foods such as fruits and vegetables, fiber and unsaturated fats, whole grains, dried beans, nuts and seeds, and unsaturated oils.

Animal Protein

Studies suggest that a high intake of animal protein may be linked to an increased risk of kidney stones and osteoporosis. Early-stage kidney disease may be worsened by dietary animal protein. Vegetarians consume less animal protein than meat eaters.

Heme Iron

A few studies have suggested a link between heme iron (iron found in animal foods) and an increased risk of heart disease and diabetes, although such links are as yet unproven.

Obesity

Although not a dietary factor itself, obesity is clearly related to diet. Obesity is linked to an increased risk of heart disease, high blood pressure, diabetes, stroke, cancer, and arthritis, to name a few. Vegetarians have a lower incidence of obesity than nonvegetarians.

Conclusion

To date, no chronic disease has been shown to have a greater incidence in vegetarians than in nonvegetarians. Research studies have typically asked how much, if any, health protection a vegetarian diet has against a particular disease.

There is, however, substantial evidence linking the typical Western diet to increases in the primary chronic disease killers of industrialized nations: namely, heart disease, cancer, diabetes, stroke, and obesity.

Given the strength of the scientific evidence, one must ask why vegetarian diets are not more commonly adopted. Undoubtedly, a host of factors play a role. These include internal factors, such as habit, fear of change, lack of good information, being taught as a child that meat is a necessary part of the diet, and thinking that many new foods or cooking methods will be required to follow a vegetarian diet. Many external factors may also play a role, including family, peer, and cultural pressures; misleading dietary guidelines; the influence of the meat and dairy industries in such things as advertising and the development of dietary guidelines; easy availability of meat-based fast foods; misinformation from health professionals who lack knowledge about vegetarian diets; and restaurant menus centered around meat.

Although the rapid increase in scientific studies related to vegetarian diets has brought enormous knowledge, many questions remain. Surely new discoveries and understandings lie ahead. More knowledge regarding the effect of vegetarian diets on various diseases will be gained; certainly, more insights into dietary factors will undoubtedly surface.

While we await these discoveries of the future, we know that what we eat today will be our future. Those consuming vegetarian diets should be sure that their diets are well balanced, taking care that those nutrients that may be more difficult to get from vegetarian diets are consumed in adequate amounts. On balance, though, there is ample evidence that the many health advantages of a vegetarian diet outweigh the many health risks that accompany the dietary excesses and deficiencies of the typical Western, meat-based diet.

Contributors

John J. B. Anderson, PhD, earned his PhD in physical biology at Cornell University in 1966. Since 1971, he has been Professor of Nutrition at the University of North Carolina at Chapel Hill. His research interests include bone metabolism as influenced by diet, exercise, and hormones, as well as other topics related to nutrition, including diet-related chronic diseases.

Dina Aronson, MS, RD, is a New Jersey-based registered dietitian, nutrition consultant, writer, and speaker specializing in plant-based nutrition and technology in dietetics. Dina is co-author of *Food Allergy Survival Guide: Surviving and Thriving with Food Allergies and Sensitivities* (Book Publishing, 2004) and *Minerals from Plant Foods: Strategies for Maximizing Nutrition* (American Dietetic Association, 2002). Dina was the recipient of the American Dietetic Association's Recognized Young Dietitian of the Year Award in 2002. Dina believes that everyone's health can benefit by moving toward a plant-based diet.

Peggy Carlson, MD, earned her medical degree from the University of Illinois Medical School. She is board-certified in emergency medicine and has practiced emergency medicine and occupational medicine for about 20 years. She authored sections in *The Clinical Practice of Emergency Medicine.* Peggy has been vegetarian for about 40 years and vegan for about 15 of these years.

James Craner, MD, MPH, received his undergraduate degree from Princeton University and his medical degree (MD) from Harvard Medical School. He completed a residency in Internal Medicine at Brown University School of Medicine, followed by a residency in Occupational and Environmental Medicine at UMDNJ/ Rutgers University, where he also completed his Master's of Public Health degree. Dr. Craner is board-certified in both Occupational Medicine and Internal Medicine, and is a fellow of both the American College of Occupational and Environmental Medicine and the American College of Physicians. He serves as an assistant clinical professor in the Division of Occupational and Environmental Medicine in the Department of Medicine at the University of California, San Francisco School of Medicine; and in the Department of Internal Medicine at the University of Nevada School of Medicine, Las Vegas. Dr. Craner has practiced occupational and environmental medicine in Nevada for 11 years. His areas of practice focus include clinical, epidemiological, and environmental investigation of problem buildings and research on sick building syndrome; medical surveillance for mining, manufacturing, and other industries; and clinical consultation for toxicological and biological exposures and related diseases.

Brenda Davis, RD, is a leader in her field and an internationally acclaimed speaker. She has worked as a public health nutritionist, clinical nutrition specialist, nutrition consultant, and academic nutrition instructor, and is a past chair of the Vegetarian Nutrition Dietetic Practice Group of the American Dietetic Association. Brenda is author of five books: the best-sellers *Becoming Vegetarian* and *Becoming Vegan*, *Dairy-free and Delicious*, *Defeating Diabetes*, and *The New Becoming Vegetarian*. She has also authored numerous professional and lay articles. Brenda is an outdoor and fitness enthusiast. She lives with her husband and family in Kelowna, British Columbia, Canada.

Simon Emms, PhD, is an associate professor of biology at the University of St. Thomas in Minnesota, where he teaches ecology and evolution and does research on plant reproductive systems. He received a BA in zoology from Oxford University (UK), an MSc in biological sciences from Simon Fraser University (Vancouver, Canada), and a PhD in ecology and evolutionary biology from Princeton University. In addition to his own research, his academic interests include human evolution, conservation biology, and the behavioral ecology of birds. He also enjoys drinking wine, playing classical guitar, and road biking, though not at the same time.

Jeanene Fogli, MS, RD, LDN, is the chief bionutritionist at the General Clinical Research Center at Beth Israel Deaconess Medical Center. She has a bachelor's degree in dietetics from the University of Delaware; a master's degree in nutrition from Marywood University in Scranton, Pennsylvania; and is currently a PhD candidate at Tufts University in Human Metabolism and Nutritional Biochemistry.

Suzanne Havala Hobbs, DrPH, MS, RD, is Clinical Assistant Professor and Director of the Executive Doctoral Program in Health Leadership (DrPH), Department of Health Policy and Administration, School of Public Health, University of North Carolina at Chapel Hill. She holds a doctorate in health policy and administration from the UNC School of Public Health. Her professional interests include health care leadership, dietary guidance policy (domestic and international), health journalism, and communication and cultural proficiency in health services delivery. She has been a faculty member at UNC since 2001, where she teaches in the doctoral and master's degree programs. Hobbs, a licensed, registered dietitian, has held clinical and administrative positions in a variety of acute-care and long-term care settings. A professional journalist and author of 10 books, she writes a weekly newspaper column on diet and health for the *News & Observer* (Raleigh) and *The Charlotte Observer*. She has served on the board of directors of the Association of Health Care Journalists and the Center for Excellence in Health Care Journalism. and is a member of the Board of Trustees of the North Carolina Writers Network.

Michael A. Klaper, MD, earned his medical degree from the University of Illinois College of Medicine in Chicago in 1972. He has post-graduate training in surgery, anesthesiology, and orthopedics from the University of British Columbia Hospitals in Vancouver and in obstetrics from the University of California at San Francisco. He serves as the founding director of the Institute of Nutrition Education and Research in Manhattan Beach, California.

Erin Kraker, MS, REHS, received her MS in environmental health and sustainable agriculture from the University of Minnesota. She has worked as an environmental health specialist with the Indian Health Service on the Hopi Reservation in northern Arizona and with remote Native villages in southwestern Alaska. She is currently pursuing a nursing degree at Northern Arizona University in Flagstaff.

Valerie Kurtzhalts, MSN, APRN, BC, has been a registered nurse for more than 30 years. Working in hospitals all over the country, she has extensive experience in critical care areas. With growing interest in illness prevention and health promotion, she completed her Master's of Science Degree in Nursing in 1995 and is now a practicing Family Nurse Practitioner in a pediatric setting. She has been a vegan for 15 years.

D. Enette Larson-Meyer, PhD, RD, FACSM, is an assistant professor at the University of Wyoming. She has a background in both nutrition and exercise physiology and is a past chair of the Vegetarian Nutrition Dietetic Practice Group. She has published numerous scientific and lay articles focusing on how nutrition and exercise influence the health and performance of active individuals. Dr. Larson-Meyer received her BS degree from the University of Wyoming,

completed her dietetic training and master's degree at Massachusetts General Hospital in Boston, and did her doctoral studies at the University of Alabama at Birmingham. She has been a serious recreational athlete for 20 years, and currently enjoys running both distance events and after her three young active vegetarians, Lindsey, Ian, and Marlena.

Reed Mangels, PhD, RD, FADA, is a nutrition advisor for the nonprofit, educational Vegetarian Resource Group and nutrition editor and a regular columnist for *Vegetarian Journal*. She co-authored the American Dietetic Association's position on vegetarian diets and has written many articles on vegetarian nutrition. She co-authored *The Dietitian's Guide to Vegetarian Diets* (2d ed.). Reed also wrote the nutrition section of *Simply Vegan* and the chapter on vegetarian diets for *The Pediatric Manual of Clinical Dietetics.* She is a past chair of the Vegetarian Nutrition Dietetic Practice Group of the American Dietetic Association.

Carol M. Meerschaert, RD, LDN, is a nutrition consultant and writer in Falmouth, Maine. She has specialized in nutrition for families and vegetarian nutrition for 20 years. She is a co-author of *Minerals from Plant Foods* (ADA, 2002) and *Eat Your Herbs* (Food and Health, 1999).

Virginia Messina, MPH, RD, is a registered dietitian with a master's degree in public health nutrition from the University of Michigan. She has taught nutrition at the university level, was a foods and nutrition specialist for the Michigan Cooperative Extension Service, and was director of nutrition services for George Washington University Medical Center in Washington, DC. She also wrote and edited the international publication *Nutrition and Health Letter*, published for five years by the School of Public Health, Loma Linda University. Ms. Messina has produced numerous publications on nutrition for professionals and is co-author of the American Dietetic Association's position on vegetarian diets. She is co-author of two popular books on nutrition—*The Vegetarian Way* and *The Simple Soybean and Your Health* (which has been translated into eight languages)—and of the first vegetarian textbook for health professionals, *The Dietitian's Guide to Vegetarian Diets*. Ms. Messina is also the co-author of three cookbooks.

Mary Helen Niemeyer, MD, MPH, FAAFP, received her medical degree from Georgetown University School of Medicine and completed a family practice residency in Greenville, SC. She served in the U.S. Public Health Service for two years, assigned to a primary care center on St. Helena's Island, SC. She earned a master's degree in public health from the University of South Carolina and has worked with the South Carolina Department of Health and Environmental Control in various capacities since 1989. Dr. Niemeyer has served on advisory boards of several animal protection organizations and has been a vegetarian since 1991 for ethical reasons, but also believes it to be the healthiest lifestyle.

Carl V. Phillips, MPP, PhD, is associate professor of public health at the University of Alberta. He received his PhD in public policy from Harvard University, a master's degree in public policy from the Kennedy School of Government at Harvard, and a BA in math and history from Ohio State University. He completed a Robert Wood Johnson Foundation postdoctoral fellowship in health policy at the University of Michigan. His research includes health science research methods, environmental and health

policy, popular communication of science, and tobacco harm reduction. He has written and spoken extensively on vegetarianism, including running the sci-veg.org e-mail list in the 1990s.

Sudha Raj, PhD, RD, is an Assistant Professor and Graduate Program Director in the Department of Nutrition and Hospitality Management in the College for Human Services and Health Professions at Syracuse University. Sudha obtained her BSc and MSc degrees in Nutrition and Dietetics from the University of Madras and Bombay University in India and her PhD in Nutrition Science from Syracuse University in 1991. Her doctoral dissertation focused on the development of processing standards for the organic/natural food industry. Her current research interests are in the areas of vegetarianism and cultural nutrition, specifically dietary acculturation among Asian Indian immigrants in the United States. Sudha served as the Chair of the Vegetarian Nutrition Dietetic Practice Group for the 2005–2006 term. She currently serves as the Chair of the American Dietetic Association's Evidence Based Analysis Project on Vegetarian Diets.

Cheryl Sullivan, MA, RD, is a past editor of the *Vegetarian Nutrition Update*, the newsletter for the Vegetarian Nutrition Dietetic Practice Group of the American Dietetic Association. She has lectured and written articles for consumers and professionals on vegetarian nutrition topics and is co-author of *Simply Soy,* a cookbook on soy foods, and *Minerals from Plant Foods*, a continuing professional education resource for dietitians. She is currently employed at the National Soybean Research Lab at the University of Illinois, where she works with the Illinois Center for Soy Foods. Ms. Sullivan also served on the Board of Directors of the Eastern Illinois Food Bank from 1997–2004.

Index

kidney disease/failure, 221–22, 257–59, 260; acute renal
    failure, 257; benefits of a low-protein diet for, 247–58;
    benefits of a vegetarian diet for, 258–59; chronic renal
    failure (CRF); and creatinine clearance, 257; end-stage
    renal disease (ESRD), 257; factors of poor renal
    function, 257; and the glomerular filtration rate (GFR),
    257–58; and renal plasma flow, 257–58
kidney stones, 254–57, 259–60; and animal protein
    intake, 255–56; composition of different types of, 254;
    diet and the recurrence of, 257; dietary factors
    affecting formation of, 254–55; and dietary potassium
    intake, 256; and dietary sodium intake, 256
Kim, Y. I., 55
Krajcovicova-Kudlackova, M., 33

lactation. *See* breast milk
Lambe, William, 3
Lanza, E., 55
Lappe, Frances Moore, 5
Laurel's Kitchen (Robertson, Flinders, and Ruppenthal),
    342
"Lectures on Diet, Regimen, and Employment" (Hitch-
    cock), 3
Lee, C., 10, 13
Leiden Intervention Trial, 125
leptin, 203
leuctrienes, 31
Lindgren, A., 188
linoleic acid (LA), 25, 31, 33, 117, 215; conversion
    of to arachidonic acid, 32; sources of, 39–40,
    282–83
Lobb, Theophile, 3
lutein, 102
lycopene, 102
Lyon heart study, 29

macular degeneration, 102
magnesium, 104–5, 243, 244, 247; food sources of, 104;
    recommended intake of, 104
Manetti, Bill, 288
manganese, 28
Mangels, R., 79, 80
Mayberry, J. F., 59
McDougall, J., 27, 171
meat (red meat), 79, 149–50, 152, 154, 347–48; con-
    sumption of, 195
Mediterranean diets, 29–30
Melina, V., 80
Messina, M., 79, 170, 292
Messina, V., 79, 80, 170, 292

Metcalf, William, 4
methane, 319, 326
methylmalonic acid (MMA), 87
Michigan State University Bread Study, 18
microalgae. *See* algae
Midgley, M., 317
molybdenum, 106, food sources of, 106; recommended
    dietary allowance (RDA) of, 106
Multiple Risk Factor Intervention Trial (MRFIT), 163,
    164, 176, 177, 188
Mussey, Reuben, 3

Nair, P., 59
National Academy of Sciences, 68
National Cancer Program, 13
National Cattlemen's Association, 8
National Cholesterol Education Program (NCEP), 166
National Dairy Council, 8–9
National Health and Nutrition Examination Survey
    (NHANES), 192, 202
National Health and Nutrition Examination Survey
    Epidemiologic Follow-up Study, 120
National Institutes of Health, 213
National Pork Producers Council, 8
National Turkey Foundation, 8
Nature Conservancy, 330
Navratilova, Martina, 288
Naylor, R. L., 324
Nestle, Marion, 8
neuropathy, 213
Nieman, D., 308
nitrocobalamin, 85
nitrogen, 325, 326; plant proteins and nitrogen balance,
    17–18
North, Milo, 3
Norway, 4
Nurses' Health Study, 56, 57, 116, 117, 120, 176, 188, 215,
    256
nuts, 37, 38–39, 44, 45, 79, 103, 205; butternuts, 37;
    cardioprotective effects of, 39; peanuts, 39; walnuts,
    37, 39, 126, 247

obesity, 59, 151, 202–4, 206, 209, 212, 348; and caloric
    imbalance, 206–7; as a cancer risk, 148; and lifestyle
    changes, 208; preobesity, 202; treatment of, 203–4.
    See also obesity, and vegetarians
obesity, and vegetarians, 204; and calorie intake, 204–5;
    dieting with a vegetarian diet, 207; and fat types, 206;
    high carbohydrate intake of vegetarians, 205; high
    fiber intake of vegetarians, 205; lower protein intake

of vegetarians, 205-6; practical suggestions for a vegetarian diet, 208

oils, 44-45; canola, 45, 247; coconut, 45, 115, 126; corn, 103; effects of heating on, 45-46; fish, 324, 325; flaxseed, 40, 126; hydrogenated, 114; olive, 37, 44; palm, 45, 115, 126; palm kernel, 45, 115, 126; peanut, 45; refined, 44; safflower, 26, 37, 45; soybean, 103, 126; storing of, 45; sunflower, 26, 37, 45; walnut, 126

Oldways Preservation & Exchange Trust, 341

olives, 37, 45

omnivores, 16, 33, 96, 138, 168, 229, 294; fat intake of, 23-24; hypertension in, 170; vitamin B12 supply in omnivore diets, 86

Ornish, Dean, 27, 123; "Reversal Diet" of, 342

osteomalacia, 79

osteoporosis, 239; and peak bone mass, 240; studies of bone density in vegetarians and vegans, 239-40. *See also* bone health, and dietary variables

oxalate. *See* urinary oxalate

oxidative stress, 30

pantothenic acid, 102

Pauly, D., 332

pellagra, 7

pernicious anemia, 86-87

Peto, R., 140

Phillips, R. L., 186

phosphate, 240

phosphorus, 104; food sources of, 104; calcium-to-phosphorus ratio (Ca:P), 242

Physicians' Health Study, 120

phytates, 65-66, 94

phytochemicals, 28, 29, 31, 111, 119, 120, 127, 148, 176, 193; as anti-cancer agents, 145-46, 154; protective properties of, 346-47

phytoestrogens, 119, 120, 127, 146, 148, 152, 152, 222

phytosterols, 26, 120, 127

Pimentel, D., 320

Pimentel, M., 320

Pixley, F., 251

Poehlman, E.T., 205

polyphenols, 66-67

potassium, 174-75, 191, 193, 195, 242, 243, 247, 306; protective properties of, 347; tomatoes as a source of, 334

pregnancy, 68, 88, 277; calcium needs during, 279; control of nausea/vomiting during, 283-84; diet guides for, 284; intake of omega-3 fatty acids during, 278; iodine needs during, 280; iron needs during, 69-70, 279; protein needs during, 278, 282; sources of

calcium for pregnant women, 283; sources of iron for pregnant women, 283; sources of linolenic acid for pregnant women, 282-83; sources of vitamin B12 and vitamin D for pregnant women, 283; vegetarian diets and pregnancy complications, 280-81; vitamin B12 needs during, 280; vitamin D needs during, 279; weight gain during, 277-78, 282; zinc needs during, 280

prostacyclins, 31

prostaglandins, 31

prostate specific antigen (PSA), 148

protein, 15, 30, 205-6, 208, 217, 222, 272, 273, 302; Acceptable Macronutrient Distribution Range for, 15; animal, 16, 348; digestibility of, 16; egg protein, 177; plant proteins and fatty acid oxidation, 206; plant proteins and nitrogen balance, 17-18; protein complementarity, 18-19; protein efficiency ratio, 17; protein intake and the urinary excretion of calcium, 254-55; protein needs of vegetarian athletes, 294-96; protein needs of vegetarians, 19-21; recommended daily allowance (RDA) of, 228, 232, 294; quality of, 16; summary of scientific literature concerning, 15-16; urinary protein loss (proteinuria), 221. *See also* soy protein

protein digestibility corrected amino acid score (PDCAAS), 17

Reddy, S., 33

Regan, T., 317

Reynolds, J. D., 332

rice, 5

Robbins, John, 5

Robertson, W. G., 254, 255

Sabaté, J., 10, 13, 39

"Science of Human Life" (Graham), 3

seeds, 39-41, 45; alfalfa sprouts, 327; chia seeds, 39; flaxseeds, 39-41, 45-46, 126, 222, 247

selenium, 29, 39, 105-6; food sources of, 105; recommended dietary allowance (RDA) of, 105

Sengupta, S., 55

Seventh-Day Adventist (SDA) Church, 4

Seventh-Day Adventists (SDAs), 100, 101, 134, 167-68, 186-87, 195, 204, 214; children of, 269; coronary heart disease (CAD) of, 112-13

Shankar, S., 55, 56-57

Shelley, Percy Bysshe, 3

Singer, Peter, 5

single-photon absorptiometry (SPA), 239

Snowdon, D. A., 187

sodium (salt), 79, 173-74, 191, 242, 306
soy, 66, 127, 222; as a protective agent against cancer, 150-51; as a source of isoflavonoids, 119
soybeans, 45, 126, 247; fermented, 85
soy flavonoids, 119
soy isoflavones, 243
soy milk, 4, 246, 268, 282
soy protein, 111, 119, 221, 243
spirulina, 37
Streptomyces griseus, 89
stroke, 162, 164, 184, 196, 232; and antioxidants, 193, 195; elevated cholesterol and risk of ischemic stroke, 188-91; embolic, 185; and fiber, 193, 195; and folate, 192, 195; and fruit and vegetable intake, 193-95; hemorrhagic, 184, 185, 195; and homocysteine, 191-93; and increased potassium intake, 191, 195; and increased sodium intake, 191; limitations of diet and stroke relationship studies, 185-86; low serum cholesterol and risk of hemorrhagic stroke, 187-88; and meat consumption, 195; problems with studies of cholesterol and stroke, 187; risk factors for, 185; studies of Seventh-Day Adventist diets and stroke, 186-87; studies of vegetarian diets and stroke, 186, 195-96; thromboembolic (ischemic), 184-85, 193; types of, 184-85
sugar, 5; refined, 7

testosterone, 148
thromboxanes, 31
Tjandra, J. J., 55
Toth, M. J., 205
triglycerides, 25, 29, 213, 223, 224, 230, 232, 289
Trock, B., 55
Truswell, A. S., 149

United Egg Association, 8
United States Department of Agriculture (USDA), 95, 300, 320; dietary guidelines of, 8; National School Lunch Program of, 269
uric acid, 254, 255, 256
urinary oxalate, 254, 255, 256
urine: acidity of, 240-41, 255, 256-57; calcium in, 255; and calcium excretion, 243, 254-55, 256; citrate in, 255, 256; and citrate excretion, 255;
Vegan Society, The, 4
vegans, 2, 4, 15, 19, 20, 23, 81, 82, 100, 102, 105, 117; average fiber intake of, 205; consumption of very-long-chain omega acids, 33;; and calcium consumption, 246-47; lower body weights among, 204; and the

need for vitamin B12, 87, 88, 345-46; zinc intake in, 94. *See also* FARM vegan community
vegetarian, first use of the term, 3-4
vegetarian athletes, 309-10: benefits of vegetarian diet for, 308-9; daily energy expenditure (DEE), 289-90; energy needs of, 289-92; energy utilization during exercise, 289; fat requirements of, 296-97, 309; female vegetarian athletes, 307-8, 310; importance of fluid intake to, 304-5, 306; importance of high-carbohydrate diets to, 292-94, 309; non-training energy expenditure, 290; nutrition after exercise, 305-6; nutrition before exercise, 304; nutrition during exercise, 304-5; optimal nutrition for, 288; pre-event meals, 305; protein needs of, 294-96, 309; recommended carbohydrate requirements for, 294; resting energy expenditure (REE), 289; sweat rate and fluid requirements of, 304, 306; training energy expenditure (TEE), 290; and weight reduction, 306-7, 310. *See also* vegetarian athletes, nutritional supplements for; vegetarian athletes, vitamin and mineral requirements of
vegetarian athletes, nutritional supplements for, 302, 309-10; caffeine, 303-4; carnatine, 303; creatine, 302-3; protein, 302
vegetarian athletes, vitamin and mineral requirements of, 297, 309; B vitamins, 300-302; calcium, 298-99; iodine, 300; iron, 299; zinc, 299-300
vegetarian diets, 107, 126-27; benefits of to diabetics, 229-31; and carbohydrates, 205; definition of, 2; fat content of, 206; high fiber content of, 205; and hypertension, 167-79; iron in, 70-71, 75-76; lacto-ovo (LOV), 167-68, 170; lifestyle factors influencing, 244-45; macrobiotic, 88; Mediterranean-style diets, 29-30; and obesity, 204-6, 207-8; research concerning, 1-2, 10, 12-13; types of, 2; worldwide, 5; very-low-fat, 27-29; very-low-fat diets compared to Mediterranean-style, 30-31; and stroke, 186-87, 195-96. *See also* children, and vegetarian diets; coronary artery disease (CAD), protections against through a vegetarian diet; coronary artery disease (CAD), treatment of through vegetarian diets; diabetes; vegetarian diets, environmental and food safety aspects of; vegetarian diets, history of; hypertension; vegetarian diets, planning of; vegetarian diets, protective factors in
vegetarian diets, environmental and food safety aspects of, 317-18, 334; aquaculture as intensive farming, 323-25, 327; chemical contamination of food, 327-29; environmental impacts of food production, 318-19;

The Food Series

The University of Illinois Press
is a founding member of the
Association of American University Presses.

─────────────────────────────────────

Composed in 11/13.5 ITC Garamond
Designed by BookComp, Inc.
Manufactured by Sheridan Books, Inc.

University of Illinois Press
1325 South Oak Street
Champaign, IL 61820-6903
www.press.uillinois.edu